SPECIES-AGE (DAYS)*

MONKEY	RAT	MOUSE	RABBIT	HAMSTER	GUINEA PIG	CHICK
166	21-22	18-20	31-34	15.5-16	64-68	20-21
4-9	3-5	3-6	2.6-6	3-4.5	4.8	
9	5-6	7	6	4.5-5	6	
18-20	9	8	6.5	7	13.5	0.25-0.75
19-21	9.5	8		7.5	13.5	1
20-21	10	8.3⁻		7.7 ⁻	14.5	1
	10	8.3		7.75	15.5 ⁻	1.5
	10.2			8. ⁻	16.5 ⁻	1.5 ⁻
	10				16.5	1.5
	10	9.1		8.5		2.75
23-24?	10.5	9	9.5	8.25	15.5	2.3 ⁻
	11-12	9.5		9	16.5	1.75
	11.3	9		8.5	16.5 ⁺	2.3 ⁻
23-24	10.5	8.6	9 ⁻	8	15.5	1.5
	11.5	9.6		8.25	16.5	2.3
	12	11			18.5	3
	10	8.5			16.5	1.8
25-26	10.5	9.3	10.5	8.25	16.5	2.2
	11.3	9.5		8.5	16.5?	3.75
1	12-13	8-10	6-9	10-14	2-3	
11	2, 5, 12, 16, 17, 18, 29	4, 8, 20	4, 5	1, 6, 23	22	9, 17

* Mid point of event except: ⁺ event beginning, ⁻ event finished (Continued on the back cover)

CATALOG OF TERATOGENIC AGENTS

CATALOG OF TERATOGENIC AGENTS

Fourth Edition

Thomas H. Shepard, M.D.

Central Laboratory for Human Embryology
Department of Pediatrics
School of Medicine
University of Washington

BIP- 94 5th ed. 1986

The Johns Hopkins University Press
Baltimore and London

First edition sponsored by the National Institute of Child Health and
Human Development, National Institutes of Health, Bethesda,
Maryland 20014

Manufactured in the United States of America

The Johns Hopkins University Press, Baltimore, Maryland 21218
The Johns Hopkins Press Ltd., London

First edition, 1973
Second edition, 1976
Third edition, 1980
Fourth edition, 1983

Library of Congress Cataloging in Publication Data

Shepard, Thomas H.
  Catalog of teratogenic agents.

  Includes bibliographical references and index.
  1. Teratogenic agents—Catalogs. I. Title.
QM691.S53   1983   616'.043   82-49063
ISBN 0-8018-3027-3

This book is dedicated with appreciation to my past and present research fellows who stimulated its production

Prasanta K. Datta
Sorrel Waxman
Pierre Ferrier
Charles P. Mahoney
Ronald J. Lemire
Ralph R. Hollingsworth
Thomas Nelson
Takashi Tanimura
Alan G. Fantel
Godfrey P. Oakley
Gerald J. Bargman
Theodore H. Regimbal
Larklyn H. Fisher
Trent D. Stephens
Philip E. Mirkes
Kohei Shiota
Margo I. Van Allen
Marlissa Campbell
John Rogers

The fourth edition is dedicated with affection and appreciation to my wife, Alice.

CONTENTS

PREFACE TO THE FOURTH EDITION

The fourth edition contains approximately 600 new additions, of which 250 are newly listed agents. A special effort has been made to obtain as much information as possible on drugs and other agents to which pregnant women may be exposed. Because of an increased awareness of the importance of negative published data, a considerable number of nonteratogenic agents have been included. Many such references are drawn from the Japanese literature and the author is, again, grateful for the help of Dr. Takashi Tanimura, who is now Professor of Anatomy at Kinki University School of Medicine. Professor A. P. Dyban from the Department of Embryology, Institute of Experimental Medicine, Leningrad, gave valuable help with the Russian literature.

Some of the advantages of using a computer program for storage and production have been realized again with this fourth edition. The originally published material does not need to be proofed; the names, references, and dosages cannot be mistakenly altered. When the program is completed, the entire final printout to be sent to the publisher can be run off within minutes. Once in the hands of the publisher, the material does not need to be typeset, a consideration that reduces the cost of the book. Finally, the computer storage tape can be used by agencies such as the National Library of Medicine to extract specific data and references on various agents and supply their many clients rapidly. Ideally, a week-to-week update of this data file could be augmented by use of a remote terminal.

There are several other sources of teratology information. James G. Wilson's text (1973) remains one of the best introductions to teratology. A comprehensive 4-volume set of books on methods and principles in teratology has been edited by J. G. Wilson and F. C. Frazer (1977). Schardein (1976) has produced *Drugs as Teratogens,* a volume containing a large number of references. Heinonen *et al.* (1977) have summarized drug exposures during more than 50,000 pregnancies and furnish useful tables of malformation-risk factors, nearly all of which are not significantly increased. The National Institute of Environmental Health Sciences maintains an Environmental Teratology Information Center (ETIC) (Staples, 1977), whose system of computerized information retrieval on teratology is available for those who require an in-depth listing of references. Their listing can be obtained directly from them or through the National Library of Medicine (TOXLINE).

Four especially useful publications on methods for detection of teratogenic agents and protection of the human population are available. The proceedings of a conference in Guadeloupe under the auspices of the Institute de la Vie addresses in vitro, pregnant animal testing, and epidemiologic methods (Shepard *et al.,* 1975). Brent and Harris (1976) edited a volume emphasizing the scientific and epidemiologic techniques useful in preventing fetal and neonatal loss. A recent volume from a conference supported by the March of Dimes Birth Defects Foundation gives detailed guidelines for studies of human populations (Bloom, 1981). The U.S. Environmental Protection Agency has published the proceedings of two conferences on techniques and risk assessment of substances that affect reproduction. Discussions of protocols for testing the effect of environmental substances on the male and female reproductive systems and the conceptus are given (Galbraith *et al.*, 1982).

REFERENCES

1. Bloom, A. D., ed.: *Guidelines for Studies of Human Populations Exposed to Mutagenic and Reproductive Hazards.* White Plains, N.Y.: March of Dimes Birth Defects Foundation, 1982.
2. Brent, R. L., and Harris, M., eds.: *Prevention of Embryonic, Fetal, and Perinatal Disease.* Bethesda, Md: DHEW (NIH) 76-853, 1976.
3. Galbraith, W. M., Voytek, P., and Ryan, M. G., eds.: *Assessment of Risks to Human Reproduction and to Development of the Human Conceptus from Exposure to Environmental Substances EPA–600/9–82–001.* Springfield, VA: National Technical Infomation Service, 1982.
4. Scharadein, J. L.: *Drugs as Teratogens.* Cleveland: CRC Press, 1976.
5. Shepard, T. H.; Miller, J. R.; and Marois, M., eds.: *Methods for Detection of Environmental Agents That Produce Congenital Defects.* New York: North Holland-American Elsevier, 1975.
6. Staples, R. E.: Environmental Teratology Information Center. (abs) Envir. Health Prospectives 20:239, 1977.
7. Wilson, J. G.: *Environment and Birth Defects.* New York: Academic Press, 1973.
8. Wilson, J. G., and Fraser, F. C., eds.: *Handbook of Teratology,* vols. 1–4. New York: Plenum Press, 1976.

ACKNOWLEDGMENTS

I wish to thank the many unnamed colleagues who have supplied me with the information included in this catalog. My students and research fellows have contributed considerably, as have other teratologists. Associates, Drs. Richard Blandau, Ronald Lemire, and David W. Smith, gave advice on the tables of comparative time periods of embryonic and fetal development in man and experimental animals. Professor Takashi Tanimura, of the Department of Anatomy at Kinki University School of Medicine (Osaka), aided with selection and translation of the Japanese literature, and Professor A. P. Dyban, Department of Embryology, Institute for Experimental Medicine, Academy of Medical Science of the USSR, Leningrad, helped with the Russian literature.

The computerization of the book was simplified by the generous help of Dr. Victor McKusick, who allowed us to make use of a program similar to that employed for production of his catalog (*Mendelian Inheritance in Man* [5th ed.; The Johns Hopkins Press, 1979]). Dr. Richard Shepard and David Bolling of The Johns Hopkins School of Medicine and James E. Peoples of the University of Arizona School of Medicine kindly helped to provide the edit-and-print programs for computerizing the body of this book.

The computerization of the material and the processing of the catalog took place in the computer center of the University of Washington under the direction of Dr. John Jacobsen. Tom Stebbins designed the figures for the tables on the endpapers.

The careful clerical work of Marceline Davis, Connie Elmendorff, and Karen Archer is appreciated. Barbara Brownfield ably assisted with the third and fourth editions.

INTRODUCTION

Defects existing at birth, irrespective of their cause, create societal problems of such magnitude that the subject needs little amplification. Approximately 3% of all human newborns have a cogenital anomaly requiring medical attention, and approximately one-third of these conditions can be regarded as life threatening. With increasing age, over twice as many congenital defects are detected. Close to one-half the number of children in hospital wards are there because of prenatally acquired malformations of one kind or another.

Our knowledge about the cause and prevention of these problems is extremely limited. About 10 percent are associated with gene mutations and another 5% with chromosomal aberrations. Less than 6% of the remaining anomalies are known to be due to a teratogenic agent. Although there are over 800 agents listed in this catalog that can produce congenital anomalies in experimental animals, only about twenty of these are known to cause defects in the human. Therefore, there exists a wide difference between our knowledge of experimental teratology and the role that external agents play in producing human malformations.

A further problem is that the teratologic literature is dispersed throughout most of the biomedical publications rather than being confined to one or two of the specialized journals. Although a number of excellent review articles have been published, a catalog such as this has not been available. Harold Kalter's (1) text deals with the teratology of the central nervous system in animals, and Josef Warkany's (2) extensive treatise is concerned with congenital defects in man. David Smith's (3) popular book on dysmorphic syndromes helps to define and extend our description of human defects. McKusick's (4) catalog of mendelian inheritance in man includes many congenital syndromes produced by gene mutations.

The main purpose of this catalog is to help link the information on experimental teratogenic agents with the congenital defects in man. The catalog should provide a source of reference for teratologists wishing knowledge of the literature dealing with a particular teratogenic agent. For the obstetrician, pediatrician, and geneticist it should help answer the often-asked question: Does this agent produce congenital defects in man or animal? Another function of this book may be to aid the scientists who protect us from our man-modified environment. Testing pharmaceutical products has become a major responsibility, and the environmental protectionist is also faced with the safety of food additives and household products. This catalog also may be useful to chemists working to develop new products. Unfortunately, because of species variability, at least in part, in teratogenic sensitivity, the ultimate testing of some products has been done in the human, with the alert clinician acting as monitor.

It is important that the presently accumulated information on teratogens be fully utilized to recognize potential teratogenic hazards and to prevent congenital malformations in man. If it happens that many anomalies are produced by the interaction of genes with a teratogenic agent, it undoubtedly will be easier to remove the agent than to alter the action of the gene. The work of producing this book will be rewarded if it contributes to the prevention of any congenital defects.

The teratogenic agents listed in this book include chemicals, drugs, physical factors, and viruses. I have attempted to make a complete listing of all agents that can produce congenital defects in animals or humans. The chemical names are, in most cases, those that appear in the *Merck Index,* but cross-indexing to alternate chemical and proprietary names has been done also. Studies carried out on species phylogenetically below the chick have been omitted. No attempt has been made to list agents that are teratogenic only when administered in combination with another agent. I have not attempted a critical exclusion of agents that are doubtful teratogens. *The presence of an agent in the catalog does not necessarily indicate that it is a teratogen* because a number of compounds, often considered teratogenic but with substantially negative teratogenic effects, have been included. When there is conflicting evidence of teratogenicity, equal representation has been attempted. An example of this is lysergic acid diethylamide (LSD).

The literature has been surveyed using the usual library aids. When possible, abstracts of work have not been utilized. Numerous excellent references dealing only with the mechanism of the defects' production have been omitted. Although some agents may have been omitted inadvertently from this listing, the method of production and printing of this type of book readily allows for easy revision. I hope that scientists in the field will feel free to send me new information or corrections for inclusion in future editions.

Each listing includes a main entry with synonyms. This is followed by a brief account of some of the work published including species, dose, gestational age at time of administration, and type of congenital defects produced. The references following each entry were chosen because of their review nature, originality, or because they are most current.

During the early planning of the book it appeared that the accumulation of the new teratologic literature could very rapidly outdate a text published in the usual manner. To obviate this partially, the catalog was constructed using a computerized system. The phrase *computerized system* has puzzled some of my associates, who initially concluded that I used some mechanical device for generating information. On the contrary, the text was compiled in the usual way and then transferred to the computer. This text was then stored on computer tape, from which a printout could be obtained. This computerized system for producing a catalog allows for easy insertion of new material or corrections during compilation and for easy production of future editions. It has the further advantage that, with the use of photocopying, the book can be printed in less than 3 months at a considerably reduced cost.

Since a teratogenic agent is defined by its ability to produce a congenital defect, it seems appropriate to provide a definition for "congenital defect" at this point. A congenital defect has its genesis during embryonic or fetal development and consists of a major or minor deviation from normal morphology or function. The border line between a minor congential defect and normal variation is most difficult to define, and this accounts for a large difference in incidence rates. David Smith (3) has offered some criteria for distinguishing the two. In general, a minor defect should be present in less than 2% or 3% of the population. This small percentage could be defined in a statistical manner as the number of observations falling outside of three standard deviations from the mean. Large morphological types of congenital defects such as cleft palate or meningomyelocele may be called anomalies or malformations, but I feel the term *defect* also includes unknown or subtle structural defects that alter function. These functional changes also could be ascribed to molecular changes, many of which are still unknown. Particularly in the nervous and endocrine systems, changes in postnatal function have become an important aspect of both experimental and human teratology. An example of this is maternal hyperphenylalaninemia, which may lead to cerebral dysfunction and mental retardation in the offspring. Another new and important teratologic area requiring long term postnatal observation is prenatally induced oncogenesis, illustrated by vaginal carcinomas produced in grown girls whose mothers were treated with diethylstilbesterol during pregnancy.

A teratogenic agent acts during pregnancy to produce a physical or functional defect in the conceptus or offspring. The definition can be made more specific by using a modification of Koch's postulates in the following manner:

Koch's postulates	Application to Teratology
1. A specific microorganism must be present in each case.	1. The agent must be present during the critical periods of development.
2. A pure culture of the organism should produce a similar disease in the experimental animal.	2. The agent should produce congenital defects in an experimental animal. The defect rate should be statistically higher in the treated group than in the control animals receiving the same vehicle or sham procedure.
3. Organisms from the experimental animal must be recovered and grown in pure culture.	3. Proof should be obtained that the agent in an unaltered state acts on the embryo-fetus either directly or indirectly through the placenta. In this area, biochemistry and organ culture are most often used instead of bacteriology.

The fulfillment of the first two conditions is sufficient to define a teratogenic agent. The third may be considered desirable but not essential. In this catalog, there are few teratogens that fit all three of these criteria. Surprisingly, teratogenic agents in the human generally do fill all three criteria—for instance, rubella virus, radiation, and androgens that masculinize the female fetus. Thalidomide, although accepted universally as a teratogen, does not fit the third criterion because the compound in its unaltered state has not been demonstrated to directly affect the conceptus. Although this third criterion may seem unnecessary to many teratologists, I believe that a more complete knowledge of these important molecular mechanisms can generate more rapidly the means for preventing malformations.

Several difficult problems face the teratologist in judging whether an agent is a teratogen. When the dosage level of a compound must be raised to near-fatal levels for the mother before defects are produced in her fetus, most workers consider the agent weakly teratogenic. However, clinicians, the Federal Drug Administration, and the pharmaceutical industry encounter difficult decisions in applying these experimental findings to man. Agents causing embryonic or fetal death in experimental animals often later prove to be teratogenic in man but are not considered to be teratogens unless physical or functional defects are produced. Similarly, an agent that can cause fetal growth retardation does not necessarily qualify as a teratogen. Retardation of fetal skeletal maturation reported as decreased ossification centers of the manubrium or immaturity of the vertebral centra is another example of a change considered physiologic but not teratogenic.

REFERENCES

1. Kalter, H. *Teratology of the Central Nervous System.* Chicago: University of Chicago Press, 1968.
2. Warkany, J. *Congenital Malformations. Notes and Comments.* Chicago: Year Book Medical Publishers, 1971.
3. Smith, D. W. *Recognizable Patterns of Human Malformations.* 2nd ed. Philadelphia: W. B. Saunders Company, 1976.
4. McKusick, V. A. *Mendelian Inheritance in Man, Catalogs of Autosomal Dominant, Autosomal Recessive, and X-linked Phenotypes,* 5th ed. Baltimore: The Johns Hopkins University Press, 1979.

NOTES FOR TABLE ON ENDPAPERS

Comparative Time Periods of Embryonic and Fetal
Development in Man and Experimental Animals

One of the main principles of teratology is that teratogenic activity is strongly dependent on exposure to an agent at a specific "sensitive" period in development. It seemed appropriate, therefore, to attempt an integration of embryonic and fetal events for man and some common experimental animals. I have tabulated events that occur in man, rhesus monkey, rat, mouse, rabbit, hamster, guinea pig, and chick. The times are given in days from copulation or ovulation for the monkey, mouse, rabbit, hamster, and guinea pig. An assumption has been made that ovulation time is approximately the same as copulation time. For man, the time is derived by subtracting 14 days from the period between the onset of the last normal mensis and time of delivery. For the rat, timing customarily has been from 9:00 A.M. of the morning following copulation, and I have chosen to follow this method. Timing in the chick is from the start of incubation.

The reader may note that the ages given for man are 2-3 days greater than the dates originally given by G. L. Streeter, who based his timing on comparable stages in the monkey. This adjustment, based on last menstrual period dates, has been drawn largely from material collected in the Central Laboratory for Human Embryology at the University of Washington (13, 24). Our data, based on North American and European specimens, agree quite well with the Japanese observations of Nishimura and Yamamura (19). Exact dating of the early somite stages is still hazardous because of the meager number of available human embryos.

A good deal of confusion exists about what the days of the pregnancy should be called. In this volume, and, I believe as a general practice among teratologists, the first 24 hours after fertilization is designated as the first day; however, if the word *day* precedes the cardinal number, this indicates that the age is at least that many days. Thus, a day-10 embryo is at least 10 days of age, but an embryo of the 10th day is between 9 and 10 days of age. Kalter (14) has eloquently discussed this problem.

Many definitions of the embryonic period have been offered. I define the end of the human embryonic period or start of the fetal period by these criteria: 54-56 gestational days, crown-rump length of 33 mm, end of Streeter's Horizon XXIII, and end of major organogenesis. Two other criteria that might help define the difference in some of the experimental animal models are the appearance of ossification and the presence of external characteristics specific for the species.

A definition of fetal growth in man and monkey is only now beginning. Tanimura *et al.* (28) designate fetal organ weights for the human, and Kerr *et al.* (15), for the monkey. Gruenwald and Minh (7) and Potter (21) give organ weight standards for fetuses over the weight of 500 gm.

The references that follow were useful in constructing the tables appearing on the front and back inside covers.

REFERENCES

1. Boyer, C. C. Chronology of the development for the golden hamster. *J. Morph.* 92: 1–37, 1953.
2. Christie, G. A. Developmental stages in somite and post-somite rat embryos, based on external appearance and including some features of the macroscopic development of the oral cavity. *J. Morph.* 114: 263–86, 1964.
3. Davies, J. *Human Developmental Anatomy.* New York: Ronald Press, 1963.
4. _____, and Hesseldahl, H. Comparative embryology of mammalian blastocysts. In Blandau, R. J. (ed.), *Biology of the Blastocyst.* Chicago: University of Chicago Press, 1971. Pp. 27–48.
5. Edwards, J. A. The external development of the rabbit and rat embryo. In Woollam, D. H. M. (ed.), *Advances in Teratology*, Vol. 3. New York: Academic Press, 1968. Pp. 239–63.
6. Graves, A. P. Development of the golden hamster *Cricetus auratus* waterhouse, during the first nine days. *Amer. J. Anat.* 77: 219–51, 1949.
7. Gruenwald, P., and Minh, H. N. Evaluation of body and organ weights in perinatal pathology. I. Normal standards derived from autopsies. *Amer. J. Clin. Path.* 34: 247–53, 1960.
8. Gruneberg, H. The development of some external features in mouse embryos. *J. Hered.* 34: 88–92, 1943.
9. Hamburger, V., and Hamilton, H. L. A series of normal stages in the development of the chick embryo. *J. Morph.* 88: 49–92, 1951.
10. Heuser, C. H., and Corner, G. W. Development horizons in embryos, description of age groups XIX, XX, XXI, XXII and XXIII being the fifth issue of a survey of the Carnegie Collection. *Contrib. Embryol.* 34: 165–96, 1951.
11. Heuser, C. H., and Streeter, G. L. Development of the macaque embryo. *Contrib. Embryol.* 29: 15–55, 1941.
12. Huber, G. C. The development of the albino rat, *Mus norvegicus albinus.* *J. Morph.* 26: 246–386, 1915.
13. Iffy, L.; Shepard, T. H.; Jakobovits, A.; Lemire, R. J.; and Kerner, P. The rate of growth in young embryos of Streeter's horizons XIII to XXIII. *Acta Anat.* (Basel) 66: 178–86, 1967.
14. Kalter, H. How should times during pregnancy be called in teratology? *Teratology* 1: 231–34, 1968.
15. Kerr, G. R.; Kennan, A. L.; Waisman, H. A.; and Allen, J. R. Growth and development of the fetal rhesus monkey. I. Physical growth. *Growth* 33: 201–13, 1969.
16. Long, J. A., and Burlingame, M. L. The development of the external form of the rat with some observations on the origin of the extraembryonic coelom and fetal membranes. *Univ. Calif. Mem. Zool.* 43: 143–83, 1938.
17. Monie, I. W. Comparative development of rat, chick and human embryos. In *Teratologic Workshop Manual* (supplement). Berkeley, California: Pharmaceutical Manufacturers Associations, 1965. Pp. 146–62.
18. Nicholas, J. S. Experimental methods and rat embryos. In Farris, E. J., and Griffith, J. Q. (eds.), *The Rat in Laboratory Investigation.* New York: Hafner Publishing, 1962. Pp. 51–67.
19. Nishimura, H., and Yamamura, H. Comparison between man and some other mammals of normal and abnormal developmental processes. In Nishimura, H., and Miller, J. R. (eds.), *Methods for Teratological Studies in Experimental Animals and Man.* Tokyo: Igaku Shoin Ltd., 1969. Pp. 223–40.

20. Otis, E. M., and Brent, R. Equivalent ages in mouse and human embryos. *Anat. Rec.* 120: 33-63, 1954.
21. Potter, E. L. *Pathology of the Fetus and Infant.* Chicago: Year Book Medical Publishers, 1961. P. 14.
22. Scott, J. P. The embryology of the guinea pig. I. Table of normal development. *Amer. J. Anat.* 60: 397-432, 1937.
23. Shenefelt, R. E. Morphogenesis of malformations in hamsters caused by retinoic acid: Relation to dose and stage of treatment. *Teratology* 5: 103-18, 1972.
24. Shepard, T. H. Growth and development of the human embryo and fetus. In Gardner, L. I. (ed.), *Endocrine and Genetic Diseases of Childhood.* Philadelphia: W. B. Saunders, 1969. Pp. 1-6.
25. Streeter, G. L. Developmental horizons in human embryos, description of age group XI, 13 to 20 somites, and age group XII, 21 to 29 somites. *Contrib. Embryol.* 30: 211-45, 1942.
26. _____. Developmental horizons in human embryos, description of age group XIII embryos about 4 or 5 millimeters long, and age group XIV, period of indentation of lens vesicle. *Contrib. Embryol.* 31: 27-63, 1945.
27. _____. Developmental horizons in human embryos, description of age groups XV, XVI, XVII and XVIII, being the third issue of a survey of the Carnegie Collection. *Contrib. Embryol.* 32: 133-203, 1948.
28. Tanimura, T.; Nelson, T.; Hollingsworth, R. R.; and Shepard, T. H. Weight standards for organs from early human fetuses. *Anat. Rec.* 171: 227-36, 1971.
29. Witschi, E. Development of the rat. In Altman, P., and Dittmer, D. S. (eds.), *Growth Including Reproduction and Morphological Development.* Washington, D.C.: Federation of American Societies for Experimental Biology, 1962. Pp. 304-414.

USE OF THE CATALOG

The text of the catalog consists of alphabetically organized entries of the agents. The chemical compounds are alphabetized without regard for single preceding letters, numbers, or Greek symbols. For instance, *l-beta-D-arabinofuranosyl-5-fluorocytosine* would be listed in the A's. The chemical name as listed in *The Merck Index* has been used most often as the main entry with trade names as synonyms. Trade names are followed by *-R.*

Certain problems are created by the computerization techniques used in producing this book. Greek symbols have been spelled out, and letters and numerals ordinarily seen as subscripts and superscripts have been placed in parentheses.

Following the catalog are the subject and author indexes for the reader's convenience. If there are various names for a single agent, the reader can locate the text entry more rapidly by consulting the subject index. For example, *irradiation* in the subject index refers the reader to the text entry under *radiation.* In both indexes, the numbers supplied refer to entries, not pages. Page numbers are given at the bottom of the page; the entry numbers appear at the top.

1   Abortion, Induced

The question does an induced abortion affect subsequent pregnancies has been debated. Pantelakis et al (1973) reported that women with previous induced abortion had double the rate of premature and stillborn children. Wright et al (1972) found an increase in second trimester spontaneous abortions in women who had previously undergone cervical dilatation. The cervical dilatation was thought to produce cervical incompetence. Critical appraisal of these and other reports on the subject (Institute of Medicine, 1975 and Lui et al 1972) suggests that further matched control studies are needed in order to fully answer the question. One such study by Daling and Emanuel (1975) carefully matched for social and other contributing factors and could find no effect on subsequent pregnancies. The congenital defect rate was also unaltered.

Bracken and Holford (1979) studied 1,427 pregnancies with previous therapeutic abortion and could detect no significant increase in malformations. Hogue et al (1982) have reviewed published data on this subject in detail and could find little indication of subsequent poor pregnancy outcome..

Bracken, M.B. and Holford, T.R: Induced abortion and congenital malformations in offspring of subsequent pregnancies. Am. J. Epidem. 109:425-432,1979.

Daling, J.R. and Emanuel, I.: Induced abortion and subsequent outcome of pregnancy: A matched cohort study. Lancet 2: 170-172, 1975.

Hogue, C.J.R.; Cates, W. and Tietze, C.: The effects of induced abortion on subsequent reproduction. Epid. Reviews 4:66-94, 1982.

Inst. of Medicine: Report of a Study on Legalized Abortion and the Public Health. Washington, D.C.: Academy of Science, 1975, pp. 47-71.

Lui, D.T.Y.; Melville, H.A.H. and Martin, T.: Subsequent gestational morbidity after various types of abortion. Lancet 2: 431 (only), 1972.

Pantelakis, S.N.; Papadimitriou, G.C. and Doxiadis, S.A.: Influence of induced and spontaneous abortions on the outcome of subsequent pregnancies. J. Obstet. Gynecol. 116: 799-805, 1973.

Wright, C.S.W.; Campbell, S. and Beazley, J.: Second trimester abortion after vaginal termination of pregnancy. Lancet 1: 1278-1279, 1972.

2   Acemetacin

Koga et al (1981) studied the effect of this non-steroidal anti-inflammatory agent during organogenesis in the rat. Oral doses of up to 8.0 mg per kg gave maternal ulcers of the small intestine of the dams and fetal growth retardation was seen. Congenital defects were not increased. At 4.0 mg per kg during the prenatal period an increase in infant mortaliy was seen (Aoki et al, 1981).

Aoki, Y.; Koga, T.; Ota, T.; Sugasawa, M.; Kobayashi, F.: Reproductive studies with acemetacin (K 708) perinatal and postnatal study in rats. Oyo Yakuri 22:777-786, 1981.

3   Acetaldehyde (see also Disulfiram)

Veghelgi et al (1978) first asked if acetaldehyde was the toxic agent in fetal alcohol syndrome. This metabolite of ethanol was administered to mice on days 7, 8 and 9 of gestation (O'Shea and Kaufman, 1979). A one or two percent solution of acetaldehyde in 0.1 ml of 0.9 percent saline per 25 gm of body weight was used. Increased resorptions and decreased embryonic protein and decreased fetal weights as compared to saline injected controls occurred. No increase in defect rate was found in the treated fetuses on day 19, but on day 10 an increased number of embryos with open anterior or posterior neural tube was reported. Campbell and Fantel (1983) studied the effect of acetaldehyde in whole embryo culture and found reduced growth at 25, 50 and 75 micromolar concentrations. Popov et al (1981) studied the effect of ethanol (6.5 - 108 mM) and its metabolite, acetaldehyde (4.5 micromolar - 45mM) in the culture of 9.5 day rat embryos. In both cases similar malformations were found. Skosyreva (1982) observed a high teratogenicity of acetaldehyde substance.

Campbell, M.A. and Fantel, A.G.: Relative teratogenicity of ethanol and acetaldehyde in vivo. Life Sciences, in press, 1983.

O'Shea, K.S. and Kaufman, M.H.: The teratogenic effect of acetaldehyde: Implications for study of the fetal alcohol syndrome. J. Anat. 128: 65-76, 1979.

Popov, V.B.; Weisman, B.L.; Puchkov, V.F. and Ignatyeva, T.V.: Embryotoxic effect of ethanol and its biotransformation products in the culture of postimplantation rat embryos. Byull, Eksp. Biol. Med. (USSR) 12:725-728, 1981.

Skosyreva, A.M.: Comparative studies of embryotoxic effects of alcohol and its metabolite, acetaldehyde during organogenesis. Akush. Ginekol. (USSR) 1:49-50, 1982.

Veghelgi, P.V.; Osztovics, M.; Kardos, G.; Leisztner, L.; Szaszovszky, S.; Igali, S. and Imrei, J.: The fetal alcohol syndrome symptoms and pathogenesis. Acta Ped. Acad. Scient. Hung. 19: 171-189, 1978.

4   Acetamide

Thiersch (1962) reported that acetamide was non-toxic to rat litters, but N-methyl acetamide and N, N-dimethyl acetamide were lethal to the embryo-fetus when 2 gm per kg were given once intraperitoneally between the 4th and 14th days of gestation. Von Kreybig et al (1969) found skeletal defects in fetuses from rats given 600 mg per kg of dimethyl or di- ethyl acetamide.

Thiersch, J.B.: Effects of acetamides and formamides on the rat litter in utero. J. Reprod. Fertil. 4: 219-220, 1962.

Von Kreybig, T.; Preussmann, R. and Von Kreybig, I.: Chemische Konstitution und teratogene Wirkung bei der Ratte. II. N-alkylharnstoffe, N-alkylsulfonamide, N,N-dialkylacetamide, N-methylthioacetamid, Chloracetamid. Arzneim. Forsch. 19: 1073-1076, 1969.

5   Acetaminophen

Heinonen et al (1976) reported on 226 infants born to mothers who took the drug during the first 4 months of preg- nancy and found no increase in malformations. Char et al (1975) reported an infant with polyhydraminos and renal failure; the nephrotoxicity was felt to be associated with acetaminophen which the mother ingested heavily during pregnancy. Collins (1981) has reviewed the subject and found no reported animal studies. In unpublished studies (Emerson, S.C. and Shepard, T.H.) rats given 750 mg per kg during organogenesis produced fetuses that were slightly underweight and had increased minor skeletal defects. No Increase in defect rate or change in liver weight occurred.

Ogawa et al (1982) gave mice an oral preparation containing 43 percent acetaminophen along with ethenzamide, caffeine and a vehicle to mice. Treatment during organogenesis with approximately 387 mg of acetaminophen produced no ill effects in the fetuses.

Char, V.C.; Chandra, R.; Fletcher, A.B.; and Avery, G.B.: Polyhydramnios and neonatal renal failure - a possible association with maternal acetaminophen ingestion. J. Ped. 86:638-639, 1975.

Collins, E.: Maternal and fetal effects of acetaminophen and salicylate in pregnancy. Obst. & Gynecol. 58:57-S-62-S, 1981.

Heinonen, O.P.; Slone, D. and Shapiro, S.: Birth Defects and drugs in Pregnancy. Publishing Sciences Group Inc.; Littleton, Mass., 1977.

Ogawa, H.; Arakawa, E.; Morobushi, A.; Yamada, H.; Ito, H.: Reproductive studies of NB-6. Kiso to Rinsho 16:683-695, 1982.

6   Acetazolamide [Diamox-R]

Layton and Hallesy (1965) produced post-axial forelimb defects in mice and rats by feeding a diet containing 0.6 percent acetazolamide. The defect was specifically localized to the forelimb and the right side was more often involved. Symmetric forelimb defects have been produced in the hamster (Layton, 1971). In monkeys, administration of 600 mg per kg for 3 to 6 embryonic days gave negative results (Wilson, 1971).

Ellison and Maren (1972) in an attempt to understand the mechanism of action of this compound produced respiratory acidosis, potassium depletion and metabolic acidosis in rats but found no forelimb defect. Maren and Ellison (1972-a) did find that replacement of potassium during acetazolamide therapy reduced the teratogenic effect. Maren and Ellison (1972-b) have also published a study comparing teratogenicity of other related thiadiazoles.

Ellison, A.C. and Maren, T.H.: The effects of metabolic alterations on teratogenesis. Johns Hopkins Med. J. 130: 87-94, 1972.

Layton, W.M.: Teratogenic action of acetazolamide in golden hamsters. Teratology 4: 95-102, 1971.

Layton, W.M. and Hallesy, D.W.: Deformity of forelimb in rats: association with high doses of acetazolamide. Science 149: 306-308, 1965.

Maren, T.H. and Ellison, A.C.: The effect of potassium on acetazolamide-induced teratogenesis. Johns Hopkins Med. J. 130: 105-115, 1972-a.

Maren, T.H. and Ellison, A.C.: The teratological effect of certain thiadiazoles related to acetazolamide, with a note on sulfanilamide and thiazide diuretics. Johns Hopkins Med. J. 130: 95-104, 1972-b.

Wilson, J.G.: Use of rhesus monkeys in teratological studies. Fed. Proc. 30: 104-109, 1971.

7   Acetohydroxamic Acid

Chaube and Murphy (1966) gave the substance on the 12th day (1000 mg per kg) and found a high incidence of encephalocele, cleft palate and skeletal defects in the rat.

Chaube, S. and Murphy, M.L.: The effects of hydoxyurea and related compounds on the rat fetus. Cancer Res. 26: 1448-1455, 1966.

8   Acetone Peroxides

Acetone peroxides are the reaction products formed by the addition of hydrogen peroxide to acetone in a mild acid solution and consist mainly of 2-2-dihydroproperoxy propane and bis-(1,1-hydroperoxy-1,1-methyl) diethyl peroxide. Oser and Morgareidge (1967) fed bread containing up to 0.045 percent to rats for 24 months and found no decrease in numbers of offspring or weanlings.

Oser, B.L. and Morgareidge, K.: Safety evaluation of flour treated with acetone peroxides. Food Cosmet. Toxicol. 5: 309-319, 1967.

9   Acetoxymethyl-methylnitrosamine

Bochert et al (1982) reported that this presumed reactive
metabolite of dimethylnitrosamine produced digital defects
in rat fetuses exposed to 5-16 mg per kg on day 11 of
gestation.

Bochert, G.; Platzek, T.; Rahm, U.: Embryotoxicity induced
by acetoxymethyl-methylnitrosamine: DNA methylation of
embryonic tissues during organogenesis as compared to
teratogenic effect in mice. (abstract) Teratology 26:14A,
1982.

10   Acetone Semicarbazone (see Semicarbazide)

11   Acetoxymethyl-methylnitrosamine

Bochert et al (1982) reported that this presumed reactive
metabolite of dimethylnitrosamine produced digital defects
in rat fetuses exposed to 5-16 mg per kg on day 11 of
gestation.

Bochert, F.; Platzek, T.; Rahm, U.: Embryotoxicity induced
by acetoxymethyl-methylnitrosamine: DNA methylation of
embryonic tissues during organogenesis as compared to
teratogenic effects in mice. (abstract) Teratology 26:14A,
1982.

12   (2-Acetyllactoyloxyethyl)trimethylammonium
      1,5-naphthalenedisulfonate

This cholinergic compound was tested in pregnant mice and
rabbits by Takai et al (1979). In mice doses of up to 7500
mg per kg orally before mating, during the first 6 days,
during days 6-15 or from day 15 through the 21st day after
birth had no effect on the fetus or offspring. In rabbit
studies 1000 mg per kg was given from the 6th through the
18th day without adverse fetal effects.

Takai, A.; Nakada, H.; Nakamura, S.; Inaba, J.; Orikawa, M.:
Toxicity test of (2-acetyl-lactoyloxyethyl)trimethylammonium
1,5- naphthalenedisulfonate (TM 723) Reproductive tests in
mice andrabbits. Oyo Yakuri 18:923-942, 1979.

13   2-Acetylaminofluorene (N-2-fluorenylacetamide)

This carcinogen and mutagen has been shown to be activated
by a liver monooxygenase in an in vitro rat culture.
Necrosis of the prosencephalon and open neural tubes were
found when the embryos were exposed to 50 micrograms per ml
of medium (Faustman-Watts et al, 1982). Two metabolites
N-hydroxy-2-acetylaminofluorene and N-Acetoxy-2-
acetylaminofluorene were teratogenic without bioactivation.

Faustman-Watts, E.; Greenaway, J.C.; Namkung, M.J.; Fantel,
A.G.; and Juchau, M.R.: Teratogenicity in vitro of
2-acetylaminofluorene: Role of biotransformation in the rat.

13

Teratology 27:19-28, 1983.

14 Acetylcholine

Beuker and Platner (1956) injected 1.2 to 2.85 mg of this compound into chick eggs during the interval 4 to 12 days of incubation and found no defects.

Beuker, E.D. and Platner, W.S.: Effect of cholinergic drugs on development of chick embryo. Proc. Soc. Exp. Biol. Med. 91: 539-543, 1956.

15 (2-Acetyllactoyloxyethyl)trimethylammonium 1,5-naphthalenedisulfonate

This cholinergic compound was tested in pregnant mice and rabbits by Takai et al (1979). In mice doses of up to 7500 mg per kg orally before mating, during the first 6 days, during days 6-15 or from day 15 through the 21st day after birth had no effect on the fetus or offspring. In rabbit studies, 1000 mg per kg was given from the 6th through the 18th day without adverse fetal effects.

Takai, A.; Nakada, H.; Nakamura, S.; Inaba, J.; Orikawa, M.: Toxicity test of (2-acetyl-lactoyloxyethyl)trimethylammonium 1,5- naphthalenedisulfonate (TM 723) reproductive tests in mice and rabbits. Oyo Yakuri 18:923-942, 1979.

16 Acetylpromazine (see Promazine and Phenothiazines)

17 3-Acetylpyrimidine

Landauer (1957) observed poorly developed musculature in 13-day chick embryos after injection of 750 microgm into the egg at 96 hours. Ackermann and Taylor (1948) found 'undersized deformed legs' in chick embryos treated with the substance.

Ackermann, W.W. and Taylor, A.: Application of metabolic inhibitor to the developing chicken embryo. Proc. Soc. Exp. Biol. Med. 67: 449-452, 1948.

Landauer, W.: Niacin antagonists and chick development. J. Exp. Zool. 136: 506-530, 1957.

18 Acetylsalicylic Acid (see Salicylate)

19 Acetylsulfanilamide (also see Sulfonamides)

Bariljak (1968) produced a 30 percent fetal mortality by giving rats 10 gm per kg on the 10th day of gestation. No abnormalities were produced.

Bariljak, I.R.: Comparison of antithyroidal and teratogenic action of some hypoglycemic sulphanylamides. Problems of

Endocrinology (Russian) 14: No. 6, 89-94, 1968.

20   N-Acetyl-L-tryptophan

This parenteral substitute for l-tryptophan was studied in rats, rabbits and mice by Maruoka, Kadota, Uesako and Ueshima and Takemoto (1980). Intraperitoneal doses of up to 600 mg per kg before conception and through day 7 were not associated with adverse effect in the rat. On days 7 through 17 the same intraperitoneal dose and up to 5.0 gm per kg daily was associated with some decrease in fetal weight but no increased malformations. Behavioral studies were carried out and no differences from controls were found. Intravenous doses in the rabbit on days 6 through 18 of up to 1000 mg per kg daily produced only fetal growth retardation at the highest dose. No effect was seen at 500 mg per kg.

Maruoka, H.; Kadota, Y.; Uesako, T.; Kakemoto, Y. and Ueshima, M.: Toxicological studies of N-acetyl-L-tryptophan 4-7. Iyakuhin Kenkyu 11:682-742, 1980.

21   Aclacinomycin A

Kamata et al (1980) studied this antineoplastic agent in rats and rabbits. Using a dose of 0.2 - 1.0 mg per kg per day on days 7 through 17 produced no ill effects in the offspring. The same doses on days 17-21 was found to have no effect on the performance of the offspring. Up to 2.0 mg per kg was given to the pregnant rabbit on days 6-18 and no adverse effects were found in the fetuses.

Kamata, K.; Tomizawa, S.; Sato, R.; Kashima, M.: Teratological studies on Aclacinomycin A. Oyo Yakuri 19:783-794, 1980.

22   Acriflavin [Trypaflavine]

Ancel (1946) used this local antiseptic dropped onto the chick embryo at 26 hours in a dose of 0.02 mg and found about 30 percent spina bifida. At 48 hours of incubation the development of the amnion was arrested by similar treatment.

Ancel, P.: Recherche experimentale sur le spina bifida. Arch. Anat. Microsc. Morphol. Exp. 36: 45-68, 1946.

23   Acrolein

This compound is one of the metabolites of cyclophosphamide. Mirkes et al (1981) added this compound to an in vitro rat embryo culture at 5 microgram per ml (equimolar to a teratogenic dose of cyclophosphamide) and found no growth retardation or increase in defects. At twice the dose the compound was lethal. Schmid, et al (1981) found growth retardation but no structural defects at 100 and 150 micromolar concentrations when rat embryos were exposed in vitro. Hales injected the compound intramniotically and at doses of 1 microgram or 0.018 micromoles per rat fetus found 85 percent defects which were similar to to those produced by cyclophosphoramide. Acrolein binds very strongly to serum proteins and this causes difficulty in assessing either in vitro or in vivo whether it is the final active metabolite in cyclophosphamide teratogenicity.

Hales, B.F.: Comparison of the mutagenicity and teratogenicity of cyclophosphamide and its active metabolites, 4-hydroxycyclophosphamide, phosphoramide mustard and acrolein. Cancer Res. 42:3016-3021, 1982.

Mirkes, P.E.; Fantel, A.G.; Greenaway, J.C. and Shepard, T.H.: Teratogenicity of cyclophosphamide metabolites: phosphoramide mustard, acrolein and 4-ketocyclophosphamide in rat embryos cultured in vivo. Toxicol. Appl. Pharm. 58:322-330, 1981.

Schmid, B.P.; Goulding, E.; Kitchin, K. and Sanyal, M.K.: Assessment of the teratogenic potential of acrolein and cyclophosphamide in a rat embryo culture system. Toxicol. 22:235-243, 1981.

24   Acrylic Acid (see methacrylate esters)

25   Acrylonitrite

Murray et al (1978) administered this compound found in plastics and fibers to rats on days 6 through 15 of gestation at doses of 25 mg per kg by mouth. Some maternal toxicity occurred and trunk and aortic anomalies were produced. Inhalation of 80 ppm produced teratogenic effects. Inhalation of 40 ppm or oral doses of 20 mg per kg caused no fetal effects.

Murray, F.J.; Nitschke, K.D.; John, J.A.; Crawford, A.A.; McBride, J.G. and Schwetz, B.A.: Teratogenic potential of acrylonitrate given to rats by gavage or inhalation. (abs) Teratoloy 17:50A (only), 1978.

26   ACTH [Adrenocorticotrophic Hormone]

Cleft palate has been produced in mice given 5 mg ACTH every 6 hours for 2 to 3 days beginning in the 13th day of gestation (Fraser et al, 1954). The subject is well summarized by Kalter and Warkany (1959).

Kotin et al (1978) injected pregnant rats with 4 and 10 units of hormone from day 11 through day 15 and observed alterations of DNA and protein biosynthesis in liver, brain and placenta of 15-day fetuses.

Fraser, F.C.; Kalter, H.; Walker, B.E. and Fainstat, T.D.: Experimental production of cleft palate with cortisone and other hormones. J. Cell Comp. Physiol. 43: Suppl. 1: 237-259, 1954.

Kalter, H. and Warkany, J.: Experimental production of congenital malformations in mammals by metabolic procedure. Physiol. Rev. 39: 69-115, 1959.

Kotin, A.M.; Chebotar, N.A. and Tishchenko, L.I.: Effect of adrenocorticotropic hormone on the synthesis and content of nucleic acids and proteins in the brain of rat embryos during early embryogenesis. Ontogenez. (USSR) 9.1:70-77, 1978.

27 Actidione

Thiersch (1971) reported that 1 mg given intraperitoneally on the 11th day was embryocidal to the rat embryo and given on the 6th day caused stunting in 24 percent of the survivors.

Thiersch, J.B.: Investigations into the differential effect of compounds on rat litter and mother. In, Tuchmann-Duplessis, H.; ed. Malformations Congenitales des Mammiferes. Paris:Masson Cie, 1971. pp. 95-113.

28 Actinobolin Sulfate

Karnofsky and Lacon (1962) list this substance as producing facial coloboma and cleft palate in the chick exposed to 5 to 10 mg. Edema and webbing of the toes also occurred.

Karnofsky, D.A. and Lacon, C.R.: Survey of cancer chemotherapy service center compounds for teratogenic effect in the chick embryo. Cancer Res. 22: 84-86, 1962.

29 Actinomycin C

Exencephaly, spina bifida and other defects have been produced in rats injected on the 6th and 10th days of gestation (Takaya, 1963). The amount injected was not stated.

Takaya, M.: Teratogenic effect of the antitumor antibiotics. (abstract) Proceedings of The Congenital Anomalies Research Association of Japan 3: 47-48, 1963.

30 Actinomycin D

Tuchmann-Duplessis and Mercier-Parot (1958) using 25 to 100 microgm per kg daily before the 10th day found in the rat various degrees of craniorachischisis, other defects of the nervous system and branchial arch malformations. The same authors (1960) found agenesis of the optic nerve, encephalocele and lumbosacral spina bifida in rabbits treated with 150 or 200 microgm per day during the 8th to 10th days of gestation. Wilson (1966) has confirmed the interesting finding that after the 10th day defects cannot be produced in the rat. Dyban and Akimova (1967) showed that 50 to 250 microgm per kg had no effect given during the 1st 4 days but given on the 9th day the embryonic ectoderm and decidual cells were affected but not the yolk sac endoderm. Baranov et al (1968) demonstrated radioautographically that the compound is localized in the embryo. Pierro (1961) has produced rumplessness in chicks with 0.06 microgm injections at 48 hours of incubation.

Baranov, V.S.; Weismann, B.L.; Nikitina, S.S.; Repina, G.V. and Repina, V.S.: Differential inhibition of serum protein synthesis in mammalian embryos by actinomycin D in various stages of liver development. Biochemistry (Russian) 33: No. 6, 1174-1182, 1968.

Dyban, A.P. and Akimova, I.M.: Some peculiarities of embryogenesis; disturbances caused by blockade of RNA synthesis in mammals. Experiments with actinomycin D in rats. Arch. Anat. (Russian) 52: No. 5, 36-50, 1967.

Pierro, L.J.: Teratogenic action of actinomycin D in the embryonic chick. J. Exp. Zool. 147: 203-210, 1961.

Tuchmann-Duplessis, H. and Mercier-Parot, L.: The terato-genic action of the antibiotic actinomycin D in Wolstenholme, G.E.W. and O'Connor, C.M. (ed.): Ciba Foundation Symposium on Congenital Malformations. Boston: Little Brown and Co.; 1960. PP. 115-128.

Tuchmann-Duplessis, H. and Mercier-Parot, L.: influence de l'actinomycine D sur la gestation et le developpement foetal du lapin. C. R. Soc. Biol. (Paris) 154: 914-916, 1960.

Wilson, J.G.: Effects of acute and chronic treatment with actinomycin D on pregnancy and the fetus in the rat. Harper Hospital Bulletin 24: 109-118, 1966.

31   Adenine (also see 2-Deoxyadenosine)

Fujii and Nishimura (1970) gave 250 and 300 mg of adenine per kg to mice on the 12th gestational day and produced cleft palate, digital defects and subcutaneous hematomas in 13 to 20 percent of the fetuses.

Fujii, T. and Nishimura, H.: Teratogenic action of adenine on mouse embryos. Jap. J. Pharmacol. 20: 445-447, 1970.

32   Adenosine (see 2-Deoxyadenosine)

33   Adenosine Monophosphate (see Adenosine Triphosphate)

34   Adenosine Triphosphate

Gordon et al (1963) studied the effect of adenosine triphosphate and its decomposition products on cortisone-induced defects in the mouse fetus. Adenosine monophosphate (29 microgm) increased the number of fetuses with hydrocephalus, spinal and eye deformity but adenosine triphosphate decreased the incidence. The mice received 2.5 mg of cortissone acetate along with these substances beginning the 11th and ending the 14th day of gestation.

Hashimoto   et   al   (1970)   injected   this   compound
intraperitoneally   into   pregnant   rats   and mice on the 7th
through the 13th day of gestation.   Doses of 400 mg   per   kg
per   day caused slight fetal growth retardation but no teratogenicity.

Gordon, H.W.; Traczyk, W.; Peer, L.A. and Bernhard, W.G.:
The effect of adenosine triphosphate and   its   decomposition
products   on   cortisone   induced   teratology.   J.   Embryol.
Exp. Morphol. 11: 475-482, 1963.

Hashimoto, Y.; Toshioka, N. and Nomura, M.: Studies on
teratogenic action of adenosine-5-monophosphate in mice   and
rats. Oyo Yakuri 4: 625-633, 1970.

35   Adrenalin (see Epinephrine)

36   Adhesives, Spray (see Spray Adhesives)

37   Adriamycin

Oguro   et   al   (1973)   gave   this   antineoplastic medication
intraperitoneally to pregnant rats and intravenously to mice
on   days   7 through 13 in amounts up to 1,000 micrograms per
day and observed no teratogenicity.   Using doses of 2 mg per
kg   intraperitoneally   and   longer treatment, Thompson et al
(1978) produced atresia of the esophagus and   intestine   and
cardiovascular   anomalies   in   rat   fetuses.   Intravenous
treatment of the rabbit with up to 0.6 mg per kg on   days   6
through 18 produced no fetal defects but abortions occurred.

Oguro, T.; Hatano, M.; Imamura, T.   and Shimizu, M.:
Toxicological   studies   on   adriamycin-HCl 4.   Teratological
study.   (Japanese) Yakubutsu Ryoho   (Medical   Treatment)   6:
1152-1164, 1973.

Thompson, D.J.; Molello, J.A.; Strebing, R.J.   and Dyke,
I.L.: Teratogenicity of adriamyin and daunomycin in the rat
and rabbit. Teratology 17:151-158, 1978.

38   Aflatoxin

Aflatoxins are products of aspergillus flavus and have   been
shown   to   be carcinogenic as well as teratogenic.   Elis and
Dipaola (1967) injected 4 mg per kg   intraperitoneally   into
hamsters   on   the   8th day of pregnancy.   Early embryos were
malformed in about   30   percent   whereas   surviving   fetuses
showed   a   defect   rate   of   6 percent.   Neural tube closure
defects, microcephaly, umbilical   hernia   and   cleft   palate
were   reported.   Fetal   liver   cell   necrosis   was   noted.
Premixing the aflatoxin B(1) with DNA reduced the teratogenic effect.   Aflatoxin feeding at 10 ppm during the last half
of gestation produced nodular hyperplasia of the   liver   in
four   and   cholangiocarcinoma   in   one   of   79 rat offspring
(Grice et al, 1973).   Yamamoto et   al   (1981)   treated   mice

intraperitoneally with 16 or 32 mg per kg for various two day consecutive periods during organogenesis. Cleft palate, open eyelid, wavy ribs and bent long bones were found after the 32 mg dose.

Elis, J. and Dipaolo, J.A.: Aflatoxin B(1) induction of malformations. Arch. Pathol. 83: 53-57, 1967.

Grice, H.C.; Moodie, C.A. and Smith, D.C.: The carcinogenic potential of aflatoxin or its metabolites in rats from dams fed aflatoxin pre- and post partum. Cancer Res. 33: 262-268, 1973.

Yamamoto, Y.; Kihara, Y. and Tanimura, T.: Effects of aflatoxin B-1 on teratogenicity of mice. (abstract) Teratology 24: 25A, 1981.

39   Afraidol Blue

This azo dye has produced malformations in rats (see trypan blue or review by Beck and Lloyd, 1966).

Beck, F. and Lloyd, J.B.: The teratogenic effects of azo dyes. In, Woollam, D.H.M. (ed.): Advances in Teratology, Vol. 1. New York, Logos and Academic Press, 1966. pp. 131-193.

40   Akabane Virus

This virus has been associated with increased rates of abortion, stillbirth and congenital malformations in cattle, sheep and goats (Kurogi et al, 1977). The major amount of study has been done in Japan. Kurogi et al (1977) isolated the virus and inoculated pregnant cattle intravenously. The two fetuses examined had myositis and some of the fall term animals had the typical syndrome with cerebral defects, hydroanencephaly and arthrogryposis.

Kurogi, H.; Inaba, Y.; Takahashi, E.; Sato, K.; Satoda, K.; Goto, Y.; Omori, T. and Matumoto, M.: Congenital abnormalities in newborn calves after inoculation of pregnant cows with Akabane virus. Infection and Immunity 17:338-343, 1977.

41   Alazopeptin A

Thiersch (1958) injected this peptide derived from streptomyces into rats on the 7th and 8th or 11th and 12th day (0.3 to 0.5 mg per kg) and produced a high litter resorption rate but no defects were found.

Thiersch, J.B.: Effect of alazopeptin (A) on litter and fetus of the rat in utero. Proc. Soc. Exp. Biol. Med. 97: 888-889, 1958.

42   Alcohol, Alcoholism (Ethanol)

Sandor (1968) injected the equivalent of 0.3 ml of ethanol into the chick air sac at 23 hours of incubation and produced neural tube and cerebral vesicle deformities along with some mesodermal defects. Sandor and Amels (1971) injected pregnant rats intravenously at 6 and 7 days of gestation with 1.0 to 2.0 gm of ethanol per kg and found embryolethality but no defects in the surviving fetuses. Chernoff (1977) fed pregnant mice before and during pregnancy with a Metracal diet containing 15 to 30 percent ethanol derived calories. At the higher concentrations resorptions occurred frequently. Neural defects and cardiac malformations were found in a significant number of offspring. Yanai and Ginsburg (1976) found increased susceptibility to audiogenic seizures in offspring of mice given alcohol. Learning is impaired in rats exposed during intrauterine life (Martin et al, 1977). Randall and Taylor (1979) showed a dose response curve between defects and dietary content of ethanol. The maternal weight changes between the sucrose fed control and ethanol group were not different and the ethanol group was supplemented with vitamins. The literature on animal models has been recently summarized (Streissguth et al, 1979).

A fetal alcohol or alcoholism syndrome has been delineated in the human. Jones et al (1973) described 8 children from mothers with chronic alcoholism. The children were characterized by small birth weight, microcephaly, reduction in width of the palpebral fissures and maxillary hypoplasia. Five had cardiac anomalies. In a subsequent report Jones and Smith (1973) estimated that about one-third of the offspring of chronic alcoholic mothers had the syndrome. Two of their children had cleft palates. All of the infants had some form of developmental delay (Jones et al, 1974). One autopsy report showing malorientation of the brain has appeared (Clarren et al, 1978). Lemoine et al (1968) in a previously obscure paper described 127 children from alcoholic mothers and found a very similar clinical picture with a 25 percent malformation rate which included, in particular, cleft palate and cardiac anomalies. Other reports of the syndrome have appeared (Palmer et al, 1974; Ferrier et al, 1973; Manzke and Grosse, 1975; Majewski, 1981). In a study of the frequency of the syndrome made in a group of 1,500 infants from middle class families, 11 newborns were judged without the examiner's knowledge to have signs compatible with the prenatal effect of alcohol (Hanson et al, 1978). Two of these had fetal alcohol syndrome and were offspring of heavy drinkers, and 9 were from the high risk group who took over two ounces of ethanol per day. Behavior studies of the at-risk newborns showed increased tremors, decreased vigorous activity and increased non-alert wake states (Landesman-Dwyer et al, 1978). The cardiac defects associated with the syndrome have been detailed (Sandor et al, 1981). A review of the clinical and animal work (Streissguth et al, 1980) indicate that the fetal alcohol syndrome may be the most commonly recognized cause of mental retardation. These authors felt that adverse fetal effects are not likely when the mother drinks less than two drinks per day (1980). Harlap and Shiono (1980), Kline et al (1980) and Streissguth et al 1981) have published data suggesting that even moderate drinking may be associated with increased spontaneous abortion in the first and-or the second trimester.

Futher studies seeking to understand the molecular pathogenesis of the syndrome were reported by Chernoff (1980) in three mouse strains. Maternal alcohol dehydrogenase levels in the three strains were related inversely to the maternal alcohol level and the number of congenital defects. Clarren and Bowden (1982) studied the effects of binge drinking in three monkeys. They gave 2.5 or 4.1 gm per kg by gavage once weekly from 40 days gestation to term. One offspring exposed to the highest dose had neurologic, developmental and facial anomalies similar to those seen in the human syndrome. One of the other two exposed to the lower dose had similar but less severe findings. Sulik and Johnston (1982) have carried out detailed embryologic studies after exposing the mouse to acute doses of alcohol. The morphologic features followed a deficiency in the neural plate. Diaz and Samson (1980) have studied the effect on brain growth of alcohol administration through intragastric cannulas to newborn rats.

The direct effects of ethanol have been studied in in vitro culures of rat embryos (Brown et al, 1979; Campbell and Fantel, 1983 and Popov et al, 1981). A growth retarding effect, especially of the central nervous system, has been shown at concentrations of 300 mg per 100 ml.

The human syndrome may not be due primarily to alcohol and other factors such as poor protein intake, pyridoxine or other B vitamin deficiency, alcohol contaminants such as lead or genetic predisposttion may play an important etiologic role. Veghelyi et al (1978) have presented the hypothesis that the syndrome is related to elevated acetaldehyde levels secondary to a defect in mitochondrial aldehyde dehydrogenase (see acetaldehyde).

Brown, N.A.; Goulding, E.H. and Fabro, S.: Ethanol embryotoxiciy: direct effects on mammalian embryos in vitro. Science 206:573-575, 1979.

Campbell, M.A. and Fantel, A.G.: The relative teratogenicity of ethanol and acetaldehyde in vitro. Life Sciences, in press, 1983.

Chernoff, G.F.: The fetal alcohol syndrome in mice. An animal model. Teratology 15:223-230, 1977.

Chernoff, G.F.: The fetal alcohol syndrome in mice: Maternal variables. Teratology 22:71-75, 1980.

Clarren, S.K.; Alvord, E.C.; Sumi, M.; Streissguth, A.P. and Smith, D.W.: Brain malformations related to prenatal exposure to ethanol. J. Pediatr. 92:64-67, 1978.

Clarren, S.K. and Bowden, D.M.: A new primate model for binge drinking and its relevance to human ethanol teratogenesis. J. Pediat. 101:819-824,1982.

Diaz, J. and Samson, H.H.: Impaired brain growth in neonatal rats exposed to ethanol. Science 208:751-753, 1980.

Ferrier, P.E.; Nicod, I. and Ferrier, S.: Fetal alcohol syndrome. Lancet 2: 1496 (only), 1973.

Hanson, J.W.; Streissguth, A.P. and Smith, D.W.: The effects of moderate alcohol consumption during pregnancy on fetal growth and morphogenesis. J. Pediatr. 92:457-460, 1978.

Harlap, S. and Shiono, P.H.: Alcohol, smoking and incidence of spontaneous abortions in the first and second trimester. Lancet 2: 173-178, 1980.

Jones, K.L. and Smith, D.W.: Recognition of the fetal alcohol syndrome in early infancy. Lancet 2: 999-101, 1973.

Jones, K.L. and Smith, D.W.: The fetal alcohol syndrome. Teratology 12: 1-10, 1975.

Jones, K.L.; Smith, D.W.; Streissguth, A.P. and Myrianthopoulos, N.C.: Outcome in offspring of chronic alcoholic women. Lancet 1: 1076-1078, 1974.

Jones, K.L.; Smith, D.W.; Ulleland, C.N. and Streissguth, A.P.: Pattern of malformation in offspring of chronic alcoholic mothers. Lancet 1: 1267-1271, 1973.

Kline, J.; Shroat, P.; Stein, Z.; Susser, M. and Warburton, D.: Drinking during pregnancy and spontaneous abortion. Lancet 2:176-180, 1980.

Landesman-Dwyer, S.; Keller, L.S. and Streissguth, A.P.: Naturalistic observations of newborns: Effects of maternal alcohol intake. Alcoholism: Clin. Exper. Res. 2:171, 1978.

Lemoine, P.; Harousseau, H.; Borteyru, J.P. and Menvet, J.C.: Les enfants de parents alcooliques: anomalies observees, a propos de 127 cas. Arch. Franc. Pediat. 25: 830-832, 1968.

Majweski, F.: Alcohol embryopathy: Some facts and speculations about pathogenesis. Neurobehavioral Toxic. and Teratology 3:129-144, 1981.

Manzke, H. and Grosse, F.R.: Incomplettes und komplettes fetal Alkoholsyndrom bei drei Kindern einer Trinkerin. Med. Wett. 26: 709-712, 1975.

Martin, J.C.; Martin, D.C.; Sigman, G. and Radow, B.: Offspring survival, development and operant performance following maternal ethanol administration. Dev. Psychobiol. 10:435-446, 1977.

Palmer, R.H.; Ovellete, E.M.; Warner, L. and Leichtman, S.R.: Congenital malformations in offspring of a chronic alcoholic mother. Pediatrics 53: 490-494, 1975.

Popov, V.G.; Weisman, B.L.; Puchkov, V.F. and Ignatyeva, T.V.: Embryotoxic effect of ethanol and biotransformation products in the culture of postimplantation rat embryos. Byull. Eksp. Biol. Med. (USSR) 12:725-728, 1981.

Randall, C.L. and Taylor, W.J.: Prenatal ethanol exposure in mice. Teratogenic effects. Teratology 19:305-312, 1979.

Sandor, G.G.S.; Smiith, D.F. and MacLeod, P.M.: Cardiac malformations in the fetal alcohol syndrome. J. Pediat. 98:771-773, 1981.

Sandor, S.: The influence of aethyl alcohol on the developing chick embryo. Rev. Roum. Embryol. Cytol. Ser. Embryol. 5: 167-171, 1968.

Sandor, S. and Amels, D.: The action of aethanol on the prenatal development of albino rats. Rev. Roum. Embryol. Cytol. Ser. Embryol. 8: 105-118, 1971.

Streissguth, A.P.; Landesman-Dwyer, S.; Martin, J.C. and Smith, D.W.: Teratogenic effects of alcohol in humans and animals. Science 209:353-361, 1980.

Streissguth, A.P.; Martin, D.C.; Martin, J.C. and Barr, H.M.: The Seattle longitudinal prospective study on alcohol and pregnancy. Neurobehavioral Toxicology and Teratology 3:223-233, 1981.

Sulik, K.K. and Johnston, M.C.: Acute ethanol administration in an animal model results in craniofacial features characteristic of the fetal alcohol syndrome. Science 214:936-938, 1982.

Veghelyi, P.V.; Osztovics, M.; Kardos, G.; Leisztner, L.; Szaszovsky, E.; Igali, S. and Imrei, J.: The fetal alcohol syndrome: symptoms and pathogenesis. Acta Paediat. Acad. Scient. Hungaricas 19:171-189, 1978.

Yanai, J. and Ginsburg, B.E.: Androgenic seizures in mice whose parents drank alcohol. J. Studies Alcohol 37:1564-1571, 1976.

43   Alcohol Sulfate (see Surfactants)

44   Aldactone-R (Spironolactone)

This diuretic and aldosterone antagonist was studied in pregnant rats and mice at intraperitoneal doses of up to 80 mg per kg during days 8 to 14 (rats) and 7 to 13 (mice). No defects were produced but at 80 mg per kg some resorptions occurred in mice (Miyakubo et al, 1977).

Miyakubo, T.; Satio, S.; Tokunaga, U.; Ando, H. and Namba, H.: Toxicological studies of SC-14266 5. Effects on the pre and postnatal development in mice and rats. (Japanese) Nichidai Igaku Zasshi 36:261-282, 1977.

45   Aldicarb (2-methyl-2(methylthio)propionaldehyde 0- (methyl-carbamoyloxime)

Reduced acetylcholinesterase activity was shown in rat fetal brain and liver for as long as 24 hours after oral administration of 0.01 or 0.10 mg per kg to the dauer (Cambon et al, 1979).

Cambon, C.; Declume, C. and Derache, R.: Effect of insecticidal carbamate derivatives (carbofuran, pirimicarb, aldicarb) on the activity of acetylcholinesterase in tissues from pregnant rats and fetuses. Toxicol. Appl. Pharmacol. 49:203-208, 1979.

46   Aldosterone

Grollman and Grollman (1962) gave 0.05 mg daily to rats during their gestation and observed increased blood pressure in the offspring at one year of age.

Grollman, A. and Grollman, E.F.: Teratogenic induction of hypertension. J. Clin. Invest. 41: 710-714, 1962.

47   Aldrin-R (see Cyclodiene Pesticides)

48   Alkylbenzene Sulfonate (also see Surfactants)

Mikami et al (1973) applied this detergent containing 13 mg of alkylbenzene sulfonate per 0.5 ml to the bare skin of pregnant rats from the 1st to the 13th day of pregnancy. The fetuses had subcutaneous bleeding, edema, cleft palate and musculo-skeletal defects. Other workers in the Japanese Ministry of Health and Welfare have not been able so far to reproduce these findings. (unpublished)

Mikami, Y.; Sakae, Y. and Miyamoto, I.: Anomalies induced by ABS applied to the skin. (abstract) Teratology 8: 98 (only), 1973.

49   Allopurinol (see Hydroxypyrazolo-(3,4-D)-pyrimidine)

50   Alloxan

Takano and Nishimura (1967) reported a 6 to 7 percent incidence of defects in the offspring of rats and mice made diabetic by alloxan. The defects were microphthalmia, exencephaly, cleft lip and palate and spina bifida. These authors in discussion of their work and that of others concluded that the diabetic state and not the alloxan was responsible for the defects. Kalter (1968) has summarized in detail the experimental literature on defects found after use of alloxan. More recent Japanese work has been summarized by Shimada, et al (1975).

Kalter, H.: Teratology of the central nervous system. Chicago: University of Chicago Press, 1968. pp. 150-152.

Shimada, T.; Endo, A. and Watanabe, G.: Lactic dehydrogenase isoenzymes in embryos of alloxan diabetic mice. Cong. Anom. 15:127-132, 1975.

Takano, K. and Nishimura, H.: Congenital malformations induced by alloxan diabetes in mice and rats. Anat. Rec. 158: 303-312, 1967.

51   17-Alpha-allyl-4-oestrene-17-beta-ol [Gestanon-R]

Jost and Moreau-Stinnakre (1970) administered 10 to 20 mg of this synthetic progestin to rats by mouth or subcutaneously from the 13th through the 21st day of gestation. Some persistence of wolffian ducts and increase in the ano-rectal distance was found in female fetuses. The males were normal. The trans-intestinal route and presence of maternal ovaries were shown experimentally to favor the occurrence of the anomalies.

Jost, A. and Moreau-Stinnakre, M.: Action d une substance progestive synthetique (17 alpha-allyl-4-oestrene-17 beta--ol) sur la differenciation sexuelle des foetus de rat. Acta Endocrinol 65: 29-49, 1970.

52   4-Allyloxy-3-chlorophenylacetic Acid [Mervan-R]

Lambelin et al (1970) found no teratogenic effects of this compound when it was given to rats in amounts of 150 mg per kg per day.

Lambelin, G.; Roba, J.; Gillet, C.; Gautier, M. and Buu-hoi, N.P.: Toxicity studies of 4-allyloxy-3-chloro-phenylacetic acid, a new analgesic, antipyretic, and anti-inflammatory agent. Arzneim. Forsch. 20: 618-630, 1970.

53   Allylthiourea (see Ethylenethiourea)

54   Allylisothiocynate (see Ethylenethiourea)

55   Alphaxalone

Esaki et al (1976) studied this anesthetic component in pregnant rats and mice. Doses of up to 30 mg per kg in mice and 12 mg in rats were given intravenously on the 8th or 12th day in mice and 9th or 13th day in rats. No adverse fetal effects occurred.

CT-1341, which is a 3 to 1 mixture of alphaxalone with alphadolone, was given subcutaneously to mice and rats during active organogenesis in doses to 5 ml per kg and no anomalies resulted (Esaki et al, 1975). Some postnatal growth retardation was found in rats. Negative studies in the monkey have been reported (Tanioka et al, 1977).

Esaki, K.; Oshio, K. and Yoshikawa, K.: Effects of intra-venous administration of alphaxalone on the fetuses of the mouse and rat (Japanese). CIEA Preclin. Rpt. 2:229-236, 1976.

Esaki, K.; Tsukada, M.; Izumiyama, K. and Oshio, K.: Influence of CT-1341 on the fetuses of the mouse and rat (Japanese) CIEA Preclin. Rpt. 1:165-172, 1975.

Tanioka, Y.; Koizumi, H. and Inaba, K.: Teratogenicity test by intravenous administration of CT-1341 in Rhesus monkeys (Japanese) CIEA Preclin. Rpt. 3:35-45, 1977.

56   Alosenn

Matsumoto et al (1981) gave rats this laxative composed of senna leaves and other vegetables during organogenesis. Oral doses of up to 2 gm per kg daily caused no adverse fetal effects.

Matsumoto, T.; Tsugitami, M.; Ouchi, M.; Tomizawa, S.; Kamata, K.: Teratological study of alosenn in rats. Kiso to Rinsho 15:36-53, 1981.

57   Alprazolam

This benzodiazepine tranquilizer was given to pregnant rats orally at doses of 0.5 to 50 mg per kg. Dosing was on the 7th through the 17th day. At the highest dose, some increase in thoracic vertebral anomalies occurred along with increased fetal death. No adverse effects were found at the other dose levels (Esaki et al, 1981).

Esaki, K.; Oshio, K. and Yanagita, J.: Effects of oral administration of alprazolam (TUS-1) on the rat fetus - experiment on drug administration during the organogenesis period. Preclin. Rep. Cent. Inst. Exp. Anim. 7:65-77, 1981.

58   Alternariol

Pero et al (1973) administered this mold toxin subcutaneously to pregnant mice on days 13 through 16 and produced an increase in unspecified malformations at a dose of 100 mg per kg. Resorptions and runts were increased at the same dose but not at 50 mg per kg.

Pero, R.W.; Posner, H.S.; Blois, M.; Harran, D. and Spalding, J.W.: Toxicity of metabolites produced by "alternaria". Env. Health Persp. 4:87-94, 1973.

59   Alum

Kanoh et al (1982) fed pregnant rats for 7 days during mid pregnancy with up to 10% of this compound in the diet. No adverse effects were noted in day 20 fetuses.

Kanoh, S.; Ema, M.; Kawasaki, H.: Studies on the toxicity of alum. Oyo Yakuri 24:65-69, 1982.

60   Aluminum

Ridgway and Karnofsky (1952) were unable to find defects in chick embryos after injecting 15 mg of AlCl (3) into the yolk sac on the 4th day. McCormack et al (1973) fed rats 0.1 percent aluminum trichloride in the drinking water from day 6 through day 19 of gestation and found no adverse fetal effects.

McCormack, K.M.; Ottosen, L.O.; Mayor, G.H.; Sanger, V.L. and Hook, J.B.: The teratogenic effects of aluminum in rats (abs) Teratology 17:50A (only), 1978.

Ridgway, L.P. and Karnofsky, D.A.: The effects of metals on the chick embryo: toxicity and production of abnormalities in development. Ann. N. Y. Acad. Sci. 55: 203-215, 1952.

61   Amantadine Hydrochloride [1-Adamantanamine Hydrochloride]

Vernier et al (1969) gave this antiviral agent to rats and rabbits and found no evidence of teratogenicity. The rats were maintained for three litters on 10 mg per kg and during one pregnancy period were given orally 32 mg per kg per day. The rabbits received up to 32 mg per kg from day 6 through day 16 of gestation. Lamar et al (1973) reported malformations in rat fetuses exposed to 50 and 100 mg per kg. These defects included edema, malrotated hindlimbs and other skeletal defects. Nora et al (1975) report that a woman taking 100 mg per day during the first trimester gave birth to a child with a single ventricle with pulmonary atresia.

Lamar, J.K.; Calhoun, F.J. and Darr, A.G.: Effects of amantadine hydrochloride on cleavage and embryonic development in the rat and rabbit. (abstract) Toxicol. Appl. Pharm. 17: 272 (only), 1970.

Nora, J.J.; Nora, A.H. and Way, G.L.: Cardiovascular maldevelopment associated with maternal exposure to amantadine. Lancet 2: 607 (only), 1975.

Vernier, V.G.; Harmon, J.B.; Stump, J.M.; Lynes, T.E.; Marvel, J.P. and Smith, D.H.: The toxicologic and pharmacologic properties of amantadine hydrochloride. Toxicol. Appl. Pharmacol. 15: 642-665, 1969.

62   Amaranth [Red Food Dye-2] [1-(4-Sulfo-1-naphthylazo-)-2-naphthol-3,6-disulfonic Trisodium Salt]

Shtenberg and Gavrilenko (1970) treated three generations of rats with this food dye in amounts of 1.5 and 15 mg per kg of body weight. The mode of oral administration was not clear. They reported decreased fertility and increased numbers of stillborn in the treated group and an unspecified number of deformed and macerated fetuses. Collins and McLaughlin (1972) administered 200 mg per kg to the rat during pregnancy and reported no increase in malformations but a small decrease in viable implants with the larger doses. Collins and McLaughlin (1973) studied the metabolites of amaranth and found an increase in sternal malformations using sodium naphthionate (100 mg per kg) and skeletal defects using the R-amino salt (200 mg per kg) in rats fed by stomach tube during gestation. The dye used by the Russian workers was obtained from Imperial Chemical Industries and that used by the American workers from H. Kohnstamm and Co.; N.Y. Holson et al (1975) in a multilaboratory study were unable to show fetotoxicity.

Collins, T.F.X.; McLaughlin, J. and Gray, G.C.: Teratology studies on food colorings. Part I. Embryotoxicity of amaranth (F.D. and C. Red No. 2) in Rats. Food Cosmet. Toxicol. 10: 619-624, 1972.

Collins, T.F.X. and McLaughlin, J.: Teratology studies on food colourings Part 11 Embryotoxicity of R salt and metabolites of amaranth (FD and C red No. 2) in rats. Food Cosmet. Toxicol. 11: 355-365, 1973.

Holson, J.F.; Gaines, T.B.; Schumacher, H.J. and Cranmer, M.F.: Is red dye No. 2 Teratogenic: A joint government-industry approach to a toxicological problem. (abstract) Toxicol. Appl. Pharm. 33: 122 (only), 1975.

Shtenberg, A.I. and Gavrilenko, E.V.: Influence of the food dye amaranth upon the reproductive function and development of progeny on albino rats. (Russian) Vopr. Pitan. 29: 66-73, 1970.

63 Ambroxol (Trans-4-[2-amino-3,5 dibromo-benzyl)amino] cyclohexanol hydrochloride)

Iida et al (1981) gave this mucolytic agent orally to rats and rabbits during organogenesis and found no evidence of teratogenesis. At the highest dose (3000 mg per kg, rats; 200 mg per kg, rabbits) maternal toxicity was present and fetal growth retardation was found.

Matsuzawa et al (1981) studied the effect of this expectorant on rats before conception, during the first 7 days of gestation and on days 17-20 of gestation. Maternal and fetal weight gain was decreased with doses of over 500 mg per kg but no adverse reproductive or postnatal changes were found.

Iida, H.; Kast, A. and Tsunenari, Y.: Teratology studies with ambroxol (NA 872) in rats and rabbits. Oyo Yakuri 21:271-279, 1981.

Matsuzawa, K.; Tanaka, T.; Enjo, H.; Mikita, I.; Hashimoto, Y.: Reproductive studies on ambroxol (NA 872) 1 and 2. Iyakuhin Kenkyu 12:358-387, 1981.

64 Amethopterin (see Methotrexate)

65 Amfepramone (see 2 diethylaminopropiophenone)

66 Amikacin (see Kanomycin)

67   Aminoacetonitrile

This nitrile compound produces the lathyrism syndrome in
fetuses (Stamler, 1955). See lathyrism.

Stamler, F.W.:   Reproduction in rats fed lathyrus peas or
aminonitriles. Proc. Soc. Exp. Biol. Med. 90: 294-298,
1955.

68   2-Aminoanthracene

Martin and Erickson (1982) fed this compound to mice
throughout pregnancy in amounts of 5 or 10 mg per kg.
Skeletal anomalies and reduced spermatogonia and oocytes
were found postnatally.

Martin, P.G.   and Erickson, B.H.:   Teratological and
reproductive effects of ingested 2-aminoanthracene in CD-1
mice (abstract) Teratology 25:61A, 1982.

69   Aminoazobenzene (and Derivatives)

Sugiyama et al, (1960) used the following derivatives :
monomethyl M-fluorodimethyl, P-chlorodimethyl and dimethyl.
In all cases the derivatives were teratogenic in mice
producing skeletal defects with a few cleft   palates.
Dosages of 200 to 700 mg per kg were used on single days
during embryogenesis.

Sugiyama, T.; Nishimura, H. and Fukui, K.: Abnormalities
in mouse embryos induced by several aminoazobenzene
derivatives. Okajimas Folia Anat. Jap. 36:195-206, 1960.

70   Aminoazotoluol

Kolesnichenko et al (1978) administered this chemical to CBA
mice intragastrically, thrice, during 4-5   day   before
delivery in sublethal doses (12 mg per kg). Numerous benign
and malignant tumors of the offspring's liver were found.

Kolesnichenko, T.S.; Popova, N.V. and Shabad, L.M.: Tumors
of the liver in mice induced by prenatal and postnatal
administration of orthoaminoazotoluol. Byull. Eksper.
Med. (USSR) 85, 2:199, 1978.

71   P-Aminobenzoic Acid

Heinonen et al (1977) reported that among 43 women who took
this drug in the first 4 lunar months, five had children
with congenital defects.

Heinonen, O.P.; Slone, D.; Shapiro, S.: Birth Defects and
Drugs in Pregnancy. Publishing Sciences Group Inc., 1977.

72   P-Aminobenzoic acid-N-xyloside-Na Salt

This antineoplastic agent was given orally by Matsumoto et al (1982) to mice and rabbits in doses of up to 1250 and 5000 mg per kg per day. No effect on fertility or postnatal function was seen and in neither species was there any adverse fetal effect.

Matsumoto, M.; Nishiyama, M.; Hayashi, H.; Ikuzawa, M.; Seto, T.; Tanaka, O.: Reproductive studies of p-aminobenzoic acid-N-xyloside Na salt. Kiso to Rinsho 16: 4029-4036, 4037-4066, 4067-4073, 4074-4099, 1982.

73   2-Amino-3-ethoxycarbonyl-6-benzyl-4,5,6,7-tetrahydro-thieno(2,3-c) pyridine Hydrochloride

Nanba et al. (1970) studied this agent in pregnant rats and mice and observed no evidence of teratogenicity. The mice received orally up to 1000 mg per kg per day from the 7th through the 12th day and the rats received 700 mg per kg per day from the 9th through the 14th day of gestation.

Nanba, T.; Hamada, Y.; Katsuhiro, I. and Imamura, H.: Studies on anti-inflammatory agents. XV. Toxicological studies of 2-amino-3-ethoxycarbonyl-6-benzyl-4,5,6,7-tetra-hydrothieno(2,3-C) pyridine hydrochloride. Yakugaku Zasshi 90: 1447-1451, 1970.

74   4-Amino Folic Acid (see Aminopterin)

75   Aminoguanidine

Neuman and McCoy (1955) produced inhibition of chick liver development by yolk sac injection with 2 to 20 mg of amino-guanidine on the 2nd through the 4th day of incubation.

Neuman, R.E. and McCoy, T.A.: Inhibition of development of chick embryo liver by aminoguanidine. Proc. Soc. Exp. Biol. Med. 90: 339-342, 1955.

76   Amino-mercaptopurine (see 6-Mercaptopurine)

77   6-Aminonicotinamide

Landauer (1957) injected 10 microgm of this niacin antagonist into chick eggs at 96 hours and observed that nearly all survivors had micromelia. This effect could be prevented by concomitant niacin administration. Since Dr. Landauer's work, 6-aminonicotinamide has become a common model for producing hydrocephalus, cleft palate and skeletal defects in the mouse (Pinsky and Fraser, 1959; Curley et al, 1968) and rat (Chamberlain and Nelson, 1963; Chamberlain, 1966). Chamberlain (1966) has reported production of cleft palate in 100 percent of rat fetuses when the mother was given 8 mg per kg on the 15th gestational day, and that defects of the urogenital and cardiovascular systems were produced by similar injections on the 10th day (Chamberlain and Nelson, 1963). Schardein et al (1967) have produced defects in the rabbit fetus. Courtney and Valerio (1968) treated monkeys from day 26 to 29 with four abortions and three normal fetuses resulting. The mechanism of action of this teratogen has been suggested by the work of of Dietrich et al (1958) who demonstrated in mouse liver insertion of 6-aminonicotinamide into the analogues of nicotinamide adenine dinucleotide (NAD) and nicotinamide adenine dinucleotide phosphate (NADP). These analogues were non-physiologic under in vitro conditions.

Chamberlain, J.G.: Development of cleft palate induced by 6-aminonicotinamide late in rat gestation. Anat. Rec. 156: 31-40, 1966.

Chamberlain, J.G. and Nelson, M.M.: Congenital abnormalities in the rat resulting from single injections of 6-aminonicotinamide during pregnancy. J. Exp. Zool. 153: 285-299, 1963.

Courtney, K.D. and Valerio, D.A.: Teratology of the macaca mulatta. Teratology 1: 163-172, 1968.

Curley, F.J.; Ingalls, T.H. and Zappasodi, P.: 6-aminonicotinamide-induced skeletal malformations in mice. Arch. Environ. Health 16: 309-315, 1968.

Dietrich, L.S.; Friedland, I.M. and Kaplan, L.A.: Pyridine nucleotide metabolism: mechanism of action of niacin antagonist, 6-aminonicotinamide. J. Biol. Chem. 233: 964-968, 1958.

Landauer, W.: Niacin antagonists and chick development. J. Exp. Zool. 136: 509-530, 1957.

Pinsky, L. and Fraser, F.C.: Production of skeletal malformations in the offspring of pregnant mice treated with 6-aminonicotinamide. Biol. Neonate 1: 106-111, 1959.

Schardein, J.L.; Woosley, E.T.; Peltzer, M.A. and Kaup, D.H.: Congenital malformations induced by 6-aminonicotinamide in rabbit kits. Exp. Mol. Pathol. 6: 335-346, 1967.

78   P-Aminophenol

P-aminophenol, a metabolic product of acetaminophen, was administered intraperitoneally or intravenously to hamsters on day 8 of gestation. At doses of 100-250 mg neural tube, eye and skeletal defects were increased. The ortho form was also teratogenic but no evidence for teratogenicity of the meta form was obtained.

Rutkowski, J.V. and Ferm, V.H.: Comparison of the teratogenic effects of isomeric forms of aminophenol in the Syrian Golden Hamster. Toxicol. Appl. Pharmacol. 63:264-269, 1982.

79   Aminophyllin (see Theophylline)

Georges and Denef (1968) reported that 100 to 200 mg per kg given subcutaneously from the 1st to the 17th day produced in the rat fetus a low but significant number of digital defects, most of which were localized to the posterior left limb.

Georges, A. and Denef, J.: Les anomalies digitales: manifestations teratogeniques des derives xanthiques chez le rat. Arch. Int. Pharmacodyn. Ther. 172: 219-222, 1968.

80   Beta-Aminopropionitrile (also see Lathyrism)

Stamler (1955) produced the lathyrus syndrome in rat fetuses by feeding diets containing 0.025 percent after the 17th day of gestation. Rosenberg (1957) injected 0.125 to 0.5 mg into the yolk sac of eggs on the 7th day and produced bowing of the long bones and scoliosis.

Rosenberg, E.E.: Teratogenic effects of beta-amino-propionitrile in the chick embryo. Nature 180: 706-707, 1957.

Stamler, F.W.: Reproduction in rats fed lathyrus peas or aminonitriles. Proc. Soc. Exp. Biol. Med. 90: 294-298, 1955.

81   Aminopterin [4-Aminopteroylglutamic Acid]

Since Thiersch and Phillips (1950) first observed the embryocidal effect of this folic acid antagonist, a large body of information has become available on the subject (see Folic acid deficiency). Thiersch (1952) induced therapeutic abortions in 12 patients in whom surgical interruption was not indicated and in three fetuses detected malformations (hydrocephalus, cleft palate and meningomyelocele). The total dosage was 6 to 12 mg given oveer several days. There are three case reports of malformed children born to mothers ingesting the drug. Small stature, abnormal cranial ossification, arched palate and reduction in derivatives of the first branchial arch were observed (Meltzer, 1956; Shaw and Steinbach, 1968; Warkany, Beaudry, and Hornstein, 1959). Shaw (1972) has given a 9 year follow-up on the amino-pterin-affected child he previously described.

Baranov (1966a) gave rats 0.1 mg per kg of body weight on the 6th day and observed defects of the eye, face, skull, brain, extremities, abdominal wall and tail. A complete mitotic block was noted in the ectotrophoblast but not the embryoblast (Baranov, 1966b). Dyban et al (1977) cultured eight-cell-blastomeres of rat embryos in Bigger's medium with the addition of 20% rat serum from animals treated with different doses of this drug. Retardation of cleavage rate, abnormalities of blastocyst formation and damage of inner cell mass was observed.

Puchkov (1967) applied aminopterin locally to different parts of the chick embryo and produced abnormalities of the head, eye, limbs and trunk.

Baranov, V.S.: The specificity of the teratogenic effect of aminopterin as compared to other teratogenic agents. Bull. Exptl. Biol. (Russian) No. 1: 77-82, 1966a.

Baranov, V.S.: Mechanism of aminopterin pathogenic effect upon embryogenesis in the albino rat. Arch. Anat. (Russian) 51: No. 8, 17-28, 1966b.

Dyban, A.P.; Sekirina, G.G. and Golinsky, G.F.: The effect of aminopterin on the preimplantation rat embryos cultivated in vitro. Ontogenez, 8.2: 121-127, 1977.

Meltzer, H.J.: Congenital anomalies due to attempted abortion with 4-aminopteroglutamic acid. J.A.M.A. 161: 1253, 1956.

Puchkov, V.F.: Teratogenic action of aminopterin and 5-fluorouracil on 4 to 23 somite chick embryos after application in ovo. Bull. Exptl. Biol. (Russian) No. 7: 99-102, 1967.

Shaw, E.B. and Steinbach, H.L.: Aminopterin-induced fetal malformation: survival of infant after attempted abortion. Amer. J. Dis. Child. 115:477-482, 1968.

Shaw, E.B.: Fetal damage due to maternal aminopterin ingestion, follow-up at age 9 years. Am. J. Dis. Child. 124: 93-94, 1972.

Thiersch, J.B.: Therapeutic abortions with folic acid antagonist 4-aminopteroylglutamic acid (4-amino P.G.A.) administered by oral route. Am. J. Obstet. Gynecol. 63: 1298-1304, 1952.

Thiersch, J.B. and Phillips, F.S.: Effect of 4-amino--pteroylglutamic acid (aminopterin) on early pregnancy. Proc. Soc. Exp. Biol. Med. 74: 204-208, 1950.

Warkany, J.; Beaudry, P.H. and Hornstein, S.: Attempted abortion with aminopterin (4-aminopteroylglutamic acid). A.M.A. J. Dis. Child. 97: 274-281, 1959.

82   4-Amino-pteroylaspartic Acid

This folic acid antagonist was used to produce defects in the mouse.

Tuchmann-Duplessis, H. and Mercier-Parot, L.: Production de malformations chez la souris par administration d'acide x-methylfolique. C. R. Soc. Biol. 151: 1855-1857, 1957.

83   Aminopyrine

Loosli et al (1964) found no deleterious effects in pregnant rats (150 mg per kg) rabbits (90 mg per kg) and mice (180 mg per kg) treated daily during most of their gestation.

Nomura et al (1977) injected mice subcutaneously on days 9 through 11 and produced defective fetuses with doses of 0.2 mg per gm of body weight. The defects were mostly ruptured omphaloceles, Sanyal et al (1981) could not demonstrate teratogenicity in vitro in the rat embryo at concentrations of 80 micrograms per ml medium.

This drug was tested in pregnant rats and mice with oral doses of 150 - 200 mg per kg together with sodium nitrate on day 21 or 16, 17 and 18 respectively and fetal pulmonary tumors, leukemia and mammary gland tumors were observed but no congenital malformations. Carcinogenic effect was eliminated by simultaneous injection of ascorbic acid.

Alexandrov, V.A. and Napalkov, N.P.: Transplacental carcinogenesis effect as a result of a combined injection of aminopyrine and nitrite in mice. Vopr. Onkol. (USSR) 25.7: 48-52, 1979.

Loosli, R.; Loustalot, P.; Schalch, W.R.; Sievers, K. and Stenger, E.G.: Joint study in teratogenicity research in some factors affecting drug toxicity. In, Proceedings of the European Society for the Study of Drug Toxicity. Cambridge: England, 1964. pp. 214-216.

Nomura, T.; Isa, Y.; Tanaka, H.; Kanzaki, T.; Kimura, S. and Sakamoto, Y.: Teratogenicity of aminopyrine and its molecular compound with barbital (abs) Teratology 16:118 (only) 1977.

Sanyal, M.K.; Kitchin, K.T. and Dixon, R.L.: Rat conceptus development in vitro: Comparative effects of alkalating agents. Toxicol. Appl. Pharm. 57:14-19, 1981.

84   2-Amino-1,3,4-thiadiazole

Beaudoin (1973) produced congenital defects in rats injected peritoneally with 25 to 200 mg per kg. The most sensitive period for defect production was during days 9 through 13. Eye defects, hydrocephalus, skeletal reduction defects and cleft palate were found. Nicotinamide supplementation diminished the teratogenic action.

Beaudoin, A.R.: Teratogenic activity of 2-amino-1,3,4-thia-diazole hydrochloride in Wistar rats and the protection afforded by nicotinamide. Teratology 7: 65-72, 1973.

85   2-Amino-1,3,4-thiadiazole-5-sulfonamide (see Acetazolamide)

86   3-Amino 1,2,4-triazole [Amitrole-R]

Landauer et al (1971) injected 20 to 40 mg of this herbicide into chick yolk sacs at 0 to 96 hours of incubation. Abnormalities of the beak and occasionally bent tibias were produced.

Landauer, W.; Salam, N. and Sopher, D.: The herbicide 3-amino-1,2,4-triazole (amitrole) as teratogen. Environ.

Res.   4: 539-543, 1971.

87   4-Amino-3,5,6-trichloropicolinic Acid (See Picloram-R)

88   Amitriptyline (Elavil-R)

Heinonen et al report that among 21 women taking this drug
in the first 4 lunar months there was no increase in
offspring with defects.

Heinonen, O.P.; Slone, D.; and Shapiro, S.:   Birth Defects
and Drugs in Pregnancy. Publishing Sciences Group, Inc.,
Littleton, Mass. 1977.

89   Ammonium Chloride

Goldman and Yakovac (1964) gave one-sixth molar ammonium
chloride to mice orally in the drinking water after day 7
during pregnancy and although the offspring were small sized
no congenital defects were found.

Goldman, A.S.   and Yakovac, W.C.: Salicylate intoxication
and congenital anomalies.   Arch.   Environ.   Health   8:
648-656, 1964.

90   Ammonium-0-sulfobenzoic Acid (see Saccharin)

91   Amniocentesis

Trasler et al, (1956) and Jost (1956) observed defects in
mice and rats respectively after amniocentesis.   The
reduction in the amount of amniotic fluid results in
contraction of the uterus with compression of the head on
the chest: this in turn lodges the tongue between the
palatine shelves and prevents closure of the palate. In
addition to cleft palate, stiff extremities, club foot,
adactyly, microstomia and short umbilical cords have
resulted from amniocentesis of the rat on days 14.5, 15.5 or
16.5.   The subject is reviewed by Kendrick and Feild (1967)
and Demyer and Baird (1969).

One might expect a higher incidence of cleft palate in
infants developing in utero with reduced amounts of amniotic
fluid (i.e.   Potter's syndrome).   The absence of this
association may be due to differences in fetal posture
between the rodent and human. Congenital defects in humans
from amniocentesis performed after the first trimester have
not been found (Parrish et al, 1957). Kennedy and Persaud
(1977) punctured the amniotic sac of the rat on day 17 and
produced fetal edema and hemorrhagge which led to limb
reduction and other compression defects.

In a multicenter study the incidence of unexplained
respiratory difficulties in newborns subjected to
amniocentesis was 1.3 percent as compared to 0.4% in matched
controls. Postural deformities were 1.0 percent as compared

to 0.2 percent (Anonymous, 1978).

Hislop and Fairweather (1982) have found significant decreases in the number of alveoli in lungs from monkey fetuses after amniocentesis of an unspecified amount of amniotic fluid. In their preliminary findings the birth weight and fixed lung volume were reduced in the fetuses exposed to amniocentesis on days 47-64 (equivalent of 14-17 weeks in the human).

Anonymous: Medical research working party. An assessment of the hazards of amniocentesis. Br. J. Obstet. Gynaecol. Suppl 2, 85, 1978.

Demyer, W. and Baird, I.: Mortality and skeletal malforma- tions from amniocentesis and oligohydramnios in rats: cleft palate, club foot, microstomia and adactyly. Teratology 2: 33-38, 1969.

Hislop, A.; Fairweather, D.V.I.: Amniocentesis and lung growth: An animal experiment with clinical implications. Lancet 2:1271-1272, 1982.

Jost, A.: The age factor in some prenatal endocrine events. Ciba Found. Coll. Ageing 2: 18-27, 1956.

Kendrick, F.J. and Feild, L.E.: Congenital anomalies induced in normal and adrenalectomized rats by amniocentesis. Anat. Rec. 159: 353-356, 1967.

Kennedy, L.A. and Persaud, T.V.N.: Pathogenesis of developmental defects induced in the rat by amniotic sac puncture. Acta Anat. 97: 23-25, 1977.

Parrish, H.M.; Lock, F.R. and Rountree, M.E.: Lack of con- genital malformations in normal human pregnancies after transabdominal amniocentesis. Science 126: 77 only, 1957.

Trasler, D.G.; Walker, B.E. and Fraser, F.C.: Congenital malformations produced by amniotic-sac puncture. Science 124: 439 only, 1956.

92   Amobarbital (see Barbituric Acid)

93   Amphetamine Sulfate (see Dextroamphetamine Sulfate)

94   Ampicillin

Bachev et al (1974) could not produce malformations in rats given 100 mg per kg during pregnancy. Korzhova et al (1981) fed rats 250 mg per kg on the 4th through the 13th or 15th through the 20th days of gestation. No teratogenic effect was found but the fetuses were smaller than the controls. Pregnancy was prolonged.

Bachev, S.; Petrova, L.; Voicheva, V.; Shishkova, M. and Kolev, N.: Experimental studies on the teratogenic effect, acute and chronic toxicity of Ampicillin. Suvrem Med.

25:28-32, 1974.

Korzhova, V.V.; Lisitsyna, N.T. and Mikhailova, E.G.: Effect of ampicillin and oxacillin on fetal and neonatal development. Bull Exp. Med (USSR) 91:169-171, 1981.

95   Anabasin Hydrochloride (alpha-piperidile-beta-pyridine-
      -hydrochloride)

Ryabchenko et al (1982) administered this compound to rats at doses up to 15 mg per kg on days 1-16 of gestation and found slight embryotoxic effect. In lower doses (5 mg per kg) no teratogenic or embryotoxic activity was found. Doses of 3 mg per kg produced no damage to rabbit embryos and did not influence postnatal development.

Ryabchenko, V.P.: Influence of anabasin hydrochloride on the embryogenesis of albino rats and rabbits. Farmakol. Toksikol. (USSR) 1:87-90, 1982.

96   Anagyrine [Lupin Alkaloids]

Keeler (1973) implicated this alkaloid found in lupins to be the compound which produces crooked calf disease, a congenital syndrome of calves which includes scoliosis, arthrogryposis and or cleft palate. The compound was found as a major alkaloid in the plant samples that were associated with the defects.

Keeler, R.F.: Lupin alkaloids from teratogenic and nonteratogenic lupins. Teratology 7: 23-30, 1973.

97   Androstenediol

Jost (1953) found masculinization of female rat fetuses when the diproprionate of methyl androstenediol was given during the last days of gestation. The diproprionate of androstenediol had less effect.

Jost, A.: Intersexualite foetale provoquee par le methyl- -Androstenediol chez le rat. C. R. Soc. Biol. (Paris) 147: 1930-1933, 1953.

98   Androstenedione

Greene et al (1939). Treated rats from before the 16th day through the 19th day with total doses of 87 to 137 mg and obtained masculinization of the external genitalia and persistence of the wolffian ducts in the female fetuses. These authors provide detailed descriptions of their experimental findings with this androgen as well as with androsterone and testosterone.

Greene, R.R.; Burrill, M.W. and Ivy, A.C.: Experimental intersexuality. The effect of antenatal androgens on sexual development of female rats. Am. J. Anat. 65: 415-470, 1939.

99   Androsterone

Greene et al (1939) using 250 to 800 mg during the latter
half of pregnancy in the rat produced masculinization of the
external genitalia and persistence of the wolffian ducts in
female fetuses.

Greene, R.R.; Burrill, M.W. and Ivy, A.C.: Experimental
intersexuality. The effect of antenatal androgens on sexual
development of female rat. Am. J. Anat. 65: 415-470,
1939.

100   Anemia, Hemorrhagic

Wilson (1953) and Moscarella et al, (1962) were unable to
produce fetal defects by hemorrhagic anemia in rats and
mice. Severe iron deficiency in the rat was associated with
a 75% resorption rate. Most embryos died on about day 12
(Shepard, et al, 1980). There were twice as many female
fetal survivors than male and no significant increase in
defects was found.

Grote (1969a and 1969b) has produced skeletal defects in
rabbits whose anesthetized mothers were bled. Immediate
treatment with salt solution reduced the number of defects.

Grote, W.: Embryonale Fehlentwicklungen bei Kaninchen nach
mutterlichem Blutverlust. Deutsch Med. Wochenschrift 94:
1120 only, 1969a.

Grote, W.: Verhutung von Skelettfehlbildungen nach
mutterlichem Blutverlust durch Elektrolytersatz. Deutsch
Med. Wochenschrift 94: 2342-2344, 1969b.

Moscarella, A.A.; Stark, R.B. and De Forest M.: Anemia,
cortisone and maternal stress as teratogenic factors in
mice. Surg. Forum 13: 469-471, 1962.

Shepard, T.H.; Mackler, B. and Finch, C.A.: Reproductive
studies in the iron-deficient rat. Teratology 22:329-334,
1980.

Wilson, J.G.: Influence of severe hemorrhagic anemia during
pregnancy on development of the offspring in the rat. Proc.
Soc. Exp. Biol. Med. 84: 66-69, 1953.

101   Anesthetics (also see Halothane, Enflurane and Nitrous
      Oxide)

Since the preliminary observations of increased spontaneous
abortion rates in anesthesiologists in Denmark and Russia,
others in the United States have confirmed the observation.
Cohen et al (1971) in a controlled study found a 38 percent
abortion rate among anesthetists and a 30 percent rate among
operating room nurses with only a 10 percent rate for the
control group of general nurses. In view of our lack of
information on the true incidence of spontaneous abortion,
it is difficult to assess reports of increased frequency of
abortion. Corbett (1972), Smith (1974) and Fink and Cullen

(1976) have reviewed the general subject of teratology as it relates to anesthesia. Corbett et al (1974) have reported a higher than expected rate of malformations among the off-spring of female anesthetists but Cote (1975) has criticized their definitions of anomalies and methods of clinical examination. Spence et al (1977) have reviewed the combined findings in Britain and the United States and believe that the increased risk of abortion in anesthetists and their wives is significantly increased over physician controls. In the combined answers from women the malformation rate in anesthetists offspring was 5.5 percent as compared to 4.4 percent in the controls (P = to 0.04). Tomlin (1978) found 4 families of 75 anesthetists to have cerebral defects in their offsping. Three had obstructive lesions of the CNS.

Cohen et al (1980) collected questionnaires from 30,650 dentists and from 30,547 of their chairside assistants. The abortion rates among the chairside assistants were 14 for light users and 19 for heavy users while rates for the non-users were 8. A heavy user was defined as being exposed for over 3,000 hours during a ten-year period. Malformation rates in the same group were 5.7 for light users, 5.2 for heavy users and 3.6 for non users. Musculo-skeletal and nervous system malformations were the categories increased. The wives of dentists did not have increased congenital defect rates but their abortion rates were 10.2 as compared to 6.7 in wives of non-users. Other disease categories among the chairside assistants of heavy users were significantly increased also.

Brackbill (1977) in studies of infants whose mothers received general anesthesia or no anesthesia during delivery found that auditory-invoked heart rate changes in the two groups differed. With repeated stimulation, infants born without anesthesia developed heart deceleration whereas those born with anesthesia shifted from initial deceleration to acceleration. Further studies are needed.

Brackbill, Y.: Long-term effects of obstetrical anesthesia on infant autonomic function. Developmental Psychobiology 10: 529-535, 1977.

Cohen, E.N.; Brown, B.W.; Wu, M.L.; Whitcher, C.E.; Brodsky, J.B.; Gift, H.C.; Greenfield, W.; Jones, T.W. and Driscoll, E.J.: Occupational disease in dentistry and chronic exposures to trace anesthetic gases. J. Am. Dent. Ass. 101:21-31, 1980.

Cohen, E.N.; Bellville, J.W. and Brown, B.W.: Anesthesia, pregnancy and miscarriage. Anesthesiology 35:343-347, 1971.

Cote, C.J.: Birth defects among infants of nurse anesthetists. Anesthesiology 42: 514-515, 1975.

Corbett, T.H.; Cornell, R.G.; Endres, J.L. and Leiding, K.: Birth defects among children of nurse anesthetists. Anesthesiology 41: 341-344, 1974.

Corbett, T.H.: Anesthetics as a cause of abortion. Fert. Steril. 23: 866-869, 1972.

Fink, B.R. and Cullen, B.F.: Anesthetic pollution: What is happening to us? Anesthesiology 45:79-83, 1976.

Smith, B.E.: Teratology in anesthesia. Clin. Obstet. Gynecol. 17: 145-163, 1975.

Spence, A.A.; Cohen, E.N.; Brown, B.W.; Knell-Jones, R.P. and Himmelberger, D.U.: Occupational hazards for operating room-based physicians. Analysis to date from the United States and United Kingdom. JAMA 238:955-959, 1977.

Tomlin, P.T.: Teratogenic effects of waste anesthetic gases. Brit. Med. J. 1:108 (only) 1978.

102 Angiotensin

Thompson and Gautieri (1969) gave angiotensin II (valyl-5) subcutaneously or intravenously to pregnant mice and produced no increase in defects. A dose of 10 mg per kg was given once on days 7 through 12 of gestation. Geber (1969) injected guinea pigs intravenously on the 8th day with 0.02 to 1.7 mg per kg and obtained 3.9 to 9.9 percent defective fetuses. The anomalies included hydrocephalus, myelocele, general and local edema and micrognathia.

Geber, W.F.: Angiotensin teratogenicity in the fetal hamster. Life Sci. 8: 525-531, 1969.

Thompson, R.S. and Gautieri, R.F.: Comparison and analysis of the teratogenic effects of serotonin, angiotensin II and bradykinin in mice. J. Pharm. Sci. 58: 406-412, 1969.

103 Anoxia (see Hypoxia)

104 Antibodies

The extensive literature on this group of agents which can be teratogenic in many species has been reviewed by Brent (1966, 1971). Ebert (1950) studied the effects of antiserum in the pre-differentiated chick embryo. McCCallion and Langman (1964) have reported that a soluble antigen from adult brain tissue caused abnormalities of the brain and eye of the chick embryo. In 1961 Brent et al, reported production of a wide spectrum of congenital defects in the rat receiving rabbit anti-kidney antiserum on the 8th day of gestation. These defects included anencephaly and other nervous system defects, anophthalmia and defects of the ventral body wall, heart, lip and urologic tract. Tuchmann-Duplessis et al, (1966) have described the facial defects found in the rat fetus when the mother received heterologous kidney antibodies on the 7th through the 11th gestational day. By careful extension of this work by Brent and co-workers an anti-placental and an anti-yolk sac antibody were shown to produce defects. They have shown that these antibodies become localized in the visceral and parietal yolk sac (Brent, 1971). This localization coupled with the finding that these antibodies are particularly teratogenic during active yolk sac nutrition may suggest that their mechanism of action is by interruption of some function played by the yolk sac.

Thyroid antibodies have been implicated in congenital athyrotic cretinism (see Thyroid antibodies). Nora et al (1974) have produced heart and other defects by treating the pregnant mouse with antiheart antibody.

New and Brent (1972) injected yolk sac antibody inside the yolk sac of explanted rat embryos and found the teratogenic effect was removed. This suggested that an interaction of the yolk sac with the antibody was necessary to produce teratogenic action.

Brent, R.L.: Immunologic aspects of developmental biology. In, Woollam, D.H.M.; Ed. Advances in Teratology, Vol. 1. London, Logos-Academic Press, 1966, pp. 81-129.

Brent, R.L.: Antibodies and malformations. In, Tuchmann-Duplessis, H.; Ed.; Malformations Congenitales Des Mammiferes. Paris: Masson and Cie, 1971, pp. 187-220.

Brent, R.L.; Averich, E. and Drapiewski, V.A.: Production of congenital malformations using tissue antibodies. 1 Kidney antisera. Proc. Soc. Exp. Biol. Med. 106: 523-526, 1961.

Ebert, J.D.: An analysis of the effect of anti-organ sera on the development in vitro of the early chick blastoderm. J. Exp. Zool. 115: 351-377, 1950.

McCallion, D.J. and Langman, J.: An immunological study on the effect of brain extract on the developing nervous tissue in the chick embryo. J. Embryol. Exp. Morphol. 12: 77-88, 1964.

Nora, J.J.; Miles, V.N.; Morriss, J.H.; Weishuhn, E.J. and Nihill, M.R.: Antiheart antibody produuction of cardiovascular malformations in the mouse: a preliminary study. Teratology 9: 143-150, 1974.

New, D.A.T. and Brent, R.L.: Effect of yolk sac antibody on rat embryos grown in culture. J. Exp. Embryol. Morph. 27: 543-553, 1972.

Tuchmann-Duplessis, H.; David, G. and Mercier-Parot, L.: Malformations de la face produites par un serum antitissulaire. Bulletin de l'association des Anatomistes, 51st Reunion: 1000-1004, 1966.

105 Anticoagulant Therapy (see Coumarin)

106 Anticonvulsants (see Diphenylhydantoin and Trimethadione)

107 Antimony

James et al, (1966) gave 2 mg per kg of antimony potassium tartrate to four sheep during the major portion of gestation

and found no fetal changes. Belyayeva (1967) exposed rats
by inhalation to a dose of 50 mg per kg. There were fewer
than expected offspring but no morphologic alterations were
seen. Ridway and Karnofsky (1952) produced no defects in
chicks given 0.10 mg on the 4th day.

Belyayeva, A.P.: The effect of antimony on reproduction.
Gig. Tr. Prof. Zabol 11:32-37, 1967.

James, L.F.; Lazar, V.A. and Binns, W.: Effects of
sublethal doses of certain minerals on pregnant ewes and
fetal development. Am. J. Vet. Res. 27: 132-135, 1966.

Ridgway, L.P. and Karnofsky, D.A.: The effects of metals
on the chick embryo: Toxicity and production of abnormalities in development. Ann. N. Y. Acad. Sci. 55:
203-215, 1952.

108 Antimycin A

Duffy and Ebert (1957) and Reporter and Ebert (1965)
observed heart-specific effects and anomalous development in
chick embryos grown on medium containing 0.03 microgm per ml
of medium. Shepard (unpublished data) was unable to produce
defects in rat embryos by intravenous injection of antimycin
A.

Reporter, M.C. and Ebert, J.D.: A mitochondrial factor
that prevents the effects of antimycin A on myogenesis.
Devel. Biol. 12: 154-184, 1965.

Duffy, L.M. and Ebert, J.D.: Metabolic characteristics of
the heart-forming areas of the early chick embryo. J.
Embryol. Exp. Morphol. 5: 324-339, 1957.

109 Apomorphine

Ancel and Scheiner (1951) report that 0.025 mg added to 2 to
3 day chick embryos produced abnormalities of the limbs and
body.

Ancel, P. and Scheiner, H.: Sur le pouvoir teratogene de
certaines substances chimiques et en particulier de l
apomorphine. Arch. Anat. Histol. Embryol. (Strasb.)
34: 19-25, 1951.

110 1-Beta-d-Arabinofuranosylaytosine (see Cytosine Arabinoside)

111 1-Beta-d-Arabinofuranosyl-5-fluorocytosine (see Cytosine
     Arabinoside)

112 Aprotinin

This trypsin inhibitor was given to rats intravenously on
days 7 through 17. At a dose of 100,000 KIU per kg,
maternal body weight was reduced and at 200,000, some fetal

death and decreased weight occurred with hypoplasia of the sternebrae (Toyoshima et al, 1976).

Toyoshima, S.; Sato, H. and Sato, R.: Effects of trasylol (aprotinin) administered to the pregnant rat during the organogenetic period (7-17 days of gestation) on the pre and postnatal development of their offspring (Japanese). Clinical Report 10: 2291-2307, 1976.

113 ARDF26SE

Iida et al (1976) treated pregnant rats and rabbits orally with this oral sulfonylurea antidiabetic medication. Doses up to 2500 mg and 250 mg per kg were used in the rat and rabbit respectively. Resorptions were increased in the rabbit at 50 and 250 mg per kg. No significant increase in defects was reported.

Iida, H.; Kast, A. and Tsunenari, Y.: Pharmacometrics. Oyo Yakuri 11:119-131, 1976.

114 Arsenic

Ridgway and Karnofsky (1952) administered sodium ortho arsenate (0.20 mg) to 4-day chick embryos and found stunting, mild micromelia, impaired feather growth and swelling of the abdomen in the resulting 18-day-old chicks. Potassium arsenate given to ewes at 0.5 mg per kg during most of pregnancy caused no defects in four fetuses (James et al, 1966). Ferm et al (1971) found that hamsters treated with 15 to 25 mg per kg of disodium arsenate on the 8th day produced fetuses with a high incidence of anencephaly and also other defects.

Hood and Bishop (1972) injected mice with a single dose of 45 mg of arsenate per kg on gestational days 6 through 11 and produced fetuses with exencephaly, agnathia, anophthalmos and a few cleft palates. Skeletal defects were present also. In preliminary experiments with sodium arsenite they were able to produce the same spectrum of defects with 10 mg per kg. More detailed studies of arsenate and arsenite teratogenicity in mice have been reported by Hood et al (1978) and Baxley et al (1981). The teratogenicity of arsenate has been reported in the rat (Beaudoin, 1974). Five women with arsenic poisoning during pregnancy have had normal offspring (Kantor & Levin, 1948).

Baxley, M.N.; Hood, R.D.; Vedel, G.C.; Harrison, W.P.; Szezech, G.M.: Prenatal toxicity of orally administered sodium arsenate in mice. Bull. Environm. Contam. Toxicol. 26:749-756, 1981.

Beaudoin, A.R.: Teratogenicity of sodium arsenate in rats. Teratology 10: 153-158, 1974.

Ferm, V.H.; Saxon, A. and Smith, B.M.: The teratogenic profile of sodium arsenate in the golden hamster. Arch. Environ. Health 22: 557-560, 1971.

Hood, R.D. and Bishop, S.L.: Teratogenic effects of sodium arsenate in mice. Arch Environ. Health 24: 62-65, 1972.

Hood, R.D.; Thacker, G.T. and Patterson, B.L.: Prenatal effects of oral versus intraperitoneal sodium arsenate in mice. J. Envir. Path. Toxicol. 1:857-864, 1978.

James, L.F.; Lazar, V.A. and Binns, W.: Effects of sublethal doses of certain minerals on pregnant ewes and fetal development. Am. J. Vet. Res. 27: 132-135, 1966.

Kantor, H.I. and Levin, P.M.: Arsenic encephalopathy in pregnancy with recovery. Am. J. Obstet. & Gynecol. 56:370-374, 1948.

Ridgway, L.P. and Karnofsky, D.A.: The effects of metals on the chick embryo: Toxicity and production of abnormalities in development. Ann. N. Y. Acad. Sci. 55: 203-215, 1952.

115 Arvin-R

Penn et al (1971) administered this defibrinating fraction of snake venom to pregnant mice and rabbits and found no significant increase in defects. A high death and resorption rate was associated at dosage ranges of 10 to 25 units per kg. Hemorrhagic placentas were observed.

Penn, G.B.; Ross, J.W. and Ashford, A.: The effects of arvin on pregnancy in the mouse and the rabbit. Toxicol. Appl. Pharmacol. 20: 460-473, 1971.

116 Artificial Insemination

Forse et al (1982) in a multicenter study of 374 liveborn children conceived by artificial insemination found 21 with major malformations and 5 with trisomies. The malformations included neural tube defects (1), congenital heart disease (5) and multiple defects (8).

Forse, R.A.; Ackman, D.G. and Fraser, F.C.: Is artificial insemination (AI) teratogenic? (Abstract) Teratology 25:40A-41A, 1982.

117 Asbestos

Schneider and Maurer (1977) fed mice up to 143 micrograms of chrysotile asbestos per ml of drinking water and found no teratogenic effects. Studies carried out with blastocyst exposure to the material found some decrease in postimplantation survival.

Schneider, U. and Maurer, R.R.: Asbestos and embryonic development. Teratology 15:273-280, 1977.

118 Ascorbic acid

118

Frohberg et al (1973) gave up to 1000 mg of ascorbic acid by
mouth to pregnant mice and rats from day 6 through day 15
and found no adverse effects on the conceptus.

Frohberg, H.; Gleich, J. and Kieser, H.:
Reproduktionstoxikologische Studien mit Ascorbinsaure an
Mausen und Ratten. Arzneim-Forsch 23: 1081-1082, 1973.

119 L-Asparaginase

Adamson et al (1970) administered intravenously 50 I.U. per
kg to rabbits on days 8 and 9 of gestation and observed 6 to
11 percent fetal defects. The defects consisted of
abdominal extrusion, spina bifida, missing tail and defects
of the lung, kidney or skeleton. No defects were produced
in the rat. The enzyme was shown to cross the rabbit
placenta and enter the fetus. Ohguro et al (1969) gave this
compound intravenously to mice and intraperitoneally to rats
in doses up to 4,000 IU per kg from the 7th through the 13th
day of gestation. Exencephaly and skeletal abnormalities
occurred in fetuses from both species when the dosage was
1000 IU or more per day.

Adamson, R.H.; Fabro, S.; Hahn, M.A.; Creech, C.E. and
Whang-Peng, J.: Evaluation of the embryotoxic activity of
L-Asparaginase. Arch. Int. Pharmacodyn. Ther. 186:
310-320, 1970.

Ohguro, Y.; Imamura, S.; Koyama, K.; Hara, T.; Miyagawa, A.;
Hatano, M. and Kanda, K.: Toxicological studies on
L-Asparaginase. (Japanese) Yamaguchi Igaku 18: 271-292,
1969.

120 L-Aspartate, Monosodium

Inouye and Murakami (1973) injected 6 m mole per kg into
pregnant mice on day 16, 17 or 18 of gestation. Pyknosis
and edema were found in the arcuate and ventromedial nuclei
of the fetal brains for 24 hours after treatment.

Inouye, M. and Murakami, U.: Brain lesions in mouse
infants and fetuses induced by monosodium aspartate. Cong.
Anom. 13: 235-244, 1973.

121 Astromycin

This aminoglycoside antibiotic was studied in rats and
rabbits by Nishikawa et al (1981). The route was
intramuscular and maximum daily doses were 500 mg per kg in
the rat and 300 mg per kg in the rabbit. No adverse fetal
changes were observed in either species. Fertility studies
and perinatal studies in the rat failed to produce any
alterations in the treated group. Some renal damage
occurred in the dams.

Nishikawa, S.; Hara, T.; Miyazaki, H.; Ohguro, Y.: Safety
evaluation of KW-1070. Chemotherapy 29:167-175, 1981.

122 Atenolol

Esaki and Imai (1980) treated rats by gavage with 20 to 2000
mg per kg daily. This beta-adrenergic blocker was
associated with some fetal loss at the highest doses but no
increase in congenital defects was found. Similar results
were found in pregnant rabbits using up to 1600 mg per kg
(Esaki, 1980).

Esaki, K.; Imai, K.:   Effects of oral atenolol on
reproduction in rats.   Preclin. Rep. Cent. Inst. Exp.
Animal 6:239-258, 1980.

Eskaki, K.:   Effects of oral administration on the rabbit
fetus. Preclin. Rep. Cent. Inst. Exp. Animal
6:259-264, 1980.

123 Atropine

Beuker and Platner (1956) injected 0.6 to 1.5 mg of atropine
into chick eggs during the interval of 4 to 12 days
incubation and produced no defects. Arcuri and Gautieri
(1973) injected pregnant mice on days 8 or 9 of gestation
with 50 mg per kg. No increase in soft tissue anomalies
occurred but skeletal abnormalities were increased when
treatment was given on day 9.

Arcuri, P.A. and Gautieri, R.F.: Morphine - induced fetal
malformations: III Possible mechanisms of action. J.
Pharm. Sci. 62:1616-1634, 1973.

Beuker, E.D. and Platner, W.S.: Effect of cholinergic
drugs on development of chick embryo. Proc. Soc. Exp.
Biol. Med. 91: 539-543, 1956.

124 AY-9944

Roux et al (1979) fed this anticholesterolemic to rats on
days 2 through 4 of gestation in amounts of 50 mg per kg.
Holoprosencephaly, ocular defects, uterohydronephrosis and
testicular ectopies occurred in a high proportion of the
fetuses.   A hypercholesterolemic diet reduced the incidence
of malformations.

Roux, C.; Horvath, C. and Dupus, R.: Teratogenic action
and embryolethality of AY-9944-R: Prevention by a
hypercholesterolemia provoking diet. Teratology 19:35-38,
1979.

125 Azacytidine

This RNA inhibitor has been shown to damage mouse fetal
brain when given intraperitoneally to the mother in doses of
2 mg per kg. (Schmahl, 1978). Takeuchi and Murakami (1978)
produced exencephaly, encephalocele and eye defects in rat
fetuses whose mothers were given 1 mg per kg
intraperitoneally on day 8.

Schmahl, W.: Different teratogenic efficacy to mouse fetal CNS of 5-Azacytidine in combination with x-irradiation depends on the sequence of successive application. Teratology 18:143 (only) 1978.

126 N-(4-Aza-endo-tricyclo[5.2.1.5]-decan-4-yl)-4-chloro-   3-sulfamoylbenzamide (TDS)

Osumi et al (1979) administered this diuretic orally to rats on days 8 through 17. At 500 mg per kg per day an increase in cleft palate occurred, but not at 2000 and 4000 mg per kg. At 4000 mg per kg there was some reduction in fetal weight. In the rabbit given up to 2000 mg per kg daily no harmful effects were noted in the fetuses (Takaya et al, 1979).

Osumi, I.; Okada, F.; Mikami, T. and Suzuki, Y.: Effects of N-(4-aza-endo-tricyclo[5.2.1.0]-decan-4-yl)- 4-chloro--3-sulfamoylbenzamide (TDS) orally administered to rats in the period of organogenesis upon the pre and postnatal development (Japanese). Yakubutsu Ryoho 12:651- 667, 1979.

Tagaya, O.; Matsubara, T.; Goto, R. and Suzuki, Y.: Effects of N-(4-aza-endo-tricyclo[5.2.1.5]-decan-4-yl)- 4-chloro-3-sulfamoylbenzamide (TDS) administered to rabbits in the period of organogenesis upon the pre and postnatal development (Japanese). Yakubutsu Ryoho 12:669-674, 1979.

Takeuchi, I. and Murakami, U.: Influence of cysteamine on the teratogenic action of 5-azacytidine (abs) Teratology 18:143 (only) 1978.

127 Azaguanine

Thiersch (1960) briefly reports that giving 500 mg per kg on days 7 and 8 caused exencephaly and stunting in rats. Waddington and Perry (1958) observed embryonic degeneration in chicks exposed in ova or in culture to the substance.

Thiersch, J.B.: In discussion of paper by M.L. Murphy, In, Wolstenholme, G.E.W. and O'Connor, C.M.; Ed.;: Ciba Foundation Symposium on Congenital Malformations. Boston: Little Brown and Co.; P. 111 only, 1960.

Waddington, C.H. and Perry, M.M.: Effects of some amino--acid and purine antagonists on chick embryos. J. Embryol. Exp. Morphol. 6: 365-372, 1958.

128 Azalomycin F

This antibiotic effective against monilia and trichomoniasis was found non-teratogenic in pregnant rats and mice (Arai, 1968). The rats received 20 mg per kg and the mice 100 mg per kg daily during the active period of embryogenesis.

Arai, M.: Azalomycin F, an antibiotic against fungi and trichomonas. Arzneim. Forsch. 18: 1396-1399, 1968.

129 Azapropazon (ssee 3-Dimethylamino-7-methyl-1,2-(N-propyl-malonyl)-1,2-dihydro-1,2,4-benzotriazine)

130 L-Azaserine [O-Diazoacetyl-1-serine]

Dagg and Karnofsky (1955) found defects of the appendicular skeleton of the chick after injecting 0.150 to 2.4 mg into the yolk on the 4th day or after. Blattner et al, (1958) studied the effect of this teratogen in the chick. D-azaserine was non-teratogenic. Murphy and Karnofsky (1956) produced skeletal and palate defects in rats receiving 2.5 mg per kg from the 8th to 12th gestational days.

Blattner, R.J.; Williamson, A.P. and Simonsen, L.: Teratogenic changes in early chick embryos following administration of antitumor agent (azaserine). Proc. Soc. Exp. Biol. Med. 97: 560-564, 1958.

Dagg, C.P. and Karnofsky, D.A.: Teratogenic effects of azaserine on the chick embryo. J. Exp. Zool. 130: 555-572, 1955.

Murphy, M.L. and Karnofsky, D.A.: Effect of azaserine and other growth-inhibiting agents on fetal development of the rat. Cancer 9: 955-962, 1956.

131 Azathioprine (Imuaran-R)

Tuchmann-Duplessis and Mercier-Parot (1968) were unable to produce defects in rats and mice but observed limb reduction deformities in rabbits given as little as 5 mg per kg per day from the 6th to 14th day. Scott (1977) found an increase in resorptions and fetal growth retardation in rats given 5 mg per kg. No defects were mentioned.

Golby (1970) studied 25 pregnancies of mothers with renal transplants treated with azathioprine and other drugs. Eighteen were normal, five had early abortions and two had prematures.

Golby, M.: Fertility after transplantation. Transplantation 10:201, 1970

Scott, J.R.: Fetal growth retardation associated with maternal administration of immunosuppressives. Am. J. Obstet. Gynecol. 128:668-676, 1977.

Tuchmann-Duplessis, H. and Mercier-Parot, L.: Foetopathes therapeutiques: production experimentale de malformations des membres. Union Med. Can. 97: 283-288, 1968.

132 5-Azauracil

Kosmachevskaya (1968) using doses of 0.5 and 4.0 mg per chick egg found 32 and 61 percent mortality respectively. Twelve of 14 survivors were defective. Anophthalmia, microphthalmia, coloboma and ectopia of the lens were

132

observed.

Kosmachevskaya, E.A.: Comparison of pathogenic activity of
5- and 6-azauracil in chick embryos. Arch. Anat.
(Russian) 3: 85-92, 1968.

133 6-Azauracil

Kosmachevskaya (1968) found that doses of 0.5 and 4.0 mg
injected on the first day of incubation caused 35 and 77
percent mortality respectively. All surviving embryos had
eye deformities indicating anophthalmia, microphthalmia,
coloboma and ectopia of the lens.

Kosmachevskaya, E.A.: Comparison of pathogenic activity of
5- and 6-azauracil in chick embryos. Arch. Anat.
(Russian) 3: 85-92, 1968.

134 6-Azauridine

Sanders et al, (1961) reported that single doses of 1 mg per
gm over 3 days from the 4th to the 6th day of gestation
interrupted all mouse pregnancies. Van Wagenen et al,
(1970) utilizing the triacetyl derivative produced abortions
and one fetus with skeletal, palate and renal defects in
Rhesus monkeys.

Vojta and Jirasek (1966) administered 7.5 to 15 gm to women
1.5 to 2.5 months pregnant and interrupted the pregnancy
within an 8-day period. Although spontaneous abortions and
congenital defects did not occur, micromolar degeneration of
the chorionic villi was seen.

Sanders, M.A.; Wiesner, B.P. and Yudkin, J.: Control of
fertility by 6-azauridine. Nature 189: 1015-1016, 1961.

Van Wagenen, G.; Deconti, R.C.; Handschumacher, R.E. and
Wade, M.E.: Abortifacient and teratogenic effects of
triacetyl-6-azauridine in the monkey. Am. J. Obstet.
Gynecol. 108: 272-281, 1970.

Vojta, M. and Jirasek, J.: 6-azauridine-induced changes of
the trophoblast in early human pregnancy. Clin. Pharmacol.
Ther. 7: 162-165, 1966.

135 Azetidine-2-carboxylic Acid

Alescio (1973) has shown that this proline analogue which
inhibits collagen accumulation in the chick embryo produces
a decrease in lung epithelial budding. Nagai et al (1978)
produced fusions of the vertebral bodies of rat fetuses
whose mothers were given 300 mg per kg intraperitoneally on
day 8. The use of 100 mg per day for 3 day periods during
organogenesis caused no ill effects in the fetuses.

Alescio, T.: Effect of a proline analogue,
azetidine-2-carboxylic acid, on the morphogenesis in vitro
of mouse embryonic lung. J. Embryol. Exp. Morph. 29:

439-451, 1973.

Nagai, H.; Kambara, K.; Sudo, H.; Yokoyama, S.; Tatsuya, T. and Nagai, N.: Teratogenic effect of proline analogue L-azetidine 2 caroxylic acid on the skeletal system of rats. Lung Anom. 18:19-23, 1978.

136 Azide

Spratt (1950) found in explanted chick embryos that sodium azide above a concentration of 10(-4)m caused degeneration. All tissues of the embryo seemed to be equally affected.

Spratt, N.T.: Nutritional requirements of the early chick embryo III the metabolic basis of morphogenesis and differentiation as revealed by the use of inhibitors. Biol. Bull. 99: 120-135, 1950.

137 Azodrin   (3-(Dimethoxyphosphinyloxyl)-N-methyl-cis-cro-tonamide)

Schom and Abbott produced teratogenicity in avian embryos with exposure levels of as little as 0.4 mg per kg.

Schom, C.B. and Abbott, U.K.: Temporal, morphological and genetic responses of avian embryos to Azodrin, an organophosphate insecticide. Teratology 15: 81-88, 1977.

138 Azoethane

Druckrey (1973) reported the transplacental production of postnatal brain tumors in rats by inhalation exposure of this gas in doses of 37 to 150 mg per kg on the 15th or 22nd day of gestation. Azoxyethane given intravenously on the 15th day (50 mg per kg) also produced a high incidence of postnatal brain tumors.

Druckrey, H.: Specific carcinogenic and teratogenic effects of indirect alkylating methyl and ethyl compounds, and their dependency on stages of ontogenic developments. Xenobiotica 3: 271-303, 1973.

139 Azoxyethane

Griesbach (1973) using 30 or 50 mg per kg subcutaneously on days 8 through 10 produced eye defects and internal hydro-cephalus in a high proportion of the rat offspring.

Griesbach, U.: Selektive erzengung von missbildungen durch Azoxyathan wahrend der Fruhenwicklung der Ratte. Naturwissenschaften 60: 555 (only) 1973.

140 Bacampicillin Hydrochloride

Noguchi and Ohwaki (1979) gavage fed this antibiotic to rats and rabbits at maximum doses of 3000 and 250 mg per kg

respectively. Treatment in both sexes before mating and
during the first week of gestation had no adverse effects.
No increase in defects occurred in rat or rabbit fetuses.
Abortion and maternal death occurred in some of the rabbit
dams at the higher doses. Treatment on days 17-21 in the
rat at 3000 mg per kg produced some maternal deaths and an
increase in stillbirths.

Noguchi, Y.; Ohwaki, Y.: Reproductive and teratologic
studies of bacampicillin hydrochloride in rats and rabbits.
Chemotherapy 27: 30-35, 1979.

141 Baclofen

This muscle relaxant was tested in pregnant mice, rats and
rabbits with negative teratogenic findings. The test was
done orally during the active periods of organogenesis.
Maximum daily dose per kg was 15, 12.5 and 4.55 mg
respectively in the mouse, rat and rabbit (Hirooka, 1976A
and B and Hirooka et al, 1976).

Hirooka, T.: Effects of baclofen (CIBA 34,647-Ba) administered orally to pregnant rats upon pre and postnatal development of their offspring. Osaka Daigaku Igaku Zasshi
28:181-194, 1976.

Hirooka, T.: Effects of baclofen (CIBA 34,647 Ba) administered orally to pregnant mice upon pre and postnatal development of the offspring. Osaka Daigaku Igaku Zasshi
28:195-203, 1976.

Hirooka, T.; Morimoto, K.; Tadokoro, T.; Takahashi, S.;
Ikemori, M.; Hirano, Y. and Miyaji, T.: Effects of
baclofen (CIBA 34647-BA) administered orally to pregnant
rabbits upon pre and postnatal development of their
offspring. Osaka Daigaku Igaku Zasshi 28:257-264, 1976.

142 Bamifylline

Georges and Denef (1968) were unable to produce defects in
rats using up to 1000 mg per kg from the 10th to 12th day.

Georges, A. and Denef, J.: Les anomalies digitales
manifestations teratogeniques des derives xanthiques chez le
rat. Arch. Int. Pharmacodyn. Ther. 172: 219-222, 1968.

143 Barbital (see Barbaturic Acid)

144 Barbituric Acid (and Derivatives)

Setala and Nyyssonen (1964) briefly reported the production
of malformations of the head and extremities in mice given
pentobarbital, but details including controls were lacking.
McColl et al, (1963) found double vertebral centra in the
offspring of mice fed 0.16 percent phenobarbital. This
skeletal finding could be due to a nutritional effect with
delayed ossification rather than representing a true congen-

ital defect. McColl et al (1967) reported skeletal and aortic arch defects in the offspring of rabbits treated with 50 mg of phenobarbitol per kg from days 8 through 16. In the rat Persaud (1965) found a low incidence of limb defects with hexobarbital and barbital given on the 4th and 8th day of gestation.

In conjunction with studies of other antiepileptic drugs and several tranqulizers prospective studies of the effect of barbiturates on pregnancy outcome have been published. Milkovich and Van den Berg (1974) in a group of about 325 women taking barbiturates during pregnancy found no increase in the defect rate. Shapiro et al (1976) studied 8,000 mothers who took phenobarbital during their pregnancies and found no evidence of fetal damage when the drug was taken for indications other than epilepsy. Fedrick (1973) studying 41 epileptic mothers taking only phenobarbital during the first trimester found no increase in congenital defects. Bethenod and Frederich (1975) studying epileptic mothers noted one one abnormal facies of six offspring exposed only to phenobarbital. Seip (1976) has described two siblings with fetal hydantoin-like syndrome from a mother treated with high doses of phenobarbital.

Bethenod, M. and Frederich, A.: Les efants des antiepileptiques. (French) Pediatrie 30:227-248, 1975.

Fedrick, J.: Epilepsy and pregnancy: A Report From the Oxford Record Linkage Study. Brit. Med. J. 2:442-448, 1973.

McColl, J.D.; Globus, M. and Robinson, S.: Drug induced skeletal malformations in the rat. Experientia 19: 183-184, 1963.

McColl, J.D.; Robinson, S. and Globus, M.: Effect of some therapeutic agents on the rat fetus. Toxicol. Appl. Pharmacol. 10: 244-252, 1967.

Milkovich, L. and Van den Berg, B.J.: Effects of prenatal meprobamate and chlordiazepoxide hydrochloride on human embryonic and fetal development. New Eng. J. Med. 291:1268-1271, 1974.

Persaud, T.V.N.: Tierexperimentelle Untersuchungen zur Frage der teratogenen Wirkung von Barbituraten. Acta Biol. Med. Ger. 14: 89-90, 1965.

Seip, M.: Growth retardation, dysmorphic facies and minor malformations following massive exposure to phenobarbitone in utero. Acta Paediatr. Scand. 65:617-621, 1976.

Setala, K. and Nyyssonen, O.: Hypnotic sodium pentobarbital as a teratogen in mice. Naturwissenschaften 51: 412 only, 1964.

Shapiro, S.; Hartz, S.C.; Siskind, V.; Mitchell, A.A.; Slone, D.; Rosenberg, L.; Monson, R.R.; Heinonen, O.P.; Idanpaan, J.; Haro, S. and Saxen, L.: Anticonvulsants and prenatal epilepsy in the development of birth defects. Lancet 1:272-275, 1976.

145 Barium

Ridgway and Karnofsky (1952) injected 20 mg of BaCl(2) into the chick yolk sac on the 8th day and observed curled toes in about 50 percent of survivors. Earlier treatment had no teratogenic effect.

Ridgway, L.P. and Karnofsky, D.A.: The effects of metals on the chick embryo: toxicity and production of abnormalities in development. Ann. N. Y. Acad. Sci. 55: 203-215, 1952.

146 Beclomethasone Diproprionate

Esaki et al (1976) administered this steroidal antiinflammatory to mice by inhalation for up to 10 minutes daily from day 6 througgh 15. The concentration in the chamber was 23 micrograms per liter. The fetuses had approximately 50 percent malformations which were mainly cleft palate but vertebral defects also occurred. Tanioka (1976) administered up to 200 micrograms per kg to monkeys on days 23 through 35 and produced no malformations in 7 fetuses.

Oral administration of up to 16 mg per kg to rats during the first week of gestation, days 7 through 17 or day 17 through 28 days after delivery was studied by Sudon et al (1979), Furuhashi et al (1979) and Hasegawa et al (1979). In the early treatment group a decrease in fetal survival and weight was associated with some maternal toxicity. During organogenesis the 1.6 and 16 mg per kg dose decreased fetal growth but no abnormalities occurred. In late gestation the treatment prolonged gestation and increased the number of dead fetuses when 1.6 or 16 mg per kg was given.

Esaki, K.; Izumiyama, K. and Yasuda, Y.: Effects of inhalant administration of beclomethasone diproprionate on the reproduction in mice (Japanese). CIEA Preclin. Rpt. 2:213-222,1976.

Furuhashi, T.; Nomura, A.; Miyoshi, K.; Ikeya, E.; Nakayoshi, H.: Teratologic and fertility studies on beclomethasone diproprionate; 2 Teratological studies by oral administration. Oyo Yakuri 18:1021-1038, 1979.

Hasegawa, T.; Nomura, A.; Nakayoshi, H.: Teratological and fertility studies on beclomethasone diproprionate; 3 Perinatal and postnatal study in rats by oral administration. Oyo Yakuri 18:1039-1054, 1979.

Sudon, S.; Sendota, H.; Yamamoto, K.; Miyoshi, K.; Nakayoshi, H.: Teratological and fertiliy studies on beclomethasone diproprionate: 1 Fertility study in rats by oral administration. Oyo Yakuri 18:1003-1019, 1979.

Tanioka, Y.: Teratogenicity test on beclomethasone diproprionate by inhalation in Rhesus monkeys. (Japanese) CIEA Preclin. Rpt 2:155-164, 1976.

147   Befunolol Hydrochloride

Yoshinaka et al (1979) and Nakamura et al (1979) and others studied this beta blocker in mice, rats and rabbits using maximal doses of 500, 200 and 100 mg per kg daily respectively. At the highest doses some delay in ossification of the fetuses was found. Stillbirths were increased in the rabbits at 100 mg per kg. Fertility and perinatal studies did not show significant differences from control in the mice.

Nakamura, K.; Yoshida, J.; Aoyama, I.; Morioka, M.; Moritoki, H.: Teratological studies in mice. Riso to Rinsho 13: 4161-4177, 1979.

Nakamura, K.; Aoyama, I.; Moritoki, H.: Teratological study in rabbits. Kiso to Rinsho 13:3715-3939, 1979.

Okuda, T.; Matubara, T.; Morioka, M.; Mortoki, H.: Perinatal and postnatal studies in mice. Kiso to Rinsho 13:3740-3759, 1979.

Yoshida, J.; Ohtani, A.; Moritoki, M.: Fertility study in mice. Kiso to Rinsho 13:3725-3739, 1979.

Yoshinka, I.; Saito, K.; Hikita, S.; Komori, A.; Iizuka, H.; Moritoki, H.: Toxicological studies of befunolol hydrochloride (BFE-60) Kiso to Rinsho 13:3678-3714, 1979.

148   Bencyclane [N-[3-(1-benzyl-cycloheptyl-oxy)-propyl]-N,N-di-methyl-ammonium-hydrogen fumarate]

Boissier (1970) gave rabbits, mice and rats oral daily doses of 5 to 100 mg per kg and found no increase in defects in the offspring.

Boissier, J.R.: Untersuchungen uber eine mogliche terato-gene Wirkung von Bencyclan. Arzneim. Forsch. 20: 1399-1402, 1970.

149   Bendectin-R (Debenex-R)

Bendectin-R which consists of equal parts doxylamine succinate, dicyclomine HCl and pyridoxine HCl was given by Gibson et al (1968) in doses of 30 mg per kg per day in the rabbit and 60 mg per kg per day in the rat during organogenesis and no increase in congenital defects was found. In 1976 dicyclomine was removed from the formulation.

Numerous epidemiologic studies on Bendectin have been published.

Milkovich and Van den Berg (1976) reported no increase in malformation rate in the offspring of 628 mothers taking the drug. Shapiro et al (1977) in over 1,000 exposed mothers found no increase in malformation rate and the offspring's intelligence at 4 years was not different from controls. Bunde et al (1963) found no increase in congenital defects

among 2000 women using Bendectin-R. Cordero et al (1981)
determined the rate of Bendectin use in the first trimester
among over 1200 pregnancies with birth defects. No
significant differences in drug exposure were found in any
of the 12 defect categories. Borderline increases were
found among the groups with amniotic band defects,
encephalocele and esophageal atresia. Mitchell et al (1981)
using a case control study method analyzed 343 infants with
facial clefts or congenital heart disease and found no
association with Bendectin. Morelock et al (1982) analyzed
1,690 mother-infant pairs and among the 375 expossed to
Bendectin no adverse fetal outcome was detected. Jick et al
(1981) linked computer stored prescriptions for Bendectin
with subsequent malformations and found no association among
over 6,800 pregnancies. MacMahon (1981) in an editorial has
pointed out that among the nine studies on Bendectin a few
significant associations have inevitably appeared but no
consistent excess of any particular malformation has been
found. If Bendectin is teratogenic at all it is only under
very rare circumstances.

Bunde, C.A. and Bowles, D.M.: A technique for controlled
survey of case records. Curr. Ther. Res. 5:245-248,
1963.

Cordero, J.F.; Oakley, G.P.; Greenberg, F. and James, L.M.:
Is Bendectin a teratogen? JAMA 245:2307-2310, 1981.

Gibson, J.P.; Staples, R.E.; Larson, E.J.; Kuhn, W.L.;
Holtkamp, D.E. and Newberne, J.W.: Teratology and
reproduction studies with an an antinauseant. Toxicol.
Appl. Pharmacol. 13:439-447, 1968.

Jick, H.; Holmes, L.B.; Hunter, J.R.; Madsen, S. and
Stergachis, A.: First trimester drug use and congenital
defects. JAMA 246:343-346, 1981.

MacMahon, B.: More on Bendectin. JAMA 246:371-372,1981.

Milkovich, L. and Van den Berg, B.J.: An evaluation of the
teratogenicty of certain antinauseant drugs. Am. J. Obst.
Gynecol. 125:244-248, 1976.

Morelock, S.; Hingson, R.; Kayne, H.; Dooling, E.;
Zuckerman, B.; Day, N.; Alpert, J.J. and Flowerdew, G.:
Bendectin and fetal development. Am. J. Obstet. Gynecol.
142:209-213, 1982.

Shapiro, S.; Heinonen, O.P.; Siskind, V.; Kaufman, D.W.;
Monson, R.R. and Slone, D.: Antenatal exposures to
perinatal mortality rate, birth weight and intelligence
quotient score. Am. J. Obstet. and Gynecol.
128:480-485, 1977.

150 Benomyl [Methyl-1-(butylcarbamoyl)-2-benzimidazolecarbamate]

This fungicide was studied in pregnant rats and when a diet
containing 0.50 percent benomyl was fed on days 6 through 15
no fetal effects or malformations resulted (Sherman et al,
1975). When the material was given by gavage (Kavlock et

al, 1982) malformations were produced in both rats and mice. The teratogenic dose in the rat was 62.5 mg per kg and in the mouse 100 mg per kg. Hydrocephalus, cleft palates, hydronephrosis and skeletal defects were found. Fetotoxicity but not teratogenicity was found when 62.5 mg per kg was administered via the diet. Shtenberg and Torchinsky (1972) have also reported teratogenicity in rats.

Kavlock, R.J.; Chernoff, N.; Gray, L.E.; Gray, J.A. and Whitehouse, D.: Teratogenic effects of Benomyl in Wistar rat and CD-1 mouse with emphasis on rate of administration. Toxicol. Appl. Pharm. 62:44-54, 1982.

Sherman, H.; Culik, R. and Jackson, R.A.: Reproduction, teratogenic and mutagenic studies with benomyl. Toxicol. Appl. Pharm. 32: 305-315, 1975.

Shtenberg, A.I. and Torchinsky, A.M.: On the interrelationship of general toxic, embryotoxic and teratogenic action of chemicals. Vestnik Akad. Nauk SSR 3:39-46, 1972.

151 Benz-a-anthracene (see Dimethylbenz-a-anthracene)

152 Benzbromarone

Soyama et al (1979) gave this drug to mice, rats and rabbits during organogenesis. The maximum oral doses were 220, 80 and 220 mg per kg in mice, rats and rabbits respectively. At the highest dose in the mouse there was embryo lethality but no adverse effects were found in the rabbit fetus. In the rat at the 80 mg per kg dose 14 percent of the fetuses were abnormal. The defects included skeletal reductions, club hands, curled tails and cleft lips.

Aoyama, T.; Terabayashi, M.; Konatru, S.; Hasegawa, T.; Shibutani, N.; Shimimura, K.: Teratologic study on benzobromarone. 1. Experiments in mice, rats and rabbits. Shinryo to Shinaku 16:1521-1545, 1979.

153 Benzene

Pushkina et al (1968) exposed pregnant rats continuously during pregnancy to benzene vapors (1 to 670 mg per cubic meter) and found no developmental malformations. The number of fetuses per liter was reduced with exxposure to the higher doses. Some reduction in ascorbic acid content of the fetuses was found. Watanabe and Yoshida (1970) injected 3.0 ml per kg of this solvent into pregnant mice on single days of gestation. Injections on the 13th day resulted in an increased incidence of cleft palate and mandible reduction. Hudak and Ungvary (1978) exposed rats to 3.3 and 1500 mg per cubic meter from day 9 through 14 and found no increase in malformations although fetal growth retardation and skeletal anomalies occurred along with some maternal mortality. Nawrot and Staples (1979) demonstrated embryolethality in the mouse gavaged with as little as 0.3 ml per kg but no teratogenicity at 1.0 mg per kg. Green et al (1978) exposed pregnant rats to 2200 ppm of the vapor and found no increase in fetal malformations. Some skeletal growth retardation was reported. Murray et al (1979) exposed rabbits and mice to 500 ppm during organogenesis and found no teratognicity. They summarized the predominantly negative findings of other workers.

Kitaev et al (1979) exposed female rats (for 4 hours daily during 30-45 days) to benzene vapors (300-1000 mg per cubic meter) and observed abnormalities in cleaving embryos.

Green, J.D.; Leong, B.K.J.; Laskin, S.: Inhaled benzene fetoxicity in rats. Toxicol. Appl. Pharm. 46:9-18, 1978.

Hudak, A. and Ungvary, G.: Embryotoxic effects of benzene and its methyl derivatives. Toxicology 11:55-63, 1978.

Kitaev, E.M.; Nikitin, A.I.; Lipovsky, S.M. and Louchikov, V.A.: Effect of benzene on some indexes of early rat embryogenesis. Akush. Ginekol. (USSR) 4:51-53, 1979.

Murray, F.J.; John, J.A.; Rampy, L.W.; Kuna, R.A. and Schwetz, B.A.: Embryotoxicity of inhaled benzene in mice and rabbits. Am. Industrial Hygiene Association Journal 40:993-998, 1979.

Nawrot, P.S. and Staples, R.E.: Embryo fetal toxicity and teratogenicity of benzene and toluene in the mouse. (abs) Teratology 19:41A, 1979.

Pushkina, N.N.; Gofmekler, V.A. and Klevtsoua, G.N.: Changes in content of ascorbic acid and nucleic acids produced by benzene and formaldehyde. Bull. Exp. Biol. Med. 66: 868-870, 1968.

Watanabe, G. and Yoshida, S.: The teratogenic effect of benzene in pregnant mice. Acta Medica Biol. 17: 285-291, 1970.

154 Benzenesulfonic Acid Hyrazide

Matschke and Fagerstone (1977) gavage fed this rodenticide to pregnant mice on days 8 through 13. Resorptions occurred at maternal toxic levels (62 mg per kg) but only delayed ossification was found in the fetuses.

Matschke, G.H. and Fagerstone, K.A.: Effects of a new rodenticide, benzensulfonic acid hydrazide, on prenatal mice. J. Toxicol. Env. Health 3:407-411, 1977.

155 Benzhydrylpiperazines (see Meclizine-R)

156 Benzimidazole

Waddington et al (1955) injecting 0.5 ml of 0.5 percent solution in eggs found a significant incidence of omphalocephalics (head reduced in size and protruding through endoderm). The teratogenic effects of three analogues (2, 5-dimethyl, 2-ethyl-5-methyl and 2-hepta-5-methylbenzimidazole) have been studied by Blackwood (1960). Doses of 0.2 to 0.7 mg injected into the egg albumen produced 53 percent defective embryos by the 14th day. The defects consisted of extruded brain and viscera and abnormal beaks.

Delatour and Richard (1976) studied this compound and 24 related chemicals in the pregnant rat. Oral doses of up to 53 mg per kg on days 8 through 12 caused neither fetal weight reduction nor malformations. Parabenzimidazole was teratogenic at doses of 10 mg per kg. The N-benzimidazolyl-2 and N-benzimidazolyl-5 carbomates were highly teratogenic. All types of defets occurred including cleft lip and palate, neural tube closure and skeletal types.

Blackwood, U.B.: Selective inhibitory and teratogenic effects of 2, 5-alkylbenzimidazole homologues on chick embryonic development. Proc. Soc. Exp. Biol. Med. 104: 373-378, 1960.

Delatour, P. and Richard, Y.: Proprietes embryotoxiques et antimitotiques en serie benzimidazole. Therapie 31:505-515, 1976.

Waddington, C.H.; Feldman, M. and Perry, M.M.: Some specific developmental effects of purine antagonists. Exp. Cell Res.; Suppl. 3: 366-380, 1955.

157 2-(N-benzl-N-methylamino)ethyl methyl 2,6-dimethyl-4-(M-nitrophenyl) 1,4-dihydropyridine-3,5-dicarboxylate Hydrochloride (YC-93)

Sato et al (1979) studied this vasodilator in pregnant rats and rabbits on day 0 through 20 and 6 through 18 respectively. The maximum daily dose in the rat was 100 mg and in the rabbit 150 mg per kg.

Sato, T.; Nagaoka, T.; Fuchigami, K.; Onsuga, F. and Hatano, M.: Reproductive studies of 2-(N-benzl-N-methyl amino) ethyl methyl 2,6-dimethyl-4-(M-nitrophenyl) 1,3-di-hydropyridine -3,5-dicarboxylate hydrochloride (YC-93) in rats and rabbits. (Japanese) Clinical Report 13:1160-1176, 1979.

158 Benzolamide

Maren and Ellison injected rats with 600 mg per kg every 6 hours starting at 4 p.m. on day 10 and ending at 10 a.m. on day 11. They found that these very large doses produced the postaxial limb defects typical of acetazolimide. Theophylline or potassium deficiency potentiated this drug's teratogenicity.

Maren, T.H. and Ellison, A.C.: The teratological effect of benzolamide, a new carbonic anhydrase inhibitor. Johns Hopkins Med. J. 130: 116-123, 1972.

159 2-(5H-[1]Benzopyrano[2-3-b]pyridin-7yl)proprionic   Acid
(Y-8004)

Hamada and Imamura (1976) studied this anti-inflammatory
agent in pregnant mice and rats. At doses of up to 25 mg
daily in the rat and 5 mg in the mouse during active
organogenesis, no adverse fetal effects occurred. Postnatal
studies were also negative.

Hamada, Y. and Imamura, H.: Teratological studies of
2-(5H-[1]Benzopyrano[2,3-b]pyridin-7yl)proprionic   acid
(Y-8004) in mice and rats. Iyakuhin Kenkyu 7:301-311, 1976.

160 Benzo[a]pyrene

Rigdon and Rennels (1964) fed rats this substance (1 mg per
gm of diet) during pregnancy and found many resorptions and
dead fetuses but only one malformed fetus from 7 litters.
MacKenzie et al (1977) observed sterility in female mice
exposed to 40-160 mg per kg on gestation days 7-16.

Shum et al (1979) studied the in-utero toxicity in relation
to the allelic difference at the Ah locus in mice. A dose
of 50-300 mg per kg was given intraperitoneally on days 7 or
10. They identified the Ah genotype of individual fetuses
by measurement of the AHH inducibility and reported that
when the mothers was Ah nonresponsive, the fetuses with Ah
responsive genotype showed decreased body weight and higher
resorption and malformation rates while the Ah nonresponsive
fetuses in the same uterus did not. The type of defect
included mainly club foot, hemangioma, cleft lip and cleft
palate. All of these defects tend to be associated with
late organogenesis. Hoshino et al (1981) using the same
general protocol and 150 or 300 mg per kg on day 8 confirmed
the findings of Shum et al (1979) for toxicity (reduced
fetal weight and increased resorptions) but they did not
find the same increase in malformations. They found only an
increase in cervical ribs and this occurred among fetuses
from Ah responsive mothers.

Hoshino, K.; Hayashi, Y.,;Takehira, Y. and Kameyama, Y.:
Influences of genetic factors on the teratogenicity of
environmental pollutants: Teratogenic susceptibility to
benzo[a]pyrene and Ah locus in mice. Congenital Anomalies
21:97-103, 1981.

MacKenzie, K.M.; Lucier, E.W. and McLachlan, J.A.:
Infertility in mice exposed prenatally to benzo-alpha-pyrene
B.P. (abs) Teratology 19:37A (only), 1979.

Rigdon, R.H. and Rennels, E.G.: Effect of feeding
benz(a)pyrene on reproduction in the rat. Experientia 20:
224-226, 1964.

Shum, S.; Jensen, N.M. and Nebert, D.W.: The murine Ah
locus: In utero toxicity and teratogenesis associated with
genetic differences in benzo(a)pyrene metabolism.
Teratology 20:365-376,, 1979.

161 5-Benzoyl-alpha-methyl-2-thiophene Acetic Acid

Hiramatsu et al (1980) gave this antiflammatory agent orally
to rabbits during organogenesis. At the highest dose (75 mg
per kg) there was maternal toxicity, implantations were
reduced and fetal ossification was delayed.

Hiramatsu, Y.; Tamura, Y.; Koniba, S.: Teratological study
of RU-15060 (5-benzoyl-alpha-methyl-2-thiophene). Yakuri to
Chiryo 8: 1773-1776, 1980.

162 Benztropine mesylate (Cogentin-Rx)

This drug given in conjunction with phenothiazines or other
drug with anticholinergic activity may be associated with
small left colon syndrome. Falterman and Richardson (1980)
reported two newborns with small left colon syndrome. Both
were exposed to maternal benztropine (2 mg or 6mg daily) and
a psychotropic drug.

Falterman, C.G. and Richardson, C.J.: Small left colon
syndrome associated with maternal ingestion of psychotropic
drugs. J. Pediat. 97: 308-310, 1980.

163 Benzydamine HCl   [1-Benzyl-3-gamma-dimethylamino-propoxy-1
H-indazole HCl]

Namba and Hamada (1969) gave this compound orally and
subcutaneously to pregnant mice and rats during
organogenesis and some growth retardation was found but no
teratogenicity. The maximum oral doses were 200 mg per kg
and for the subcutaneous they were 100 (mice) and 150 mg per
kg per day (rats). Silvestrini et al (1967) found no fetal
effects in long term studies in the mouse.

Namba, T. and Hamada, Y.: Teratogenic tests with
benzydamine hydrochloride. Oyo Yakuri 3: 271-281, 1969.

Silvestrini, B.; Barcellona, P.S.; Garau, A. and Catanese,
B.: Toxicology of benzydamine. Toxicol. Appl. Pharm.
10: 148-159, 1967.

164 Benzyl Alcohol

Duraiswami (1954) injected 0.01 or 0.02 ml of benzyl alcohol
into the yolk sac of the chick from before incubation up to
the 7th day. Meningoceles and skeletal defects were
produced.

Duraiswami, P.K.: Experimental teratogenesis with benzyl
alcohol. Johns Hopkins Hospital Bull. 95: 57-67, 1954.

165 Benzylpenicillin Sodium (Sodium penicillin G) (see
Penicillin)

166 Beryllium

No defects were produced in the chick embryo by administration of up to 113 micromoles of BE(SO)4 by Ridgway and Karnofsky (1952).

Ridgway, L.P. and Karnofsky, D.A.: The effect of metals on the chick embryo: toxicity and production of abnormalities in development. Ann. N. Y. Acad. Sci. 55: 203-215, 1952.

167 Betamethasone [9-Alpha-fluoro-16-Beta-methylprednisolone]

This steriod is a glucocorticoid with a prominent sodium retaining ability. Walker (1971) produced cleft palate in the rat and mouse using 0.05 - 0.3 mg daily for 3 to 4 days during organogenesis.

Walker, B.F.: Induction of cleft palate in rats with antiinflammatory drugs. Teratology 4:39-42, 1971.

168 Bidrin-R [3-Hydroxy-N,N-dimethyl-cis-crotonamide Dimethyl Phosphate]

This organophosphate insecticide was injected into chick eggs and amounts of 30 microgm or more per egg produced parrot beaks, micromelia, straight legs, abnormal feathering and edema.

Nicotinic acid, nicotinamide and certain of their precursors alleviated this teratogenic action. Injection on the 4th day of incubation gave the maximum response.

Roger, J.C.; Upshall, D.G. and Casida, J.E.: Structure-activity and metabolism studies on organophosphate teratogens and their alleviating agents in developing hen eggs with special emphasis on bidrin. Biochem. Pharmacol. 18: 373-392, 1969.

169 Biodiastase

Tsutsumi et al (1979) administered up to 2500 mg per kg orally to mice and rats during organogenesis and produced no ill effects in the fetuses.

Tsutsumi, S.; Sakuma, N. and Fukiage, S.: Invetigations on the possible teratogenicity of biodiastase in mice and rats. (Japanese) Clinical Report 11:1335-1343, 1979.

170 Biotin

Giroud et al, (1956) were unable to produce malformations in rat fetuses after maternal dietary deficiency of this substance. The dietary deficiency was augmented either by oral succinyl sulfathiazole or by mixture with the biotin antagonist avidin. Watanabe et al (1982) found cleft palates and micromelia in the offspring of mice maintained on a diet of egg whites. Simultaneous feeding of 10 mg of biotin prevented the defects.

Giroud, A.; Lefebvres, J. and Dupuis, R.: Carence en
biotine et reproduction chez la ratte. C. R. Soc. Biol.
(paris) 150: 2066-2067, 1956.

Watanabe, T.; Hoshi, E.; Sato, F. and Endo, A.:
Teratogenicity of maternal biotin deficiency in mice.
(abstract) Teratology 26:17A, 1982.

171 Biphenyl

Khera et al, 1979, administered this fungicide by gavage to
rats at doses up to 500 mg per kg on days 6-15 and found no
teratogenicity.

Khera, K.S.; Whalen, C.; Angers, G. and Trivett, G.:
Assessment of the teratogenic potential of piperonyl
butoxide, biphenyl, and phosalone in the rat. Toxicol.
Appl. Pharmacol. 47:353-358, 1979.

172 Birth Control Pills (see Oral Contraceptives)

173 Bismark Brown

Gillman et al (1951) could find no congenital defects after
treating the pregnant rat with this substance.

Gillman, J.; Gilbert, C.; Spence, I. and Gillman, T.: A
further report on congenital anomalies in the rat produced
by trypan blue. S. Afr. J. Med. Sci. 16: 125-135,
1951.

174 Bis-(beta-chloethyl)-methylamine (HN2) [Mustargen-R]

Murphy et al (1958) found that this alkylating agent given
on the 12th day to the rat (about 0.7 mg per kg) caused
cleft palate and defects of the central nervous and skeletal
systems. They also produced defects in the chick embryo.

Murphy, M.L.; Moro, A.D. and Lacon, C.R.: The comparative
effects of five polyfunctional alkylating agents, with
additional notes on the chick embryo. Ann. N. Y. Acad.
Sci. 68: 762-781, 1958.

175 Bismuth

Ridgway and Karnofsky (1952) found no defects in chick
embryos receiving 20 mg of BiCi(3) via yolk sac on either
the 4th or 8th day. James et al, fed 5 mg per kg to sheep
daily for extended periods of gestaton and found one of the
four fetuses to be stunted, hairless and exophthalmic.

James, L.F.; Lazar, V.A. and Binns, W.: Effects of
sublethal doses of certain minerals on pregnant ewes and
fetal development. Am. J. Vet. Res. 27: 132-135, 1966.

Ridgway, L.P. and Karnofsky, D.A.: The effects of metals

175

on the chick embryo: toxicity and production of abnormalities in development. Ann. N. Y. Acad. Sci. 55: 203-215, 1952.

176 Bisphenol A

Hardin et al (1981) carried out preliminary studies injecting 85 or 125 mg per kg intraperitoneally into rats on days 0 through 14 of gestation. At the higher dose very few rats became pregnant. At the lower dose there was a significant increase in dilated cerebral ventricles and growth retardation.

Hardin, D.D.; Bond, G.P.; Sikov, M.R.; Andrew, F.D.; Beliles, R.P. and Niemeier, R.W.: Testing of selected workplace chemicals for teratogenic Potential. Scand. J. Work Environ. Health 7:Suppl. 4 66-75, 1981.

177 Bladex-R

Lu et al (1982) gavaged pregnant rats on days 12 and 15 with 25 mg per kg and found maternal and fetal weight decrease along with some minor skeletal variations.

Lu, C.C.; Tang, B.S. and Chai, E.Y.: Teratogenicity evaluations of technical Bladex-R in Fisher-344 rats. Teratology 25:59A-60A, 1982.

178 Bleeding (also see Anemia)

Vaginal bleeding during early pregnancy with its multitude of causes is considered by most obstetricians to be associated with a higher than normal abnormality rate in the conceptus. However. Nishimura et al, (1966) in comparing 2,328 embryos obtained by therapeutic abortion from mothers without vaginal bleeding could not show a significant difference in malformation rate as compared to 427 embryos from mothers who did have vaginal bleeding before therapeutic abortion.

For the effect of major maternal hemorrhage on the embryo see the heading anemia.

Nishimura, H.; Takano, K.; Tanimura, T.; Yasuda, M. and Uchida, T.: High incidence of several malformations in the early human embryos as compared with infants. Biol. Neonate 10: 93-107, 1966.

179 Bluetongue Vaccine Virus

This virus can produce encephalopathy followed by cystic cavities in the subcortical tissues of the cerebrum and cerebellum in lambs after the mother is injected with live virus around the 40th day (Young and Cordy, 1964). The fetuses exposed after 70 gestational days are less susceptible to encephalopathy. The subject is reviewed briefly by Kalter (1968).

Kalter, H.: Teratology of the central nervous system. Chicago: University of Chicago Press, 1968. P. 177 only.

Young, S. and Cordy, D.R.: An ovine fetal encephalopathy caused by bluetongue vaccine virus. J. Neuropathol. Exp. Neurol. 23: 635-659, 1964.

180 Bonaphthon

Proinova et al (1980) treated rats with 400 mg per kg of this antiviral drug (on days 10-13 of pregnancy) and found neither embryotoxic and teratogenic effect nor any postnatal morphological and functional deviations.

Proinova, V.A.; Pershin, G.N.; Shashkina, L.F.; Nechushkina, L.V. and Fedorova, E.A.: Postnatal development of rats after exposure to bonaphthon. Farmakol. Toksikol. (USSR) 4:404-408, 1980.

181 Boric Acid

Landauer (1952) produced rumplessness, curled toe and facial palate defects in chicks using injections of 2.5 mg. Rumplessness was common following treatment at 24 hours incubation while the facial and palate defects appear after treatment at 4 days. Dousset (1971) has reported that boric acid is metabolized differently when the rat becomes pregnant. The chemical begins to appear first in the spinal fluid. Weir and Russell (1972) gave boric acid or borax to pregnant rats at 350 ppm given during pregnancy. No reduction in liveborn or physical defects were found.

Heinonen et al (1977) reported on 253 offspring of mothers using boric acid in the first 4 lunar months and observed 13 major malformations when only 7 were expected. The increase was still within the 95 percent confidence levels.

Dousett, G.: Penetration du bore organique dans le liquide cephaloachildien de la ratte gestante. Compt. Rendu (Paris) 165:722-724, 1971.

Heinonen, O.P.; Slone, D. and Shapiro, S.: Birth Defects and Drugs In Pregnancy. Publishing Sciences Group, Inc.; Littleton, Mass.; 1977.

Landauer, W.: Malformations of chicken embryos produced by boric acid and the probable role of riboflavin in their origin. J. Exp. Zool. 120: 469-508, 1952.

Weir, R.J. and Fisher, R.S.: Toxicologic study on borax and boric acid. Toxicol. Appl. Pharm. 23:351-364, 1972.

182 Botulinum Toxin

Drachman and Sokoloff (1966) paralyzed chick embryos with this material and inhibited joint cavity production.

Drachman, D.B. and Sokoloff, L.: The role of movement in

182

embryonic joint development. Dev. Biol. 14: 401-420,
1966.

183 Bovine Albumen Anaphylaxis

Takayama (1981) immunized mice to purified bovine albumen
and then administered 0.05 to 0.5 mg intraperitoneally or
intravenously on day 8.5 of gestation. A significant
increase in defects mainly exencephaly and omphalocele
occurred in about 3 percent of the fetuses. No defects
occurred in the non-immunized controls receiving the same
dose. Bovine serum albumen intraperitoneally in a dose of
50 mg did produce similar defects.

Takayama, Y.: Teratogenic effects of anaphylactic immune
reaction in mice. Cong. Anom. 21:175-186, 1981.

184 Bovine Viral Diarrheal-Mucosol Disease (BVD-MD)

This mild diarrheal disease occurring in pregnant cattle has
been associated with ataxia in the newborn calf. Kahrs et
al (1970) injected the attenuated virus into pregnant cows
between 100 to 200 days of gestation and observed ataxia
with cerebellar hypoplasia in the newborn calves. Optic
atrophy and lenticular opacities were found in some.

Kahrs, R.F.; Scott, F.W. and De Lahunta, A.: Congenital
cerebellar hypoplasia and ocular defects in calves following
bovine viral diarrhea-mucosol disease infection in pregnant
cattle. Am. Vet. Med. Assoc. 156: 1443-1450, 1970.

185 Bradykinin

Thompson and Gautieri (1969) injected synthetic bradykinin
into pregnant mice once on gestational days 7 through 12.
When they used 25 microgm intravenously they found an
increased incidence of fetal hydronephrosis. Fetal growth
retardation and defects in ossification were found also. An
increased transfer rate of radioactive sodium from the
mother to the placentas was shown to occur during the
treatment.

Thompson, R.S. and Gautieri, R.F.: Comparison and analysis
of the teratogenic effects of serotonin, angiotensin II and
bradykinin in mice. J. Pharm. Sci. 58: 406-412, 1969.

186 Bredinin
(4-Carbamoyl-1-Beta-D-ribofuranosylimidazolium-5-olate)

This immunosuppressive agent was given intraperitoneally to
rats on day 8, 9, 10 or 11 in amounts of 5 mg per kg and
produced anophthalmos, hydrocephaly and other visceral
defects as well as some skeletal defects. Day 9 was teratogenically the most susceptible.

Okamoto, K.; Kobayashi, Y.; Yoshida, K.; Nozaki, Y.; Kawai,
Y.; Kawano, H.; Mayumi, T. and Hama, T.: Teratogenic

effects of bredinin, a new immunosuppressive agent, in rats. Cong. Anom. 18:227-233, 1978.

187   Bromide

Opitz et al (1972) have reported short stature and small cranium in two children born to a mother ingesting large amounts of bromide. One of these children had congenital heart disease.

Opitz, J.M.; Grosse, F.R. and Haneberg, B.: Congenital effects of bromism? . Lancet 1: 91-92, 1972.

188   5-Bromo-1-(2-deoxy-beta-d-ribofuranosyl)-5-fluoro-6-methoxy-O-hydrouracil

Chaube and Murphy (1968) report production of brain, palate and skeletal defects in the rat with 75 to 300 mg per kg injected on the 11th or 12th day.

Chaube, S. and Murphy, M.L.: The teratogenic effects of the recent drugs active in cancer chemotherapy. In, Woollam, D.H.M. (ed.): Advances in Teratology, Vol. 3. New York: Academic Press, 1968. pp. 204-205.

189   5-Bromodeoxyuridine

Dipaolo (1964) produced polydactylous offspring by injecting pregnant mice with 124 mg per kg. Chaube and Murphy (1965) produced defects of the nervous system, palate and skeleton in rat fetuses whose mothers were injected with 100 to 800 mg per kg on the 11th or 12th day. In the hamster Ruffolo and Ferm (1965) produced mostly nervous system defects with 400 mg per kg given on the 8th day. No deleterious effects on 6.5 day rabbit blastocysts from mothers treated with 50 to 80 mg per kg were noted by Adams et al, (1961).

Adams, C.E.; Hay, M.F. and Lutwak-Mann, C.: The action of various agents upon the rabbit embryo. J. Embryol. Exp. Morphol. 9: 468-491, 1961.

Chaube, S. and Murphy, M.L.: The teratogenic effects of the recent drugs active in cancer chemotherapy. In, Woollam, D.H.M. (ed.): Advances in Teratology, Vol. 3. New York: Academic Press, 1968. pp. 204-205.

Dipaolo, J.A.: Polydactylism in the offspring of mice injected with 5-bromodeoxyuridine. Sciennce 145: 501-503, 1964.

Ruffolo, P.R. and Ferm, V.H.: The embryocidal and teratogenic effects of 5-bromodeoxyuridine in the pregnant hamster. Lab. Invest. 14: 1547-1553, 1965.

190   Brovanexine Hydrochloride

This expectorant was given by Tsuruzaki et al (1982) to rats orally in maximum doses of 5000 mg per kg during organogenesis and no adverse fetal effects were found.

Tsuruzaki, T.; Naki, H.; Shimo, T.; Noguchi, Y.; Kato, H.; Ito, Y.; Yamamoto, M.: Reproductive studies of brovanexine hydrochloride in rats. Kiso to Rinsho 16:7179-7195, 1982.

191 5-Br-2-phenyl-indan 1,3-dione [Uridion-R]

This uricosuric drug was tested in pregnant rats and rabbits with oral doses of 15 and 40 mg per kg during active organogenesis and resorptions and fetal growth were observed but no congenital defects. (Fanelli, et al, 1974).

Fanelli, D.; Mazzoncini, V. and Ferri, S.: Toxicological and teratological study of 5-Br-2-phenyl-indan-1,3 dione, a uricosuric drug. Arzneim Forsch. 24:1604-1613, 1974.

192 Buclizine (also see Meclizine)

This antihistamine belongs to the benzhydrylpiperazine series of compounds and has been used to produce cleft palate in the rat. It is more fully described under meclizine.

193 Bucloxic Acid (4-(3-Chloro-4-cyclohexyl-phenyl)-4-oxo--butyric Acid)

Mazue et al (1974) gave rabbits, rats and mice 25 mg per kg during active organogenesis and found no fetal damage.

Mazue, G.; Landsmann, F. and Brunaud, M.: Study of possible teratogenicity of bucloxic acid (804 CB). Arzneim Forsch 24: 1413-1425, 1974.

194 Budralazine (1-(2-(1,3-dimethyl-2-butenylidene)-hydrazino)phthalazine)

Shimada et al (1981) carried out fertiliy and teratogenicity studies in rats with this antihypertensive. Fertility was not altered by dietary doses of 80 mg per kg daily. At 100 mg per kg during days 7-17 no adverse fetal effects occurred. Perinatal and postnatal studies by Watanabe et al (1981) found some weight reduction but development and function were not affected. Studies in the rabbit during organogenesis with doses of 80 mg per kg did not produce teratogenic effects (Nagaoka et al, 1981).

Nagaoka, T.; Narama, I.; Oshima, Y.: Reproductive studies of budralazine; perinatal and postnatal studies in rats. Oyo Yakuri 21:343-350, 1980.

Shimada, H.; Ohura, K.; Mochida, K.; Arauchi, T.; Morita, H.: Reproductive studies of budralazine in rats. Oyo Yakuri 21:313-330, 1981.

Watanabe, T.; Ohura, K.; Michida, K.; Arauchi, T.; Morita,

H.: Reproductive studies of budralazine, perinatal and postnatal studies in rats. Oyo Yakuri 21:331-341, 1981.

195 Bunitrolol (0-[-2-hydroxy-3-(tert-butylamine)propyl] benzonitrile hydrochloride]

Matsuo et al (1981) gave rats up to 300 mg per kg and rabbits up to 50 mg per kg daily during organogenesis. Although there was maternal toxicity in both species at the higher doses, no adverse effects on reproduction were found. Behavioral studies in the offspring were not different from controls. This drug is a beta-adrenoceptor blocker. Studies before breeding and during the postnatal period were also done. Only an increase in neonatal death was found at 300 mg per kg dose levels (Matsuo et al, 1981).

Matsuo, A.; Kast, A.; Tsunenari, Y.: Fertility and reproduction studies with bunitrolol hydrochloride (KOE 1366 Cl) in rats. Iyakuhin Kenkyu 12:976-987, 1981.

Matsuo, A.; Kast, A. and Tsunenari, Y.: Teratological studies on bunitrolol hydrochloride (Koe 1366 Cl) in rats and rabbits (Japanese) Iyakuhin Kenkyu 12:12-24, 1981.

196 Buprenorphine

Mori et al (1982) studied the effect of this analgesic in rats on days 7 through 17 and 17-21. With doses over 0.05 mg per kg per day fetal growth retardation was found but no defects were produced up to 5 mg per kg. In the late treatment group at 5 mg per kg the offspring had a reduced survival rate.

Mori, N.; Sakanoue, M.; Kamata, S.; Takeuchi, M.; Shimpo, K.; Tamagawa, M.: Toxicological studies of buprenorphine teratogenicity, perinatal and postnatal studies in the rat. Iyakuhin Kenkyu 13: 509-544, 1982.

197 Busulfan (1-4-Butanedioldimethanesulfonate) [Myleran-R]

Murphy et al, (1958) have produced cleft palate, stunting and digital defects in the fetuses of rats treated on the 12th gestational day with 18 to 34 mg per kg. Heller and Jones (1964) produced ovarian dysgenesis in the rat fetus by treating the mother intraperitoneally on day 13 of gestation with 10 mg per kg. Diamond et al, (1960) reported a stunted infant with cleft palate, eye defects and generalized cytomegaly of cells born to a pregnant mother who received 6-mercaptopurine, X-ray treatments and busulfan. These authors attributed the effects to busulfan because of a previous pregnancy in which 6-mercaptopurine and X-rays alone caused no fetal defects. Vanhems and Bousquet (1972) gave 10 mg per kg intraperitoneally to rats on the 13th day of gestation and found destruction of the seminiferous tubules of the surviving male fetuses.

Diamond, I.; Anderson, M.M. and McCreadie, S.R.: Transplacental transmission of busulfan (Myleran) in a mother with leukemia: production of fetal malformations and cytomegaly.

Pediatrics 25: 85-90, 1960.

Heller, R.H. and Jones, H.W.: Production of ovarian dysgenesis in the rat and human by busulphan. Am. J. Obstet. Gynecol. 89: 414-420, 1964.

Murphy, M.L.; Delmoro, A. and Lacon, C.R.: The comparative effects of polyfunctional alkylating agents in the rat fetus with additional notes on the chick embryo. Ann. N. Y. Acad. Sci. 68: 762-781, 1958.

Vanhems, E. and Bousquet, J.: Influence du misulban sur le Developpement du testicule du rat. Ann. Endocrin. 33: 119-128, 1972.

198 Butalamine   [3-Phenyl-5-dibutylaminoethylamino-1,2,4-oxa-diazole HCl]

This vasodilator was tested in pregnant rats by Fujimura et al (1975) in oral doses as high as 300 mg per kg during the 7th to the 14th day. No teratogenicity was found.

Fujimura, H.; Hiramatsu, Y.; Tamura, Y. and Suzuki, T.: Effect of butalamine administered to pregnant rats on pre- and post-natal development of their offspring. Oyo Yakuri 9: 727-731, 1975.

199 Butoctamide   semisuccinate
    (N-(2-ethylhexyl)-3-hydroxybutyramide   hydrogen succinate)
    (M-2H)

Kuraishi et al (1979) gave this hypnotic orally to rats during organogenesis in doses up to 1500 mg per kg daily. Although maternal weight gain was less than controls no adverse fetal effects were found.

Kuraishi, K.; Nabeshima, J.; Haresaku, M.; Inoue, S.: Teratologic study with N-(2-ethylhexyl)-3-hydrobutyramide hydrogen succinate (M-2H) in rats. Oyo Yakuri 17:315-324, 1979.

200 Butorphanol

In a series of papers Takahashi et al (1982) studied the effect of this analgesic on rat and rabbit reproduction. In the rat up to 25 mg per kg daily subcutaneously before mating, during organogenesis or late in gestation caused no reproductive problems, teratogenicity or postnatal behavioral defects. Some decrease in viability was found three days postpartum after treatment on days 17-20 of gestation. Intravenously administered doses of up to 5 mg on days 7-17 of gestation in the rat produced some increase in fetal deaths but no increase in defects. Doses of up to 10 mg per kg subcutaneously in the rabbit on days 6-18 of gestation produced no teratogenic effect.

Takahashi, N.; Kai, S.; Kohmura, H.; Ishikawa, K.;
Karoyangai, K.; Hamajimma, Y.; Kadota, T.; Kawano, S.;
Yamada, K.; Koike, M.: Reproductive studies of butorphanol
tartrate 1-5. Iyakuhin Kenkyu 13:390-467, 1982.

201 Butoxybenzyl Hyoscyamine Bromide

Suzuki et al (1974) studied this drug in pregnant mice and
rats with maximum oral doses of 500 mg per kg per day and
maximum intraperitoneal doses of 40 mg per kg. The dams
evidenced autonomic reactions. No increase in fetal death
or congenital defects were found in fetuses exposed during
active organogenesis.

Suzuki, Y.; Okada, F.; Kondo, S.; Asano, F.; Chiba, T. and
Wakabayashi, T.: Teratological study with butoxybenzyl
hyoscyamine bromide in rats and mice. Oyo Yakuri 8:
319-337, 1974.

202 P-Butoxyphenylacethydroxamic Acid [Droxaryl-R]

This non-steroidal antiinflammatory drug has been given to
pregnant rats and rabbits and no teratogenicity found (Roba

et al, 1970). Doses up to 750 mg per kg in the rat and 500
mg per kg in the rabbit were administered by mouth during
active organogenesis.

Roba, J.; Lambelin, G. and Buu-hoi, N.P.: Teratological
studies of P-butoxyphenylacethydroxamic acid (CP 1044j3) in
rats and rabbits. Arzneim. Forsch 20:565-569, 1970.

203 1-(Tert-butylamino)-3-(2-chloro-5-methylphenoxy)-2-propanol
HCl

Kagiwada et al (1973) studied the effect of this beta-
-adrenergic blocker in pregnant mice and rats giving maximum
oral doses of 100 mg per kg in mice and 150 mg per kg per
day in rats. No teratogenic effects were found.

Kagiwada, K.; Ishizaki, O. and Saito, G.: Effects of beta-
-receptor blocking agent, 1-(tert-butylamino)-3-(2-chloro-
-5-methylphenoxy)-2-propanol hydrochloride (Kl 255), on pre-
and post-natal development of the offsprings in pregnant
mice and rats. (Japanese) Oyo Yakuri 7: 65-74, 1973.

204 1-Tert-butylamino-3-(2-Nitrilophenoxy)-2-propanol
[KO-1366-Cl]

Fuyuta et al (1973) injected this beta adrenergic blocker
into pregnant rats from the 7th to the 13th day of pregnancy
and found no increase in malformation rate. Doses up to 7.5
mg per kg were given orally and to 10 mg per kg per day
intraperitoneally.

Fuyuta, M.; Fujimoto, T. and Kaihara, N.: Examination of
the teratogenic effect of an adrenergic beta receptor

blocking agent KO-1366-Cl in rats. (abstract). Teratology 8: 92 (only), 1973.

205 Butylated Hydoxyanisole [3-Tertbutyl-4-hydroxyanisole]

Clegg (1965) administered by mouth 500 to 1000 mg per kg to several strains of mice and rats for various periods of time during gestation and observed no increase in fetal congenital malformations.

Clegg, D.J.: Absence of teratogenic effect of butylated Hydoxyanisole (BHA) and butylated hydoxytoluene (BHT) in rats and mice. Food Cosmet. Toxicol. 3: 387-403, 1965.

206 Butylated Hydroxytoluene [3-Tert-butyl-4-hydroxyanisole]

Brown et al (1959) reported that three out of 30 litters from rats receiving this material at levels of 0.5 percent of the diet contained fetuses with anophthalmia. The dose was approximately 250 mg per kg per day. Clegg (1965) was unable to confirm their findings using 500 to 1000 mg per kg in several strains of mice and rats.

Clegg, D.J.: Absence of teratogenic effect of butylated hydoxyanisole (BHA) and butylated hydoxytoluene (BHT) in rats and mice. Food Cosmet. Toxicol. 3: 387-403, 1965.

Brown, W.D.; Johnson, A.R. and Halloran, M.W.: The effect of the level of dietary fat on toxicity of phenolic antioxidants. Aust. J. Exp. Biol. Med. Sci. 37: 533-548, 1959.

207 Butylflufenamate   (Butyl-2-((3-(trifluouromethyl)phenyl) amino)benzoate)

Isuruzaki et al (1979) studied this nonsteroidal antiinflammatory agent in rats orally before mating and during the first 7 days, on days 7-17 and days 17-20 of gestation. No effects on reproduction were noted after giving up to 60 mg per kg. Up to 120 mg per kg was given during organogenesis without adverse fetal effects. Perinatal administration of up to 45 mg per kg produced no abnormal postnatal changes.

Isuruzaki, T.; Kubo, S.; Shimo, T.; Yamazaki, M.; Kato, H.; Yamamoto, M.: Reproductive studies of butyl-2-((3-trifluoromethyl) phenyl)amino)benzoate (HF-264) in rats. Kiso to Rinsho 13:3279-3287, 3288-3301, 3302-3313, 1979.

208 2-Sec-butyl-4,6-dinitrophenol (see Dinoseb) [Premerge-R]

209 Butylene Glycol Adipic Acid Polyester

Fancher et al (1973) found no adverse effects of a diet with 10,000 PPM fed to 3 generations of rats.

Fancher, O.E.; Kennedy, G.L.; Plank, J.B.; Lindberg, D.C.; Hunt, W.H. and Calandra, J.C.: Toxicology of a butylene glycol adipic acid polyester. Toxicol. Appl. Pharmacol. 26: 58-62, 1973.

210 Butylhydroquinone (TBHQ)

Tertiary butylhydroquinone was fed to pregnant rats during active organogenesis and no deleterious fetal effects were found (Krasavage, 1977). The highest dietary dose was 0.5 percent.

Krasavage, W.J.: Evaluation of the teratogenic potential of tertiary butylhydroquinone (TBHQ) in the rat. Teratology 16: 31-34, 1977.

211 Butyl-malonic   Acid-mono-(1,2-diphenylhydrazine)   Calcium [Bumadizone-Ca] [Eumotol-R]

Konig et al (1973) found no teratogenicity in mice, rats and rabbits. Oral doses of 80 (mouse) or 100 mg per kg (rat and rabbit) were used before and during gestation. A two generation study was done.

Konig, J.; Knoche, C. and Schafer, H.: Der Einfluss von Butyl-malonsaure   -mono-(1,2-diphenyl-hydrazid-calcium) (bumadizon-calcium)   auf   die Reproduktion und die pranatale Entwicklung. Arzneim-Forsch 23: 1246-1251, 1973.

212 9-Butyl-6-mercaptopurine (see 6-Mercaptopurine)

213 1-Butyryl-4-cinnamylpiperazine HCl

This analgesic was studied in pregnant rabbits, mice and rats by Irikura et al (1972) using oral or subcutaneous routes of up to 180 mg per kg daily during organogenesis. No congenital defects resulted but some reduction in fetal weight was found in all species at the highest doses.

Irikura, T.; Sugimoto, T.; Suzuki, H. and Hosomi, J.: Studies on analgesic agents. Part 2 Teratogenic studies of 1-butyryl-4-cinnamylpiperazine hydrochloride (AP237). Oyo Yakuri 6: 271-277, 1972.

214 Cadmium

Ferm and Carpenter (1967) reported mid-line facial and palate defects in hamsters after maternal intravenous injection of 2 mg per kg of cadmium sulfate on the 8th day of gestation. Mulvihill et al (1970) have described the embryonic events contributing to these defects. Barr (1973) using 16 micromoles of cadmium per kg intraperitoneally in rats on days 9, 10 or 11 of gestation produced eye defects, hydrocephaly, thinning of the abdominal wall with undescended testes, and other defects. Subcutaneous admin- istration was not teratogenic. Chernoff (1973) produced

214

weight reduction in the developing fetal lungs of maternally treated rats. Dencker (1975) has shown that CD-109 enters the hamster and mouse embryo via the yolk sac and then through the primitive gut. Golden (Ph.D. thesis, 1975, University of Michigan) using 100 ppm in the drinking water during pregnancy found an increase in blood pressure in the postnatal period. Levin and Miller (1981) found a decrease in placental blood flow associated with placental necrosis and fetal death after administration of 40 micromoles of cadmium chloride subcutaneously in rats. The acute distribution of cadmium in the rat has been studied (Samarawickrama and Webb, 1981).

Although Cvetkova (1970) reported that the weights of newborns of women employed in the cadmium industry were significantly lower than controls, Nomiyama in a personal communication to Thuerauf et al (1975) stated that no fetal damage could be detected in Itai- itai disease, a syndrome associated with high cadmium exposure.

Barr, M.: The teratogenicity of cadmium chloride in two stocks of Wistar rats. Teratology 7: 237-242, 1973.

Chernoff, N.: Teratogenic effects of cadmium in rats. Teratology 8: 29-32, 1973.

Cvetkova, R.P.: Materials on the study of the influence of cadmium compounds on the generative function. Gig. Tr. Prof. Zabol. 14:31, 1970.

Dencker, L.: Possible mechanisms of cadmium fetotoxicity in golden hamsters and mice: uptake by the embryo, placenta and ovary. J. Reprod. Fert. 44: 461-471, 1975.

Ferm, V.H. and Carpenter, S.J.: Teratogenic effect of cadmium and its inhibition by zinc. Nature 216: 1123 only, 1967.

Levin, A.A. and Miller, R.K.: Fetal toxicity of cadmium in the rat: Decreased utero-placental blood flow. Toxicol. Appl. Pharm. 58:297-306, 1981.

Mulvihill, J.E.; Gamm, S.H. and Ferm, V.H.: Facial formation in normal and cadmium-treated golden hamsters. J. Embryol. Exp. Morphol. 24: 393-403, 1970.

Samarawickrama, G.P. and Webb, M: The acute toxicity and teratogenicity of cadmium in the pregnant rat. J. Appl. Toxicol. 1:264-269,1981.

Thuerauf, J.; Schaller, K.H.; Engelhardt, E. and Gossler, K.: The cadmium content of the human placenta. Int. Arch. Occup. Environ. Healh 36:19-27, 1975.

215 Ca-DTPA (Calcium Trisodium Diethylenetriaminepentacetate)

Fisher et al (1976) injected 1,440 micromoles subcutaneously into mice daily from 2 to 6 or from 7 to 11 days and produced neural tube closure defects in the fetuses.

Fisher, D.R.; Calder, S.E.; Mays, C.W. and Taylor, G.N.: Ca-DTPA-induced fetal death and malformations in mice. Teratology 14:123-128, 1976,

216 Caerulein

This decapeptide with gastrin-like activity was not terato-genic in rabbits and rats. Doses of 25 (rabbit) and 50 mg (rat) per kg were given subcutaneously during pregnancy (Chieli et al, 1972).

Chieli, T.; Bertazzoli, C.; Ferni, F.; Delloro, I.; Capella, C. and Solci, E.: Experimental toxicology of caerulein. Toxicol. Appl. Pharm. 23: 480-491, 1972.

217 Caffeine

Nishimura and Nakai (1960) using single injections of 250 mg per kg to mice on days 10 through 14 found fetuses with predominantly digital defects but also with subcutaneous hemorrhage and cleft palate. Knoche and Konig (1964) found only seven different defects among over 700 mouse fetuses whose mothers received 50 mg per day during gestation. Loosli et al (1964) reported no defects in rats, mice or rabbits treated with 100 mg per kg during organogenesis. Bertrand et al (1965) could not produce significant numbers of defects in the mouse with 100 mg per kg but in rats gavaged with 75 to 150 mg per kg per day during gestation found digital defects and associated hemorrhages. The rate of ectrodactyly in the fetuses was dose dependent and there was a predilection for the left posterior extremity. They estimate that the amount of caffeine that could be ingested by a person drinking one liter per day would be approximately 20 to 25 mg per kg. Bertrand et al (1970) produced ectrodachtyly in rabbit fetuses by administration of doses of 100 mg per kg. Mulvihill (1973) has reviewed the teratogenicity and mutagenicity of this chemical.

Fujii and Nishimura blocked the teratogenic effects of caffeine by preadministration of the beta-adrenergic blocker, propranolol. Caffeine administered directly to the chick embryo has produced aortic arch anomalies (Gilbert et al, 1977).

Weathersbee (1977) and Borlee et al (1978) have carried out studies on caffeine and coffee in pregnancy. Weathersbee et al studied 489 households in the Utah area and in 16 where the mothers ingested 600 mg or more per day, it was found that 15 had fetal loss or prematurity. A coffee serving is estimated at 75 mg of caffeine. In the study by Borlee et al, 202 malformed children and 175 controls were included. In the group of mothers of malformed offspring, the overconsumers (more than 8 cups per day) were 44 while in the control there were only 21. (P was less than 0.05). Hydrocephalus, intraventricular septal defect and cleft lip were the most commonly found malformations. Both studies are subject to criticism since the matching of controls was either not detailed or not performed. Sociological variables could have accounted for the differences.

Heinonen et al (1977) list 5,000 pregnancies where caffeine exposure was present and did not find an increase in defect rate over matched controls.

Linn et al (1982) have published a carefully controlled analysis of the coffee drinking (and smoking) habits of over 12,000 pregnant women. After controlling for smoking, other habits, demographic characteristics and medical history, no relationship was found between coffee consumption and low birth weight or malformation in the offspring. In a case-control study of 2,030 women giving birth to offspring with selected congenital defects no malformation group was found in which caffeine consumption was significantly increased (Rosenberg et al, 1982).

Bertrand, M.; Giroud, J. and Rigaud, M.F.: Ectrodachtylie provoquee par la cafeine chez les rongeurs. Role des facteurs specifiques et genetiques. C. R. Soc. Biol. (Paris) 164: 1488-1489, 1970.

Bertrand, M.; Schwam, E.; Frandon, A.; Vagne, A. and Alary, J.: Sur un effet teratogene systematique et specifique de la cafeine chez les rongeurs. C. R. Soc. Biol. (Paris) 159: 2199-2202, 1965.

Borlee, I.; Lechat, M.F.; Bouckaert, A. and Misson, C.: Coffee, risk factor during pregnancy? (French) Louvain Med. 97:279-284, 1978.

Fujii, T. and Nishimura, H.: Reduction in frequency of fetopathic effects of caffeine in mice by pretreatment with propranolol. Teratology 10: 149-152, 1974.

Gilbert, E.F.; Bruyere, H.J.; Ishikawa, S.; Cheung, M.O. and Hodach, R.J.: The effects of methylxanthines on catecholamine-stimulated and normal chick embryos. Teratology 16: 47-52, 1977.

Heinonen, O.P.; Slone, D.; and Shapiro, S.: Birth Defects and Drugs in Pregnancy. Publishing Science Group Inc.; Littleton, Mass.; 1977.

Knoche, C. and Konig, J.: Zur pranatelen Toxizitat von Diphenylpyralin-8-theophyllinat unter Berucksichtigung von Erfahrungen mit Thalidomid und Coffein. Arzneim. Forsch. 14: 415-424, 1964.

Linn, S.; Schoenbaum, S.C.; Monson, R.R.; Rosner, B.; Stabblefield, P.G. and Ryan, K.J.: No association between coffee consumption and adverse outcomes of pregnancy. New Eng. J. Med. 306:141-145, 1982.

Loosli, R.; Loustalot, P.; Schalch, W.R.; Sievers, K. and Steager, E.G.: Proceedings European Society for Study of Drug Toxicity 4: 214-216, 1964.

Mulvihill, J.J.: Caffeine as teratogen and mutagen. Teratology 8: 69-72, 1973.

Nishimura, H. and Nakai, K.: Congenital malformations in offspring treated with caffeine. Proc. Soc. Exp. Biol.

Med. 104: 140-142, 1960.

Rosenberg, L.; Mitchell, A.A.; Shapiro, S. and Slone, D.: Selected birth defects in relation to caffeine-containing beverages. JAMA 247:1429-1432, 1982.

Weathersbee, P.S.; Olsen, L.K. and Lodge, J.R.: Caffeine and pregnancy. Postgraduate Med. 62: 64-69, 1977.

218 Calcium Carbonate

Heinonen et al (1977) in a survey of 1007 women taking calcium compounds in the first trimester found 10 defects of the central nervous system while 4.7 were expected. The type of defect was not confined to any specific deformity.

Heinonen, O.P.; Slone, D.; Shapiro, S.: Birth Defects and Drugs in Pregnancy. Publishing Sciences Group, Inc., 1977.

219 Calcium Cyclamate (see Cyclamate)

220 Calcium   D-(+)-4-(2,4-dihydroxy-3,3-dimethylbutramide) butyrate hemihydrate (HOPA)

Asano et al (1980) gave rats up to 60 mg per kg on days 17-21 of gestation. An increase in stillbirths and a decrease in postnatal survival was found at the highest dose. Reproduction by the offspring was not adverrsely affected.

Asano, Y.; Ariyuki, F.; Higaki, K.: Pre and postnatal studies of calcium D(+)-4-(2,4-dihydroxy-3,3-dimethyl-butramide) butyrate hemihydrate (HOPA) (HOPA) in rats. Oyo Yakuri 19:1011-1017, 1980.

221 Cannabis (see Marihuana)

222 Captan   [N-Trichloromethylthio-4-cycloh   ex-ane-1-2-dicarboximide]

Fabro et al (1965) fed 80 mg per kg daily to rabbits on days 7 through 12 and found no congenital defects in the fetuses. Kennedy et al (1968) found no teratogenicity using rats and hamsters. Verrett et al (1969) injected 3 to 20 mg per kg into the air cell or yolk of chick eggs before incubation and observed defects of the nervous or skeletal system in 7.8 percent. Phocomelia and amelia were especially noteworthy.

Negative studies with this compound have been reported in the pregnant beagle (Kennedy et al 1975) and non-human primate (Vondruska et al, 1971).

Fabro, S.; Smith, R.L. and Williams, R.T.: Embryotoxic activity of some pesticides and drugs related to phthalimide. Food Cosmet. Toxicol. 3: 587-590, 1966.

Kennedy, G.L.; Fancher, O.E. and Calandra, J.C.: An investigation of the teratogenic potential of Captan, Folpet and Difolatan. Toxicol. Appl. Pharmacol. 13: 420-430, 1968.

Kennedy, G.L.; Fancher, O.E. and Calandra, J.C.: Non-teratogenicity of Captan in Beagles. Teratology 11: 223-226, 1975.

Verrett, M.J.; Matchler, M.K.; Scott, W.F.; Reynaldo, E.F. and McLaughlin, J.: Teratogenic effects of Captan and related compounds in the developing chicken embryo. Ann. N. Y. Acad. Sci. 160: 334-343, 1969.

Vondruska, J.F.; Fancher, O.E. and Calandra, J.C.: An investigation into the teratogenic potential of Captan, Folpet and Difolatan in non-human primates. Toxicol Appl. Pharmacol. 18: 619-624, 1971.

223 Carbamazepine (Tegretol-R)

Although the pharmaceutical companay distributing this compound reports 2 malformations in 135 rat fetuses whose mothers were exposed to 250 mg per kg daily, there is very little recorded experience regarding human teratogenic potential. Millar and Nevin (1973) report one infant exposed to phenobarbital and carbamazepine with myelomenigocele and Schardein (1977) lists references which reported malformed offspring generally exposed to several anticonvulsants.

Millar, J.H.D. and Nevin, N.C.: Congenital malformations and anticonsulsant drugs. Lancet 1: 328 (only), 1973.

Schardein, J.L.: Drugs as Teratogens, CRC Press, Cleveland, 1976, p. 116.

224 Carbaryl [1-Naphthyl N-Methylcarbamate]

This carbamate cholinesterase inhibitor used as a pesticide was studied by Robens (1969) in the guinea pig, hamster and rabbit. Only in the guinea pig were defects produced. Using a near lethal dose for the mother (300 mg per kg) from day 11 to day 20 she found vertebral anomalies in about one-half of the surviving fetuses. Weil et al (1973) found no teratogenicity in the rat (200 mg per kg orally).

Smalley et al (1968) fed 3.1 to 50 mg per kg to Beagles during pregnancy. At levels of 6.25 and above the defect rate was increased in the offspring. Midline abdominal wall defects and skeletal defects were the most common type. Reduced conception was found at the 50 mg per kg level.

Smalley, H.E.; Curtis, J.M.; Earl, F.L.: Teratogenic action of carbaryl on Beagle dogs. Toxicol. Appl. Pharmacol. 13:392-403, 1968.

Robens, J.F.: Teratologic studies of carbaryl, diazinon, norea, disulfiram and thiram in small laboratory animals.

Toxicol. Appl. Pharmacol. 15: 152-163, 1969.

Weil, C.S.; Woodside, M.D.; Bernard, J.B.; Condra, N.I.; King, J.M. and Carpenter, C.P.: Comparative effect of carbaryl on rat reproduction and guinea pig teratology when fed either in the diet or by stomach intubation. Toxicol Appl. Pharm. 26: 621-638, 1973.

225 Carbazochrome Sodium Sulfonate [1-Methyl-5-semi-carbazo-ono-6-oxo-2,3,5,6-tetrahydroindole-3-sulfonate sodium]

Fujii and Kowa (1970) gave this adrenochrome derivative to pregnant mice and rats on the 7th through the 14th day of gestation. Both the intraperitoneal and oral routes were used and the dosages were as high as 3,000 mg per kg orally and 1,600 mg per kg intraperitoneally. No increase in malformations was found.

Fujii, T.M. and Kowa, Y.: Teratological studies of carbazochrome sodium sulfonate in mice and rats. Oyo Yakuri 4: 39-46, 1970.

226 Carbofuran
(dihydro-2,2-dimethyl-7-benzofuranolN-Methylcarbamate)

McCarthy et al (1971) reported that although no increase in defects occurred in the offspring of treated rats, rabbits and dogs, a reduced survival rate was seen in rat offspring exposed to 100 ppm in the diet. Wolfe and Esher (1980) repeated this dietary dose level in mice and found a reduced survival rate but the difference was not significant. Fetal weights were not reduced. Postnatal plasma corticosterone levels were elevated in the offspring of mice exposed in utero to 0.01 or 0.50 mg per kg per day (Cranmer et al, 1978). A transplacental effect on activity of acetylcholinesterase of the day 18 rat fetus has been shown. (Cambon et al, 1979).

Cambon, C.; Declume, C. and Derache, R.: Effect of the insecticidal carbamate derivatives (carbofuran, pirimicard, aldicarb) on the activity of acetylcholinesterase in tissues from pregnant rats and fetuses. Toxicol. Appl. Pharmacol. 49:203-208, 1979.

Cranmer, J.P.; Avery, D.L.; Grudy, R.R. and Kitay, J.I.: Endocrine dysfunction resulting from prenatal exposure to carbofuran, diazinon and chlordane. J. Envir. Path. Toxicol. 2:357-369, 1978.

McCarthy, J.F.; Fancher, O.E.; Kennedy, G.L.; Keplinger, M.L. and Calandra: Reproduction and teratology studies with the insecticide Carbofuran (abs) Toxicol. Appl. Pharmacol. 19:370 (only) 1971.

Wolfe, J.L. and Esher, R.J.: Toxicity of carbofuran and lindane to the Old-Field mouse (P. gossypinus). Bull. Environ. Contam. Toxicol. 24:894-902, 1980.

227   Carbon Dioxide

Haring (1960) has exposed rats during a single gestational day to 6 percent CO_2 20 percent oxygen and 74 percent nitrogen and observed 23 percent cardiac malformations in the offspring as compared to 6.8 percent in controls. The highest incidence of the defect occurred on the 10th day. The cardiac lesions were characterized as due to overgrowth. The majority of these lesions were partial transposition or ventricular outflow stenosis but intraventricular septal defects also were observed.

Grote (1965) administered 10 to 13 percent CO_2 to rabbits between the 7th and 12th day of gestation and found 16 fetuses of 67 to have defects of the vertebral column. Only one abnormal animal was found in the 30 controls. He was not able to determine the role of indirect O_2 deficiency in this experiment. Storch and Layton (1971) were unable to mimic the teratogenic effect of acetazolamide in hamsters by giving 10 percent carbon dioxide in the atmosphere.

Grote, W.: Storung der Embryonalentwicklung bie erhohtem CO_2 und O_2 - partial Druck und bie Unterdruck. 2. Morphol. Anthropol. 56: 165-194, 1965.

Haring, O.M.: Cardiac malformations in rats induced by exposure of the mother to carbon dioxide during pregnancy. Circ. Res. 8: 1218-1227, 1960.

Storch, T.G. and Layton, W.M.: The role of hypercapnia in acetazolamide teratogenesis. Experientia 27: 534-535, 1971.

228   Carbon Monoxide

Carbon monoxide poisoning of the mother has resulted in impaired development of the central nervous system of the fetus. Longo (1977) has reviewed the biologic effects of carbon monoxide on pregnancy.

Warkany (1972) in his review of the subject could not detect any clear correlation between time of exposure and symptomatology of the children. Beaudoin et al (1969) have also reviewed the subject. Schwetz et al (1979) found no teratogenicity from 250 ppm exposure for 7 of 24 hours between days 6 through 15 in mice and 6 through 18 in rabbits. Some increase in minor skeletal anomalies was associated in mice with the exposure. Astrup and colleagues (1972) exposed rabbits during pregnancy to 180 ppm carbon monoxide. Perinatal death occurred in 43 of 123 treated offspring but in only one of a comparable control group. The birth weight was approximately 10 gm less in the treated group and 3 had defects of their extremities. A group of rabbits exposed to 90 ppm gave birth to smaller offspring but the increase in perinatal death was less dramatic. Fechter and Annau (1977) reported behavioral changes in the offsping of rats exposed to concentrations of carbon monoxide producing only 15 percent maternal carboyhemoglobin concentrations. Acute exposure studies in late fetal monkeys produced hemorrhagic necrosis of the fetal cerebral hemispheres at levels which were tolerated by the mothers

(Ginsberg and Myers, 1974). Robkin et al (1975) could not produce alteration in fetal heart or viability in explanted rat embryos exposed to as much as 10 percent carbon monoxide. Robkin and Cockroft (1978) have shown that carbon monoxide causes a shift toward anerobic glucose metabolism in exposed rat embryos.

Astrup, P.; Trolle, D.; Olsen, H.M. and Kjeldsen, K.: Effect of moderate carbon-monoxide exposure on fetal development. Lancet 2: 1220-1222, 1972.

Beaudoin, A.; Gachon, J.; Butin, L-P. and Bost, M.: Les consequence foetales de l'intoxication oxycarbonee de la mere. Pediatrie 24: 459-461, 1969.

Fechter, L.D. and Annau, Z.: Toxicity of mild prenatal carbon monoxide exposure. Science 197: 680-682, 1977.

Ginsberg, M.D. and Myers, R.E.: Fetal brain damage following maternal carbon monoxide intoxication: an experimental study. Acta Obstet. Gynec. Scand. 53: 309-317, 1974.

Longo, L.D.: The biological effects of carbon monoxide in the pregnant woman, fetus and newborn infant. Am. J. Obstet. Gynecol. 129:69-103, 1977.

Robkin, M.A.; Beachler, D.W. and Shepard, T.H.: Effect of carbon monoxide on early rat embryo heart rates. Environ. Res.12:32-37, 1976.

Robkin, M.A. and Cockroft, D.L.: The effects of carbon monoxide on glucose metabolism and growth of rat embryos. Teratology 18: 337-342, 1978.

Schwetz, B.A.; Smith, F.A.; Leong, K. J. and Staples, R.E.: Teratogenic potential of inhaled carbon monoxide in mice and rabbits. Teratology 19: 385-392, 1979.

Warkany, J.: Congenital Malformations Notes and Comments. Chicago: Year Book Medical Publishers, 1971. P. 128 only.

229 Carbon Tetrachloride

Wilson (1954) administered carbon tetrachloride on 2 or 3 days of gestation by mouth (0.3cc) or subcutaneously (0.8cc) and caused no congenital defects in the rat offspring. Adams et al (1961) noted some degeneration of embryonic discs from rabbit blastocysts exposed in vivo to 1.01 ml per kg.

Schwetz et al (1974) exposed pregnant rats to 300 and 1000 ppm for 7 hours on days 6 through 15 of gestation. Fetal size was reduced but neither resorptions nor malformations were increased over the control.

Transplacental passage has been shown in the pregnant mouse (Roschlau and Rodenkirchen, 1969) rat (Tsirel'nikov and Dobrovol'ska, 1973) and human (Dowty and Laseter, 1976).

Adams, C.E.; Hay, M.F. and Lutwak-Mann, C.: The action of various agents upon the rabbit embryo. J. Embryol. Exp. Morphol. 9:468-491, 1961.

Dowty, B.J. and Laseter, J.L.: The transplacental migration and accumulation in blood of volatile organic constituents. Pediat. Res. 10:696-701, 1976.

Roschlau, G. and Rodenkirchen, H.: Histologische untersuchungen uber die diaplazentare Wirkung von Tetrachlorkohlenstaff and ally-alkohol auf Mausefeten. Exp. Path. 3:255-263, 1969.

Schwetz, B.A.; Leong, B.K.; Gehring, P.J.: Embryo and fetotoxicity of inhaled carbon tetrachloride, 1,1-dichloroethane and methyl ethyl ketone in rats. Toxicol. Appl. Pharmacol. 28:452-464, 1974.

Tsirel'nikov, N.I.; Dobrovol'ska, S.G.: Morphohistochemical investigation of the embryonic liver after CCl4 administration at various stages of ontogeny. Bull Expt. Biol. & Med. 76:1467-1469, 1973.

Wilson, J.G.: Influence on the offspring of altered physiologic states during pregnancy in the rat. Ann. N.Y. Acad. Sci. 57:517-525, 1954.

230 Carboxyethylgermanium sesquioxide (GE-132)

Nagari et al (1980) gave this compound intraperitoneally at 500 and 1000 mg per kg per day in a 3 generation study and found no adverse effects. Shimpo and Mori (1980) gave rabbits intravenously up to 1000 mg per kg during organogenesis without fetal ill effects.

Nagari, H.; Hasegawa, K.; Shimpo, K.: Reproductive study of rats intraperitoneally treated with carboxyethylgermanium sesquioxide (GE-132) Oyo Yakuri 20:271-280, 1980.

Shimpo, K.; Mori, N.: Teratogenicity test of carboxyethylgermanium sesquioxide (GE-132) given during the period of organogenesis in rabbits. Oyo Yakuri 20:675-679, 1980.

231 S-Carboxymethyl Cysteine

Ito et al (1977 A and B) studied this expectorant in pregnant rats and rabbits during active organogeneis. No harmful effects were noted with maximum daily doses of 500 mg and 250 mg per kg in the rat and rabbit.

Kawabata and Sugimoto (1979) gave this expectorant by mouth to rats on day 17-21 of gestation and for 21 days after birth. No adverse effects on postnatal development were found.

Ito, R.; Toida, S.; Matsuura, S.; Tanihata, T.; Hidano, T.; Miyamoto, K.; Matsuura, M. and Nakai, S.: A safety study in reproduction and teratology of S- carboxymethyl cysteine, a new organogenesis, perinatal and lactation in rats (Japanese). J. Med. Soc. Toho, Japan 24:62-662, 1977A.

Ito, R.; Toida, S.; Tanihata, T.; Matsuura, S.; Miyamoto, K.; Matsuura, M. and Nakai, S.: A safety study of teratogenicity in organogenesis in rabbits of S- carboxymethyl cysteine, A new expectorant (Japanese). J. Med. Soc. Toho, Japan 24:663-666, 1977B.

Kawabata, R.; Sugimoto, T.: Perinatal and postnatal study of S-CMC in rats. Effect on function behavior reproductive function of the offspring. Kiso to Rinsho 18:1311-1317, 1979.

232 N-[N-(4-Carboxyphenyl)glycyl]aminoacetonitrile

This drug used for chronic hepatitis was given by Irikura et al (1975) orally to mice and rabbits during organogenesis and no teratologic effects were seen. The maximum dose in the mouse was 2,500 mg per kg and 1500 in the rabbit.

Irikura, T.; Sugimoto, T.; Hosomi, J. and Suzuki, H.: Teratological studies on N-[N(-4-carboxyphenyl)glycyl]amino-acetonitrile in mice and rabbits. (Japanese) Oyo Yakuri 9: 523-534, 1975.

233 Carbutamide [1-Butyl-3-sulfanilylurea]

Demeyer and Isaac-Mathy (1958) found cleft palate, eye defects and generalized edema in rat fetuses whose mothers received 500 mg per day for 1, 2 or 3 days during the embryonic period. Tuchmann-Duplessis and Mercier-Parot (1959a) using 800 mg per kg from the 1st through 12th day in rats produced 10 to 33 percent malformed fetuses. The majority of the defects involved the eye and included absence of the optic nerve. Some nervous system defects were reported. The same authors (1959b) noted that carbutamide sulfylurea was more teratogenic in rats than other hypoglycemia sulfylureas. Demeyer (1961) has cauused cleft palates and hydrocephalus with this substance in rats. Bariljak (1967) found that sodium carbonate reduced this drug's teratogenic and lethal action in the rat.

Bariljak, I.R.: The influence of natrium hydrocarbonate on teratogenic activity of oranil (carbutamide). Pharmacol. Toxicol. (Russian) No. 5: 631-633, 1967.

Demeyer, R.: Etude experimentale de la glycoregulation gravidique et de l'action teratogene des perturbations du metabolisme glucidique. Arcia, Bruxelles: Paris, Masson Et Cie, 1961. pp. 175-183.

Demeyer, R. and Isaac-Mathy, M.: A propos de l'action teratogene d'un sulfamide hypoglycemiant. Ann. Endocrinol. 19: 167-172, 1958.

Tuchmann-Duplessis, H. and Mercier-Parot, L.: Sur l'action teratogene d'un sulfamide hypoglycemiant. etude experimentale chez la ratte. J. Physiol. 51: 65-83,

1959a.

Tuchmann-Duplessis, H. and Mercier-Parot, L.: Influence de divers sulfamides hypoglycemiants sur le developpement de l'embryon. Etude experimentale chez le rat. Acad. Nat. Med. (Paris) 143: 238-241, 1959b.

234 Carcinogens

There are a large number of- carcinogenic chemicals which are also teratogenic. Dipaolo and Koten (1966) reviewed this subject comprehensively. Several reviews on the subject of transplacental carcinogenesis have appeared (Alexandrov, 1973; Druckery, 1973; Rice, 1973).

Alexandrov, V.A.: Embryotoxic and teratogenic effects of chemical carcinogens In, Tomatis, 1. and Mohr, U. (eds) Transplacental Carcinogenesis. International Agency For Research in Cancer (IARC Scientific Publication No. 4) (Lyons), 1973, pp. 112-126.

Dipaolo, J.A. and Kotin, P.: Teratogenesis-oncogenesis: a study of possible relationships. Arch. Pathol. 81: 3-23, 1966.

Druckrey, H.: Chemical structure and action in transplacental carcinogenesis and teratogenesis In, Tomatis, 1. and Mohr, U. (eds) Transplacental Carcinogenesis. International Agency For Research in Cancer (IARC Scientific Publication No. 4). (Lyons), 1973, pp. 45-57.

Rice, J.M.: An overview of transplacental chemical carcinogenesis. Teratology 8: 113-126, 1973.

235 Carcinolipin [Cholesteryl-14-methylhexadecanoate]

Shabad et al (1973) gave this compound intraperitoneally during the last one-third of rat pregnancy in total doses of 5 to 18 mg. A fourfold increase in lung tumors was found in the postnatal animals.

Shabad, L.M.; Kolesnichenko, T.S. and Savluchinskaya, L.A.: Transplacental effect of carcinolipin in mice. Neoplasma 20: 347-348, 1973.

236 Cargutocin (Deamino-dicarba-[gly-7]oxytocin)

This oxytocin-like drug was given intravenously to pregnant rats and rabbits in maximum daily doses of 100 and 10 units respectively in the rat and rabbit. Treatment during major organogenesis was not associated with any fetal ill effects (Hamada et al, 1979).

Hamada, Y.; Imanishi, M.; Onishi, R. and Hashiguchi, M.: Teratogenicity study of cargutocin in rats and rabbits Iyakuhin Kenkyu 10:26-40, 1979.

237 Carmine

Schluter (1970) injected lithium or sodium carmine into mice
on the 8th gestational day and produced fetuses with malformation of the ribs and vertebral column as well as
exencephalies. He demonstrated that the carmine was
localized in the visceral yolk sac epithelium.

Schluter, G.: Uber die embryotoxische Wirkung von Carmin
bei der Maus. Z. Anat. Entivicklungsgesch. 131: 228-235,
1970.

238 L-Carnosine

Akatsuka et al (1974) gave this chemical to pregnant rats
intraperitoneally on the 8th through the 14th day and to
mice intravenously on the 7th through the 13th day of
gestation. Maximum doses of 3,000 mg per kg gave some
increases in resorptions but no increase in defects.
Postnatal studies were negative.

Akatsuka, K.; Hashimoto, T.; Takeuchi, K.; Miyame, Y. and
Horisaka, K.: Effects of L-carnosine on the development of
their fetuses and offspring in the pregnant mice and rats.
Oyo Yakuri 8: 1219-1228, 1974.

239 Carotene (see hypervitaminosis A and Palm Oil)

240 Cartap HCl [,3-Bis(Carbamoylthio)-2-(N,N-dimethylamino-
)-propane Hydrochloride]

Mizutani et al (1971) studied this insecticide in pregnant
mice, rats and hamsters. Doses up to 100 mg per kg given
during organogenesis caused only minor skeletal changes
which were ascribed to the maternal toxicity which occurred.

Mizutani, M.; Ihara, T.; Kanamori, H.; Takatani, D.;
Matsokawa, J.; Amano, T. and Kaziwara, K.: Teratogenesis
studies with cartap hydrochloride in the mouse, rat and
hamster. J. Takeda Res. Lab. 30: 776-785, 1971.

241 Carteolol

This beta-adrenergic blocker was given orally to pregnant
mice in doses of up to 150 mg per kg daily. Resorptions
were increased at 75 and 150 mg levels but the rate of
congenital defects was not increased (Tanaka et al (1979).
Perinatal and postnatal studies were also negative (Tamagawa
et al, 1979).

Tamagawa, M.; Namoto, T.; Tanaka, N.; Hishino, H.:
Reproduction study of carteolol hydrochloride in mice; part
2 Perinatal and postnatal toxixity. J. Toxicol. Sci.
4:59-78, 1979.

Tanaka, N.; Shingai, F.; Tamagawa, M.; Nakatsu, I.:
Reproductive study of carteolol hydrochloride in mice. Part

241

1 Fertility and reproductive performance. J. Toxicol. Sci. 4:47-58, 1979.

242 Carzinophilin

Takaya (1965) injected this antibiotic into rats at doses of 0.01 to 0.03 mg per kg on the 6th through 10th day and produced 10 percent defective offspring. The defects were micro(an)opthalmia and hydronephrosis.

Takaya, M.: Teratogenic effects of antibiotics (Japanese) Journal Osaka City Medical center 14: 107-115, 1965.

243 Cassava Root

Rats fed the powder of this root as 80 percent of their diet during the first 15 days of gestation had fetuses with limb reduction defects and microcephaly (Singh, 1981). Cyanide is known to be released from this food by hydrolysase.

Singh, J.D.: The teratogenic effects of dietary cassava on the albino rat: A preliminary report. Teratology 24:289-291, 1981.

244 Cefachlor

This cephalosporin antibiotic was given orally by Nomura et al (1979) to mice, rats and rabbits. No increase in defects was found among the rat and mouse fetuses exposed daily to up to 2000 mg per kg daily during organogenesis and no adverse fetal effects observed. Prenatal or perinatal administration of up to 2000 mg per kg to rats was not associated with reproductive or postnatal changes (Furuhashi et al, 1979).

Furuhashi, T.; Nomura, A.; Uehara, M.; Komuro, E.; Nakayoshi, H.: Fertility and perinatal study of cefachlor in rats. Chemotherapy 27: 865-880, 1979.

Nomura, A.; Furuhashi, T.; Ikega, E.; Sawaki, A.; Nakayoshi, H.: Fertility and perinatal study of cefaclor in mice, rats and rabbits. Chemotherapy 27:846-864, 1979.

245 Cefadroxil

Tauchi et al (1981) gave this antibiotic to rats and rabbits orally in amounts of up to 2300 and 100 mg per kg daily respectively. No significant increase in defects was seen in either species. Fetal weight was reduced in the rabbit when 100 mg per kg was used. Postnatal studies in the rat were done and no differences from controls were found.

Tauchi, K.; Kawanishi, H.; Igarashi, N.; Maeda, Y.; Maekama, Y.; Ebino, K.; Suzuki, K.; Imamichi, T.: Studies of the reproductive toxicity of cefadroxil. Japanese J. of Antibiotics 33:478-486, 487-496, 497-502, 503-509, 1981.

246   Cefatrizine (S-640-P)

Matsuzaki et al (1976A) carried out teratogenicity studies in the rat and mouse at 3,200 mg per kg orally during active organogenesis. Except for weight reduction in the treated rat fetuses, no ill effects were observed. In the rabbit at doses of 400 and 800 mg per kg, an increase in fetal death and reduction in fetal weight was found (Matsuzaki et al, 1976B).

Matsuzaki, A.; Akutsu, S.; Shimamura, T. and Honda, H.: Studies on the possible teratogenicity of cefatrizine (S-640-P). (Japanese) Japanese J. of Antibiotics 29: 812-825, 1976A.

Matsuzaki, A.; Akutsu, M.; Mukaikawa, H. and Kobayashi, K.: Studies of the possible teratogenicity of cefatrizine (S-640-P) 2. Effects on the embryos when administered to pregnant rabbit. (Japanese) Japanese J. of Antibiotics 29:144-152, 1976.

247   Cefmetazole

Esaki et al (1980) administered this antibiotic to pregnant beagle dogs on the 18th through the 35th day in doses of up to 1000 mg per kg. No adverse effects were noted.

Esaki, K.; Nomura, G.; Iwaki, T.: Effects of intravenous administration of cefmetazole (CS -1170) on the fetus of the beagle dog. Preclin. Rep. Cent. Inst. Exp. Animal 6:289-292, 1980.

248   Cefmetrazol

Masuda et al (1978) gave this antibiotic in doses of up to 1000 mg per kg to rats for 14 days after mating and found no adverse reproductive effects. On days 6-15 up to 2000 mg per kg was given intravenously without teratogenic changes. Perinatal and postnatal studies using 2000 mg per kg intravenously in rats on days 17-21 were carried out and no changes were found in behavior or reproductive ability of the offspring.

Masuda, H.; Kimura, K.; Hirose, K.: Toxicological studies of CS-1170 2. Reproductive studies of CS 1170 in mice and rats. Sankyo Kenkyasho Nenpo (Ann. Rep. Sankyo Res. Lab) 30:148-167, 1978.

249   Cefoperazone

Tanioka and Koizumi (1979) injected this antibiotic intravenously into pregnant monkeys on days 23-47 at doses of up to 400 mg per kg per day. No teratogenic effect was found in 9 pregnancies.

Nakada et al (1980) administered this drug subcutaneously to rats in amounts of up to 1000 mg per kg daily on days 17-21 or 7-17 of gestation. No adverse fetal effects were seen and postnatal function was not changed. Administration of 500 mg per kg before mating in both sexes and during the first 7 days was done with no adverse effect.

Nakada, H.; Nakamura, S.; Inaba, J.; Komae, N.; Takai, A.: Toxicity test of cefoperazone (T-1551) Reproductive study in rats. Chemotherapy 28:268-291, 1980.

Tanioka, Y.; Koizumi, H.: Effects of T-1551 on the fetus of rhesus monkeys. Preclin. Rept. Cent. Inst. Exp. Animal 5: 145-156, 1979.

250 Cefotaxime

This cephalosporin antibiotic was studied in mice and rabbits by Sugisaki et al (1981A). Intravenous doses of up to 2000 were used prenatally and perinatally and subcutaneous doses of up to 6000 mg per kg were used for studies during organogenesis. No adverse effects on fertility, the fetuses or the behavior of the offspring were found. Pregnant rabbits received up to 50 mg intravenously on days 6-18 of gestation and the fetuses were not different from controls (Sugisaki et al, 1981B)

Sugisaki, T.; Kitatani, T.; Takagi, S.; Akaike, M.; Hayashi, S.: Reproductive studies of cefotaxime in mice. Oyo Yakuri 21:351-373, 1981A.

Sugisaki, T.; Akaike, M.; Hayashi, S.: Teratological study of cefotaxime given intravenously in rabbits. Oyo Yakuri 21:375-384, 1981B.

251 Cefotetan

This antibiotic was given intraperitoneally to rats before mating and during the first 7 days of gestation in doses of up to 2000 mg per kg and no adverse reproductive changes were found (Odami and Nakata, 1982). Uchida and Odani (1982) gave rats intravenously doses of up to 2000 mg per kg on days 17-21. Some growth retardation was found but no behavioral effects were observed.

Shibata and Tamada (1982) gave up to 2000 mg per kg intravenously to rats on days 7-17 and produced no adverse fetal effects.

Odani, Y. and Nakata, M.: Reproduction study of cefotetan (Y.M. 09330) Fertility study in rats when administered intraperitoneally. Oyo Yakuri 23:641-649,1982.

Shibata, M.; Tamada, H.: Teratological evaluation of cefotetan (YM 09330) administered intravenously to rats. Chemotherapy 30:278-294, 1982.

Uchida, T. and Odani, Y.: Reproductive studies of cefotetan (Y.M. 09330) Perintal and postnatal study in rats by intravenous administration. Oyo Yakuri 23:767-783, 1982.

252 Cefroxadin

This antibiotic was given to rabbits orally in doses of up to 10 mg per kg on days 6-18 of gestation and no significant fetal changes were found (Hirooka et al, 1980). With oral doses of up to 1000 mg per kg in the rat no adverse effects on reproduction were reported (Hirooka et al, 1979)

Hirooka, T.; Tadokoro, T.; Takahashi, S.; Katagawa, K.K.; Kitagawa, S.: Reproductive tests of cefroxadin (CGP-9000) in rats. Iyakuchin Kenkyu 10:802-824, 1979.

Hirooka, T.; Takahashi, S.; Tadokoro, T.; Kitagawa, S.: Reproductive studies of cefroxadin (CGP-9000) a new oral antibiotic. 4. Teratological tests in rabbits. Oyo Yakuri 19:669-679, 1980.

253 Ceftezole

Niki et al (1976) studied this antibiotic in mice and rats using the intravenous and subcutaneous routes and found no increase in fetal defects. The mice received 4000 and 2000 mg per kg by the subcutaneous and intravenous routes respectively and the rats received 1000 mg by each route. Treatments were given during mid gestation.

Niki, R.; Shiota, S.; Usami, M.; Noguchi, G.; Sugiyama, O.; Ohkawa, H. and Takagaki, Y.: Studies of toxicity and teratogenicity of ceftezole (Japanese) Chemotherapy 24:671-702, 1976.

254 Ceftizoxime Sodium

This cephalosporin antibiotic was given to rats subcutaneously by Fukuhara et al (1981) in amounts of up to 1000 mg per kg daily. Dosing was either before mating and during the first 17 days, during days 7-17 or on days 17-21. No adverse effects were found in the fetuses or offspring.

Fukuhara, K.; Fujii, T.; Kado, Y.; Watanabe, N.: Reproductive studies on ceftizoxime sodium in rats. Japanese J. Antibiotics 34:466-476, 1981.

255 Cefuroxine

Furuhashi et al (1979) administered this cephalosporin antibiotic to rabbits subcutaneously or intravenously on days 6 through 18 of gestation. Doses of up to 150 mg per kg had no adverse effects on the fetuses.

Furuhashi, T.; Nomura, A.; Ikeya, E.; Nakazawa, M.: Teratological studies on cefuroxine in rabbiits. Chemotherapy 27:245-292, 1979.

256 Cephalexin

Aoyama et al (1969) found no teratogenicity in the offspring of mice and rats given oral doses of up to 800 (mice) and 4,000 mg per kg (rats) during organogenesis.

Aoyama, T.; Furuoka, R.; Hasegawa, N. and Nemoto, K.: Teratologic studies of cephalexin in mice and rats. Oyo Yakuri 3: 249-263, 1969.

257 Cerium

Ridgway and Karnofsky injected 8 mg of Ce(No-3)3 into chick eggs on the 4th day and found no defects.

D'Agostino et al (1982) injected cerium chloride subcutaneously into mice on day 7 or 12 of gestation at a dose of 80 mg (Ce) per kg. Except for an increased frequency of rearings in the open field of the adult offspring exposed in utero, there was no apparent effect on behavioral parameters. Other reproductive effects were not reported in the paper.

D'Agostino, R.B.; Lown, B.A.; Morganti, J.B.; Massaro, E.J.: Effects of in utero or suckling exposure to cerium (citrate) on the postnatal development of the mouse. J. Toxicol. Environ. Health 10:449- 458, 1982.

Ridgway, L.P. and Karnofsky, D.A.: The effects of metals on the chick embryo: Toxicity and production of abnormalities in development. Ann. N. Y. Acad. Sci. 55: 203-215, 1952.

258 Cesium

Lemeshevskaya and Silaev (1979) exposed rats by inhalation with concentrations of 4.6 and 0.43 mg per m squared during the entire gestation and observed different types of congenital malformations. The non-toxic dose for females (0.003 mg per m squared) produced no embryotoxic activity.

Lemeshevskaya, E.M. and Silaev, A.A.: Embryotoxic studies of cesium arsenate at the inhalation action. Gigiena tr. prof. zabol. (USSR) 9:56, 1979.

259 Cesium-137

Hirata (1964) injected mice intravenously with 2 to 4 microcuries per gm of body weight on day 4, 8, 10, 12 or 15. A small number of cleft palates or tail anomalies were detected. Treatment on day 8 for instance produced 7 abnormal fetuses of the 157 examined.

Hirata, M.: Experimental study on fetal disorders in mice due to radioactive cesium. Fetal disorders due to CS(137) irradiation. J. Hiroshima Obstet. Gynecol. Soc. 3: 224, 1964.

260 Alpha-Chaconine

This glycoalkaloid constituent of potato tubers given in doses of 16 mg per kg to mice on days 8 or 9 produced skeletal defects and midline facial defects (Pierro et al, 1977).

Pierro, L.J.; Haines, J.S. and Osman, S.F.: Teratogenicity and toxicity of purified alpha-chaconine and alpha solanine. (abs) Teratology 15:31A (only), 1977.

261 Chenodeoxycolic Acid

Kitao et al (1982) gave rats orally up to 360 mg per kg on days 7-17 and found no fetal ill effects.

Kitao, T.; Kamishita, S.; Yoshikawa, H.; Sakaguchi, M.: Teratogenicity studies of chenodeoxycolic acid in rats. Yakuri to Chiryo 10:3887-3901, 1982.

262 Cherry, Wild Black

Selby et al (1971) reported an epidemic of six malformed pigs from nine mothers who fed on wild black cherries during the 16th to 28th day of gestation. Defects did not occur in sows pastured nearby in a field without black cherries. The one defective piglet described in detail was very similar to the human form of sirenomelia with absence of the anus, plantar-flexed hind legs, rudimentary external genitalia and a blindly-ending colon.

Selby, L.A.; Menges, R.W.; Houser, E.C.; Flatt, R.E. and Chase, A.C.: An outbreak of swine malformations associated with wild black cherry, Prunus serotina. Arch. Environ. Health 22: 496-501, 1971.

263 Chicken Pox (see Varicella)

264 Chlorambucil [Alpha-(N-N-di-2-chlorethyl)aminophenylbutyric Acid]

This alkylating agent used in treating malignancy produces defects of the nervous system, palate and skeleton in rat fetuses when given to the mother in doses of 8 to 12 mg per kg on the 11th or 12th day. Chaube and Murphy (1968) have summarized the effects of these agents. Monie (1961) provides a detailed account of the defects this substance produces in the urogenital system of the rat. Soukup et al (1967) found about 10 percent abnormal metaphase figures in rat embryos after maternal treatment with 8 mg per kg. Mirkes and Greenaway (1982) produced defects of the prosencephalon in rat embryos grown in vitro with as little as 1.5 microgram per ml of medium. The toxic activity was enhanced by the presence of a liver monooxygenase system.

Shotton and Monie (1963) have described a human fetus of 120 mm crown-rump length with unilateral absence of a ureter and kidney. The mother had received 6 mg of chlorambucil daily during early pregnancy.

Chaube, S. and Murphy, M.L.: The teratogenic effects of the recent drugs in cancer chemotherapy. In, Woollam, D.H.M.; Ed.: Advances in Teratology, Vol. III. Academic Press, New York, 1968. pp. 194-196.

Mirkes, P.E. and Greenaway, J.C.: Teratogenicity of chlorambucil in rat embryos in vitro. Teratology 26:135-143, 1982.

Monie, I.W.: Chlorambucil-induced abnormalities of the urogenital system of rat fetuses. Anat. Rec. 139: 145-153, 1961.

Shotton, D. and Monie, I.W.: Possible teratogenic effect of chlorambucil on a human fetus. J.A.M.A. 186: 74-75, 1963.

Soukup, S.; Takacs, E. and Warkany, J.: Chromosome changes in embryos treated with various teratogens. J. Embryol. Exp. Morphol. 18: 215-226, 1967.

265 Chloramphenicol [Chloromycetin-R]

In chick embryos chloramphenicol inhibits protein synthesis and growth but only infrequent defects of the splanchnopleure and neural tube have been reported (Blackwood, 1962 and Billett et al, 1965). In the rabbit (Brown et al, 1968) and monkey (Courtney and Valerio, 1968) no congenital defects were produced. Generalized edema was found in the rat in 12 to 71 percent of fetuses whose mothers received 2 to 4 percent chloramphenicol in the diet during the latter half of gestation (Mackler et al, 1975). Prochazka et al (1964) have reported no defects in the rat fetuses whose mothers received 100 to 200 mg per kg during pregnancy. Fritz and Hess (1971) using the rat, mouse and rabbit found little evidence of teratogenicity.

Dyban and Chebotar (1971) administering very large doses (2500 mg per kg) by stomach tube on the 9th through the 11th day produced eventration, hydrocephalus, cleft lip and defects of the diaphragm.

Billet, F.S.; Collini, R. and Hamilton, L.: The effects of D and L threo-chloramphenicol in the early development of the chick embryo. J. Embryol. Exp. Morphol. 13: 341-356, 1965.

Blackwood, U.B.: The changing inhibition of early differentiation and general development in the chick embryo by 2-ethyl-5-methyl-benzimidazole and chloramphenicol. J. Embryol. Exp. Morphol. 10: 315-336, 1962.

Brown, D.M.; Harper, K.H.; Palmer, A.K. and Tesh, S.A.: Effect of antibiotics upon the rabbit. (abstract) Toxicol. Appl. Pharmacol. 12: 295, only, 1968.

Courtney, K.D. and Valerio, D.A.: Teratology in the Macaca

mulatta. Teratology 1: 163-172, 1968.

Dyban, A.P. and Chebotar, N.A.: Can cleft palate be induced by chloramphenicol? Arch. Anat. (Russian) 60: No. 5, 25-29, 1971.

Fritz, H. and Hess, R.: The effect of chloramphenicol on the prenatal development of rats, mice and rabbits. Toxicol. Appl. Pharm. 19:667-674, 1971..

Mackler, B.; Grace, R.; Tippit, D.F.; Lemire, R.J.; Shepard, T.H. and Kelley, V.C.: Studies of the development of congenital anomalies in rats. 3. Effects of inhibition of mitochondrial energy systems on embryonic development. Teratology 12:391-396, 1975.

Prochazka, J.; Simkova, V.; Havelka, J.; Hejzlar, M.; Viklicky, J.; Kargerova, A. and Kubikova, M.: Concerning the penetration of the placenta by chloramphenicol. (Russian) Pediatriia 19:311-314, 1964.

266 2-Chlor-4-azaphenthiazine [Cloxypendyl-R]

Gross et al (1968) gave 5 mg per kg to rats from the 8th through the 20th day and found no evidence of teratogenicity.

Gross, A.; Thiele, K.; Schuler, W.A. and Schlichtegroll, A.: 2-chloro-4-azaphenthiazine Synthese und Pharmakologische eigenschafter von Cloxypendyl. Arzneim. Forsch. 18: 435-442, 1968.

267 Chlorcyclizine [1-(P-Chloro-alpha-phenylbenzyl)-4-methyl--piperizine] (see Meclizine)

This antihistamine belongs to the benzhydrylpiperazine series of compounds and has been used to produce cleft palate in the rat. It is more fully discussed under meclizine.

268 Chlordan [1,2,4,5,6,7,8,8-Octachloro-4-7-methano-3alpha, 4,7,7,alpha-tetrahydroindane]

Ingle (1952) found normal offspring of rats fed 150 to 300 PPM chlordan during and after gestation. Maintained with their lactating mothers, these young developed excitability and tremors. If they were transferred to foster mothers on normal diets, their development was normal.

Crammer et al (1979) treated mice throughout pregnancy and with 8.0 mg per kg per day the offspring were shown to have a defect in cell-mediated immune response.

Cranmer, J.S.; Avery, D.L. and Barnett, J.B.: Altered immune competence of offspring exposed during development to the chlorinated hydrocarbon pesticide chlordane (abs) Teratology 19:23A only (1979).

268

Ingle, L.: Chronic oral toxicity of chlordan to rats. Archives of Industrial Hygiene and Occupational Medicine 6: 357-367, 1952.

269 Chlordiazepoxide [Librium-R] (see Meprobamate)

In a study of 136 women taking this drug in the first 13 weeks of pregnancy, Crombie et al (1975) found only three offspring with congenital defects. Hartz et al (1975) in a followup of 50,000 pregnancies could not associate an increased defect rate in the 501 pregnancies where the drug was taken in the first trimester. Milkovich and Van den Berg (1974) using a computer linkage between prescriptions given to mothers and the outcome of their pregnancies found four congenital defects among 35 women taking the drug in the first 42 days.

Crombie, D.L.; Pinsent, R.J.; Fleming, D.M.; Rumeau-Rouquette, C.; Goujard, J. and Huel, G.: Fetal effects of tranquilizers in pregnancy. New. Eng. J. Med. 293: 198-199, 1975.

Hartz, S.C.; Heinonen, O.P.; Shapiro, S.; Siskind, V. and Slone, D.: Antenatal exposure to meprobamate and chlordiazepoxide in relation to malformations, mental development and childhood mortality. New Eng. Med. 292:726-728, 1975.

Milkovich, L. and Van den Berg, B.J.: Effects of prenatal meprobamate and chlordiazepoxide hydrochloride on human embryonic and fetal development. New Eng. J. Med. 291:1268-1271, 1974.

270 Chlorguanide [Cyclamide-R]

Bariljak (1965) gave pregnant rats 2000 mg per kg of body weight on days 9 and 10 and caused 46 percent embryonic death but no abnormalities.

Bariljak, I.R.: Comparison of teratogenic action of carbutamide and cyclamide in rat embryos. Pharmakol. Toxicol. (Russian) No. 5: 616-621, 1965.

271 Chlormadinone Acetate

Takano et al. (1966) reported that this progestin produced defects in mice and rabbits. The mice were given 3 to 50 mg per kg orally during the latter two-thirds of pregnancy; cleft palate and club foot were the main defects observed. In rabbits with administration of 10 mg per day from the 8th through the 17th gestational day skeletal and palate defects occurred along with a relatively high incidence of abdominal wall defect. Masculinization of the female mouse and rabbit fetuses was not produced. Chambon et al. (1966) have reported a similar type of teratogenicity in the rabbit and rat, but the dose in the rabbit was 0.5 mg per day, considerably less than that used by Takano.

Chambon, Y.; Depagne, A. and Leveve, Y.: Malformations et deformations foetales par insuffisance hormonale gestative chez le lapin et chez le rat. Comptes Rendus De l'association Des Anatomistes 131: 270-279, 1966.

Takano, K.; Yamamura, H.; Suzuki, M. and Nishimura, H.: Teratogenic effect of chlormadinone acetate in mice and rabbits.

Proc. Soc. Exp. Biol. Med. 121: 455-457, 1966.

272 Chloroacetamide

Thiersch gave pregnant rats 20 mg per kg on single days (7th, 11th or 12th) and found no effects on litter size or fetuses.

Thiersch, J.B.: Investigations into the differential effect of compounds on rat litter and mother. In, Tuchmann-Duplessis, H. (ed.): Malformations Congenitales Des Mammiferes. Paris: Masson et Cie, 1971. pp. 95-113.

273 4-Bis(2-Chlorobenzyl aminomethyl) Cyclohexane (AY-9944)

This inhibitor of cholesterol synthesis has been studied by Roux et al (1972) in rats giving 50 mg per kg on the second through fourth gestational days. Ocular anomalies were found in 42 percent of the Wistar rat fetuses but none were seen in the Sprague-Dawley strain. Both groups of fetuses had hydronephrosis and ectopia of the testes.

Roux, C.; Taillemite, J.L.; Aubry, M. and Dupuis, R.: Effets teratogenes compares du chlorhydrate du [Trans-1, 4-bis(2-chlorobenzyl aminomethyl)cyclohexane] (AY-9944) chez le rat Wistar et le rat Sprague-Dawley. C.R.. Soc. Biol. 166: 1233-1236, 1972.

274 O-Chlorobenzylidene Malononitrile [CS]

Upshall (1973) studied this irritant which is used for dispersing unruly crowds. Five minute exposures of up to 60 mg per cubic meter were used on days 6 through 15 in rats and day 6 through 18 in rabbits. No adverse fetal effects were found. Rats given 20 mg per kg intraperitoneally on days 6, 8, 10, 12 and 14 gave birth to normal fetuses.

Upshall, D.G.: Effects of o-chlorobenzylidene malononitrile (CS) and the stress of aerosol inhalation upon rat and rabbit embryonic development. Toxicol. Appl. Pharm. 24: 45-59, 1973.

275 Chlorobiphenyls (see Kanechlor also)

Maternal ingestion of chlorobiphenyls from contamination of a brand of cooking oil in Japan was responsible for dark-brown staining of the skin of the newborn babies (Miller, 1971). This syndrome called the cola-colored baby

275

was associated frequently with intrauterine growth
retardation but no defects were recorded and the skin
discoloration faded in a few months (Taki et al.; 1969).
Funatsu et al. (1972) reported four newborns with the
syndrome and noted that three had exophthalmus and two had
teeth present at birth. Shiota (1976) gives some data on
polychlorinated biphenyl concentrations in human fetuses.
Rogan (1982) has reviewed the clinical aspects.

Kato et al (1972) demonstrated that the compound crosses the
rat placenta but found no defects in the fetuses. Marks et
al (1981) gavaged hexachlorobiphenyl on days 6 through 15 of
pregnancy in the mouse. At doses of 0.1 and 1 mg per kg no
significant increase in defects was produced but at 2, 4, 8
and 16 mg per kg one was found. Cleft palate and
hydronephrosis were the most common types found. Maternal
toxicity was found at 8 mg per kg. From study of other
isomers they concluded that the 3, 3 prime, 4 and 4-prime
positions seemed essential for teratogenicity.

Funatsu, H.; Yamashita, F.; Ito, Y.; Tsugawa, S.; Funatsu,
T.; Yoshikane, T.; Hayoshi, M.; Kato, T.; Yakashiji, M.;
Okamoto, G.; Yamasaki, S.; Arima, T.; Kuno, T.; Ioe, H. and
Ide, I.: Polychlorbiphenyls (PCB) induced fetopathy. I.
Clinical observation. Kurume M. J. 19: 43-50, 1972.

Kato, T.; Yakushiji, M.; Tuda, H.; Arimi, A.; Takahashi, K.;
Shimomura, M.; Miyahara, M.; Adachi, M.; Tashiro, Y.;
Matsumoto, M.; Funatsu, I.; Yamashita, F.; Ito, Y.; Tsugawa,
S.; Funatsu, T.; Yoshikane, T. and Hayashi, M.: Polychlorobiphenyls (PCB) induced fetopathy. II. Experimental
studies: Possible placental transfer of polychlorobiphenyls
in rats. Kurume M. J. 19: 53-59, 1972.

Marks, T.A.; Kimmel, G.L.; Staples, R.E.: Influence of
symmetrical polychlorinated biphenyl isomers on embryo and
fetal development. Toxicol. Appl. Pharm. 61:269-276,
1981.

Miller, R.W.: Cola-colored babies. Chlorobiphenyl
poisoning in Japan. Teratology 4: 211-212, 1971.

Rogan, W.J.: PCBs and cola-colored babies: Japan, 1968, and
Taiwan Teratology 26:259-261, 1982.

Shiota, K.: Fetal accumulation of polychlorinated biphenyls
(PCB's). A consideration on the problem of human
pollutants. Cong. Anom. 16: 9-16, 1976.

Taki, I.; Hisanaga, S. and Amagase, Y.: Report on Yusho (-
chlorobiphenyls poisoning). Pregnant women and their
fetuses. Fukuoka Acta Med. 60: 471-474, 1969.

276 3-Chloro-5-[3-(4-carbamyl-4-piperidinopiperidino)propyl-
]-10,11-di hydro-5H-dibenz [B,F] Azepine Dihydrochloride
Monohydrate

Hamada (1970) gave this compound orally to pregnant rats and
mice on several or more days during midgestation. At the
highest dose in the mouse (200 mg per day) fetal growth

retardation and cleft palates were increased. In the rats
at doses up to 250 mg per kg,no fetal changes occurred.

Hamada,   Y.:   Studies   on   psychotropic   drugs.   14
Toxicological   studies   of   3-chloro-
-5-[3-(4-carbamyl-4-piperidinopiperidino)-propyl]-10,11-d
dihydro-5H-dibenz [B,F] azepine dihydrochloride monohydrate.
Oyo Yakuri 5: 663-668, 1970.

277   0-Chloro-alpha-(tert-butylaminomethyl)-benzylalcohol Hydro-
      chloride

Tsurusaki   et   al   (1977)   tested   this   bronchodilator   in
pregnant   rats   and   with   oral   doses   of   up   to   75   mg per   kg
during organogenesis produced no ill effects in the fetuses.
Kawana   et   al   (1977)   found   no   teratogenic   effect   of   oral
doses of 40 mg per kg in the rabbit.

Kawana,   S.;   Watanabe,   G.;   Ito,   T.;   Yamamoto,   M.   and
Kamimura, K.: Effects of the bronchodilator C-78 on fetal
development   in rabbits.   Acta Medica et Biologica 25:67-73,
1977.

Tsurusaki,   T.; Shita, T.; Yamasaki, M.; Kubo, N.; Yamamota,
M.   and Vemura, K.:   Effects of 0-chloro- alpha-(tert-butylaminomethyl)benzylalcohol   on   the   reproductive function of
rats.   (Japanese) Clinical Report 11:439-453, 1977.

278   6-Chloro-3-carbomethoxy-3,4-dihydro-2-methyl-
      -2H-1,2,4-benzothiadiazine-7-sulfonamide-1-dioxide

Takai   et   al   (1973)   gave   this   antihypertensive   drug to
pregnant   mice   and   rats   orally   in   amounts   up   to   3,000   mg   per
kg per day during active organogenesis. Although some delay
in fetal ossification was seen, no increase in gross malformations   occurred.   The neonates were also followed for 3
weeks   after   birth   without   appearance   of   significant
differences from the control group.

Takai,   A.;   Nakada,   H.   and Yoneda,   T.:   A   pharmacological
study   on   6-chloro-3-carbomethoxy-3,4-dihydro-2-methyl-
-2H-1,2,4-benzothiadi

iazine-7-sulfonamide-1,1-dioxide   (DU   5747),   a   new
antihypertensive-diuretic agent.   5 Teratological Studies of
DU 5747. (Japanese) Oyo Yakuri 7: 267-274, 1973.

279   10-Chloro-11b-(2-chlorophenyl)-2,3,5,6,7,11b-hexahydro-
      benzo[6,7] -1,4-dibenzepino[5,4-b]oxazol-6-one

Tanase   et   al   (1971)   treated   mice   and   rats   with   this
tranquilizer during active organogenesis with up to 600 mg
per   kg   per   day   by   mouth.   No fetal defects or postnatal
effects were found.

Tanase,   H.;   Hirose,   K.   and Suzuki, Y.:   2.   Effects of
CS-370 upon the development of pre- and post-natal offspring
of experimental animals. (Japanese) Ann. Sankyo Res. Lab.

23: 180-191, 1971.

280   Chlorocholine   Chloride   [(2-Chloroethyl)trimethylammonium
      Chloride]

      Juszkiewicz et al. (1970) administered 25 to 400 mg per kg
      orally to hamsters on the 8th gestational day. With doses
      of 300 and 400   mg   5.9 and 8.8 percent of the fetuses
      respectively were abnormal. The defects were polymorphic
      but   included   encephaloceles,   anophthalmia   and
      microphthalmia. Ackermann et al. (1970) found no terato-
      genicity in the rat.

      Ackermann, H.; Proll, J. and Luder, W.: Untersuchungen zur
      Toxikologischen beurteilung von chlorcholinclorid.   Arch.
      Experiment. Veterin. 24: 1049-1057, 1970.

      Juszkiewicz, T.; Rakalska, Z. and Dzierzawski, A.:   Effet
      embryopathie du chlorure de chlorocholine (CCC) chez le
      hamster dore. European Journal of Toxicology 3: 265-270,
      1970.

281   Chlorocyclamide-R

      This oral hypoglycemic used in a dose of 1000 mg per kg in
      rats on the 9th and 10th days of pregnancy resulted in 29
      percent abnormal fetuses. The defects included hydro-
      cephalus, microcephaly, hydronephrosis and heart malforma-
      tions (Bariliak, 1968).

      Bariliak, I.R.: Comparison of antithyroidal and teratogenic
      activity of some hypoglycemic sulphanylamides. Problems of
      Endocrinology (Russian). 14: No. 6, 89-94, 1968.

282   5-Chloro-2-deoxyuridine

      Chaube and Murphy (1964) produced defects of the nervous
      system, palate and skeleton in rats treated with 125 to 1000
      mg per kg on the 12th day. Thymidine protected the fetus
      against the teratogenic effects of this compound.

      Chaube, S. and Murphy, M.L.:   Teratogenic effects of 5-
      chlorodeoxyuridine   on   the   rat   fetus; protection by
      physiological pyrimidines.   Cancer Res.   24: 1986-1989,
      1964.

283   P-Chlorodimethylaminobenzene (see Aminoazobenzene)

284   Chloroisopropamide

      Bariliak (1968) using 1000 mg per kg on the 9th and 10th
      gestational days of the rat produced 30 to 45 percent fetal
      mortality but no congenital defects were found.

      Bariliak, I.R.: Comparison of antithyroidal and teratogenic
      activity of some hypoglycemic sulphanylamides. Problems of

Endocrinology (Russian) 14: No. 6, 89-94, 1968.

285 N-[4-(2-(5-Chloro-2-methoxybenzamido)-ethyl-
)phenylsulfonyl]-N-cyclohexylurea (HB-419)

Miyamoto et al (1970) fed this compound to pregnant rats and
mice in maximal doses of 2,000 mg per kg per day and found
no fetotoxicity or teratogenicity. The rats were fed from
the 6th through the 15th day and the mice from the 4th
through the 13th day of gestation.

Miyamoto, M.; Ohtsu, M.; Kumai, M.; Takayama, K. and
Sakaguchi, T.: Influence of N-[4-(2-(5-chloro-2-methoxy-
benzamido)-ethyl)phenylsulfonyl] N-cyclohexylurea (HB-419)
on embryos (Japanese). Oyo Yakuri 4: 271-283, 1970.

286 Chloromethylenecycline (see Chlorotetracycline)

287 3-Chloro-2-[N-methyl-N-[morpholino-carbonyl]methyl]

Iida et al (1974) gave pregnant rabbits and rats up to 1,000
mg per kg by mouth and 20 mg per kg by intravenous route and
observed no teratogenic activity. The compound was given in
rats from the 9th to the 14th day and in rabbits from the
8th to 16th day.

Iida, H.; Kast, A. and Tsanenari, Y.: Studies on the teratogenicity of 3-chloro-2-[N-methylN-[(morpholino-carbonyl)-
methyl] aminomethylbenzanilide (PB 89) in rats and rabbits.
Oyo Yakuri 8: 1073-1087, 1974.

288 4-Chloro-2-methylphenoxyacetic Acid Ethylester (MCPEE)

Yasuda and Maeda (1972) tested this herbicide in pregnant
rats. It was given (with the diet at levels of 40, 500,
1000 and 2000 PPM) on days 8 through 15 of gestation. At
the highest dose which was equivalent to approximately 100
mg per kg per day, congenital malformations including cleft
palate, ventricular septal defect and kidney defects were
found. At this high level there was maternal weight loss.
Their report contains a summary of teratologic testing of
other phenoxyalkanoic acid herbicides.

Yasuda, M. and Maeda, H.: Teratogenic effects of 4-chloro-
-2-methylphenoxyaceticacetic acid ethylester (MCPEE) in
rats. Toxicol. Appl. Pharm. 23: 326-333, 1972.

289 2-Chloro-11-(4-methyl-1-piperazinyl)-dibenzo
[b,f][1,4]oxazepine

Mineshita et al (1970) administered this neuroleptic orally
to pregnant rats and mice during organogenesis. At the dose
level of 12 mg per kg per day fetal survival was decreased
and a low incidence of exencephaly was found. All of these
abnormal fetuses occurred in one litter of the 20 treated at
that level. No defects were found in the rat offspring.

The thiazepine derivative of this drug was similarly studied and no teratogenicity was found.

Mineshita, T.; Hasegawa, Y.; Inoue, Y.; Kozen, T. and Yamamato, A.: Teratological studies on fetuses and suckling young of mice and rats of S-805. Oyo Yakuri 4:305-316, 1970.

290 4[(5-Chloro-2-oxo-3-benzothiazolinyl)acetyl]-1-piperazine Ethanol Hydrochloride (Tiaramide Hydrochloride-R)

This antiinflammatory compound was given to mice, rats and rabbits in maximum daily oral doses of 250, 1000 and 250 mg per kg. (Watanabe et al, 1973). No defects or fetal effects of significance were found.

Watanabe, N.; Takashima, T.; Ito, N.; Fujii, T. and Miyazaki, K.: Toxicological and teratological studies of 4[(5-chloro-2-oxo-3-benzothiazolinyl)acetyl]-1-piperazine ethanol hydrochloride (tiaramide hydrochloride), an anti-inflammatory drug. Arzneim Forsch 23: 504-508, 1973.

291 8-[3-(2-Chloro-10-phenothiazinyl)propyl-]-3-oxo-1-thia-4,8-diazas piro[4,5]decane HCl

Hamada et al (1970) studied the effect of this drug on the pregnant rat and mouse. They gave up to 100 mg per kg per day to mice and 200 mg per kg per day to rats during organogenesis. Some minor abnormalities of the cervical vertebrae and sternum were found in fetuses from both species but no gross defects or change in survival occurred.

Hamada, Y.; Namba, T.; Okada, T. and Izaki, K.: Studies on psychotropic drugs. 9 Teratological studies of APY-606. Oyo Yakuri 4: 497-504, 1970.

292 O-Chloro-beta-phenyl-ethlhydrazine   Dihydrogen   Sulfate (WL-27)

Poulson and Robson (1964) found that this amineoxidase inhibitor prevented implantation in mice. When they gave 20 mg per kg per day on the 6th through 11th days, five litters were examined and no defects noted. Rabbits receiving 27 mg per kg on day 7 to 11 of pregnancy gave birth to 30 fetuses, one of which exhibited unusual facial, skull and limb defects.

Poulson, E. and Robson, J.M.: Effect of phenelzine and some related compounds on pregnancy and sexual development. J. Endocrinol. 30: 205-215, 1964.

293 Chlorophenols (see Pentachlorophenol)

294 1-(3-Chlorophenyl)-3-N,N-dimethylcarbamyl-5- methoxypyrazole (PZ-177)

This antiinflammatory analgesic agent was given to rats and rabbits during active organogenesis in maximum daily doses of 250 mg and 200 mg per kg in the rat and rabbit respectively. No ill effects were observed except in the rat fetus at 250 mg per kg, there was slight osseous retardation.

Yamamoto, H.; Miyake, J.; Miyake, H.; Nakamura, Y.; Kawase, Y.; Ohhata, H. and Yamada, S.: The effects of 1-(3-chlorophenyl)-3-N,N-dimethylcarbamoyl-5-methoxypyrazole (PZ-177) on reproduction in rats. (Japanese) Iyakuhin Kenkyu 9:538-548, 1978.

Yamamoto, H.; Miyake, J.; Miyake, H. and Asada, M.: A teratological study of 1-(3-chlorophenyl)3-N,N- dimethylcarbamoyl-5-methoxypyrazole (PZ-177) in rabbits. Iyakuhin Kenkyu 9:558-562, 1978.

Schwetz et al (1974a) report studies with 2,3,4,6-tetrachlorophenol in the rat using 30 mg and 50 mg per kg respectively orally on days 6 through 15 of gestation. Although some fetal edema and delay in ossification occurred no defects were produced.

For pentachlorophenol Schwetz et al (1974b) found embryotoxicity when oral doses above 5 mg per kg were given. No teratogenic activity was found.

Schwetz, B.A.; Keeler, P.A. and Gehring, P.J.: Effect of purified and commercial grade tetrachlorophenol on rat embryonal and fetal development. Toxicol. Appl. Pharm. 28: 146-150, 1974a.

Schwetz, B.A.; Keeler, P.A. and Gehring, P.J.: The effect of purified and commercial grade pentachlorophenol on rat embryonal and fetal development. Toxicol. Appl. Pharm. 28: 151-161, 1974b.

295   4-(P-Chlorophenyl)-2-phenyl-5-thiazoleacetic Acid

Shimazu et al (1979) studied this antiinflammatory during organogenesis in rats and rabbits. No ill effects were produced with oral doses up to 50 mg and 100 mg per kg daily in the rat and rabbit respectively. In the rabbit maternal weight gain was reduced at 100 mg per kg.

Shimazu, H.; Ichikara, T.; Matuura, M. and Kajima, N.: Effects of 4-(P-chlorophenyl)-2-phenyl-5-thiazoleacetic cetic acid in the reproduction tests in rats and rabbits. (Japanese) Clinical Report 13:1929-1945, 1979.

296   Chlorophos

This agent was given to pregnant hamsters and mice during active organogenesis (300 mg per kg daily). Low incidence of cleft palate and some skeletal defects in hamster fetuses were found. All of these abnormal fetuses occurred in hamsters treated on day 8. Neither embryotoxicity nor teratogenicity was found in mice.

296

Martson, L.V.: Teratological studies on chlorophos in golden hamsters and white mice. Gigiena i Sanitariya (USSR) 7:70-72, 1979.

297 Beta-Chloroprene (2-Chlorobutadiene-1,3)

Culik et al (1978) exposed rats by inhalation to 25 ppm for 4 hours daily on days 3 through 20 and found no adverse fetal effects.

Culik, R.; Kelley, D.P. and Clary, J.J.: Inhalation studies to evaluate the teratogenic and embryotoxic potential of Beta-chloroprene (2-chlorobutadiene-1,3) Toxicol. Appl. Pharm. 44:81-88, 1978.

298 6-Chloropurine

Tuchmann-Duplessis and Mercier-Parot (1959) produced circular body constrictions of rat fetuses treated with 5 mg doses on the 9th and 10th gestational day of the rat. Amniotic bands were present also. Murphy and Chaube (1962) gave 100 to 400 mg per kg to rats and produced cleft palate and skeletal defects. Thiersch (1957) used 100 mg per kg in rats and found that this dose on the 11th and 12th day caused defects in 53 percent of the fetuses. He commented that the placenta was more resistent than the fetus to this drug.

Murphy, M.L. and Chaube, S.: Teratogenic effects of abnormal purines and their ribosides in the rat. (abstract) Proc. Amer. Ass. Cancer Res. 3: 347, only, 1962.

Thiersch, J.B.: Effect of 2-6 diaminopurine (2-6 DP): 6-chloropurine (CLP) and thioguanine (THG) on rat litter in utero. Proc. Soc. Exp. Biol. Med. 94: 40-43, 1957.

Tuchmann-Duplessis, H. and Mercier-Parot, L.: Sur l'action abortive et teratogene de la 6-chloropurine. C. R. Soc. Biol. (Paris) 153: 1133-1136, 1959.

299 Chloroquine

Smith (1966) cites the case of a woman who during four of her eight pregnancies was given chloroquine (250 mg daily from the 6th week after conception); two of these children were congenitally deaf with instability of gait. One of these children had chorioretinitis of the type associated with chloroquine toxicity in the adult. A 3rd exposed child had hemihypertrophy and developed a Wilm's tumor. The family was reported by Hart and Naunton (1964).

Udalova (1967) using 1000 mg per kg on the 9th day induced embryonic death in 27 percent and eye abnormalities in 47 percent of the surviving rat fetuses. Anophthalmia and microphthalmia were the only defects found. Dencker et al (1975) using an I-125 labeled chloroquine analogue showed transplacental passage and concentration in the monkey fetus. The adrenal cortex and retina were found to concentrate the isotope.

Dencker, L.; Lindquist, N.G. and Ulberg, S.: Distribution of an I-125 labeled chloroquine analogue in a pregnant macaca monkey. Toxicology 5:255-264, 1975.

Hart, C.W. and Naunton, R.F.: The ototoxicity of chloroquine phosphate. Arch. Otolaryngol. 80: 407-412, 1964.

Smith, D.W.: Dysmorphology (teratology). J. Pediatr. 69: 1150-1169, 1966.

Udalova, L.D.: The effect of chloroquine on the embryonal development of rats. Pharmacol. Toxicol. (Russian) No. 2: 226-228, 1967.

300 Chlorosil

Boikova et al (1981) studied this agent in pregnant rats. At doses of up to 100 mg taken orally during 14 days of gestation, no adverse fetal effects occurred.

Boikova, V.V.; Golikov, S.N.; Korkhov, V.V. and Mots, M.N.: Reproductive studies with a new cholinolytic chlorosil in rats. Farmakol. Toksikol. (USSR) XLIV, 1:03-95, 1981.

301 Chlorotetracycline [Aureomycin-R]

Tubaro (1964) produced skeletal defects in chicks receiving 1 mg via the yolk sac on the 8th day. Chlormethylenecycline was non-teratogenic. This author reports negative findings in pregnant rabbits and rats receiving 10 mg per kg per day of chlorotetracycline.

Tubaro, E.: Possible relationship between tetracycline stability and effect on foetal skeleton. Br. J. Pharmacol. 23: 445-448, 1964.

302 8-Chlorotheophylline

This drug constitutes about 45 percent of the commonly used anti-motionsickness compound Dramamine-R. In 319 exposed pregnancies, Heinonen et al (1976) found no general increase in malformations. Five children with congenital heart disease were identified but this was not statistically significant.

Heinonen, O.P.; Slone, D. and Shapiro, S.: Birth Defects and Drugs in Pregnancy. Publishing Sciences Group Inc.; Littleton, Mass.; 1977.

303 Chlorothiazide

Grollman and Grollman (1962) reported persistent hypertension in rat offspring after maternal treatment with 166 mg daily from day 15 until birth. Chlorothiazide and hydrochlorothiazide were injected into the pregnant rat in amounts of 250 mg per kg on day 10 and 11 and no defects resulted (Maren and Ellison, 1972). Heinenon et al (1977) reported no increase in defect rate among 5,283 exposed infants.

Grollman, A. and Grollman, E.F.: Teratogenic induction of hypertension. J. Clin. Invest. 41: 710-714, 1962.

Heinonen, O.P.; Slone, D.; Shapiro, S.: Birth Defects and Drugs in Pregnancy. Publishing Sciences Group, Inc., 1977.

Maren, T.H. and Ellison, A.C.: The teratogenic effect of certain thiadiazoles related to acetazolamide with a note on sulfamilamide and thiazide diuretics. Johns Hopkins Med. J. 130: 95-104, 1972.

304 Chlorphenesin Carbamate

Jacobs (1971) produced profound muscular flaccidity in rat fetuses given 500 mg per kg on day 15.3 of gestation. This flaccidity did not interfere with normal closure of the palate.

Jacobs, R.M.: Failure of muscle relaxants to produce cleft palate in mice. Teratology 4: 25-30, 1971.

305 Chlorphentermine

Lullmann-Rauch (1973) reported that injection of 40 mg per kg of body weight given to pregnant rats from day 10 through day 21 produced a lipidosis characterized by cytoplasmic inclusions in the fetal cardiac and pulmonary cells. This drug is used as an anorexigenic in humans.

Lullmann-Rauch, R.: Chlophentermine-induced ultrastructural alterations in foetal tissues.. Virchows Arch. Abt. B. Zellpath. 12: 295-302, 1973.

306 Chlorproguanil (see Cycloguanil)

307 Chlorpromazine (also see Phenothiazines, Thorazine-R)

This phenothiazine compound is of doubtful teratogenicity: the literature on its teratogenicity is critically surveyed by Kalter (1968). Chambon (1955) found an increased fetal mortality when rats were given 10 mg per kg, but no defects. Sobel (1960) reviewed 52 instances where the mother was treated and found no increase in defects or wastage but he did observe respiratory distress in newborns from three women receiving very high doses (500 to 600 mg daily) up to parturition. Radioactive S(35) from the drug accumulates in the fetal mouse and monkey retina (Lindquist et al.; 1970).

Clark et al (1973) injected 3 mg per kg into rats from days 12 through 15 of gestation and then subjected the offspring to several types of behavior tests. Although the latencies were shorter than controls, the treated group made significantly more errors in the maze and took longer to learn the bar-press response. Reversal in the T-maze or extinction of operant response were not altered.

Vince (1969) commented on the reports of others indicating that phenothiazines are not teratogenic in humans. His experience with one patient who had transposition of the great vessels and the reported myocardial damage from phenothiazines raised his question about embryonic or fetal myocardial toxicity.

Chambon, Y.: Action de la chlorpromazine sur l'evolution et l'avenir de la gestation chez la ratte. Ann. Endocrinol. 16: 912-922, 1955.

Clark, C.V.H.; Gorman, D. and Vernadakis, A.: Effects of prenatal administration of psychotropic drugs on behavior of developing rats. Developmental Psychobiology 34: 225-235, 1970.

Kalter, H.: Teratology of the central nervous system. Chicago: University of Chicago Press, 1968. P. 164 only.

Lindquist, N.G.; Sjostrand, S.E. and Ullberg, S.: Accumulation of chorio-retinotoxic drugs in the foetal eye. Acta. Pharmacol. Toxicol. 28: 64 only, 1970.

Sobel, D.E.: Fetal damage due to ECT, insulin, coma, chlorpromazine or reserpine. A.M.A. Gen. Psych. 2: 606-611, 1960.

Vince, D.J.: Congenital malformations following phenothiazine administration during pregnancy. Canad. Med. Assoc. J. 100: 223 (only), 1969.

308 Chlorpropamide

This oral hypoglycemic sulfylurea compound was found not to be teratogenic in rats when Tuchmann-Duplessis and Mercier-Parot (1959) gave 200 mg per day from the 1st through 12th day of gestation. Brock and Kreybig (1965) found 'disrupted' 13-day embryos in one strain of rats after injecting 10 mg per kg on the 4th day.

Although Jackson et al (1962) initially reported an unusually high fetal mortality, subsequent studies and review of other work have tended to indicate that the poor fetal outcome was due to the diabetes rather than the drug (Sutherland et al, 1974).

Brock, N. and Kreybig, T.V.: Experimentelles Beitrag zur prufung teratogener Wirkungen von Arzneimitteln an der Laboratoriumratte. Naunyn-Schmeidebergs Arch. Pharmakol. Exp. Pathol. 249: 117-145, 1964.

Jackson, W.P.U.; Campbell, G.D.; Notelovitz, M. and Blumsohn, D.: Tolbutamide and chlorpropamide during pregnancy in humans. Diabetes 11: 98-101, 1962.

Sutherland, H.W.; Brewsher, P.D.; Cormack, J.D.; Hughes,

C.R.T.; Reid, A.; Russell, G. and Stowers, J.M.: Effect of moderate dosage of chlorpropamide in pregnancy on fetal outcome. Arch. Dis. Child. 49: 283-291, 1974.

Tuchmann-Duplessis, H. and Mercier-Parot, L.: Action de la chlorpropamide, sulfamide hypoglycemiant, sur la gestation et le developpement foetal du rat. C. R. Acad. Sci. (Paris) 249: 1160-1162, 1959.

309 Cholestyramine

Koda et al (1982) gave this anion exchange resin by mouth to rats and rabbits in amounts of up to 2 gms per kg daily. No adverse fetal or fertility effects were found. Postnatal studies in rats were done and no changes were found in function.

Koda, S.; Anabuki, K.; Miki, T.; Kahi, S.; Takahoshi, N.: Reproductive studies on cholestyramine. Kiso to Rinsho 16: 2040-2049, 2050-2069, 2070-2077, 2078- 2094, 1982.

310 Choline

A deficiency of choline in the pregnant mouse did not produce congenital defects (Meader and Williams, 1957).

Meader, R.D. and Williams, W.L.: Choline deficiency in the mouse. Am. J. Anat. 100: 167-204, 1957.

311 Chondroitin Sulfate

Kamei (1961) injected 1 cc of a 2 percent solution into mice on the 9th, 10th and 11th gestational days. Cleft palates or kinky tails were produced in some of the offspring.

Kamei, T.: The teratogenic effect of excessive chondroitin sulfate in the DDN strain of mice. Med. Biol. 60: 126-129, 1961.

312 Chromium

Ridgway and Karnofsky (1952) reported mild achondroplasia in chicks after adding 2.5 mg sodium dichromate to the chorioallantoic membrane on the 8th day. Gale and Bunch (1979) injected hamsters intravenously on day 7, 8 or 9 with 8 mg per kg of chromium trioxide and produced cleft palates and resorptions.

Gale, T.F. and Bunch, J.D.: The effect of the time of administration of chromium trioxide on the embryotoxic response in hamsters. Teratology 19:81-86, 1979.

Ridgway, L.P. and Karnofsky, D.A.: The effects of metals on the chick embryo: toxicity and production of abnormalities in development. Ann. N. Y. Acad. Sci. 55: 203-215, 1952.

313   Chromomycin A-3

This substance has been reported to be teratogenic in rats (Takaya, 1963). Tanimura and Nishimura (1963) injected 0.5 to 2.0 mg per kg into mice on day 10, 11 or 12 and found 36 to 51 percent of the fetuses to have kinky tails, hydrops or abnormal head shapes.

Takaya, M.: Teratogenic effect of the antitumor antibiotics. (abstract) Proceedings of the Congenital Anomalies Research Association of Japan 3: 47-48, 1963.

Tanimura, T. and Nishimura, H.: Effects of antineoplastic agents especially chromomycin A-3 administered to pregnant mice upon the development of their offspring. Acta Anat. Nippon 38: 1, 1963.

314   Cianidanol

Yokoi et al (1982) gave up to 5000 mg per kg orally before and during the first 7 days of gestation or on days 7-17 of gestation in the rat. Some fetal growth inhibition was found at the highest dose but no increased defect rate. Rabbits received up to 500 mg per kg during gestation with no adverse fetal effects.

Yokoi, Y.; Yoshida, H.; Mitsumori, T.; Nagano, M.; Hirano, K.; Terasaki, M.; Nose, T.: Reproductive studies of cianidanol (KB-53) Oyo Yakuri 24:383-390, 495-507, 521-529, 1982.

315   Cigarette Smoking

In 1941 Schoeneck showed that rabbits exposed to the equivalent of 20 cigarettes per day gave birth to fetuses that were 17 percent less in weight than controls. Since Simpson (1957) identified increased prematurity rates in fetuses from smoking mothers, several reports documenting reduced birth size have appeared (Lowe, 1959; Herriot et al.; 1962; Ravenholt and Applegate, 1965). There have been reports that the proportion of male newborns was reduced (Ravenholt and Levinski, 1965). The neonatal mortality and incidence of congenital defects are not increased by smoking (Lowe, 1959; Underwood et al.; 1965; Frazier et al.; 1961; Yerushalmy, 1964). Underwood et al. (1965) did report that premature ruptured membranes were significantly increased in heavy smokers. Nicotine and cigarette smoking in animals has been studied also and reduced fetal weight recorded (see Nicotine). Miller and Gardner (1981) reported that the cadmium content of placentas from smokers was nearly three times that of non-smokers.

Boue et al (1975) have studied a large number of spontaneous abortions and found a significant reduction in chromosome aberrations among women who inhaled cigarettes. This rate was 50 percent as compared to the noninhalers rate of 62 percent. This increase in abortuses with normal karyotype may be explained by an increase of the incidence of abortions in chromosomally normal embryos as a result of

315

cigarette smoking. Himmelberger et al (1978) using a mail survey of operating room personnel reported significant increases in spontaneous abortion and congenital defects in the offspring of smoking mothers. Although all systems were involved, the cardiovascular and urogenital were most often affected.

The important question of whether or not cigarette smoking causes a change in intellectual function in the intrauterine exposed child has been studied in detail by Davie et al (1972) who reported a 3 to 4 month delay in reading achievement after carefully factoring out the many other related variables. Hardy and Mellitis (1972) could find no intellectual impairment in another study of the offspring of heavy smokers. Dunn et al (1977) found reduced neurological and intellectual maturation in 6 year-olds whose mothers smoked during pregnancy. Some increase in the incidence of "minimal brain dysfunction" was also found. The authors give a balanced discussion of the other characteristics of smokers that might contribute to differences in their off-spring. In rats injected with 3 mg of nicotine daily during pregnancy a learning deficit was found in the offspring (Martin and Becker, 1971). Miller and Hassanein (1974) reported evidence that the reduced birth weight in smokers offspring was not due to decreased nutritional intake.

Naeye (1978) reported that white cigarette smokers in a large collaborative study gave birth to anencephalics with a frequency of 1.72 per 1000 while non-smokers had a rate of 0.1 per 1000. A difference in the social class of the two groups could account for some of this increase since smoking and anencephaly are both higher in the lower social classes.

The subject has been recently reviewed (Landesman- Dwyer and Emanuel, 1979).

Boue, J.; Boue, A.; Lazar, P.: Retrospective and prospective epidemiological studies of 1500 karyotyped spontaneous human abortions. Teratology 12: 11-26, 1975.

Davie, R.; Butler, N. and Goldstein, H.: From birth to seven: A Report of the National Child Development Study, London: Longman and the National Children's Bureau, 1972, pp. 175-177.

Dunn, H.G.; Karaa, A.; Ingram, S. and Hunter, C.M.: Maternal cigarette smoking during pregnancy and the child's subsequent development II Neurological and intellectual maturation to the age of 6 and one-half years. Canad. J. Public Health 68:43-49, 1977.

Frazier, T.M.; Davis, G.H.; Goldstein, H. and Goldberg, I.D.: Cigarette smoking and prematurity: A prospective study. Am. J. Obstet. Gynecol. 81: 988-996, 1961.

Hardy, J.B. and Mellitis E.D.: Does maternal smoking have a long-term effect on the child? Lancet 2: 1332-1336, 1972.

Herriot, A.; Billewicz, W.Z. and Hytten, F.E.: Cigarette smoking in pregnancy. Lancet 1: 771-773, 1962.

Himmelberger, D.U.; Brown, B.W.; Cohen, W.N.: Cigarette smoking during pregnancy and the occurrence of spontaneous abortion and congenital abnormality. Am. J. Epid. 108:470-479, 1978.

Landesman-Dwyer, S. and Emanuel, I.: Smoking during pregnancy. Teratology 19:119-126, 1979.

Lowe, C.R.: Effect of mothers smoking habits on birth weight of their children. Br. Med. J. 2: 673-676, 1959.

Martin, J.C. and Becker, R.F.: Effects of maternal nicotine absorption or hypopoxic episodes upon appetitive behavior of rat offspring. Devel. Psychobiol. 4: 133-147, 1971.

Miller, H.C. and Hassanein, K.: Maternal smoking and fetal growth of full term infants. Pediat. Res. 8: 960-963, 1974.

Miller, R.K.; Gardner, K.A.: Cadmium in the human placenta: relationship to smoking (abstract) Teratology 23:51A, 1981.

Naeye, R.L.: Relationship of cigarette smoking to congenital anomalies and perinatal death. Am. J. Path. 90:289-293, 1978.

Ravenholt, R.T. and Levinski, M.J.: Smoking during pregnancy. Lancet 1: 961 Only, 1965.

Schoeneck, F.J.: Cigarette smoking in pregnancy. N. Y. State J. Med. 41: 1945-1948, 1941.

Simpson, W.J.: A preliminary report in cigarette smoking and the incidence of prematurity. Am. J. Obstet. Gynecol. 73: 808-815, 1957.

Underwood, P.; Hester, L.L.; Tucker, L. and Gregg, K.U.: The relationship of smoking to the outcome of pregnancy. Am. J. Obstet. Gynecol. 91: 270-276, 1965.

Yerushalmy, J.: Mother's cigarette smoking and survival of infant. Am. J. Obstet. Gynecol. 88: 505-518, 1964.

316 Cimetidine [Tagamet-R]

Hirakawa et al (1980) gave this anti-ulcer agent to rats and rabbits by mouth in maximum daily doses of 2000 and 100 mg per kg respectively. No adverse fertility effects were found in rats. The fetuses from both species were not adversely affected and postnatal development and function in the rat were not altered.

Leslie and Walker (1977) gave oral doses of 950 mg per kg daily to rabbits, rats and mice during organogenesis. They found no adverse fetal effects. Postnatal studies in rats indicated some delay in pinna opening and onset of nocturnal activity. In the F-2 generation females had lower numbers of corpora lutea of pregnancy. No effect on the male phallus was found after in utero exposure but some delay in development of the prostate and seminal vesicles was observed.

Case reports of liver impairment have been reported in offspring of mothers treated in late pregnancy (Glade et al, 1980).

Glade, G.; Saccar, C.L.; Pereira, G.R.: Cimetidine in pregnancy: apparent transient liver impairment in the newborn. Am. J. Dis. Child. 134:87-88, 1980.

Hirakawa, T.; Suzuki, T.; Hayashizaki, A.; Nishimura, N.; Sano, Y.; Nishikawa, M.; Nagashima, Y.; Seki, K.; Kihara, T.: Reproductive studies of cimetidine. Kiso to Rinsho 14:2819-2831, 1980.

Leslie, G.B.; Walker, T.F.: Toxicological profile of cimetidine in Burland, W.L. and Simkins, M.A., eds., Cimetidine, Proceedings of the Second International Symposium of Histamine H-2 Receptor Antagonists, Excerpta Medica Amsterdam, 1977, pp. 30-31.

317 Cinepazide Maleate [1-(1-pyrrolidinylcarbonyl) methyl]-4-(3,4,5-trimethoxy-cinnamoyl) priperazine maleate

Ino et al (1979) gave up to 1,060 mg per kg daily by mouth to mice on days 6 through 15 and observed no malformations. Some reduction in fetal weight occurred at the highest dose. Shimada et al (1979) gave 200 mg orally to rabbits on days 6 through 18 and found no alterations in the fetuses.

Ino, T.; Kobayashi, H. and Morita, H.: Reproduction studies of cinepazide maleate (2) teratogenicity study in mice. (Japanese) Iyakuhin Kenkyu 10:546-558, 1979.

Shimada, H.; Tashiro, K.; Morita, H. and Akimoto, T.: Reproduction studies of cinepazide maleate (4) teratogenicity study in rabbits. (Japanese) Iyakuhin Kenkyu 10:572-578, 1979.

318 Cinoxacin

Sato et al (1980) gave rats orally up to 200 mg per kg daily before mating, during organogenesis or on days 17-21. Increased mortalty of the dams was seen at 200 and 300 mg per kg. No effects on fertility were found and no increase in defects occurred. In the perinatal studies at 200 mg per kg there was an increase in stillbirths and neonatal deaths. Rabbit studies during organogenesis using 800 mg per kg did not show adverse effects (Sato and Kobayashi, 1980).

Sato, T.; Keneko, Y.; Saegusa, T.; Kobayashi, F.: Reproductive studies of cinoxacin in rats. Chemotherapy 28:484-507, 1980.

Sato, T.; Kobayashi, F.: Teratological study on cinoxacin in rabbits. Chemotherapy 28:508-575, 1980.

319 Cisplatin (cis-Platinum diamine dichloride)

Nagaoka et al (1981) gave this antineoplastic agent intravenously to rats and rabbits in maximum doses of 0.54 and 0.3 mg per kg respectively. No ill effects were found in the rabbit fetuses exposed during organogenesis. In the rat some embryolethality and decreased body weight occurred at 0.375 mg per kg during organogenesis and in the perinatal period.

Anabuki et al (1982) administered this antineoplastic platinum compound intraperitoneally to rats and rabbits in maximum daily doses of 0.5 mg per kg. With rats treated before mating and during the first 7 days of gestation resorptions were increased at 0.25 mg per kg and above. At the highest dose some lethality and growth retardation was seen when rats were treated during organogenesis. Postnatal studies showed decreased viability and exploratory behavior in rat offspring exposed to 0.25 and 0.5 mg per kg. Teratologic studies were also negative in the rabbit except for increased embryolethality over 0.125 mg per kg.

Anabuki, K.; Kitazima, S.; Koda, S.; Takahashi, N.: Reproductive studies on cisplatin. Yakuri to Chiryo 10:659-671, 673-694, 695-701, 1982.

Nagaoka, T.; Nanama, I.; Konoha, N.: Reproductive studies on cislatin. Kiso to Rinsho 15:5769-5781, 5782-5800, 5801-5808, 1981.

320 Citrinin

Hood et al (1976) injected mice intraperitoneally with up to 40 mg per kg on days 7 through 10 and produced no malformations. Prenatal survival was decreased as was birth weight.

Hood, R.D.; Hayes, A.W. and Cammell, S.: Effects of prenatal administration of citrinin and viriditoxin in mice. Fd. Cosmet. Toxicol. 14:175-178, 1976.

321 Clebopride Malate

Kawano et al (1982) gave this anti-ulcer agent orally to rats and rabbits in amounts up to 100 mg per kg daily. In the rats there was no effect on fertility or postnatal function. No adverse fetal effect was seen in either species.

Kawana, K.; Katoh, M.; Akutsu, S.; Simamura, T.; Komatsu, H.; Matsuyama, K.; Matsuzaki, M.: Effect of clebopride malate (LAs) on reproduction. Kiso to Rinsho 16: 5649-5660, 5661-5669, 5670-5680, 5681- 5687, 1982.

322 Clindamycin

Bollert et al (1974) administered this antibiotic to rats and mice on days 6 through 15 and observed no adverse fetal effects. Doses up to 180 mg per kg per day were given subcutaneously.

Bollert, J.A.; Gray, J.E.; Highstrete, J.D.; Moran, J.; Purmalis, B.P. and Weaver, R.N.: Teratogenicity and neonatal toxicity of clindamycin 2-phosphate in laboratory animals. Toxicol. Appl. Pharm. 27: 322-329, 1974.

323 Clobetasone 17-butyrate

Shinpo et al (1980) studied this topical steroid in rats giving up to 3.0 mg per kg by subcutaneous route. Cleft palates and omphaloceles were produced at the higher doses (1.0 and 3.0 mg). Some decrease in pregnancy rate and resorptions was found in females treated before pregnancy and during the first week of gestation. Pregnancy was prolonged when 1.0 mg per kg was given on days 17-21. In rabbits at 60 micrograms per kg during organogenesis cleft palates and joint contractures were increased.

Shinpo, D.; Mori, N.; Takahashi, M.; Togashi, H.; Tanabe, T.: Reproductive studies of clobetasone 17-butyrate (SN-203). Kiso to Rinsho 14:333-342, 343-358, 359-372, 373-379, 1980.

324 Clobutinol [1-(4-Chlorophenyl)-2,3-dimethyl-4-dimethylamino--2-butanol HCl]

This antitussive was studied in rats and mice and no fetal or postnatal effects were observed. Treatment was from the 8th through the 14th day and oral doses to 75 mg per kg per day were used.

Kataoka, M.; Yuizono, T.; Kase, Y.; Miyata, T.; Kito, G. and Ishihara, T.: Teratological studies of clobutinol in mice and rats. (Japanese) Oyo Yakuri 4: 981-989, 1970.

325 Clofezone

This antiinflammatory agent was given orally to mice and rats during organogenesis in maximum doses of 600 mg and 240 mg respectively. No teratogenic effects were observed but the rat fetuses at the maximal dose were retarded in growth (Kamada and Tomizawa, 1979).

Kamada, K. and Tomizawa, S.: Influences of clofezone on fetuses of mice and rats. Oyo Yakuri 18:235-246, 1979.

326 Clomiphene [Clomid-R] [Chloramiphene] [2-[p-(2-Chloro--1,2-diphenylvinyl)phenoxyl]-triethylamine]

Eneroth et al. (1971) produced hydraminios and cataracts in rat fetuses by injecting maternal rats with this substance from the 6th to the 14th day of gestation. The hydraminios was found from dose levels of 2 mg per kg and the cataracts appeared at 50 mg per kg. Courtney and Valerio (1968) treated 18 monkeys with 1 to 4 mg per kg per day for several days during the embryonic period and found no defects in the fetuses. Suzuki (1970a and b) has treated pregnant rats and mice with amounts up to 128 mg per kg orally and in both species found a dose dependent increase in fetal mortality but no gross malformations. McCormack and Clark (1979) injected 2 mg per kg into rats on day 5 or 12 of pregnancy and produced multiple abnormalities in the genital tract of the female offspring. Some of the changes were reminiscent of the vaginal adenosis seen in young girls whose mothers had received diethylstilbestrol.

Oakley and Flynt (1972) report that in a group of women receiving clomiphene or menotropins a total of 6 Down's syndrome infants occurred when the age corrected expectation was only 2. They proposed that the increased risk might be the underlying abnormal physiology of the women rather than the medication. Nevin and Harley (1976) and James (1977) have noted an increase in neural tube defects among the offspring of women using the drug. They note that these women may have been subject to a higher neural tube defect risk for other reasons. Schardein (1980) has reviewed the clinical aspects.

Courtney, K.D. and Valerio, D.A.: Teratology in the Macaca mulatta. Teratology 1: 163-172, 1968.

Eneroth, G.; Eneroth, V.; Forsberg, U.; Grant, C.A. and Gustafsson, J.A.: Clomiphene-induced hydraminios and fetal cataracts in rats inhibited by progesterone. (abstract) Teratology 4: 487, only, 1971.

James, W.H.: Clomiphene, anencephaly and spina bifida. Lancet 1:603 only, 1977.

McCormack, S. and Clark, J.H.: Clomid administration to pregnant rats causes abnormalities of the reproductive tract in offspring and mothers. Science 204:629- 631, 1979.

Nevin, N.C.; Harley, J.M.G.: Clomiphene and neural tube defects. Ulster Med. J. 45:59-64, 1976.

Oakley, G.P. and Flynt, J.W.: Increased prevalence of Down's syndrome (mongolism) among the offspring of women treated with ovulation-inducing agents. (abstract) Am. J. Hum. Gen. 24: 20a (only), 1972.

Schardein, J.: Congenital abnormalities and hormones during pregnancy; A clinical review. Teratology 22: 251-270, 1980.

Suzuki, M.R.: Effects of oral cyclofenil and clomiphene, ovulation inducing agents on pregnancy and fetuses in rats. (Japanese) Oyo Yakuri 4: 635-644, 1970a.

Suzuki, M.R.: Effects of oral cyclofenil and clomiphene, ovulation inducing agents on pregnancy and fetuses in mice. Oyo Yakuri 4: 645-651, 1970b.

327 Clonazepam

Takeuchi et al (1977) administered this benzodiazipine

derivative to rabbits orally on days 6 through 18 in doses
up to 20 mg per kg and found no fetal ill effects.

Takeuchi, Y.; Shiozaki, U.; Noda, A.; Shimizu, M. and
Udaka, K.: Studies on the toxicity of clonazepam. Part 3
Teratogenicity tests in rabbits. (Japanese) Yakuri to
Chiryo 5:2457-2466, 1977.

328 Cloxacillin

Brown et al. (1968) reported negative teratogenic results
after giving 100 mg per kg to rabbits during pregnancy.

Brown, D.M.; Harper, K.H.; Palmer, A.K. and Tesh, S.A.:
Effect of antibiotics upon pregnancy in the rabbit.
(abstract) Toxicol. Appl. Pharmacol. 12: 295, only, 1968.

329 Clozapine [8-Chloro-11-(4-methyl-1-piperazinyl)5-H dibenzo-
-[1,4]-diazepine]

Lindt et al. (1971) gave up to 40 mg per kg daily to
pregnant rabbits and rats during active organogenesis and
observed no deleterious effects in the offspring.

Lindt, S.; Lauener, E. and Eichenberger, E.: The
toxicology of 8-chloro-11-(4-methyl-1-piperazinyl)-5H-di-
benzo[1,4]diazepine (cl clozapine). Farmaco (Sci.) 26:
585-602, 1971.

330 Coal Products

Andrew et al (1982) used solvent, refined coal solvent and
heavy distillate by gavage on days 12-16 of rat gestation
and observed increased perinatal mortality.

Andrew, F.D.; Lytz, P.S.; Buschbom, R.L.; Springer, D.L.:
Postnatal effects following prenatal exposure of rats to
solvent refined coal (SRC) hydrocarbons. (abstract)
Teratology 25:26A, 1982.

331 Cobalt

Kury and Crosby (1968) injected the chick yolk sac on the
4th day with 0.4 to 0.5 mg of cobaltons chloride and
observed anemia in the surviving 20 day chicks. Some
thyroid epithelial hyperplasia was observed in three
embryos. Nadeenko et al (1980) demonstrated that cobalt was
embryotoxic to rat fetuses when it was administered during
the entire gestation (dose of 0.05 mg per kg). The dose of
0.005 mg per kg was non-toxic to females, however the
progeny of treated females had a reduced weight.

Kury, G. and Crosby, R.J.: Studies on the development of
chicken embryos exposed to cobaltons chloride. Toxicol.
Appl. Pharmacol. 13: 199-206, 1968.

Nadeenko, V.G.; Lenchenko, V.G.; Saichenko, S.P.;

Arkhipenko, T.A. and Radovskaya, T.L.: Embryotoxic action of cobalt administered per os. Gigiena i Sanitariya (USSR) 2:6-8, 1980.

332 Cocaine

In the mouse and rat 60 mg and 50 mg per kg respectively given intraperitoneally caused no congenital defects (Fantel and MacPhail, 1982). Treatment days were 8 through 12 for the rat and days 7 through 16 for the mouse. Hayasaka et al (1976) reported that cocaine (20 mg per kg) potentiated the teratogenic effects of caffeine in mice.

Fantel, A.G.; MacPhail, B. J.: The teratogenicity of cocaine. Teratology 26: 17-19, 1982.

Hayasaka, I.; Sasaki, H. and Fujii, T.: Potentiation of the fetopathic effects of caffeine in mice by modification of catecholamine turnover: 2 by cocaine, an uptake inhibitor. (abs) Teratology 14:239- 240, 1976.

333 Cocodylic Acid

This organic arsenical herbicide was tested in rats and mice on days 7-16 (Rogers et al, 1981). Gavage feedings of 200 - 600 mg per kg and 7.5 - 60 mg per kg were administered to mice and rats respectively. At doses of 400 mg or more, cleft palate occurred in mice; this dose was above the maternal toxic dose. Irregular palatine rugae were found in rat fetuses at doses of 15 mg per kg.

Rogers, E.H.; Chernoff, N. and Kavlock, R.J.: The teratogenic potential of cocodylic acid in the rat and mouse. Drug and Chemical Toxicology 4:49-61, 1981.

334 Codeine

Heinonen et al (1976) reported on 563 pregnancies where codeine was used during the first four lunar months and found no increase in defect rates. Eight respiratory malformations were reported while only 3 were expected. This increase was not statistically significant. Geber and Shramm (1975) injected hamsters on day 8 subcutaneously with 73 to 360 mg per kg and found 6 to 8 percent cranioschisis in the offspring. No dose response was found and not a single malformation occurred in over 1400 saline injected controls.

Geber, W.F. and Schramm, L.C.: Congenital malformations of the central nervous system produced by narcotic analgesics in the hamster. Am. J. Obstet. Gynecol. 123:705-713, 1975.

Heinonen, O.P.; Slone, D. and Shapiro, S.: Birth Defects and Drugs in Pregnancy. Publishing Sciences Group Inc.; Littleton, Mass.; 1977.

335 Colchicine

In most experiments desacetylmethylcolchicine has been employed. Morris et al (1967) in rabbits using 0.1 to 5.0 mg per kg,found the higher dosages after the 9th day to be highly lethal to fetuses. With dosage levels of 0.1 to 0.5 mg per kg a small incidence of gastroschisis and failure of neural tube closure was found. The same authors used 1 to 2 mg per kg in monkeys on single days over a wide gestational period and obtained four normal fetuses. Embryocidal effects of the compound have been shown in rabbits (Didock et al.; 1965) and in rats (Tuchmann-Duplessis and Mercier-Parot, 1958; Thiersch, 1962). Adams et al. (1961) have shown arrested cleavage in ova and degeneration of rabbit blastocysts after administering 2 to 8 mg per kg. Sieber et al (1978) injected mice with 0.5 or 1.0 mg per kg intraperitoneally on day 6, 7 or 8 and producd a low but significant increase in defective fetuses. These defects included microphthalmia, microtia, exencephaly and other defects.

An unusual experiment was performed by Chang (1944) who suspended sperm in 0.1 percent colchicine and artificially inseminated females. Thirty-three young resulted; one had an open fontanelle and very small philtrum. One was otocephalic and the third had microcephaly with enlarged eyes. Doses of similar origin were artifically inseminated and gave 425 normal young.

Ferreira and Frota-Pessoa (1969) reported that two persons under colchicine therapy were found among 54 parents of Down's syndrome patients. Zemer et al, 1976 reported 3 normal offspring from fathers on therapy and one normal from a mother treated during the entire pregnancy. Of four mothers who discontinued the medication when pregnancy was detected, one aborted and the other three gave birth to normal infants.

Adams, C.E.; Hay, M.F. and Lutwak-Mann, C.: The action of various agents on the rabbit embryo. J. Embryol. Exp. Morphol. 9: 468-491, 1961.

Chang, M.C.: Artificial production of monstrosities in the rabbit. Nature 154: 150 only, 1944.

Didock, K.; Jackson, D. and Robson, J.M.: The action of some nucleotoxic substances on pregnancy. Br. J. Pharmacol. 11: 437-441, 1965.

Ferreira, N.R. and Frota-Pessoa, O.: Trisomy after colchicine therapy. Lancet 1: 1160-1161, 1969.

Morris, J.M.; Van Wagenen, G.; Hurteau, G.D.; Johnston, D.W. and Carlsen, R.A.: Compounds interfering with ovum implantation and development: alkaloids and antimetabolites. Fert. Steril. 18: 7-17, 1967.

Sieber, S.M.; Whang-Peng, J.; Botkin, C. and Knutsen, T.: Teratogenic and cytogenetic effects of some plant-derived antitumor agents (vincristine, colchicine, maytansine,

VP 16-213 and VM-26) in mice. Teratology 18:31-48, 1978.

Thiersch, J.B.: Effect of N-desacetyl-thio-colchicine (TC) and N-desacetyl-methyl-colchicine (MC) on the rat fetus and litter in utero. Proc. Soc. Exp. Biol. Med. 98: 479-485, 1958.

Tuchmann-Duplessis, H. and Mercier-Parot, L.: Sur l'action teratogene de quelques substances antimitotiques chez le rat. C. R. Acad. Sci. (Paris) 247: 152-154, 1958.

Zemer, D.; Pras, M.; Sohar, E. and Gofni, J.: Colchicine in familial Mediterranean fever. New Eng. J. Med. 294:170-171, 1976.

336 Colistin Sodium Methanesulfonate

Tomizawa and Kamada (1973) administered this compound intraperitoneally to pregnant mice and rats during active organogenesis. The maximum dose in the mouse was 150 mg per kg per day and 40 mg in the rat. At the highest doses some fetal deaths occurred in the mouse fetuses but no gross or skeletal defects occurred in either species.

Saitoh et al (1981) gave mice intravenously up to 500 mg per kg before mating and during the first 7 days of gestation. No changes in fertility, defect rate or postnatal behavior were found. Rats were given up to 25 mg per kg daily before mating and during the first 7 days, on days 7-17 or on days 17-21. No changes in fertility, defect rate or postnatal behavior were reported (Tsujitani et al, 1981A). Rabbits received up to 80 mg per kg on days 6-18 and no adverse fetal effects were found (Tsujitani et al, 1981B).

Saitoh, T.; Tsujitani, M.; Ohuchi, M.; Matsumoto, T.: Reproductive studies of sodium colistin methanesulfonate. Chemotherapy 29:887-890, 1044-1050, 1051-1061, 1981.

Tomizawa, S. and Kamada, K.: Colistin sodium methanesulfonate on fetuses of mice and rats. Oyo Yakuri 7: 1047-1060, 1973.

Tsujitani, M.; Ohuchi, M.; Saitoh, T.; Matsumoto, T.: Reproductive studies of sodium colistin methanesulfonate in rabbits. Chemotherapy 29: 300-305, 1981B.

Tsujitani, M.; Oyama, M.; Kadoya, K.; Ohuchi, M.; Saitoh, T.; Matsumoto, T.: Reproductive study of sodium colistin methane sulfonate in rats. Chemotherapy 29:149-163, 1981A.

337 Compazine (see Prochlorperazine)

338 Concanavalin A

Desesso (1979) gave 4 micrograms of this material intraperitoneally to rabbit embryos on days 12,13,14 or 15 and produed craniofacial trunk and limb anomalies. In some cases the limbs were fused to the head or body. Hayasaka

338

and Hoshino (1979) injected 3 and 5 mg per kg intravenously into mice and on day 7 produced exencephaly. They postulated that the mechanism was via an effect on the surface coat material of the neural tube.

Desesso, J.M.: Lectin teratogenesis. Defects produced by concanavalin A in fetal rabbits. Teratology 19: 15-26, 1979.

Hayasaka, I. and Hoshino, K.: Teratogenicity of concanavalin A in the mouse. Cong. Anom. 19;125-128, 1979.

339 Congo Red

Beaudoin (1964) reported that a single 20 mg dose of this substance on the 8th day of gestation produced hydro-nephrosis, hydrocephalus or microphtalmia in about 15 percent of rat offspring. Wilson (1955) using 10 mg on 3 days found only one rat fetus with hydrocephalus out of over 100 examined specimens.

Beaudoin, A.R.: The teratogenicity of congo red in rats.

Proc. Soc. Exp. Biol. Med. 117: 176-179, 1964.

Wilson, J.G.: Teratogenic acitivity of several azo dyes chemically related to trypan blue. Anat. Rec. 123: 313-334, 1955.

340 Conine

Keeler and Balls (1978) produced arthrogryposis and 'pinal curvature in calves whose mothers were gavaged with the plant, Conium maculatum, between days 50-75 of gestation. The active principle was 15 conine. A number of analogs of conine were not teratogenic.

Keeler, R.F. and Balls, L.O.: Teratogenic effects in cattle of conium maculatum, conium alkaloids and analogs. Clinical Toxicol. 12:2, 1978.

341 Contraceptives, Oral (see Oral Contraceptives)

342 Copper (Deficiency and Excess)

Copper deficiency during pregnancy has been associated with swayback, a degeneration of the nervous system in lambs (Innes and Saunders, 1962). Kalter (1968) has summarized the relatively negative teratogenic findings in the rat and the cerebellar dysgenesis in guinea pig fetuses (Everson et al.; 1968). O'dell et al. (1961) have reported edema, hemorrhage and abdominal hernias in offspring of rats on a copper-deficient diet.

Ridgway and Karnofsky (1952) administered 0.6 mg of Cu Cl-2 to chicks on the 4th day and observed no abnormalities. James et al. (1966) treated four sheep with 10 mg per kg daily throughout gestation and found three normal fetuses and one abortion. DiCarlo (1980) administered 2.7 mg per kg intrapertoneally to hamsters on the morning of the eighth day of gestation. A high percentage of the embryos were edematous and had various cardiovascular defects.

To study the mechanism of action of copper intrauterine devices Brinster and Cross (1972) carried out in vitro tests on mouse ova and found that copper wire or exposure to concentrations of CuCl-2 above 2.5x10-4 m were lethal at the blastocyst stage. Webb (1973) found embryo lethality in rats during the late preimplantation period. This could be due to either a direct action of copper or a secondary effect from the inflammatory reaction of endometrial tissue.

Brinster, R.L. and Cross, P.C.: Effect of copper on the preimplantation mouse embryo. Nature 238: 398-399, 1972.

DiCarlo, F.J.: Syndromes of cardiovascular malformations induced by copper citrate in hamsters. Teratology 21:89-101, 1980.

Everson, G.J.; Shrader, R.E. and Wang, T.: Chemical and morphological changes in brains of copper-deficient guinea pigs. J. Nutr. 96: 115-125, 1968.

Innes, J.R.M. and Saunders, L.Z.: Comparative neuropathology. New York: Academic Press, 1962. pp. 577-590.

James, L.F.; Lazar, V.A. and Binns, W.: Effects of sublethal doses of certain minerals on pregnant ewes and fetal development. Am. J. Vet. Res. 27: 132-135, 1966.

Kalter, H.: Teratology of the central nervous system. Chicago: University of Chicago Press, 1968. pp. 45-46.

O'dell, B.L.; Hardwick, B.C. and Reynolds, G.: Mineral deficiencies of milk and congenital malformations in the rat. J. Nutr. 73: 151-157, 1961.

Ridgway, L.P. and Karnofsky, D.A.: The effects of metals on the chick embryo: toxicity and production of abnormalities in development. Ann. N. Y. Acad. Sci. 55: 203-215, 1952.

Webb, F.T.G.: Contraceptive action of the copper IUD in the rat. J. Reprod. Fert. 32: 429-439, 1973.

343 Cortisone

This compound has been used extensively by teratologists as a tool for the study of mechanisms which produce cleft lip and palate in experimental animals (see Reviews by Fraser et al.; 1954; Giroud and Tuchmann-Duplessis, 1962). Cortisone acts on the multifactorial system which has been shown by Fraser and colleagues to produce cleft palate in the mouse

(Fraser, 1969). Cortisone has an effect on the growth and intrinsic movement of the palatine shelves (Larsson, 1962) and an additional action possibly through reduction of the amount of amniotic fluid resulting in contraction of the uterus with compression of the head on the chest, thus lodging the tongue between the palatine shelves and preventing their closure. Walker (1965) using 2.5 mg of the acetate form on the 11th through 14th days could not associate the amount of amniotic fluid with production of cleft palate. Fainstat (1954) has produced cleft palate ·in the rabbit. Grollman and Grollman (1962) produced hypertension in the offspring of rats treated with cortisone.

Walker (1967, 1971) has compared a number of the glucocorticoid steroids for their abiliy to produce cleft palate in the mouse, rat and rabbit. In the rat, high doses of methylprednisolone, prednisolone and cortisone produced no cleft palate while triamcinolone, betamethasone and dexamethasone produced clefts. Methylprednisolone, beta-methasone, dexamethasone and triamcinolone produced cleft palate in the mouse. Walker compared the same six drugs in pregnant rabbits and found methylprednisolone ineffective in producing cleft palate.

In 260 pregnant women treated with corticoids during preg-nancy, Bongiovanni and McPadden (1960) found reports of only two newborns with cleft palate and Serment and Ruf (1968) identified among 428 treated cases three clefts of the palate or lip and a small number of defects of other systems. Although this does not exclude the possibility of human teratogenicity, it indicates that this compound is not highly dangerous.

Bongiovanni, A.M. and McPadden, A.J.: Steroids during pregnancy and possible fetal consequences. Fertil. Steril. 11: 181-186, 1960.

Fainstat, T.D.: Cortisone-induced congenital cleft palate in rabbits. Endocrinology 55: 502-508, 1954.

Fraser, F.C.: Gene-environment interactions in the production of cleft palate. In, Nishimura, H. and Miller, J.R. (eds.): Methods For Teratological Studies in Animals and Man. Tokyo: Igaku Shoin Ltd, 1969. pp. 34-49.

Fraser, F.C.; Kalter, H.; Walker, B.E. and Fainstat, T.D.: The experimental production of cleft palate with cortisone and other hormones. J. Cell. Comp. Physiol. Suppl. 43:237-259, 1954.

Giroud, A. and Tuchmann-Duplessis, H.: Malformations Con-genitales: role des facteurs exogenes. Pathol. Biol. (Paris) 10: 119-151, 1962.

Grollman, A. and Grollman, E.F.: Teratogenic induction of hypertension. J. Clin. Invest. 41: 710-714, 1962.

Kalter, H. and Warkany, J.: Experimental production of congenital malformations in mammals by metabolic procedure. Physiol. Rev. 39: 69-115, 1959.

Larsson, K.S.: Studies on the closure of the secondary palate. IV. Autoradiographic and histochemical studies of mouse embryos from cortisone-treated mothers. Acta Morphol. Neerl. Scand. 4: 369-386, 1962.

Serment, H. and Ruf, H.: Corticotherapie et grossesse. Bull. Fed. Soc. Gynecol. Obstet. Lang. Fr. 20: 77-85, 1968.

Walker, B.E.: Amniotic fluid measurement in cortisone-treated and x-irradiated mice. Proc. Soc. Exp. Biol. Med. 118: 606-609, 1965.

Walker, B.: Induction of cleft palate in rabbits by several glucocorticoids. Proc. Soc. Exp. Biol. Med. 125:1281-1284, 1967.

Walker, B.: Induction of cleft palate in rats with antiinflammatory drugs. Teratology 4:39-42, 1971.

344 Coumarin Derivatives [Dicumerol-R] [Coumadin] (Sodium-Warfarin) [Phenindione]

Since Kerber et al (1968) reported nasal hypoplasia in the offspring of a woman treated with warfarin during pregnancy an association has been made between the use of coumarin derivatives and Conradi syndrome which consists of nasal hypoplasia with calcific stippling of the secondary epiphyses (Becker et al, 1975; Holmes et al, 1972; Pettiflor and Benson, 1975 and Shaul et al, 1975). The dose given to the mother was from 2.5 to 10 mg per day during the first trimester. One patient received coumadin during only the first 8 weeks and another took phenindione. Nasal obstruction complicated the neonatal course of these infants who were of low birth weight. Three of the children were reported to be blind but their long term development is still unknown. Eleven reported cases have appeared in the literature. (see summaries by Shaul and Hall, 1977 and Pauli et al, 1976). Warkany (1976) has summarized the clinical data and cites 5 offspring with central nervous system problems including hydrocephalus. Pauli and Hall (1982) report 13 patients with nervous system defects after 2nd and 3rd trimester treatment. The pathology of a human fetus exposed to warfarin has been reported (Barr and Burdi, 1976). Congenital defects following maternal use of heparin have not been reported. In 1965, Villasanta reviewed 38 pregnancies where heparin was employed and reported no mal-formations. The pregnancy loss rate with heparin is on the order of 20-30% (Pauli and Hall, 1982).

In experimental animals Kronick et al (1974) found no significant malformations in mice whose mothers were given up to 4 mg per kg on days 8 through 11. On days 3 through 11 placental hemorrhage and subsequent fetal loss occurred. Grote and Weinmann (1973) treated rabbits intravenously on the 6th through the 18th day with up to 100 times the therapeutic dose and found no effect on resorption rate or the fetus (including skeletal studies).

Barr, M. and Burdi, A.R.: Warfarin - associated

embryopathy in a 17 week abortus. Teratology 14:129- 134, 1976.

Becker, M.H.; Genieser, N.B.; Finegold, M.; Miranda, D. and Spackman, T.: Chondrodysplasia punctata. Is warfarin therapy a factor? Am. J. Dis. Child. 129: 365-359, 1975.

Grote, W. and Weinmann, I.: Uberprufung der wirkstoffe Cumarin und Rutin im teratologischen Versuch an Kaninchen. Arzneim-Forsch 23: 1319-1320, 1973.

Holmes, B.; Moser, H.W.; Halldorsson, S.; Mack, C.; Pant, S.S. and Matzilevich, B.: Mental retardation: An atlas of disease with associated physical abnormalities. New York, Macmillan Co.; 1972, pp. 136-137.

Kerber, I.J.; Warr, O.S. and Richardson, C.: Pregnancy in a patient with prosthetic mitral valve. J.A.M.A. 203: 223-225, 1968.

Kronick, J.; Phelps, N.E.; MCallion, D.J. and Hirsh, J.: Effects of sodium warfarin administered during pregnancy in mice. Am. J. Obstet. Gynecol. 118: 819-823, 1974.

Pauli, R.M.; Hall, J.G.: Warfarin embryopathy. Am. J. Med. 68:122-144, 1980.

Pauli, R.M.; Madden, J.D.; Kranzler, K.J.; Culpepper, W. and Port, R.: Warfarin therapy initiated during pregnancy and phenotypic chondrodysplasia punctata. J. Ped. 88:506-508, 1976.

Pettiflor, J.M. and Benson, R.: Congenital malformations associated with the administration of oral anticoagulants during pregnancy. J. Pediatr. 459-462, 1975.

Shaul, W.L.; Emery, H. and Hall, J.G.: Chondrodysplasia punctata and maternal warfarin during pregnancy. Am. J. Dis. Child. 129: 360-362, 1975.

Shaul, W.L. and Hall, J.G.: Multiple congenital anomalies associated with oral anticoagulants. Am. J. Obstet Gynecol. 127:191-198, 1977.

Villasanta, U.: Thromboembolic disease in pregnancy. Am. J. Obstet. Gynecol. 93: 142-160, 1965.

Warkany, J.: Warfarin embryopathy. Teratology 14:205-209, 1976.

345 Coxiella burnetii [Q Fever agent]

Giroud et al. (1968) administered this live agent to rats on the 9th gestational day and found cataracts in 46 of 133 fetuses. Histologic changes were present in the retina or optic nerves of 105 of these fetuses. The maternal rats had no evidence of illness except for antibody rises.

These authors review the serological studies of women with

spontaneous abortions and defective offspring (Giroud and
Giroud, 1964). Positive serologic values for different
rickettsial antigens were found in eight of 16 mothers who
gave birth to anencephalics. In three there was a positive
reaction to C. burnetii. A 1 percent incidence of positive
rickettsial serums was reported in controls.

Giroud, P. and Giroud, A.: Anencephalie et rickettsioses
maladies inapparentes. Bull. Acad. Nat. Med. (Paris)
148: 621-626, 1964.

Giroud, A.; Giroud, M.; Martinet, M. and Deluchat, C.H.:
Inapparent maternal infection by Coxiella burnetii and fetal
reprocussions. Teratology 1: 257-262, 1968.

346 Coxsackie virus B

Although this virus has been reported to produce
meningoencephalitis and carditis in newborn infants (Kibrick
and Benirschke, 1958) no clear-cut association with teratogenicity are known to the author. Evans and Brown (1963)
have carried out a prospective study of antibodies to four
coxsackie strains during pregnancy and found a statistically
significant increase in the overall congenital defect rate
in those mothers who had a rise in titer.

Evans, T.N. and Brown, G.C.: Congenital anomalies and
virus infections. Am. J. Obstet. Gynecol. 87: 749-758,
1963.

Kibrick, S. and Benirschke, K.: Severe generalized disease
encephalohepatomyocarditis occurring in the newborn period
and due to infection with coxsackie virus, group B.:
Evidence of intrauterine infection with this agent.
Pediatr. 22: 857-875, 1958.

347 CT-1341 (see Alphaxalone)

348 Curare (see D-Tubocurarine)

349 Cyanide (see Cassava root and Laetrile)

Spratt (1950) found in explanted chick embryos that sodium
cyanide above a concentration of 5 x 10(-3)m inhibited
development of the central nervous system with less effect
on heart development. Doherty, et al (1982) administered
0.126 to 0.1295 millimoles per kg per hour intravenously to
hamsters between days 6 and 9 of gestation. Neural tube,
heart and limb defects occurred. Sodium thiosulfate given
concurrently prevented the defects.

Doherty, P.A.; Ferm, V.H. and Smith, R.P.:Congenital
malformations induced by infusion of sodium cyanide in the
golden hamster. Toxicol. Appl. Pharmacol. 64:456-464,
1982.

Spratt, N.T.: Nutritional requirements of the early chick

349

embryo. III. The metabolic basis of morphogenesis and differentiation as revealed by the use of inhibitors. Biol. Bull. 99: 120-135, 1950.

350 Cyanox-R

This compound was given in doses of 10 mg per kg to pregnant rats on days 9 through 14 and no teratogenic activity was detected (Yamamoto et al, 1972).

Yamamoto, H.; Yano, I.; Nishino, H.; Furuta, H. and Masuda, M.: Teratological studies on Cyanox-R in rats. Oyo Yakuri 6:523-528, 1972.

351 Cyclamate

Tuchmann-Duplessis and Mercier-Parot (1970) administered 100 to 500 mg per kg by stomach tube to rats on the 12th or else 6th through 14th day of pregnancy and found neither an increase in resorptions nor congenital defects in the off-spring. Perinatal and postnatal studies were done and no effect of early cyclamate treatment was found. Negative teratologic studies in the rat and rabbit were reported in an abstract by Vogin and Oser (1969). Long term studies using 5 percent sodium cyclamate for the diet of mice showed no teratogenicity (Kroes et al, 1977).

Although there are reports of teratogenic findings in the chick (Taylor, 1969), these publications have eluded the author.

Kroes, R.; Peter, D.W.J.; Berkvens, J.M.; Verschuuren, T.D. and Van Esch, G.J.: Long term toxicity and reproduction study (including a teratogenicity study) with cyclamate, saccharin and cyclohexylamine. Toxicology 8:285-300, 1977.

Taylor, G.: Cyclamates. Lancet 2: 1189, only, 1969.

Tuchmann-Duplessis, H. and Mercier-Parot, L.: Influence du cyclamate de sodium sur la fertilite et le developpement pre- et post-natal du rat. Therapie 25: 915-928, 1970.

Vogin, E.E. and Oser, B.L.: Effects of cyclamate: saccharin mixture on reproduction and organogenesis in rats and rabbits. Fed. Proc. 28:2709 (only), 1969.

352 Cyclazocine

This narcotic antagonist has been given to pregnant rats and rabbits in maximal oral doses of 30 and 10 mg per kg respectively during active organogenesis and no fetal effects or anomalies were found (Nuite et al, 1975).

Nuite, J.A.; Smith, S.; Kennedy, G.L.; Keplinger, M.L. and Calandra, J.C.: Reproductive, teratogenic, perinatal and postnatal studies with cyclazocine. Toxicol. Appl. Pharm. 31: 534-543, 1975.

353 Cyclizine (also see Meclizine)

This antihistamine belongs to the benzhydrylpiperazine series of compounds. It has been used as a teratogen in the rat. The details are discussed under meclizine. Milkovich and Van den Berg (1976) reported no increased malformation rate among 111 offspring of mothers taking the drug during the first 84 days of pregnancy.

Milkovich, L. and Van den Berg, B.J.: An evaluation of the teratogenicity of certain antinauseant drugs. Am. J. Obstet. Gynecol. 125:244-248, 1976.

354 Cyclocytidine [2,2-Anhydro-1-beta-d-arabinofuranosylcytosine HCl]

Ohkuma et al (1974) studied this antitumor agent in rats and rabbits. A dose of 50 mg per kg intraperitoneally in the rat from days 7 through 14 of pregnancy produced reduction defects of the extremities. In the rabbit an intravenous dose of 6.0 mg per kg on days 7 through 16 resulted in cleft palate, open eye and reduction defects of the extremities.

Ohkuma, H.; Hikita, J.; Kiyota, K.; Tsuyama, S. and Hirayama, H.: Teratogenic evaluation of cyclocytidine a new antitumor agent in rat and rabbit. Oyo Yakuri 8: 1681-1691, 1974.

355 Cyclodiene Pesticides [Aldrin-R] [Dieldrin-R] [Endrin]

This group of chlorinated cyclodiene pesticides was studied by Ottolenghi et al (1974) in hamsters and mice. Single oral doses of approximately one-half the respective LD-50 doses were given on days 7, 8 or 9 in the hamster and on day 9 in the mouse. A significant number of defects were produced in both species on all the days treated. The malformations in both species were open eye, webbed feet and cleft palate.

Ottolenghi, A.D.; Haseman, J.K. and Suggs, F.: Teratogenic effects of aldrin, dieldrin, and endrin in hamsters and mice. Teratology 9: 11-16, 1974.

356 Cyclofenil [bis-(p-Acetoxyphenyl)cyclohexylidenemethane]

Suzuki (1970a) gave pregnant rats this ovulation inducing agent during the middle stages of gestation (days 9 through 14) in amounts up to 128 mg per kg orally. An increase in fetal death occurred but no teratogenic action was detected. The same type of result was found using clomiphene. In the mouse the findings for both drugs were essentially the same (Suzuki, 1970b).

Suzuki, M.R.: Effects of oral cyclofenil and clomiphene, ovulation inducing agents on pregnancy and fetuses in rats. (Japanese) Oyo Yakuri 4: 635-644, 1970a.

Suzuki, M.R.: Effects of cyclofenil and clomiphene,

ovulation inducing agents on mouse fetuses. (Japanese) Oyo
Yakuri 4: 645-651, 1970b.

357 Cycloguanil

This antimalarial drug given by gavage at 4 hour intervals
at 30 mg per kg to pregnant rats on the first day of
gestation caused 90 percent of the embryos to die.
Treatment on the 9th and 13th days had no harmful effect on
the fetuses. Two analogues chlorproguanil and proguanil in
similar doses and periods of gestation had no effect on the
segmenting embryo or fetus.

Chebotar, N.A.: Embryotoxic and teratogenic action of
proguanil, chlorproguanil and cycloguanil on albino rats.
(Russian). Byulleten Eksperimentalnoi Biologii Meditsing
77: 56-57, 1974.

358 Cycloheximide

Zimmerman et al. (1970) used this inhibitor of protein
synthesis to study glucocorticoid teratogenicity. In
experiments with 10 mg per kg in mice on day 11.5 they found
29 percent resorptions but no cleft palates. Eighty mg per
kg was embryolethal. Lary et al (1982) produced skeletal
defects includng polydactyly and oligodactyly in the
offspring of mice treated with 30 mg per kg
intraperitoneally on day 9.

Lary, J.M.; Hood, R.D.; Lindahl, R.: Interactions between
cycloheximide and T-locus alleles during mouse
embryogenesis. Teratology 25:345-349, 1982.

Zimmerman, E.F.; Andrew, F. and Kalter, H.: Glucocorticoid
inhibition of RNA synthesis responsible for cleft palate in
mice: a model. Proc. Nat. Acad. Sci. 67: 779-785, 1970.

359 Cyclohexylamine

Becker and Gibson (1970) injected pregnant mice
intraperitoneally with 61 to 122 mg per kg on day 12 and
produced no increase in congenital defects. Tanaka et al
(1975) gave up to 36 mg per kg on days 7 through 13 of
gestation and observed no fetal changes. Takano and Suzuki
(1971 found no teratogenic effect after feeding mice 100 mg
per kg per days on days 6 through 11 of gestation.

Becker, B.A. and Gibson, J.E.: Teratogenicity of
cyclohexylamine in mammals. Toxicol. Appl. Pharmacol.
17: 551-552, 1970.

Takano, K. and Suzuki, M.: Cyclohexylamine, a
chromosome-aberration producing substance: No teratogenicity
in the mouse. (Japanese) Cong. Anomalies 11:51-57, 1971.

Tanaka, S.; Nakaura, S.; Kawashima, K.; Nagao, S.; Kuwamura,
T. and Omori, Y.: Teratogenicity of food additives. 2
Effect of cyclohexylamine and cyclohexylamine sulfate on

fetal development in rats. Shokuhin Eiseigaku Zasshi
14:542, 1973.

360 6-Cyclohexyl-1-Hydroxy-4-methyl-2(1h)-pyridone Ethanolamine
Salt (HOE 296)

Miyamoto et al (1975) studied this new antimitotic agent in
mice and rats. The maximal subcutaneous dose was 10 mg per
kg and for the oral route it was 100 mg per kg. No teratogenic effects were seen with treatment during organogenesis.

Miyamoto, M.; Ohtsu, M.; Sugisaki, T. and Takayama, K.:
Teratological studies of 6-cyclohexyl-1-Hydroxy-4-methyl-
-2(1h)-pyridone ethanolamine salt (HOE 296) in mice and
rats. Oyo Yakuri 9: 97-108, 1975.

361 Cyclopamine

This compound derived from the plant Veratrum californicum
has been shown to be teratogenic in ruminants (Binns et al.;
1963). Natural epidemics of cyclopian sheep with cleft
palates and cerebral defects were observed when the ewes
grazed on Veratrum californicum. Doses of 0.8 to 2.0 gm of
the purified substance on the 8th gestational day produced
the cyclopian defects in newborn sheep. Jervine and
veratrosine, two alkaloids prepared from Veratrum
californicum, were similarly teratogenic (Keeler and Binns,
1968). By buffering the material to prevent its conversion
to the inactive form veratramine, Keeler (1970) was able to
produce similar defects in rabbit offspring.

Binns, W.; James, L.F.; Shupe, J.L. and Everett, G.: A
congenital cyclopian-type malformation in lambs induced by a
maternal ingestion of a range plant, Veratrum californicum.
Am. J. Vet. Res. 24: 1164-1175, 1963.

Keeler, R.F.: Teratogenic compounds of Veratrum
californicum (Durand): x. Cyclopia in Rabbits Produced By
Cyclopamine. Teratology 3: 175-180, 1970.

Keeler, R.F. and Binns, W.: Teratogenic compounds of
Veratrum californicum (Durand) v. Comparison of cyclopian
effects of steroidal alkaloids from plant and structurally
related compounds from other sources. Teratology 1: 5-10,
1968.

362 Cyclophosphamide (Cytoxan-R)

Chaube et al. (1967) administered 7 to 10 mg per kg to rats
and with treatment on the 11th or 12th day the fetuses
developed skeletal defects, cleft palates and exencephaly or
encephalocele. This compound was shown to be relatively
more embryolethal than chloroambucil when the fetal-maternal
toxicity ratios of the two were compared. Brock and Kreybig
(1964) have examined the early embryonic effects of the
teratogen in the rat. Gibson and Becker (1968) have shown
the compound to be teratogenic in mice. In the rabbit Fritz
and Hess (1971) have found a high incidence of cleft lip

and-or palate and reduction defects of the extremities using intravenously 30 mg per kg on single days 11, 12 or 13. In the rhesus monkey, 10 mg per kg on days 27 through 29 produced facial clefts and when given on days 32 through 40, meningoencephalocele was observed. (Wilk et al ,1978).

Greenberg and Tanaka (1964) have reported that a treated mother gave birth to a 1900 gm infant with multiple anomalies including 4 toes on each foot, flattening of the nasal bridge and a hypoplastic 5th finger. The clinical picture was compatible with fetal injury occurring during an intensive course of intravenous therapy (1,800 mg) given at about the 77th to 82nd day of gestation. Scott (1977) has summarized some human exposure experience.

A number of studies of the metabolism of cyclophosphamide and its products in in vitro cultures with rat embryos have shown that the compound must be bioactivated by a liver monofunctional oxygenase system in order to be teratogenic (Fantel et al, 1979, Popov, 1981, Popov et al, 1981 and Kitchin et al, 1981).   The morphologic changes found in vitro were very similar to those seen in vivo (Greenaway et al, 1982). Phosphoramide mustard in equimolar doses caused effects similar to those of bioactivated cyclophosphamide in vitro (Mirkes et al, 1981) and when given intraamnioticaly (Hales, 1982).   Acrolein was toxic but its effect was difficult to assess because of protein binding (see Acrolein).   The   other   stable   metabolite, 4-ketocyclophosphoramide, was only weakly teratogenic in vitro (Mirkes et al).   Spielmann and Jacob-Muller (1981) concluded   that   phosphoramide   mustard was the active teratogenic metabolite in a mouse blastocyst system.

Brock, N.   and Kreybig, T.V.: Experimentelles Beitrag zur prufing teratogener Wirkungen von Arzneimitteln an der Laboratoriumsratte. Naunym-Schmiedelbergs Arch. Pharmakol. Exp. Pathol. 249: 117-145, 1964.

Chaube, S.; Kury, G. and Murphy, M.L.: Teratogenic effects of cyclophosphamide (NCA-26271) in the rat.   Cancer Chemother. Rep. 51:363-376, 1967.

Fantel, A.G.; Greenaway, J.C.; Juchau, M.R.; Shepard, T.H.:: Teratogenic bioactivation of cyclophosphamide in vitro. Life Sciences 25:67-72, 1979.

Fritz, H.   and Hess, R.: Effects of cyclophosphamide on embryonic development in the rabbit.   Agents and Actions 2:83-86, 1971.

Gibson, J.E.   and   Becker,   B.A.:   Teratogenicity of cyclophosphamide in mice. Cancer Res. 28: 475-480, 1968.

Greenaway, J.C.; Fantel, A.G.; Shepard, T.H.; Juchau, M.R.: The in vitro teratogenicity of cyclophosphamide in the rat. Teratology 25:335-342, 1982.

Greenberg, L.H. and Tanaka, K.R.: Congenital anomalies probably induced by cyclophoshphamide.   J.A.M.A.   188: 423-426, 1964.

Hales, B.F.: Comparison of the mutagenicity and teratogenicity of cyclophosphamide and its active metabolites, 4-hydroxycyclophosphamide, phosphoramide mustard and acrolein. Cancer Res. 42:3016-3021, 1982.

Kitchin, K.T.; Schmid, B.P.; Sanyal, M.K.: Teratogenicity of cyclophosphamide in a coupled microsomal activating embryo culture system. Biochem. Pharmacol 30:59-64, 1981.

Mirkes, P.E.; Fantel, A.G.; Greenaway, J.C.; Shepard, T.H.: Teratogenicity of cyclophosphamide metabolites: phosphoramide mustard, acrolein and 4-ketocyclophosphamide in rat embryos cultured in vitro. Toxicol. Appl. Pharm. 58:322-330, 1982.

Popov, V.B.: A study of the effect of cyclophophamide in the culture of postimplantation rat embryos. Ontogenez (USSR) 12.3: 251-256, 1981.

Popov, V.B.; Weisman, B.L. and Puchkov, V.F.: Embryotoxic effect of cyclophosphamide after biotransformation in the culture of postimplantation rat embryos. Byull. Eksper. Biol. i Med. (USSR) 5:613-615, 1981.

Scott, J.R.: Fetal growth retardation associated with maternal administration of immunosuppressive drugs. Am. J. Obstet. Gynecol. 128; 668-676, 1977.

Spielmann, H.; Jacob-Muller, U.: Investigations on cyclophosphamide treatment during the preimplantation period. 2 In vitro studies on the effects of cyclophosphamide and its metabolites 4-OH-cyclophosphamide, phosphoramide mustard, and acrolein on blastulation of four-cell and eight-cell mouse embryos and on their subsequent development during implantation. Teratology 23:7-13, 1981.

Wilk, A.L.; McClure, H.M. and Horigan, E.A.: Induction of craniofacial malformations in the rhesus monkey with cyclophosphamide (abs). Teratology 17:24A, only, (1978).

363 Cyclosiloxanes

Le Feure et al (1972) administered an equilibrated copolymer of mixed cyclosiloxanes represented by cylic [(Phmesio)2] (PMXMMY) orally to rabbits and rats. Before implantation in both species it proved lethal to zygotes or prevented implantation. Maternal rats given 220 mg per kg per day on day 16 gave birth to female pups with a urogenital structural anomaly associated with urinary incontinence.

Le Feure, R.; Coulston, F. and Goldberg, L.: Action of a copolymer of mixed phenylmethylcyclosiloxanes on reproduction in rats and rabbits. Toxicol. Appl. Pharm. 21: 29-44, 1972.

364 Cyproterone Acetate [1,2 Alpha-Methyl-ene-chlor-delta-(4,6)-pregnadeine-17-alpha-01-3,20-di one-acetate]

Neuman et al. (1966) produced vaginas in male rat fetuses using 10 mg per day from the 13th to the 22nd gestational day. Forsberg and Jacobsohn (1969) reproduced this work. Similar results have been described in the rabbit (Elger, 1966; Jost, 1966). Jost has emphasized that although this anti-androgenic compound suppressed the masculinizing effects of the fetal testis, it did not prevent the inhibitory action on the mullerian ducts. Early differentiation of the testes was not prevented by this compound (Jost, 1966). Eibs et al (1982) have shown in the mouse that the time of treatment determines whether the malformations are in the urinary tract, lung or palate. During preimplantation 30 micrograms was lethal and 3 micrograms inhibited inner cell mass growth in vitro (Eibs et al, 1982B)

Goldman (1973) and Neumann, et al (1970) have reviewed the enzymatic mechanism of action of this and related compounds. A non-competitive binding of androgen biosynthesizing enzymes has been reported.

Eibs, H.G.; Spielmann, H. and Hagele, M.: Teratogenic effects of cyproterone acetate and medroxyprogesterone treatment during the pre- and postimplantation period of mouse embryos. Teratology 25:27-36, 1982A.

Eibs, H.G.; Spielman, H.; Jacob-Muller, U.; Klose, J.: Teratogenic effects of cyproterone acetate and medroxyprogesterone treatment during the pre- and postimplantation period of mouse embryos II Cyproterone acetate and medroxyprogesterone acetate treatment before implantation in vivo. Teratology 25:291-299, 1982B.

Elger, W.: Die Rolle der fetalen Androgene in der Sexualdifferenzierung des Kaninchens und ihre Abgrenzung gegen andere Hormonale und somatische Faktoren durch Anwendung eines starken Antiandrogens. Arch. Anat. Microsc. Morphol. Exp. 55: 658-743, 1966.

Forsberg, J.G. and Jacobsohn, D.: The reproductive tract of males delivered by rats given cyproterone acetate from days 7 to 21 of pregnancy. J. Endocrinol. 44: 461-462, 1969.

Goldman, A.S.: Sexual programming of the rat fetus and neonate studied by selective biochemical testosterone-depriving agents. In, Raspe, G. and Berhnard, S. (eds): Advances in the Biosciences, 13, Oxford: Pergamon Press, 1973, pp. 17-40.

Jost, A.: Steroids and sex differentiation of the mammalian foetus. In, Proceedings of The Second International Congress on Hormonal Steroids. Milan: Excerpta Medica International Congress Series No. 132, 1966. pp. 74-81.

Neumann, F.; Elger, W. and Kramer, M.M.: Development of a vagina in male rats by inhibiting androgen receptors through an anti-androgen during the critical phase of organogenesis. Endocrinology 78: 628-632, 1966.

Neumann, F.; Von Berswordt-Wallrabe, R.; Elger, W.;

Steinbeck, H.; Hahn, J.D. and Kramer, M.: Aspects of androgen-dependent events as studied by antiandrogens. Recent Progr. Horm. Res. 26: 337-410, 1970.

365   Cysteamine Hydrochloride

Adams et al. (1961) exposed rabbits to 70 to 160 mg per kg during preimplantation and recovered normal 6-day blastocysts.

Adams, C.E.; Hay, M.F. and Lutwak-Mann, C.: The action of various agents upon the rabbit embryo. J. Embryol. Exp. Morphol. 9: 468-491, 1961.

366   Cysteine

Olney et al (1972) treated pregnant mice and rats subcutaneously with 1.2 mg per gm on the last day of pregnancy and observed brain degeneration one day later in the fetus. Oral dosing did not produce lesions.

Olney, J.W.; Ho, O.L.; Rhee, V. and Schainker, B.: Cysteine-induced brain damage in infant and fetal rodents. Brain Res. 45: 309-313, 1972.

367   Cytochalasin B

Linville and Shepard (1971) exposed explanted pre-somite chick embryos to 0.5 to 1.0 microgm of this naturally-occurring fungal metabolite and observed a high incidence of neural tube closure defects.

Greenaway et al (1977) found cytochalasins A,D and E to prevent neural tube closure in the chick but at different concentrations. Ruddick et al (1974) fed 1 mg per kg to rats on days 6 through 15 and produced no defects. Wiley (1979) produced exencephaly in hamsters using 7.5 mg per kg intraperitoneally. Snow (1973) and Niemierko (1973) have produced polyploidy in the mouse embryo by blocking polar body formation or later cleavage.

Greenaway, J.C.; Shepard, T.H. and Kuc, J.: Comparison of cytochalasins (A,B,D and E) in chick explant teratogenicity and tissue culture systems. Proc. Soc. Exp. Biol. Med. 155:239-242, 1977.

Linville, G.P. and Shepard, T.H.: Neural tube closure defects due to cytochalasin B. Nature 236: 246-247, 1972.

Niemierko, A.: Induction of triploidy in the mouse by cytochalasin B. J. Embryol. Exp. Morph. 34:279-289, 1975.

Ruddick, J.A.; Harwig, J. and Scott, P.M.: Non- teratogenicity in rats of blighted potatoes and compounds contained in them. Teratology 9:165:-168, 1974.

Snow, M.H.L.: Tetraploid mouse embryos produced by

367

cytochalasin B during cleavage. Nature 244: 513-515, 1973.

Wiley, M.J.: Ultrastructural analysis of cytochalasin-induced neural tube defects in vivo. (abs) Teratology 19:53A (only), 1979.

368 Cytochalasin D

Shepard and Greenaway (1977) injected intraperitoneally 0.4 to 0.9 mg per kg on days 7 through 11 and produced exencephaly, hypognathia and skeletal reduction defects in C-57 and BALB-C strain mice but not in Swiss Webster mice. Wiley (1979) produced exencephaly in hamsters treated on the 8th day with 1.5 mg per kg intraperitoneally. Although non-teratogenic in vivo in the rat, 3 nanograms per ml of medium in vitro is associated with open neural tubes (Fantel et al, 1981).

Fantel, A.G.; Greenaway, J.C.; Shepard, T.H.; Juchau, M.R.; Selleck, S.B.: The teratogenicity of cytochalasin D and its inhibition by drug metabolism. Teratology 23:223-231, 1981.

Shepard, T.H. and Greenaway, J.C.: Teratogenicity of cytochalasin D in the mouse. Teratology 16:131-136, 1977.

Wiley, M.J.: Ultrastructural analysis of cytochalasin-induced neural tube defects in vivo (abs) Teratology 19: 53A (only), 1979.

369 Cytochalasin E

Austin et al (1982) using 0.9 to 2.0 mg per kg intraperitoneally in two strains of mice produced neural tube defects, cleft lip and palate and other skeletal defects.

Austin, W.L.; Wind, M.; Brown, K.S.: Differences in toxicity and teratogenicity of cytochalasins D and E in various mouse strains. Teratology 25:11-18, 1982.

370 Cytomegalovirus (CMV)

This virus with a DNA core and estimated molecular weight of 65 million is classified as a herpes virus. The entire subject has been comprehensively reviewed by Hanshaw (1970) and Weller (1971).

There is evidence that about 5 percent of pregnant women become infected with CMV virus (Sever et al.; 1962) and approximately 1.3 percent of newborns have positive urine cultures for the virus (Hanshaw, 1970). The virus may cross the placenta during the last two trimesters or the fetus could be infected while in the birth canal (Alexander, 1967). The virus has not been shown to cause spontaneous a-bortions. The syndrome produced by the virus, cytomegalic inclusion disease (CID), is characterized by intrauterine growth retardation associated with or followed by microcephaly. The ependymal area of the nervous system is

primarily affected and may contain calcified areas.
Chorioretinitis, seizures, blindness and optic atrophy may
be associated with the syndrome. In the neonatal period,
hepatospleenomegaly with jaundice and thrombocytopenia can
be the presenting symptoms. Although deafness may occur it
is not a common feature. Serological or virus culture
methods for diagnosis are available. Although this
infection plays a significant role in about 25 percent of
children with microcephaly, the true spectrum of the
clinical syndrome is only beginning to appear (Emanuel and
Kenny, 1966). Pass et al (1980) have given results of
follow-up of 34 symptomatic newborns.

Benirschke, et. al. (1974) have described the varied fetal
and placental pathology. Melish and Hanshaw (1973) surveyed
3,800 newborns and found 20 with positive cultures.
Seventeen of the 20 were asymptomatic and of the remaining
3, one had deafness, one possible brain damage and the third
had slow development following premature birth.

Alexander, E.R.: Maternal and neonatal infection with
cytomegalovirus in Taiwan. (abstract) Pediatr. Res. 1:
210, only, 1967.

Benirschke, K.; Mendoza, G.R. and Bazeley, P.L.: Placental
and fetal manifestations of cytomegalovirus infection.
Virchows Arch. B Cell Path. 16: 121-139, 1974.

Emanuel, I. and Kenny, G.E.: Cytomegalic inclusion disease
in infancy. Pediatrics 38: 957-965, 1966.

Hanshaw, J.B.: Developmental abnormalities associated with
congenital cytomegalovirus infection. In, Woollam, D.H.M.
(ed.): Advances in Teratology, Vol. 4. New York: Academic
Press, 1970. pp. 62-93.

Melish, M.E. and Hanshaw, J.B.: Congenital cytomegalovirus
infection: developmental progress of infants detected by
routine screening. Am. J. Dis. Child. 126: 190-194,
1973.

Pass, R.F.; Stagno, S.; Myers, G.J.; Alford, C.A.: Outcome
of symptomatic congenital cytomegalovirus infection: Results
of long-term longitudinal follow-up. Pediat. 66:758-762,
1980.

Sever, J.L.; Huebner, R.J.; Castellano, G.A. and Bell,
J.A.: Serological diagnosis 'en masse' with multiple
antigens. Am. Rev. Resp. Dis. Suppl. 88: 342-359,
1962.

Weller, T.H.: The cytomegalo viruses: ubiquitous agents
with protean clinical manifestations (second of two parts).
N. Engl. J. Med. 285: 267-274, 1971.

371 Cytosine Arabinoside [1-Beta-d-arabinofaranosylcytosine]

Karnofsky and Lacon (1966) produced facial and skeletal
defects in the chick, Chaube and Murphy (1965) skeletal and
palate defects in the rat and Fischer and Jones (1965)

cerebellar hypoplasia in the hamster. Chaube and Murphy in their review (1968) report that 20 to 800 mg per kg to rats or mice produced cleft palate and skeletal defects in the offspring and that the analogue, 1-beta-d-arabino furanosyl-5-fluorocytosine was teratogenic at 50 to 200 mg per kg given to the rat on the 12th day. Chaube and Murphy (1965) were able to nullify the teratogenic effect of cytosine arabinoside by simultaneous injection of deoxycytidine.

Percy (1975) treating rats and mice for 3 days toward the end of gestation produced cerebella hypoplasia, microcystic renal changes and retinal dysplasia. Doses of 50 mg per kg produced retinal dysplasia.

Wagner et al (1980) reported that limb reduction and small ears with atresia of the canals occurred in the offspring of a leukemia mother treated with this drug alone.

Chaube, S. and Murphy, M.L.: Teratogenic effects of cytosine arabinoside (CA) in the rat fetus. (abstract) Proc. Amer. Ass. Cancer Res. 6: 11, only, 1965.

Chaube, S. and Murphy, M.L.: The teratogenic effects of the recent drugs active in cancer chemotherapy. In, Woollam, D.H.M. (ed.): Advances in Teratology, Vol. 3. New York: Academic Press, 1968. pp. 204-205.

Fischer, D.S. and Jones, A.M.: Cerebellar hypoplasia resulting from cytosine arabinoside treatment in the neonatal hamster. (abstract) Clin. Res. 13: 540, only, 1965.

Karnofsky, D.A. and Lacon, C.R.: The effects of 1-beta-
-d-arabinofuransylcytosine on the developing chick embryo.

Biochem. Pharm. 15: 1435-1442, 1966.

Percy, D.H.: Teratogenic effects of pyrimidine analogues 5-iododeoxyuridine and cytosine arabinoside in late fetal mice and rats. Teratology 11: 103-118, 1975.

Wagner, V.W.; Hill J.S.; Weaver, D.; Baehner, R.L.: Congenital abnormalities in a baby born to cytarabine treated mother. Lancet 2:98-100, 1980.

372 Cytoxan-R (see Cyclophosphamide)

373 Dactinomycin (see Actinomycin D)

374 Dalmane-R (see Flurazepam)

375 Dantrolene

Nagaoka et al (1977A and B) gave up to 60 mg per kg daily by mouth to pregnant rats and rabbits during days 7 to 17 and 6 to 18 respectively. At the highest dose, minor skeletal variations occurred in both species and in the rat, both maternal and fetal weights were reduced.

Nagaoka, T.; Osuka, F.; Shigemura, T.; and Hatano, M.: Reproductive test of dantrolene. Teratogenicity test on rats. (Japanese) Clinical Report 11:2218- 2230, 1977A.

Nagaoka, T.; Osuka, F. and Hatano, M.: Reproductive studies of dantrolene. Teratogenicity study in rabbits. (Japanese). Clinical Report 11:2212-2217, 1977B

376 Daunomycin

Chaube and Murphy (1968) injected this antibiotic into pregnant rats once on the 5th through 12th day and produced no congenital defects in survivors. Maternal doses of 20 mg per kg were not lethal to the fetus.

Thompson et al (1978) using 1-4 mg per kg in rats for various periods during organogenesis produced atresia of the alimentary canal, urogenital defects and cardiovascular anomalies.

Chaube, S. and Murphy, M.L.: The teratogenic effects of the recent drugs active in cancer chemotherapy. In, Woollam, D.H.M. (ed.): Advances in Teratology, Vol. 3. New York: Logos and Academic Press, 1968. pp. 181-237.

Thompson, D.J.; Molello, J.A.; Strebing, R.J. and Dyke, I.L.: Teratogenicity of adriamycin and daunomycin in the rat and rabbit. Teratology 17:151- 158, 1978.

377 Daraprim-R (see 2,-Diamino-5-chlorophenyl-6-ethylpyrimidine)

378 Darvan-R (see Propoxyphene Napsylate)

379 2-4,D (see Dichlorophenoxyacetic Acid)

380 DDT [1,1,1-Trichloro-2,2-bis(p-chlorophenyl)ethane Chlorophenothane]

Although the thickness of egg shells of birds is reduced by chlorinated hydrocarbons (Hickey and Anderson, 1968), no reports of teratogenicity in the chick, mouse (Ware and Good, 1967) or rat (Ottoboni, 1969) have been identified. In Ottoboni's publication a significant increase in ringtail, a constriction of the tail followed by amputation, occurred in the offspring of mothers whose diets contained 200 p.p.m. Ware and Good (1967) showed reduced fertility in mice maintained for long periods on diets of 7 P.P.M. Hart et al. (1971) using 50 mg per kg in the rabbit on day 7, 8 and 9 of gestation noted premature delivery, increased fetal resorptions and reduced intrauterine growth but no congenital defects were produced.

Fabro (1973) reported a reduction in the brain weights of rabbit fetuses given 1 mg orally on days 4 through 7.

DDT may disrupt the early developing hypothalamic-gonadotropin mechanism according to the experiments by Heinricks et al, (1971) who showed persistent estrus in rats following injection of 1 mg on the 1st 3 postnatal days.

O'Leary et al (1970) measured the DDT and DDE levels in the serum of patients having spontaneous abortions and found no difference from serums drawn from women with normal pregnancies.

Fabro, S.: Passage of drugs and other chemicals into uterine fluids and preimplantation blastocyst, In, Fetal Pharmaology, edited by L. Boreus, Raven Press, New York, 1973, pp. 443-461.

Hart, M.M.; Adamson, R.H. and Fabro, S.: Prematurity and intrauterine growth retardation induced by DDT in the rabbit. Arch. Int. Pharmacodyn. Ther. 192: 286-290, 1971.

Heinrichs, W.L.; Gellert, R.J.; Bakke, J.L. and Lawrence, N.L.: DDT administered to neonatal rats induces persistent estrus syndrome. Science 173: 642-643, 1971.

Hickey, J.J. and Anderson, D.W.: Chlorinated hydrocarbons and eggshell changes in raptorial and fish-eating birds. Science 162: 271-273, 1968.

O'Leary, J.A.; Davies, J.E. and Feldman, M.: Spontaneous abortion and human pesticide residues of DDT and DDE. Am. J. Obstet. Gynecol. 108:1291- 1292, 1970.

Ottoboni, A.: Effect of DDT on reproduction in the rat. Toxicol. Appl. Pharmacol. 14: 74-81, 1969.

Ware, G.W. and Good, E.E.: Effects of insecticides on reproduction in the laboratory mouse II mirex, telodrin and DDT.

Toxicol. Appl. Pharmacol. 10: 54-64, 1967.

381 Decachlorooctahydro-1-3-4-metheno-2h-cyclo-buta-(6d)-pentalen- one 2-one (see Kepone)

382 Decamethonium Bromide

Drachman and Sokoloff (1966) paralyzed chick embryos with intravenous infusions of this material after the 9th day and for several days joint cavity formation was inhibited.

Drachman, D.B. and Sokoloff, L.: The role of movement in emmbryonic joint development. Devel. Biol. 146 401-420, 1966.

383 Dehydration

Brown et al (1974) produced isolated cleft palate in A-J
mice by depriving them of water for 72 hours or by depriving
them for 48 hours in the presence of dehumidified air. This
treatment was started during day 12 of gestation. Schwetz
et al (1977) thirsted CF-1 mice for 48 hours during periods
of organogenesis and found up to 28 percent of the litter
contained fetuses with cleft palate. The water deprivation
on days 12 and 13 caused a reduction in food intake which by
itself produced malformations. Twenty- five percent of the
litters had fetuses with cleft palate and 5 percent of the
litters had a fetus with exencephaly.

Brown, K.S.; Johnston, M.C. and Murphy, P.F.: Isolated
cleft palate in A-J mice after transitory exposure to
drinking-water deprivation and low humidity in pregnancy.
Teratology 9: 151-158, 1974.

Schwetz, B.A.; Nitschke, K.D. and Staples, R.E.: Cleft
palates in CF-1 mice after deprivation of water during pregnancy. Toxicol. Appl. Pharm. 40:307-315, 1977.

384 Dehydroepiandrosterone

Greene et al. (1939) produced masculinization of female
fetuses by treatment of the maternal rat with a total dose
of 100 to 280 mg. They found regression of the wolffian
ducts was inhibited by treatment. Before the 16th day
masculinization of the external genitalia was associated.

Greene, R.R.; Burrill, M.W. and Ivy, A.C.: Experimental
intersexuality. The effect of antenatal androgens on sexual
development of female rats. Am. J. Anat. 65: 415-470,
1939.

385 Delayed Fertilization

Since the early work of Blandau and Young (1939), there has
been little doubt that a delay in fertilization of an egg
once ovulated may lead to abnormal development of the ovum
and embryo. Several summaries of this experimental field
have been published (Austin, 1970; Carr, 1971; Witschi,
1970). There is evidence that the delayed fertilization
leads to abnormalities in chromosome complement which in
some cases may be the result of polyspermy (Vickers, 1969;
Shaver and Carr, 1969). Triploidy is the most common abnormality found. The mouse, rat, guinea pig, rabbit, pig
and frog have been studied and in general after
fertilization delay of 4 to 7 hours abnormal blastocysts
appear and with further delay the recovery rate of embryos
drops sharply.

In the human Jongbloet (1971) has collected information on
conditions which might lead to delayed fertilization of the
ovum. He reported the incidence of pathologic progeny to be
increased to 50 percent when conception occurred in the
first month after marriage of couples without prenuptial
contact. Based on small numbers he found that couples

conceiving while practicing the safe period of birth control
experienced a higher incidence of abortion and pathologic
offspring when their planned period of abstinence was
increased.

Guerrero and Rojas (1975) studied 965 women who recorded
their basal temperatures and coital history and observed
that the probability of abortion diminished significantly at
the time of ovulation. At ovulation, the chance was 7.5
percent while three days later it was 24 percent.

Boue et al (1975) found that polyploid human abortuses were
more common when the mother's ovulation occurred after the
14th day. The average presumed day of ovulation determined
by temperature curves was 15 for trisomic and normal
abortuses and 17 for those with polyploidy.

Austin, C.R.: Ageing and reproduction: post-ovulatory
deterioration of the egg. J. Reprod. Fertil. Suppl. 12:
39-53, 1970.

Boue, J.; Boue, A. and Lazar, P.: Retrospective and
prospective epidemiological studies of 1500 karyotyped
spontaneous human abortions. Teratology 12: 11-26, 1975.

Blandau, R.J. and Young, W.C.: The effects of delayed
fertilization on the development of the guinea pig ovum.
Am. J. Anat. 64: 303-329, 1939.

Carr, D.H.: Chromosome abnormalities in the preimplanting
ovum. In, Blandau, R.J. (ed.): The Biology of The
Blastocyst. Chicago: University of Chicago Press, 1971.
pp. 355-357.

Guerrero, R. and Rojas, O.I.: Spontaneous abortion and
aging of human ova and spermatozoa. N. Eng. J. Med.
293:573-575, 1975.

Jongbloet, P.H.: Mental and physical handicaps in
connection with overripeness ovopathy. H.E. Stenfert
Kroese N.V. - Leiden, 1971, pp. 22-61.

Shaver, E.L. and Carr, D.H.: Chromosome abnormalities in
rabbit blastocysts following delayed fertilization. J.
Reprod. Fertil. 14: 415-420, 1967.

Vickers, A.D.: Delayed fertilization and chromosomal anomalies in mouse embryos. J. Reprod. Fertil. 20: 69-76,
1969.

Witschi, E.: Teratogenic effects from overripeness of the
egg. In, Fraser, F.C. and McKusick, V.A. (ed.): Congenital Malformations. Amsterdam: Excerpta Medica, 1970. pp.
157-169.

386 Demeton-R

This organophosphorus insecticide was given
intraperitoneally to mice on a single day between days 7 and
12 in doses up to 14 mg per kg. The higher doses produced

fetal growth retardation (Budreau and Singh, 1973). A few minor skeletal malformations were found when dosing was carried out daily during 3 day periods of organogenesis.

Budreau, C.H. and Singh, R.P.: Teratogenicity and embryotoxicity of demeton and fenthion in CF No. 1 mouse embryos. Toxicol. Appl. Pharm. 24: 324-332, 1973.

387   Dengue II Virus

London et al (1979) injected an attenuated form of this virus intraamniotically on day 100 of the Rhesus pregnancy and found hemorrhagic necrosis and hydrocephalus in 3 of 20 exposed fetal brains.

London, W.T.; Levitt, H.H.; Martinez, A.J.; Palmer, A.E.; Curfman, B.L.; Sever, J.L.: Hydrocephalus and necrotic encephalopathy in Rhesus fetuses caused by Dengue II virus. (abstract) Fed. Proc. 38: 911, only, 1979.

388   2-Deoxyadenosine

Karnofsky and Lacon (1961) reported that chick embryos injected on the 4th day with 0.5 to 4 mg of this substance developed skeletal and palate defects. Seven percent of embryos given adenine (2 to 8 mg) were abnormal but none receiving adenosine (2 to 8 mg) were defective.

Karnofsky, D.A. and Lacon, C.R.: Effects of physiological purines on the development of the chick embryo. Biochem. Pharmacol. 7: 154-158, 1961.

389   Deoxycorticosterone Acetate (DOCA)

Grollman and Grollman (1962) administered 1 mg per day from day 4 through pregnancy and found that the rat offspring had hypertension which persisted for at least one year.

Walker (1965) injecting 0.1 to 1.25 mg of this compound in mice on days 11 through 14 found no cleft palates and only one spina bifida out of 69 fetuses.

Grollman, A. and Grollman, E.F.: Teratogenic induction of hypertension. J. Clin. Invest. 41: 710-714, 1962.

Walker, B.E.: Cleft palate produced in mice by human-equivalent dosage with triamcinolone. Science 149: 862-863, 1965.

390   2-Deoxyglucose

Demeyer (1961) gave 120 mg per day from the 9th through the 20th gestational day of the rat. Resorptions were 69 percent and the surviving fetuses were all malformed. Anophthalmia, cleft lip and palate and lesions of the extremities were observed. Spielmann et al (1973) gave 1 gm per kg on days 8, 9, 10 or 11 and found no malformations in the surviving rat fetuses.

Demeyer, R.: Etude experimentale de la glycoregulation gravidigne et de l'action teratogene des perturbations du metabolisme glucidigne. Bruxelles: Editions Arscia S.A.; 1961. pp. 184-189.

Spielmann, H.; Meyer-Wendecker, R. and Spielmann, F.: Influence of 2-deoxy-D-glucose and sodium fluoraetate on respiratoy metabolism of rat embryos during organogenesis. Teratology 7:127-134, 1973.

391   2-Deoxyguanosine

Karnofsky and Lacon (1961) reported coloboma, cleft palate and skeletal defects in chicks receiving 0.25 to 1.0 mg via the yolk sac on the 4th day. Guanine had no effects but a few defects were found when guanosine was used.

Karnofsky, D.A. and Lacon, C.R. : Effects of physiological purines on the development of the chick embryo. Biochem. Pharmacol. 7: 154-158, 1961.

392   2-Deoxyinosine

Karnofsky and Lacon (1961) found some facial colobomas and skeletal defects in chicks after injecting 0.5 to 4 mg into the yolk sac on the 4th day. Hypoxanthine was non-terato-genic in doses of 2 to 8 mg per egg. An occasional defect was seen in chicks receiving 2 to 8 mg of inosine.

Karnofsky, D.A. and Lacon, C.R.: Effects of physiological purines on the development of the chick embryo. Biochem. Pharmacol. 7: 154-158, 1961.

393   Desacetylaminocolchicine (also see Colchicine)

Greene et al. (1967) reported that in a very limited set of experiments it caused litter destruction in the rabbit at dose levels of 0.5 to 5.0 mg per kg given on single days after implantation.

394   Desacetylmethylcolchicine [Colcemid-R] (also see colchicine)

Sokal and Lessmann (1960) cite two reports where pregnant women given 1.5 to 7.5 mg per day from early in gestation produced normal infants.

Sokal, J.E. and Lessmann, E.M.: Effects of cancer chemotherapeutic agents on the human fetus. J.A.M.A. 172: 1765-1771, 1960.

395   Desatrine [Protoverine]

Keeler and Binns (1968) gave 0.3 to 0.8 gm to ewes and found in four instances normal lambs.

Keller, R.F. and Binns, W.: Teratogenic compounds of Veratrum californicum (Durand): v. Comparison of cyclopian effects of steroidal alkaloids from plant and structurally related compounds from other sources. Teratology 1: 5-10, 1968.

396 Deserpidine [11-desmethoxyreserpine]

Tuchmann-Duplessis and Mercier-Parot (1961) gave large doses (1.8 mg per kg) from the 6th through the 16th day of gestation and found rat fetuses with reduced weight and multiple subcutaneous hemorrhages associated with some necrosis of the extremities and skeletal defects.

Tuchmann-Duplessis, H. and Mercier-Parot, L.: Malformations foetales chez le rat traite par de fortes doses de deserpidine. C. R. Soc. Biol. 155: 2291-2293, 1961.

397 4-Desoxypyridoxine Hydrochloride (also see Pyridoxine Deficiency)

This antagonist to pyridoxine has been used to augment a pyridoxine deficient diet and produce anomalies in rats (Davis et al.; 1970). Fetuses from mothers maintained during pregnancy on a B-6 deficient diet and 2.3 mg of desoxypyridoxine developed digital defects, cleft palates and omphaloceles and occasionally exencephaly. Based on splenic and thymus hypoplasia, the authors raised the question of defective development of the immune system. The syndrome could be prevented by supplementation with pyridoxine.

Davis, S.D.; Nelson, T. and Shepard, T.H.: Teratogenicity of vitamin B-6 deficiency: omphalocele, skeletal and neural defects with splenic hypoplasia. Science 169: 1329-1330, 1970.

398 Detralfate

Towizawa et al (1972) gave this anti-ulcer agent orally to pregnant mice and rats during active organogenesis in amounts up to 4.0 gm per day and observed no teratogenicity or post-natal effects.

Towizawa, S.; Kamata, K. and Yoshimari, M.: Effects of detralfate administered to pregnant mice and rats on pre- and post-natal development of their offsprings. Oyo Yakuri 6: 599-611, 1972.

399 Dexamethasone (also see Cortisone)

This potent glucocorticoid has the same general teratogenic action as cortisone. Buck et al. (1962) produced neural tube closure defects in rabbits. Pinsky and DiGeorge (1965) found that dexamethasone when compared to hydrocortisone had a much greater cleft palate producing activity than would be expected by comparison of their glucocorticoid activities.

Esaki et al (1981) applied the 17-valerate form to rabbits dermally at doses of up to 0.1 mg per kg and no adverse fetal effects were found.

Buck, P.; Clavert, J. and Rumpler, Y.: Action teratogenique des corticoides chez la lapine. Ann. Chir. Infant 3: 73-87, 1962.

Esaki, K.; Shikata, Y.; Yanagita, T.: Effect of dermal administration of dexamethason-17-valerate in rabbit fetuses. Preclin. Rep. Cent. Inst. Exp. Anim. 7:245-256, 1981.

Pinsky, L. and DiGeorge, A.M.: Cleft palate in the mouse: A teratogenic index of glucocorticoid potency. Science 147: 402-403, 1965.

400 Dextroamphetamine Sulfate

Nora et al. (1968) using 50 mg per kg of body weight on the 8th day in two strains of mice produced a significant increase in ventricular and atrial septal defects. Yasuda et al. (1967) gave amphetamine sulfate (50 mg per kg) from gestational day 0 to 17 in the mouse and found five cleft palates in 274 fetuses as compared to 1 in 127 controls. Fetal weight was not reduced in the treated group. Kasirsky and Tansy (1971) using methamphetamine, a derivative of dexamphetamine, treated pregnant mice and rabbits. In the mice with a dose of 10 mg per kg on days 9 through 15 13.6 percent of the fetuses had exencephaly, cleft palate or eye defects. In the rabbit treated with 1.5 mg per kg for 3 or 18 days during organogenesis a significant increase in brain and eye defects was found.

Clark et al (1973) injected rats with 1 mg per kg on days 12 through 15 of gestation and performed behavior tests on the offspring. The treated animals had low activity test scores early in testing and were delayed in reaching adult activity levels. No differences were found in T-maze learning or reversal or in performance or extinction of the operant response. Seliger (1973) found that 5 mg doses during day 5 through 9 in rat gestation was associated with higher activity in the offspring. Adams et al (1982) reported deficits of acquisition of escape in rat offsprng whose mothers received 0.5 to 2.0 mg per kg on days 12-15 of gestation. Increased sensitivity to postnatal d-amphetamine challenge was also seen in the females.

Some significant increase in the incidence of congenital heart disease following amphetamine ingestion was reported by Nora et al (1970). They found 20 of 184 mothers of children with congenital heart disease had taken the drug during the vulnerable period as opposed to 3 of 108 control mothers (P less than 0.025). Levin (1971) reported that among 11 mothers of children with biliary atresia 4 took amphetamines during the second or third month of gestation. Milkovich and Van den Berg (1977) in a prospective study found no increase in the malformation rate among 1824 exposed children followed until their 5th birthday. Facial clefts occurred in 3 of 175 offspring exposed during the

first 56 days after the last menses. The authors state that
this could have occurred by chance. They did not find an
increase in congenital heart defects.

Adams, J.; Buelke-sam, J.B.; Kimmel, C.A. and LaBorde,
J.B.: Behavioral alterations in rats prenatally exposed to
low doses of d-amphetamine. Neurobehavioral Toxicol. and
Teratol. 4:63-70, 1982.

Clark, C.V.H.; Gorman, D. and Vernadakis, A.: Effects of
prenatal administration of psychotropic drugs on behavior of
developing rats. Devel. Psychobiol. 34: 225-235, 1970.

Kasirsky, G. and Tansy, M.F.: Teratogenic effects of
methamphetamine in mice and rabbits. Teratology 4: 131-134,
1971.

Levin, J.N.: Amphetamine ingestion with biliary atresia.
J. Pediat. 79: 130-131, 1971.

Milkovich, L. and Van den Berg, B.J.: Effects of antenatal
exposure to anorectic drugs. Am. J. Obstet. and Gynecol.
129:637-642, 1977.

Nora, J.J.; Vargo, T.A.; Nora, A.H.; Love, K.E. and
McNamara, D.G.: Dexamphetamine: a possible environmental
trigger in cardiovascular malformations (letter). Lancet 1:
1290 (only), 1970.

Nora, J.J.; Sommerville, R.J. and Fraser, F.C.: Homologies
for congenital heart diseases: murine models, influenced by
dextroamphetamine. Teratology 1: 413-416, 1968.

Seliger, D.L.: Effect of prenatal maternal administration
of D-amphetamine on rat offspring activity and passive
avoidance learning. Physiol. Psych. 1: 273-280, 1973.

Yasuda, M.; Ariyuki, F. and Nishimura, H.: Effect of
successive administration of amphetamine to pregnant mice
upon the susceptibility of the offspring to the teratogen-
scity of thio-tepa. Congenital Anomalies 7: 66-73, 1967.

401 DFP (Diisopropyl Phosphorofluoridate)

Fish (1966) administered this material intraperitoneally to
rats in amounts of 1 to 4 mg per kg on days 8, 9 or 12 and
found no defects, but perinatal mortality was increased and
weight gain postnatally was reduced. Treatment on days 7,
8, 9 and 10 did not increase the resorption rate.

Fish, S.A.: Organophosphorus cholinesterase inhibitor and
fetal development. Am. J. Obstet. Gynecol. 96:
1148-1154, 1966.

402 Diabetes

There is controversy about whether diabetes contributes to a
general increase in human congenital defects. Warkany
(1971) has carefully reviewed this evidence. Rubin and

402

Murphy (1958) showed that the increased incidence of defects
in the diabetic offspring can be explained by intensified
scrutiny of these children either during hospitalization or
at autopsy examination. Farquhar (1965) was to show
an increased rate of defects but Hagbard (1961) and Pedersen
et al. (1964) give reports with small increases. Comess et
al. (1969) in an Indian population reported a 38 percent
incidence of anomaly in the offspring of diabetics diagnosed
before 25 years of age. Crane and Wahl (1981) have studied
spontaneous abortion in 154 diabetics and found no increase.

Although there is doubt about the overall incidence of congenital defects, most authors have observed a significant
number of offspring with caudal dysplasia or caudal
regression syndrome. The defect may appear in as high as
0.2 to 1 percent of diabetic offspring and consists of
varying amounts of sacral and femoral agenesis sometimes
associated with defects of the palate and branchial arches
(Kucera et al, 1965); Passarge, 1965: Rusnak and Driscoll,
1965 and Kucera, 1971). The role of insulin, oral
hypoglycemics and other physiologic changes of diabetes is
difficult to evaluate. It is of interest that an early
report of 439 diabetic offspring by White (1949) cites only
one patient with congenital skeletal defects. A small left
colon syndrome has also been described in these children
(Davis and Campbell, 1975). Milunsky et al (1982) using
serum alpha-fetoprotein for diagnosis found a 10-fold
increase in nerual tuube defects among 411 pregnant
diabetics.

Stehbens et al (1977) studied the intellectual function of
diabetic offspring and found that the presence of acetone in
the urine during gestation was associated with a significant
reduction in IQ at 3 and 5 years of age.

An interesting model using streptozotocin-treated rats has
been used to show that with isulin treatment the incidence
of caudal dysplasia is reduced (Eriksson et al, 1982) and
Baker et al, 1981). Sadler (1980) has studied the effect of
serum from streptozotocin- treated rats on mouse embryos
grown in vitro. Neural closure defects were found.

Baker, L.; Egler, J.M.; Klein, S.H.; Goldman, A.S.:
Meticulous control of diabetes during organogenesis prevents
congental lumbosacral defects in rats. Diabetes 30:955-959,
1981.

Comess, L.J.; Bennett, P.H.; Man, M.B.; Burch, T.A. and
Miller, M.: Congenital anomalies and diabetes in the Pima
Indians of Arizona. Diabetes 18: 471-477, 1969.

Crane, J.P; Wahl, N.: The role of maternal diabetes in
reproductive spontaneous abortion. Fertility and Sterility
36:477-479, 1981.

Davis, W.S. and Campbell, J.B.: Neonatal small left colon
syndrome. Am. J. Dis. Child 129:1024-1027, 1975.

Ericksson, W.; Dahlstrom, E.; Larsson, K.S.; Hellerstrom,
C.: Increased incidence of congenital malformations in the
offspring of diabetic rats and their prevention by maternal

insulin therapy. Diabetes 31:1-6, 1982.

Farquhar, J.W.: The influence of maternal diabetes on the fetus and child. Gairdner, D. (ed.): Recent Advances in Pediatrics. Boston: Little Brown and Company, 1965 (3rd Ed.). pp. 126-129.

Hagbard, L.: Pregnancy and Diabetes. Springfield, Ill.: Charles C. Thomas, 1961. pp. 21-25.

Kucera, J.; Lenz, W. and Maier, W.: Missbildungen der beine und der Kaudalen Wirbelsaule bei kindern Diabetischer mutter. Dtsch. Med. Wochenschr. 90: 901-905, 1965.

Kucera, J.: Rate and type of congenital anomalies among offspring of diabetic women. J. Reprod. Med. 7: 61-70, 1971.

Milunsky, A.; Alpert, E.; Kitzmiller, J.L.; Younge, M.D.; Neff, R.K.: Prenatal diagnosis of neural tube defects 8 The importance of serum alpha-fetoprotein in diabetic pregnant women. Am. J. Obst. Gynecol. 142:1030-1032, 1982.

Passarge, E.: Congenital malformations and maternal diabetes. Lancet 1: 324-325, 1965.

Pedersen, L.M.; Tygstrup, I. and Pedersen, J.: Congenital malformations in newborn infants of diabetic women. Correlation with maternal diabetic vascular complications. Lancet 1: 1124-1126, 1964.

Rubin, A. and Murphy, D.P.: Studies in human reproduction. 3. The frequency of congenital malformations in the off-spring of nondiabetic and diabetic individuals. J. Pediatr. 53: 579-585, 1958.

Rusnak, S.L. and Driscoll, S.G.: Congenital spinal anomalies in infants of diabetic mothers. Pediatrics 35: 989-995, 1965.

Sadler, T.W.: Effects of maternal diabetes on early embryogenesis: I. The teratogenic potential of diabetic serum. Teratology 21:339-347, 1980.

Stehbens J.A.; Baker, G.I. and Mitchell, M.: Outcome at ages 1,2 and 5 years of children born to diabetic women. Am. J. Obstet. Gynecol. 127:408, 1977.

Warkany, J.: Congenital Malformations: Notes and comments. Chicago: Year Book Publishers, 1971. pp. 124-125.

White, P.: Pregnancy complicating diabetes. Am. J. Med. 7: 609-616, 1949.

403 2,4-Diamino-5-chlorophenyl-6-ethylpyrimidine   [Daraprim-R] [Chloridin-R] [Ethlpyrimidine] [Primethamine]

This antimalarial drug which is also a folic acid antagonist was used by Dyban et al (1965) to produce defects in the rat. By using 3 to 10 mg per animal on gestational days 9,

10 or 13 a high incidence of cleft palate, mandibular
hypoplasia and limb defects was found. Neural tube closure
defects were also recorded. When 0.6 mg was given by mouth
on days 9, 10 and 11 a defect rate of 36 percent was
produced. Anderson and Morse (1966) have produced similar
defects in the rat. Sullivan and Takacs (1971) reported a
low incidence of congenital defects in guinea pigs after 20
mg on day 9. These authors point out that the teratogenic
dose of 0.5 mg per day in the rat does not differ greatly
from the 25 mg daily dose being used in humans for treatment
of toxoplasmosis. Thiersch (1954) used the methyl
pyrimidine form and found defects in the rat with 0.5 mg per
kg. Kotb (1972) found that the methyl form in amounts of 75
mg per kg on the first day of gestation caused mortality in
nearly all embryos. Folinic acid has been shown to
antagonize the action of ethyl pyrimidine (Sullivan and
Takacs, 1971). Stanzheuskaya (1966) has shown that the
compound is teratogenic in the chick.

Dyban and Udalova (1967) induced various chromosomal
aberrations in 5-day rat embryos when the mother received
the drug 8 hours after insemination.

Pyrimethamine was given by gavage (2 or 5 mg per kg) to the
adult female rat just before ovulation. A significant
dose-dependent decrease in the rate of cleavage was
observed. In a dose of 2 mg per kg no chromosomal
aberrations were observed in 5 day rat embryos. Five mg per
kg induced chromosomal aberrations in 14 percent of all
5-day rat embryos. In the control group only 6% of the
embryos had chromosmal aberrations. Pyrimethamine induced
mostly trisomy or chromosomal mosaicism in rat embryos
(Baranov and Chebotar, 1980).

Male rats were treated with pyrimethamine (10 mg per kg once
every day by gavage during 1-3 weeks) before mating with
normal females. In these experiments no increased embryonic
mortality was found (Udalova, 1976).

This drug was given to rats on 9 or 10 days of gestation and
severe damage of decidual tissue was observed. It was shown
that this effect resulted from the direct inhibition of
dihydrofolate reductase not only in embryonic but also in
decidual cells. Different sensitivity of mesometral and
antimesometral parts of the decidua was observed. Under the
effect of pyrimethamine differences in DNA synthesis between
the mesometral and antimesometral regions were manifested
which were connected with differences in thymidine
monophosphate synthesis in the two populations of decidual
cells (Dyban et al, 1976a).

Pyrimethamine given intragastricaly (50 mg per kg) to female
rats on the 13th day of pregnancy induced typical severe
malformations in all embryos. It was shown that
pyrimethamine inhibited DNA and RNA synthesis within 15 to
20 minutes following the administration of the drug. The
rate of 14C-thymidine incorporation in DNA of abnormal
embryos did not change within 4 hours following the
administration of pyrimethamine. The data presented agree
with the earlier results which suggested that the mechanism
of teratogenic action of pyrimethamine on rat embryonic

development was due to the primary inactivation of dihydrofolate reductase and the inhibition of folate cycle in the embryonic cells (Kotin and Repin, 1973).

Pyrimethamine (50 mg per kg given by gavage on the 1st day of pregnancy) did not induce any disturbances in preimplantation development of CBA mouse embryos while a single dose of 25 mg per kg on the first day of pregnancy caused death of all cleaving rat embryos. The cleavage of mouse embryos cultured in medium containing blood serum from rats treated with pyrimethamine was abnormal and significant numbers of embryos died. It was concluded that mouse and rat embryos had the same sensitivity to pyrimethamine in culture in vitro but not during the development in the maternal organism because of a barrier function of the oviduct to this drug in mice (Dyban et al, 1976b).

Female rats were treated on the 10th day of pregnancy with pyrimethamine (25 mg per kg intragastrically) and after different time intervals (from 15 minutes to 24 hours) animals were sacrificed, embryos removed from the uterus and cultured in vitro in blood serum from control (non-treated) rats. It was shown that teratogenic action of pyrimethamine became irreversible 6 hours after exposure of pregnant rats to this drug. In the other experiments embryos from intact control females were cultured (1-4 hours) in the serum from rats treated with the same dose of pyrimethamine. In these conditions the irreversible teratogenic action of pyrimethamine was observed after culturing rat embryos 3 hours in this serum. These data supported the conclusion that to produce embryotoxic and teratogenic action the presence in blood of pyrimethamine and-or its metabolites for at least 5-6 hours is needed (Popov, 1982).

The teratogenic and embryotoxic effects of the following 6 derivatives of 2,4-diamino-5-phenylpyrimidine with different length of the alkyl radical in the 6 position of pyrimidine ring was studied in rats (2,4-diamino-5-phenylpyrimidine: 2,4-diamino-5-phenyl-6- methylpyrimidine; 2,4-5-phenyl- -6-ethylpyrimidine; 2,4-diamino-5- phenyl-6-propyl- pyrimidine; 2,4-diamino-5-phenyl-6-butylpyrimidine). It was found that among these analogues of pyrimidine the highest teratogenic and embryotoxic activity was the substance with an ethyl group and the lowest the H-radical (Dyban et al, 1976d). The mitotic activity of liver cells in rat embryos from treated animals and corneal epithelium in adult rats obtained after administration of these substances was studied. A definite correlation was established between antimitotic, embryotoxic and teratogenic activities of previously mentioned pyrimethamine analogues (Dyban et al, 1976c).

Anderson, I. and Morse, L.M.: The influence of solvent on the teratogenic effect of folic acid antagonist in the rat. Exp. Mol. Pathol. 5: 134-145, 1966.

Baranov, V.S.; Chebotar, N.A.: Mutagenic effect of pyrimethamine injection before ovulation on preimplantational rat embryos. Tsitol. i. Genet. (USSR) 14.6:20-24, 1980.

Dyban, A.P.; Akimova, I.M. and Svetlova, V.A.: Effect of 2-4-diamino-5-chlorophenyl-6-ethylpyrimidine on the embryonic development of rats. Akad. Nauk. S.S.S.R. 163: 455-458, 1965.

Dyban, A.P. and Udalova, L.D.: Study of chromosome aberrations at the early stages of mammalian embryogenesis. I. The experiments with the effect of 2,4-diamino, 5-p-chlorphenyl, 6-ethyl pyrimidine (pyrimethamine) on Rats. Genetika (Russian) No. 4: 52-65, 1967.

Dyban, A.P.; Samoshkina, N.A.; Weisman, B.L. and Golinsky, G.F.: Pattern of DNA synthesis in antimesometral and mesometral regions of the decidual tissue in rats. Ontogenez. (USSR) 7.4:323-332, 1976a.

Dyban, A.P.; Sekirina, G.G. and Golinsky, G.F.: Sensitivity of the early mouse embryos to antifolic preparation chloridine (pyrimethamine). Byull. Eksper. Biol. Med. (USSR) 82:10:1247-1250, 1976b.

Dyban, A.P.; Barilyak, I.R.; Tichodeeva, I.I. and Chebotar, N.A.: On correlation of teratogenic and antimitotic activity of some derivatives of 2,4-diaminopyrimidine. Ontogenez. (USSR) 7.1: 58-63, 1976c.

Dyban, A.P.; Bariljak, I.R. and Tichodeeva, I.I.: The teratogenic and embryotoxic activity of some 2,4-diaminopyrimidine derivatives. Arkh. Anat. Gistol. Embryol. (USSR) 7:29-35, 1976d.

Kotb, M.M.: Peculiarities of damage effect of the structural analogue of antimalarial drug chloridine (lem-687) on different stages of embryogenesis in the rat. Arch. Anat. (Russian) 63: No. 8, 88-96, 1972.

Kotin, A.M. and Repin, V.S.: Effect of pyrimethamine on nucleic acid metabolism in white rat embryos. Ontogenez. (USSR) 4.2:128-137, 1973.

Popov, V.B.: Study into the time of realizing embryotoxic action of cyclophophamide and chloridine in vivo and in vitro. Farmakol. Toksikol. (USSR) 45.1:79-83, 1982.

Stanzheuskaya, T.L.: Effect of chloridin on chick embryogenesis. Bull. Exp. Biol. Med. 61: 427-429, 1966.

Sullivan, G.E. and Takacs, E.: Comparative teratogenicity of pyrimethamine in rats and hamsters. Teratology 4: 205-210, 1971.

Thiersch, J.B.: The effect of substituted 2,4-diamino--pyrimidines on the rat fetus in utero. Proceedings of the International Congress on Chemotherapy 3: 367-372, 1954.

Udalova, L.D.: postimplantation development of rat embryos after the action of some chemical agents on male gametes. Arkh. Anat. Gistol. Embriol. (USSR) 1:46-50, 1976.

404   2,4-Diamino-5-(3,4-dichlorophenyl)-6-methylpyrimidine   (see

2,4 Diamino-5-p-chlorophenyl-6-ethylpyrimidine)

405 2,5-Diaminotoluene [Hair Dye]

This hair-dye constituent was given in single dose subcutaneously to mice on days 7 through 14. Using 50 mg per kg on day 8, eighteen percent of the fetuses were malformed with vertebral and rib abnormalities most common but exencephaly and prosoposchisis also seen (Inoye and Murakami, 1977). Reproductive studies in rats have given negative studies (Burnett et al, 1976 and Wernick et al, 1975).

Inouye and Murakami () gave 75 mg or 50 mg per kg by subutaneous or intraperitoneal route, respectively to mice on day 8 and noted some maternal deaths and a low incidence of exencephaly in the fetuses.

Burnett, C.; Goldenthal, E.I.; Harris, S.B.; Wazeter, F.X.; Strausburg, J.; Kopp, R. and Voelker, P.: Teratology and percutaneous toxicity studies on hair dyes. J. Toxicol. Envir. Health 1:1027, 1976.

Inouye, M. and Murakami, U.: Teratogenicity of 2,5-diaminotoluene, a hair dye component in mice. (abs) Teratology 14:241-242, 1976.

Inouye, M. and Murakami, U.: Teratogenicity of 2,5-diaminotoluene a hai-dye constituent in mice. Fd. Cosmet. Toxicol. 15:447-451, 1977.

Wernick, T.; Lanman, B.M. and Fraux, J.L.: Chronic toxicity, teratologic and reproductive studies with hair dyes. Toxicol. Appl. Pharmacol. 32:450 1975.

406 2-6-Diaminopurine

Chaube and Murphy (1968) report that this purine analogue has a fetal LD-100 of 200 mg per kg of maternal weight. No congenital defects were found. Thiersch (1957) using 50 mg per kg found a high incidence of resorption when rats were treated on the 4th and 5th days and a few stunted fetuses when the same dose was injected on the 7th and 8th days.

Chaube, S. and Murphy, M.L.: The teratogenic effects of the recent drugs active in cancer chemotherapy. In, Woollam, D.H.M. (ed.): Advances in Teratology, Vol. 3. New York: Logos and Academic Press, 1968. pp. 181-237.

Thiersch, J.B.: Effect of 2-6 diaminopurine (2-6 DPP), 6-chlorpurine (CLP) and thioguanine (THG) on rat litter in utero. Proc. Soc. Exp. Biol. Med. 94: 40-43, 1957.

407 Diathermy (see Microwave Radiations)

408 Diazepam [Valium-R]

Aarskog (1975) questioned 130 mothers of children with oral clefts and found that seven of 111 had first trimester exposure. Only four out of 362 women controls questioned by another method had exposures. Czeizel found that 15 percent of mothers with children having facial clefts had taken the drug and this rate was the same for the mothers of infants with neural tube closure defects.

Saxen (1975) and Saxen and Saxen (1975) reported a significant increase in incidence of cleft palate and cleft lip and palate among mothers ingesting antineurotics (mostly diazepam) during the first trimester. She viewed these observations as mostly prospective because prescriptions were required for the use of these drugs. Safra and Oakley (1975) also found a four-fold increase in the ingestion of this drug among mothers giving birth to children with cleft lip or cleft lip and palate. Safra and Oakley (1976) point out that a four-fold increase in oral clefts if confirmed would imply only a 0.4 percent risk for cleft lip with or without cleft palate and a 0.2 percent risk for having a child with cleft palate. Crombie et al (1975) in a study of 64 women who took this drug in pregnancy found no offspring with defects.

Beall (1972) reported no teratogenicity in the rat exposed to as much as 200 mg per kg given orally from day 6 through 15. Diazepam and N-demethyl-diazepam produced cleft palate in mice treated with 40 mg per kg by mouth on day 14 (Miller and Becker, 1973). Erkkola et al (1974) have shown that this medication is transfered easily to the early human fetus. Miller and Becker (1975) treated pregnant mice with diazepam orally on days 11, 12 and 13 and at the dosage level of 140 mg per kg found an increase in cleft palates in the fetuses. Kellog et al (1980) reported that rats exposed prenatally on days 13 to 20 to 2.5 to 10 mg per kg of maternal weight exhibited delayed locomotion and acoustic startle reflexes that normally appear in the third postnatal week.

Aarskog, D.: Association between maternal intake of diazepam and oral clefts. Lancet 2:29 (only), 1975.

Beall, J.R.: Study of the teratogenic potential of diazepam and SCH 12041. Can. Med. Assoc. J. 106: 1061, only, 1972.

Crombie, D.L.; Pinsent, R.J.; Fleming, D.M.; Rumeau-Rouquette, Goujard, J. and Huel, G.: Fetal effects of tranquilizers in pregnancy. New Eng. J. Med. 293: 198-199, 1975.

Czeizel, A.: Diazepam, phenytoin and etiology of cleft lip and-or cleft palate. Lancet 1:810 (only), 1976.

Erkkola, R.; Kanto, J. and Sellman, R.: Diazepam in early human pregnancy. Acta Obstet. Gynec. Scand. 53: 135-138, 1974.

Kellogg, C.; Tervo, D.; Ison, J.; Parisi, T.; Miller, R.K.: Prenatal exposure to diazepam alters behavioral development in rats. Science 207:205-207, 1980.

Miller, R.P. and Becker, B.A.: The teratogenicity of diazepam metabolites in Swiss-Webster mice (abstract) Toxicol. Appl. Pharm. 25: 453 (only) 1973.

Miller, R.P. and Becker, B.A.: Teratogenicity of oral diazepam and diphenylhydantoin in mice. Toxicol. Appl. Pharm. 32: 53-61, 1975.

Safra, M.J. and Oakley, G.P.: An association of cleft lip with or without cleft palate and prenatal exposure to valium. Lancet 2: 478-479, 1975.

Safra, M.J. and Oakley, G.P.: Valium: an oral cleft teratogen? Cleft Palate Journal 13:198-200, 1976.

Saxen, I.: Associations between oral clefts and drugs taken during pregnancy. Int. J. Epid. 4: 37-44, 1975.

Saxen, I. and Saxen, L.: Association between maternal intake of diazepam and oral clefts. Lancet 2: 498 (only), 1975.

409 Diazinon (0,0-diethyl 0-[2-isopropyl-6-methyl-4-pyrimidinyl] phosphorothioate)

This organo phosphorus pesticide was given to rats in doses of 100 to 200 mg per kg intraperitoneally on the 11th day of gestation (Kimbrough and Gaines, 1968). At 200 mg per kg some maternal mortality occurred along with limb reduction and hydrocephalus in surviving fetuses. At 150 mg per kg only fetal weight reduction was found. Robens (1969) studied rabbits and guinea pigs at doses up to 30 and 0.25 mg per kg respectively and reported no malformations.

Kimbrough, R.D.; Gaines, T.B.: Effect of organic phosphorus compounds and alkalating agents on the rat fetus. Arch. Environ. Health 16:805-808, 1968.

Robens, J.F.: Teratologic studies of carbaryl, diazinon, Norea, disulfiram and thiram in small laboratory animals. Toxicol. Appl. Pharm. 15:152-163, 1969.

410 O-Diazoacetyl-l-serine (see Azaserine)

411 6-Diazo-5-oxo-l-norleucine (DON)

Chaube and Murphy (1968) have reviewed the teratogenic information on this tumor inhibiting glutamine analogue. Murphy (1960) produced lip or palate defects in the rat by using a lethal dose (0.5 mg per kg) of DON modified by addition of adenine or guanine (100 mg per kg). Friedman (1957) produced cleft palate in the dog fetus by giving DON in amounts of 0.15 mg per kg on days 20, 21 and 22. Greene and Kochhar (1975) gave mice intramuscularly 0.5 mg per kg on day 10 or 11 of gestation and produced median cleft lip and skeletal defects in the offspring. Friedman (1975) has studied the drug in pregnant dogs.

411

Chaube, S. and Murphy, M.L.: The teratogenic effects of the recent drugs active in cancer chemotherapy. In, Woollam, D.H.M. (ed.): Advances in Teratology, Vol. 3. New York: Logos and Academic Press, 1968. pp. 181-237.

Friedman, M.H.: The effect of 0-diazoacetyl-1-serine (azaserine) on the pregnancy of the dog - A preliminary report. J. Am. Vet. Med. Assoc. 130: 159-162, 1957.

Greene, R.M. and Kochhar, D.M.: Limb development in mouse embryos: protection against teratogenic effects of 6-diazo--5-oxo-norleucine (DON) in vivo and in vitro. J. Embryol. Exp. Morph. 33: 355-370, 1975.

Murphy, M.L.: Teratogenic effects of tumor inhibiting chemicals in the rat. In, Wolstenholme, G.E.W. and O'Connor, C.M. (eds.): A Ciba Foundation Symposium on Congenital Malformations. London: J. and A. Churchill Ltd.; 1960. pp. 92-95.

412 Dibromochloropropane (DBCP)

Ruddick and Newsome (1979) gave up to 50 mg per kg daily to rats by gavage on days 6-15 of gestation. Some maternal toxicity, fetal weight decrease and decreased fetal viability was found but no increase in malformations.

Ruddick, J.A.; Newsome, W.H.: A teratogenicity and tissue distribution study on dibromochloropropane in the rat. Bull. Environ. Contam. Toxicol. 21:483-487, 1979.

413 Di-n-butyl Phthalate (see Phthalate esters)

414 Dichloralphenazone

McColl et al. (1965) reported no teratogenic effect of 500 mg per kg fed daily during the entire pregnancy of the rat.

McColl, J.D.; Globus, M. and Robinson, S.: Effect of some therapeutic agents on the developing rat fetus. Toxicol. Appl. Pharmacol. 7:409-417, 1965.

415 Bis(Dichloracetyl)diamine (Win 18,446, N-N-bis(dichloro-acetyl)-1,8-octamethylenediamine)

416 N-N-bis(Dichloroacetyl)-1,8-octamethylenediamine (WIN-18,446)

Oster et al (1974) studied this male antifertility agent in pregnant rats and found the drug to be highly embryocidal. When they used 200 mg per kg per day on days 11 and 12 a high incidence of fetal edema, cleft lip and microcephaly was found. In a later publication these authors also detailed septal heart defects, diaphragmatic hernias and small irregular thymuses (Taleporos et al, 1978). More detailed studies were published in 1982 (Kilburn et al).

416

Kilburn, K.H.; Hess, R.A.; Lesser, M.; Oster, G.: Perinatal death and respiratory apparatus dysgenesis due to bis (dichloroacetyl) diamine. Teratology 26:155-162, 1982.

Oster, G.; Salgo, M.P. and Taleporos, P.: Embryocidal action of bis(dichloroacetyl)diamine: an oral abortifacient in rats. Am. J. Obstet. Gynecol. 119: 583-588, 1974.

Taleporos, P.; Salgo, M.P. and Oster, G.: Teratogenic action of a Bis(dichloroacetyl)diamine on rats: Patterns of malformations produced in high incidence at time- limited periods of development. Teratology 18:5-16, 1978.

417 3,3-Dichloro-5,5-dinitro-0,0-biphenol [Distolon-R]

This compound used to treat liver flukes in sheep was given by Juszkiewicz et al (1971) to hamsters by mouth on the 8th day of gestation. With 20 mg per kg a 4 percent incidence of skeletal retardation was found. One meningomyelocele occurred among 77 examined fetuses.

Juszkiewicz, T.; Rakalska, Z. and Dzierzawski, A.: Effet embryopathique du 3,3-dichloro-5,5-dinitro-0,0-biphenol (Bayer 9015) chez le hamster dore. Eur. J. Toxicol. 4: 523-528, 1971.

418 1,2-Dichloroethane (Ethylene Chloride, Ethylene Dichloride)

Alumot et al (1976) administered 250 or 500 ppm in feed mash to rats for a two year period. Approximately 60-70% of the dose was consumed. No significant decrease in fertility, litter size or fetal weight was observed. Rao et al (1980) exposed rats to vapor at 100 and 300 ppm for 7 hours daily during days 6-15 of gestation. Ten of the 16 rats at 300 ppm died and only one rat had an implanted pregnancy with total resorption. With 100 ppm there was neither increased resorption nor decrease in fetal weight. Lane et al (1982) administered up to 1,000 mg per kg in drinking water and found no adverse reproductive effects.

Vozovaya (1976) and Vozovaya and Malyarova (1975) have reported preimplantation reproductive failure and accumulation of the material in fetal rat liver.

Alumot, E.; Nachtomi, E.; Mandel, E.; Holstein, P.: Tolerance and acceptable daily intake of chlorinated fumigants in the rat diet. Fd. Cosmet. Toxicol. 14:105-110, 1976.

Lane, R.W.; Riddle, B.L.; Borzelleca, J.F.: Effect of dichloroethane 1,1,1-trichloroethane in drinking water on reproduction and development in mice. Toxicol. Appl. Pharmacol. 63:409-421, 1982.

Rao, K.S.; Murrary, J.S.; Deacon, M.M.; John, J.A.; Calhoun, L.L.; Young, J.T.: Teratogenicity and reproduction studies in animals inhaling ethylene dichloride in Banbury Report 5 ethylene dichloride: A potential health risk, edited by B. Ames, P. Infante and R. Reitz, Cold Spring Harbor

418

Laboratory 149-161, 1980.

Vozovaya, M.A.: TThe effect of small concentrations of
benzene and dichloroethane separately and combined on the
reproductive function of animals. Gig. Sanit. 6:100,
1976.

Vozovaya, M.A.; Malyarova, L.K.: Mechanism of action of
ethylene dichloride on the fetus of experimental animals.
Gig. Sanit. 6:94, 1975.

419 1,1-Dichloroethylene (Vinylidene chloride)

Murray et al (1979) exposed rats and rabbits by inhalation
to concentrations of up to 160 ppm for 7 hour period during
days 6 through 18 and 6 through 15 of gestation. Maternal
toxicity was demonstrated in both species. No increased
general malformation rate was found but wavy ribs and
delayed ossification were increased in rat fetuses exposed
to 80 and 160 ppm. Rats were fed 200 ppm in their drinking
water on days 6 through 15 of gestation and no differences
from the fetal controls were found. Alumot et al (1976) fed
rats up to 500 ppm over a two year period and found no
alteration in fetal mortality or weight. Approximately
60-70 percent of the substance was actually consumed.

Anderson et al (1977) exposed male mice to 50 ppm 6 hours
daily for 5 days and found no evidence of dominant
lethality. Short et al (1977) had similar findings in the
rat.

Alumot, E.; Nachtomi, E.; Mandel, E.; Holstein, P.:
Tolerance and acceptable daily intake of chlorinated
fumigants in the rat diet. Fd. Cosmet. Toxicol.
14:105-110, 1976.

Anderson, D.; Hodge, M.C.E.; Purchase, I.F.H.: Dominant
lethal studies with halogenated olefins vinyl chloride and
vinylidene dichloride in male CD-1 mice. Envir. Health
Persp. 21:71-78, 1977.

Murray, F.J.; Nitschke, K.D.; Rampy, L.W.; Schwetz, B.A.:
Embryotoxicity and fetotoxicity of inhaled or ingested
vinylidene chloride in rats and rabbits. Toxicol. Appl.
Pharmacol. 49:189-202, 1979.

Short, R.D.; Minor, J.L.; Winston, J.M.; Lee, C.C.: A
dominant lethal study in male rats after repeated exposure
to vinyl chloride or vinylidene chloride. J. Toxicol.
Envir. Health 3:965-968, 1977.

420 Dichloroisocyanurate sodium (Sodium 3,5-chloro-1,3,5-trizime
2,4,6-trione)

Tani et al (1981) gave mice up to 400 mg per kg on days 6-15
of gestation. No adverse fetal effects were found.

Tani, I.; Shibata, H.; Ninomiya, M.; Taniguchi, J.; Fuyita,
I.: Effect of SD (SDIC) on the embryonic development and

newborns given orally in the period of organogenesis in
mice. Yakubutsu Ryoho (Medical Treatment 13:353-363, 1981.

421 Dichloromethane (methylene chloride)

Schwetz et al (1975) exposed pregnant mice and rats to this
vapor in concentrations of 1225 ppm. Both species were
exposed for 7 hour daily periods on days 6 through 15 of
gestation. No fetal toxicity or teratogenicity was found.
Hardin and Manson (1980) exposed rats to 4500 ppm for 6
hours per day before and during the first 17 days of
gestation. Some fetal weight reduction occurred but no
malformation increase was found. In the same treatment
group as above behavioral studies were done (Bornschein et
al, 1980). Post natal growth activity and avoidance
learning were not impaired but behavioral habituation was
more rapid in the exposed group.

Bornschein, L.; Hastings, L.; Manson, J.M.: Behavioral
toxicity in the offspring of rats following maternal
exposure to dichloromethane. Toxicol. Appl. Pharmacol.
52:29-37, 1980.

Hardin, B.D.; Manson, J.M.: Absence of dichloromethane
teratogenicity with inhalation exposure in rats. Toxicol.
Appl. Pharmacol. 52:22-28, 1980.

Schwetz, B.A.; Leong, B.K.J.; Gehring, P.J.: The effect of
maternally inhaled trichloroethylene, perchlorethylene,
methyl chloroform and methylene chloride on embryonal and
fetal development in mice and rats. Toxicol. Appl.
Pharmacol. 32:84-96, 1975.

422 Dichloromethatrexate (see Methatrexate)

423 2,4-Dichlorophenol (see Nitrofen)

424 2,4-Dichlorophenoxyacetic Acid [2-4-D]

Schwetz et al. (1971) gave rats up to 87.5 mg per kg on
days 6 through 15 of gestation. With doses above 25 mg per
kg subcutaneous edema, wavy ribs, delayed ossification and
lumbar ribs were observed. Similar findings were reported
following administration of the butyl ether and isooctyl
esters of the compound.

Konstantinova et al (1978) studied the action of this agent
in rats at the doses of 0.5-1.0 mg per kg and found that
this herbicide is highly embryotoxic. Aleksashina et al
(1979) injected rats with one-twentieth LD-50 on the
4,5,6,9,10,11,12,13,14 and 15th day of pregnancy and noted
strong embryotoxic effects.

Aleksashina, Z.A.; Buslovich, S.Yu. and Kolosovskaya, V.M.:
Embryotoxical activity of herbicides derivatives
2,4-dichlorophenoxyacetic acid. Gigiena i Sanitaria (USSR)
4:70-71, 1979.

424

Konstantinova, T.K.; Efimenko, L.P.; Antonenko, T.A.;
Nechkina, M.A. and Shilov, V.N.: Data for hygienic
standardization of herbicides 2,4-D in the environmental
objects. Gigiena i Sanitariya (USSR) 11:9-13, 1978.

Schwetz, B.A.; Sparschu, G.L. and Gehring, P.J.: The
effect of 2,4-dichlorophenoxyacetic acid (2,4-d) and esters
of 2,4-d on rat embryonal, foetal and neonatal growth and
development. Food Cosmet. Toxicol. 9: 801-817, 1971.

425 2,2-Dichlorphenoxy-gamma-Butyric Acid

Sokolova (1976) observed increased fetal mortality, growth
retardation and behavioral abnormalities in the offspring of
rats receiving herbicide in amounts of 0.1 mg per kg on days
4,5,7,9,10,11 and 14 or during the entire gestation (0.1 - 3
mg per kg).

Sokolova, L.A.: Studies of herbicide 2,4D effect on
gestation, embryognesis and gonads of white rats. Gigena i
Saitariya (USSR) y:20-23, 1976.

426 2,4-Dichlorophenyl-nitrophenyl Ether

Kimbrough et al (1973) studied the high neonatal death rate
in the offspring of rats gavaged with 50 mg per kg per day
on days 7 through 15 and found poor expansion of the lungs
with less well developed lamellar bodies. Nakao et al
(1981) fed 500 ppm to pregnant rats and found either
diaphragmatic hernia or under development of the lungs.

Kimbrough, R.D.; Gaines, T.B. and Linder, R.E.: The ffect
of 2,4-dichlorophenyl-p-nitrophenyl ether on the rat fetus
(abstract) Toxicol. Appl. Pharm. 25: 456, only, 1973.

Nakao, Y.; Ueki, R.; Tada, T.; Iritani, I.; Kishimoto, H.:
Experimental model of congenital diaphragmatic hernia
induced chemically. (abstract) Teratology 24:11A, 1981.

427 Dichlorphenamide

Hallesy and Layton (1967) reported that this carbonic
anhydrase inhibitor produced postaxial defects of the right
upper extremity in rats. The drug was given in the diet
providing 350 mg per kg per day. The defect appeared to be
the same as that caused by acetazolamide, a compound of
quite different chemical structure.

Purichia and Erway (1972) produced fetal otolith deficits by
injecting pregnant mice with a single dose (2.4-3.6 mg)
between days 13 to 18 of pregnancy.

Landauer and Wakasogi (1968) found that ADP reduced the
teratogenic effect of this compound in the chick.

Hallesy, D.W. and Layton, W.M.: Forelimb deformity of offspring of rats given dichlorphenamide during pregnancy.
Proc. Soc. Exp. Biol. Med. 126: 6-8, 1967.

Landauer, W. and Wakasugi, N.: Teratological studies with sulphonamides and their implications. J. Embryol. Exp. Morphol. 20: 261-284, 1968.

Purichia, N. and Erway, L.C.: Effect of dichlorophenamide, zinc and manganese on otolith development in mice. Dev. Biol. 27: 395-405, 1972.

428 Dichlorvos (Dimethyl-2,2-dichlorovinyl PO4)

Thorpe et al (1972) exposed pregnant rats and rabbits to this active principle of various vapor insecticides and found no teratogenic effect even at levels toxic to the mother. The highest dose used was 6.25 microgram per liter of air during the entire gestation. Schwetz et al (1979) reported lack ot teratogenic effect in the mouse and rabbit given 60 and 5 mg per kg per day respectively. Inhalation studies were also negative at 4 micrograms per liter.

Schwetz, B.A.; Ioset, H.D.; Leong, B.K.J.; Staples, R.E.: Teratogenic potential of dichlorvos given by inhalation and gavage to mice and rabbits. Teratology 20:383-388, 1979.

Thorpe, E.; Wilson, A.B.; Dix, K.M. and Blair, D.: Teratologic studies with dichlorvos vapour in rabbits and rats. Arch. Toxikol. 30: 29-38, 1972.

429 Dicloxacillin

Brown et al. (1968) report briefly that giving 100 mg per kg to rabbits during pregnancy caused no fetal loss or congenital defects.

Brown, D.M.; Harper, K.H.; Palmer, A.K. and Tesh, S.A.: Effect of antibiotics upon the rabbit. Toxicol. Appl. Pharmacol. 12: 295, only, 1968.

430 Dicumarol [Bishydroxycoumarin] (see Coumarin Derivatives)

431 Dicyclomine [see Bendectin-R]

Bendectin-R which consists of equal parts doxylamine succinate, dicyclomine HCl and pyridoxine HCl was given by Gibson et al (1968) in doses of 30 mg per kg per day in the rabbit and 60 mg per kg per day in the rat during organogenesis and no increase in congenital defects was found. In 1976 dicyclomine was removed from the formulation. Numerous epidemiologic studies on Bendectin have been published.

Gibson, J.P.; Staples, R.E.; Larson, E.J.; Kuhn, W.L.; Holtkamp, D.E. and Newberne, J.W.: Teratology and reproduction studies with an antinauseant. Toxicol. Appl. Pharmacol. 13: 439-447, 1968.

432 3,4-Dideoxykanamycin B

432

Koeda and Moriguchi (1973) gave rats and mice doses of 400 and 300 mg per kg respectively and produced no gross or skeletal defects. The doses were given daily during organogenesis by intraperitoneal or intramuscular route.

Koeda, T. and Moriguchi, M.: Teratological studies of 3,4-dideoxykanomycin B (DKB) in rats and mice. Jap. J. Antibiotics 26: 40-48, 1973.

433 Dieldrin (also see Cyclodiene Pesticides)

This chlorinated hydrocarbon pesticide was administered orally to pregnant sows during periods in the last month of gestation. Doses up to 15 mg per kg produced no fetal changes but the compound was detectable in the fetal tissues (Uzoukwu and Sleight, 1972). Oral doses of 4.0 mg per kg per day of this active organochlorine produced no teratogenic effects in mice (Dix et al, 1977).

Dix, K.M.; Van der Pauw, C.L. and McCarthy, W.V.: Toxicity studies with dieldrin: Teratological studies in mice dosed orally with HEOD. Teratology 16:57-62, 1977.

Uzoukwu, M. and Sleight, S.D.: Effects of dieldrin on pregnant sows. J.A.V.M.A. 160: 1641-1643, 1972.

434 1-(2-Diethylaminoethyl)phenobarbital (see Barbituric acid)

435 2-Diethylaminopropiophenone

Cahen et al. (1964) reported that this drug was non-teratogenic in the rat and mouse. The treatment period was during the entire gestation and the dose in the mouse was 16 to 50 mg per kg and in the rat 7 to 20 mg per kg.

Cahen, R.L.; Sautai, M.; Montagne, J. and Pessonnier, J.: Recherche de l'effet teratogene de la 2-diethylamino-propiophenone. Medicine Experimentale 10: 201-224, 1964.

436 N-N-Diethylbenzene Sulfonamide

Leland et al. (1972) administered this proposed mosquito repellant to pregnant rats on days 5 through 10 or 13 of gestation in doses up to 500 mg per kg. The material was given by stomach tube or intraperitoneally. Tail defects, umbilical hernias and reduction defects of the extremities were found, especially following treatment on day 9.

Leland, T.M.; Mendelson, G.F.; Steinberg, M. and Weeks, M.: Studies on the prenatal toxicity and teratology of N-N diethylbenzene sulfonamide. (abstract) Toxicol. Appl. Pharm. 22: 315 only, 1972.

437 Diethylcarbamazine

This antifilariasis drug was tested orally in pregnant rats

at 100 mg per kg from day 8 through 16 and in rabbits at 200 mg per kg on days 8 through 16 and no adverse fetal effects were found. (Fraser, 1972).

Fraser, P.J.: Diethylcarbamazine: lack of teratogenic and abortifacient action in rats and rabbits. Indian J. Med. Res. 60: 1529-1532, 1972.

438   Diethyl-1-(2-4-dichlorophenyl)-2-chlorovinyl Phosphate

Ambrose et al. (1970) fed rats diets with up to 300 PPM of this organophosphate ester pesticide during several generations and found no increase in congenital defects.

Ambrose, A.M.; Larson, P.S.; Borzelleca, J.F. and Hennigar, G.R.: Toxicologic studies on diethyl-1-(2,4-dichlorophenyl)2-chlorovinyl phosphate. Toxicol. Appl. Pharmacol. 17: 323-336, 1970.

439   Di(2,ethylhexyl) Phthalate (see phthalate Esters)

440   1,2-Diethylhydrazine [Hydrazines]

Druckrey (1973) and Druckrey et al (1972) have reviewed the extensive work with the transplacental carcinogenicity of the hydrazines. Twelve to 33 percent of the LD-50 of diethylhydrazine on the 15th day by any route produced postnatally a very high incidence of tumors of the nervous system. Administration before the 11th day produced no tumors. The doses used ranged from 10 to over 50 mg per kg. On the 10th day, the development of the eyes and optic nerves was inhibited completely. Later in gestation hydrocephalus and malformations of the paws was produced. 1-methyL-2-benzyl-Hydrazine also had transplacental carcinogenicity (15-20 mg subcutaneously on the 15th and 21st day).

Druckrey, H.: Specific carcinogenic and teratogenic effects of indirect alkylating methyl and ethyl compounds, and their dependency on stages of ontogenic developments. Xenobiotica 3: 271-303, 1973.

441   Diethyl-0-4-nitrophenyl Phosphorothiote (see Parathion)

442   Diethylnitrosamine

Druckrey (1973) has summarized his work with indirect alkylating compounds. Giving 70 mg per kg intravenously on the 15th day to the rat produced no postnatal tumors but a few were found when the dose was given on the 22nd day. After oral administration a very high incidence of liver carcinomas, nephroblastomas and neurogenic tumors was found postnatally. Dimethylnitrosamine given on the last day of pregnancy produced only a few uncharacteristic tumors. Dimethylnitrosamine was not teratogenic in rats when 30 mg was given orally in single days during gestation (Napalkov and

442

Alexandrov, 1968).

Diethylnitrosamine in doses of 70 mg per kg was not found to be teratogenic in the rat.

Druckrey, H.: Specific carcinogenic and teratogenic effects of indirect alkylating methyl and ethyl compounds, and their dependency on stages of ontogenic developments. Xenobiotica 3: 271-303, 1973.

Napalkov, N.P. and Alexandrov, V.A.: On the effects of blastomogenic substances on the organism during embryogenesis. Z. Krebsforsch 71: 32-50, 1968.

443 Diethylstilbestrol [Stilbestrol-R]

Greene et al. (1940) used this compound and produced feminization of male fetuses but partial retention of wolffian bodies in female fetuses. The maternal rats were treated with a total of 10 to 42 mg from the 12th to 19th gestational day.

Bongiovanni et al. (1959) reported clitoromegaly in female newborns whose mothers were treated with diethylstilbestrol (5 to 50 mg per day during the first trimester).

Herbst et al. (1971) have reported that adenocarcinoma of the vagina occurring in relatively young women was associated in 7 out of 8 instances with Stilbesterol-R treatment of the mother of the patients during the first trimester of pregnancy. A high incidence of benign adenosis of the vagina was found in these girls. The authors comment that their prenatal exposure to the synthetic estrogen may have increased the amount of benign tissue subsequently at risk for malignant change. This is a remarkable delay in teratogenic response and has obvious implications.

Further studies of this problem (Herbst et al, 1975a; Herbst et al, 1975b) based on many more cases indicate that the precancerous vaginal adenosis occurs in 73 percent of women exposed before the 9th week of gestation but in only 7 percent of those exposed after the 17th week. Clear-cell carcinoma has not occurred in women who were exposed in utero after the 18th week. Over 90 percent of the cancers occurred after age 14 years. The total dose of diethyl-stilbestrol received by cancer patients had varied from 1.5 mg to 225 mg. Two other non-steroidal estrogens (dienestrol and hexestrol) may have the same effect. It is estimated that the risk of development of adenocarcinoma after in utero exposure is exceedingly small at least in the population under 25 years. O'Brien et al (1979) in a prospective study of 2,940 intrauterine exposed women found that both time in gestation and amount of administered drug were related to incidence of vaginal adenosis. Exposure starting at 4 weeks was associated with adenosis in 56 percent of the offspring while at 16 and 20 weeks the figure was 30 and 10 percent respectively. The vaginal changes from DES decreased as the age of the exammined woman increased. Not a single subject with clear cell carcinoma was identified from 1,340 participants identified from

record review. Herbst et al (1975a) suggest that the drug
produced adenosis by either inhibiting upward growth of the
vaginal plate or stimulating mullerian epithelium resulting
in its persistence in the developing vagina.

The reproductive histoy of intrauterine exposed women has
been studied by Barnes et al (1980). Miscarriages and
absence of full term infants were significantly more common.
Nineteen percent of these women had no full term infants as
compared to a matched control of 4.9 percent.

Gill et al (1976) studied 134 males exposed in utero and
found that 27 percent had genital lesions (epididymal cysts,
hypotrophic testes or capsular induration of the testes).
In 29 percent pathologic changes were found in spermatozoa.
No signs of malignancy were found.

A Comprehensive review of the experimental models and the
human clinical experience is given by McLachlan and Dixon
(1977).

Barnes, A.B.; Colton, T.; Gundersen, J.; Noller, K.L.;
Tilley, B.C.; Strama, T.; Townsend, D.E.; Hatab, P.;
O'Brien, P.C.: Fertility and outcome of pregnancy in women
exposed in utero to diethylstilbestrol. N. Eng. J.   Med.
302:609-613, 1980.

Bongiovanni, A.M.; DiGeorge, A.M. and Grumbach, M.M.:
Masculinization of the female infant associated with
estrogenic therapy alone during gestation. Four cases.   J.
Clin. Endocrinol. Metab. 19: 1004-1011, 1959.

Gill, W.B.; Schumacher, G.F.B. and Bibbo, M.:   Structural
and functional abnormalities in the sex organs of male offspring of mothers treated with diethylstilbestrol (DES). J.
Reprod. Med. 16:147-153, 1976.

Greene, R.R.; Burrill, M.W. and Ivy, A.C.:   Experimental
intersexuality. The effects of estrogens on the antenatal
sexual development of the rat. Am. J. Anat. 67: 305-345,
1940.

Herbst, A.L.; Ulfelder, H.   and Poskanzer, D.C.:
Adenocarcinoma of the vagina: association of maternal
stilbestrol therapy with tumor appearance in young women.
N. Engl. J. Med. 284: 878-881, 1971.

Herbst, A.L.; Scully, R.E. and Robboy, S.J.:   Effects of
maternal DES ingestion on the female genital tract.
Hospital Practice, October: 51-57, 1975a.

Herbst, A.L.; Poskanzer, D.C.; Robboy, S.J.; Friedlander, L.
and Scully, R.E.:   Prenatal exposure to stilbestrol: A
prospective comparison of exposed female offspring with
unexposed controls. New Eng. J. Med. 292: 334-339,
1975b.

McLachlan, J.A. and Dixon, R.L.: Teratologic comparisons
of experimental and clinical exposures to diethylstilbestrol
during gestation, In, Regulatory Mechanisms Affecting
Research, edited by J. A. Thomas and R.L. Singhal,

University Park Press, Baltimore, 1977, pp. 309-336.

O'Brien, P.C.; Noller, K.L.; Robboy, S.J.; Barnes, A.B.;
Kaufman, R.H.; Tilley, B.C. and Townsend, D.E.: Vaginal
epithelial changes in young women enrolled in the National
Cooperative Diethylstilbestrol Adenosis (DESAD) Project.
Obstet. Gynecol. 53:300-308, 1979.

444 Diethylsulfoxide

Caujolle et al. (1965) were unable to demonstrate teratogenicity in mice, rats or rabbits. The mice were injected
daily during gestation with 2 gm per kg and the rabbits 4 gm
per kg. Celosomia and limb defects were produced in the
chick embryo with as little as 0.1 percent of the LD-100.

Caujolle, F.M.E.; Caujolle, D.H.; Cros, S.B.; Calvet, M.J.
and Tollon, Y.: Pouvoir teratogene du dimethylsulfoxyde et
du diethylsulfoxyde. C. R. Acad. Sci. (d) (Paris) 260:
327-330, 1965.

445 Diethyl-triazene (see 1-Phenyl-3,3 Dimethyl Triazine)

446 Diflucortolone Valerate

Ezumi et al (1977A and B and 1978A and B) made studies of
this steroid in mice, rats and rabbits. No defects were
produced in the rat at 0.1 mg per kg but cleft palate
occurred in the mouse and rabbit fetuses at subcutaneous
doses of 0.01 and 0.05 mg per kg given during organogenesis.
In all 3 species the fetal weight decreased and fetal
mortality increased.

Ezumi, Y.; Tomoyama, J. and Kodama, N.: Effects of
diflucortolone valerate subcutaneously injected into rats in
mid gestation (period of organogenesis) or late gestation on
the pre and postnatal development of their offspring
(Japanese). Yakubutsu Ryoho 10:1357-1365, 1977A.

Ezumi, Y.; Tomoyama, J. and Kadama, N.: Teratogenicity
especially on the formation of cleft palate in mouse embryos
of diflucortolone valerate by a single administration.
(Japanese) Yakubutsu Ryoho 10;1585-1594, 1977B.

Ezumi, Y.; Tomoyama, J. and Kodama, N.: Effects of
diflucortolone valerate subcutaneously injected to mice in
mid gestation (period of organogenesis) or late gestation on
the pre and postnatal development of the offspring.
Yakubutsu Ryoho 11: 237-256, 1978A.

Ezumi, Y.; Tomoyama, J. and Kodama, N.:Effects of
diflucortolone valerate subcutaneously injected to rabbits
in midgestation on the prenatal development of their offspring. (Japanese) Yakabutsu Ryoho 11:229-236, 1978B.

447 Diflunisol (5-(2,4 difluorophenyl) Salicylic acid)

Nakatsuka and Fujii (1979) treated rats orally with up to 100 mg per kg on days 7 through 17. The dams gained less weight than controls but no adverse fetal effects were found.

Nakatsuka, T.; Fujii, T.: Comparative teratogenicity study of diflunisol (MK-647) and aspirin in the rat. Oyo Yakuri 17: 551-557, 1979.

448 Difolatan-R   [N-Tetrachloroethyl-
thio-4-cyclohexene-1-2-dicarboximide]

Verrett et al. (1969) injected 3 to 20 mg per kg into the air cell or yolk sac of the chick egg before incubation and found 6.7 percent abnormal embryos. The defects included those of the central nervous and skeletal system with phocomelia and amelia being particularly noteworthy. The epoxide form was even more teratogenic.

Verrett, M.J.; Mutchler, M.K.; Scott, W.F.; Reynaldo, E.F. and McLaughlin, J.: Teratogenic effects of captan and related compounds in the developing chicken embryo. Ann. N. Y. Acad. Sci. 160: 334-343, 1969.

449 Digitalis

Many human pregnancies in which digitalis has been used are complicated by heart failure and the use of other drugs, particularly warfarin. Laros et al (1970) reviewed 24 pregnancies associated with heart prostheses and except for the presence of two infants with warfarin embryopathy, the offspring were healthy.

Laros, R.K.; Hage, M.L. and Hayashi, R.H.: Pregnancy and heart valve prostheses. Obst. Gynecol. 35:241-247, 1970.

450 Digoxin

Singh and Mirkin (1978) demonstrated that digoxin crosses the rat fetal placenta.

Nagaoka et al (1976) gave up to 1.75 mg of methyldigoxin orally to rats on days 7 through 17. Except for variation in lumbar ribs at 0.5 mg per kg, no fetal changes occurred. In the rabbit, the same workers found an increase in fetal lethality at 10 mg per kg when the drug was given orally. There were no other adverse fetal changes.

Hatano, M.: Reproduction studies of beta-methyldigoxin 1. Teratogenicity study in rats. (Japanese). Clinical Report 10:579-593, 1976.

Nagaoka, T.; Osuka, F.; Shigemura, T. and Hatano, M.: Teratogenicity test of beta-methyldigoxin (Beta-MD) (Japanese) Clinical Report 10:405-411, 1976.

Singh, S. and Mirkin, B.L.: Placental transfer and tissue localization of digoxin in the pregnant rat. Toxicol.

450

Appl.   Pharm.   46: 395-403, 1978.

451   5,11-Dihydro-11-[(4-methyl-1-piperazinyl)acetyl]6H-pyrido
       [2,3-B] [1,4] benzodiazepin-6-on Dihydrochloride

       This antigastric ulcer drug was given in oral doses as high
       as 1000 mg to rats and 125 mg to rabbits during pregnancy
       and although maternal toxicity occurred no teratogenicity
       was found (Iida, et al, 1975).

       Iida, H.; Kast, A. and Tsunenari, Y.: Reproductive studies
       of   5,11-dihydro-11-[(4-methyl-
       -1-piperazinly)acetyl]-6H-pyrido   [2,3-b   b]   [1,4]
       benzodiazepin-6-dihydrochloride (LS519Cl(2)) on rats and
       rabbits 1. Teratological study.   Oyo Yakuri 9: 377-386,
       1975.

452   Dihydrostreptomycin (also see Streptomycin)

       The dihydro form of streptomycin has been injected into rats
       and mice at 200 to 800 mg per kg daily during pregnancy
       (Suzuki and Takeuchi, 1969).   The 800 mg dose level was
       lethal in all the mothers and lower doses caused reduction
       in fetal size.   A large number of surviving fetuses were
       tested and responded to sound.

       Varpela et al.   (1969) found normal hearing in 50 children
       who   were   exposed   in utero to dihydrostreptomycin or
       streptomycin.

       Suzuki, Y.   and Takeuchi, S.:   Etude experimentale sur
       l'influence de la streptomycine sur l'appareil audit du
       foetus apres administration de doses variees a la mere
       enceinte. Keio J. Med. 10: 31-41, 1961.

       Varpela, E.; Hietalahti, J. and Aro, M.J.T.: Streptomycin
       and dihydrostreptomycin medication during pregnancy and
       their effect on the child's inner ear. Scand. J. Resp.
       Dis. 50: 101-109, 1969.

453   Diisopropyl Phosphofluoridate (see DFP)

454   Dilantin-R (see Diphenylhydantoin)

455   Diltiazem Hydrochloride

       This coronary dilator was injected intraperitoneally during
       organogenesis in pregnant mice, rats and rabbits (Ariyuki,
       1975).   At 80 mg and 12.5 mg per kg respectively in rats and
       rabbits, malformations of the limbs and tail were found.   No
       malformations occurred in the mouse.

       Ariyuki, F.:   Effects of diltiazem hydrochloride on
       embryonic   development: species   differences   in   the
       susceptibility and stage specificity in mice, rats and
       rabbits. Okajimas Fol. Anat. Jap. 52:103-107, 1975.

456 Dimenhydrinate

McColl et al. (1965) reported no teratogenic effect of 75 mg per kg per day of this material fed during the entire pregnancy of the rat.

McColl, J.D.; Globus, M. and Robinson, S.: Effect of some therapeutic agents in the developing rat fetus. Toxicol. Appl. Pharmacol. 7: 409-417, 1965.

457 Dimercaprol [2,3-Dimercapto-1-propanol] [BAL]

Nishimura and Takagaki (1959) injected mice subcutaneously with 0.001 ml per gm of body weight once on the 9th, 11th or 12th day of gestation. Reduction defects of the fetal extremities occurred in many of the fetuses with the highest incidence (69 percent) following treatment on the 12th day. A few cases of cleft palate and brain hernia were reported.

Nishimura, H. and Takagaki, S.: Developmental anomalies in mice induced by 2,3-dimercaptopropanol (bal). Anat. Rec. 135: 261-268, 1959.

458 Dimetacrine [Istonyl-R]

Aoyama et al (1970) administered this compound orally to rats in amounts up to 100 mg per kg and found no teratogenicity. Taoka et al (1971) gave the compound intraperitoneally to rats and mice in maximum doses of 60 and 90 mg per kg respectively and found no adverse fetal effects.

Aoyama, J.; Nakai, K.; Ogura, M.; Saito, K. and Iwaki, R.: Acute toxicity and teratological studies of dimetacrine in mice and rats. Oyo Yakuri 4: 855-869, 1970.

Taoka, K.; Nakamura, T.; Mitarai, H.; Tsuchiya, S. and Honda, K.: Teratological studies on demetracine. Oyo Yakuri 5: 129-139, 1971.

459 N-(3-4-dimethoxycinnamoyl)anthranilic Acid

Nakazawa et al (1978) found no effect of 600 mg per kg given orally to rats on days 7 through 17. No adverse effects on the rabbit fetus were observed after oral doses of 750 mg per kg on days 6 through 18. (Iwadare et al, 1978).

Nakazawa, M.; Ooba, M.; Imai, K. and Iwadare, M.: Effects of N-(3-4-dimethoxycinnamoyl)anthranilic acid (N-5) administered orally on reproductive performance of rats 2. Teratogenicity test. (Japanese) Iyakuhin Kenkyu 9:161-172, 1978.

Iwadare, M.; Ooba, M.; Tsukamoto, T.; Imai, K. and Nakazawa, M.: Effects of N-(3-4-dimethoxycinnamoyl) anthranilic acid (N-5) administered orally on reproductive performance in rabbits. Teratogenicity test. (Japanese) Iyakuhin Kenkyu 9:187-193, 1978.

460

460 Dimethylacetamide

Thiersch (1971) found that giving pregnant rats 1.5 ml per
kg on gestational day 4 or 7 led to over 60 percent
resorptions. The survivors were stunted but no defects were
found. Painting the tails for weekly periods caused no
effect on the litters.

Thiersch, J.B.: Investigations into the differential effect
of compounds on rat litter and mother. In,
Tuchmann-Duplessis. H. (ed.): Malformations Congenitales
Des Mammiferes. Paris: Masson et Cie, 1971. pp 95-113.

461 0,0-Dimethyl-s-(2-acetylaminoethyl) Dithiophosphate

Hashimoto et al (1972) gave this pesticide to mice orally in
maximal daily doses of 40 mg per kg from day zero through
day 14 of gestation and found no increase in defects but
some reduction in fetal survival was seen at the highest
dose.

Hashimoto, Y.; Makita, T. and Noguchi, T.: Teratogenic
studies of 0,0-dimethyl-S-(2-acetylaminoethyl)
dithiophosphate (DAEP) in ICR strain mice. Oyo Yakuri 6:
621-626, 1972.

462 Dimethylaminoazobenzene (see Aminoazobenzene)

463 3-Dimethylamino-7-methyl-1-2-[N-propylmalonyl[-1-,2-dihydro-
-1,2,4 4 benzotriazine [Azapropazone - Dihydrate]
[Prolixan-R]

Adrian (1973) found no fetal changes in the offspring of
rats treated with 100 mg per kg per day during the entire
period of pregnancy.

Adrian, R.W.: Reproduktionstoxikolische unter such ungen
mit azapropazon an ratten. Arzneim Forsch 23: 658-660,
1973.

464 7-12-Dimethylbenz-(a)-anthracene [DMBA]

This potent carcinogen which has adrenolytic properties has
been shown to be teratogenic in the rat (Currie et al.;
1970). Injection of 25 mg per kg on day 8 or 13 produced a
high incidence of incomplete neural tube closure and other
defects in the fetuses. Also, cleft palate, eye and kidney
defects were found. A monohydroxymethyl product of
metabolism of DMBA, 7-hydroxymethyl-12-methyl-
benz(a)anthracene was teratogenic, but two other products
lacking adrenolytic acitivity were non-teratogenic. For
adrenolytic and teratogenic activity benz(a)anthracene must
possess two active side chains situated at C-7 and C-12; an
active methyl group at C-12 was mandatory and at C-7 one of
several substitutions was possible. Currie et al. (1970)
report that if the maternal adrenal is inhibited at the time
of exposure to these compounds teratogenicity is abolished.

Lambert and Nebert (1977) using this compound and 3-methyl-
cholanthrene at doses of 25-50 mg and 70 mg per kg
respectively on single days between day 7 and 13 in the
mouse produced stillbirths and resorptions in mouse strains
whose bioactivating liver systems were inducible. A few
malformations, mostly club foot, were found.

Lambert, G.H. and Nebert, D.W.: Genetically mediated
induction of drug-metabolized enzymes associated with congenital defects in the mouse. Teratoloy 16: 147-154, 1977.

Currie, A.R.; Bird, C.C.; Crawford, A.M. and Sims, P.:
Embryopathic effects of 7,12-dimethylbenz(a)anthracene and
its hydroxymethyl derivatives in the Sprague-Dawley rat.
Nature 226: 911-914, 1970.

465   2,5-Dimethylbenzimidazole (see Benzimidazole)

466   1,1-Dimethylbiguamide (see Metformin)

467   0,0-Dimethyl-0-cyanophenyl Phosphorothioate

Yamamoto et al (1972) gave this compound orally to rats from
the 9th through the 14th day. The maximum doses of 10 mg
per kg produced no fetal changes.

Yamamoto, H.; Yano, I.; Nishino, H.; Furuta, H. and Masuda,
M.: Teratological studies on Cynox-R in rats. (Japanese)
Oyo Yakuri 6: 523-528, 1972.

468   Dimethyldioxane

Smirnov et al (1978) treated rats for 4 months with 0.01 and
0.004 mg per cubic meter of this substance and found a
prolongated oestrus phase and slight embryolethal effect.
Treatment during gestation with the same doses caused both
pre- and postimplantation embryonic death.

Smirnov, V.T.; Dubrovskaya, F.I. and Kiseleva, T.I.:
Action of dimethyldioxane on the generative function of
experimental animals. Gigiena i Sanitariya (USSSR) 9:16-18,
1978.

469   Dimethylforamide

Thiersch (1971) reports that unlike methylforamide 0.5 to
2.0 ml of dimethylforamide per kg had no litter effects in
the rat.

Thiersch, J.B.: Investigations into the differential effect
of compounds on rat litter and mother. In,
Tuchmann-Duplessis (ed.): Malformations Congenitales Des
Mammiferes. Paris: Masson and Cie, 1971. pp 95-113.

470   1,1-Dimethyl-5-methoxy-3-(dithien-2-ylmethyl-

ene)-piperidinium bromi

Fujisawa et al (1973) gave this drug intraperitoneally and orally to pregnant mice and rats during organogenesis. Orally the maximum doses were 160 mg per kg daily. The maximum intraperitoneal dose was 40 mg per kg per day in mice and 20 mg per kg per day in rats. No increase in defects was found and no post-natal differences were observed in the 4 week post-natal study.

Fujisawa, Y.; Fujii, T.M. and Kowa, Y.: The effects of 1,1dimethyl-5-methoxy-3-(dithien-2-ylmethylene) piperidinium Bromide (SA-504) upon offsprings of mice and rats administered maternally during critical period of pregnancy. (Japanese) Oyo Yakuri 7: 1293-1304, 1973.

471 3-3-Dimethyl-1-phenyl-triazene (Triazene)

Murphy et al. (1957) summarized theiir work with this compound in the chick and the rat. Skeletal defects in the chick were reversed partially by nicotinamide. Treatment at 11 days in the rat produced major skeletal defects and at 12 days cleft palate and absence of the mandible became predominant. The single daily dose was 30 mg per kg.

Murphy, J.L.; Dagg, C.P. and Karnofsky, D.A.: Comparison of teratogenic chemicals in the rat and chick embryos: An exhibit with additions for publication. Pediatrics 19: 701-714, 1957.

472 Dimethyl-0-4-nitrophenyl Phosphorothioate (see Methyl Parathion)

473 2-Dimethylsulfamido-10-(2-dimethylaminopropyl)phenothiazine

Tanaka and Matsuura (1970) gave this antihistamine to pregnant rabbits from day 8 through 16 of gestation in doses up to 60 mg per kg per day and observed no teratogenicity.

Tanaka, O. and Matsuura, M.: Effect of 8599RP administered to pregnant rabbits on pre- and post-natal development of their offspring. Oyo Yakuri 4: 373-379, 1970.

474 Dimethyl Sulfoxide [DMSO]

Ferm (1966) using hamsters reported that DMSO injected on the 8th ay day (0.5 to 8.0 gm per kg) of gestation produced exencephaly in a high proportion of fetuses. Rib fusions, microphthalmia, limb abnormalities and cleft lip were found also. Thiersch (1971) using 4.0 ml per kg on days 4 and 5 or tail painting on days 11 through 18 caused no defects in rat fetuses. Caujolle et al. (1967) could produce only a few defects using 8 gm per kg in the mouse and rat. When they used 10 to 12 mg per egg, a 22 percent incidence of limb defects was seen in chicks. At doses between 10 and 30 gm per kg, Juma and Staples (1967) found increased resorptions in the rat.

474

Bariljak et al (1978) showed that the peritoneal injection
of 5.0 ml per kg on 13-day rat pregnancy reduced teratogenic
and embryolethal action of pyrimethamine (50 mg per kg).

Bariljak, I.R.; Neumerzhitskaja, L.V. and Turkevich, A.N.:
Studies on the antimutagenic and antiteratogenic
characteristics of dimexide (DMSO). Tsitol. i Genet.
(USSR) 12:50-56, 1978.

Caujolle, F.M.E.; Caujolle, D.H.; Cros, S.B. and Calvet,
M.J.: Limits of toxic and teratogenic tolerance of dimethyl
sulfoxide. Ann. N. Y. Acad. Sci. 141: 110-125, 1967.

Ferm, V.H.: Congenital malformations induced by dimethyl
sulphoxide in the golden hamster. J. Embryol. Exp.
Morphol. 16: 49-54, 1966.

Juma, M.B. and Staples, R.E.: Effect of maternal administration of dimethylsulfoxide on the development of rat
fetuses. Proc. Soc. Exp. Biol. Med. 125:567-569,1967.

Thiersch, J.B.: Investigations into the differential effect
of compounds on rat litter and mother. In,
Tuchmann-Duplessis, H. (ed.): Malformations Congenitales
Des Mammiferes. Paris: Masson et Cie, 1971. pp 95-113.

475 N,N-Dimethylthiourea (see Ethylenethiourea)

476 5-(3,3-Dimethyl-1-triazeno)imidazole-4-carboxamide

Chaube (1973) studied rats by giving this antineoplastic
compound intraperitoneally in doses of 200 to 1000 mg per
kg. On days 11 or 12 a single dose of 800 or 1000 mg per kg
produced skeletal reduction defects and some cleft palates
and encephaloceles.

Chaube, S.: Protective effects of thymidine, 5-amino-
imidazolecarboxamide and riboflavin against fetal abnormalities produced in rats by 5-(3,3-dimethyl-
-1-triazeno)imidazole-4-carboxamide. Cancer Res. 33:
2231-2240, 1973.

477 Dimethyl Tubocurarine Chloride (see Tubocurarine)

478 Dinitrophenol

Goldman and Yakovac (1964) produced fetal growth inhibition
but no defects in rat fetuses after maternal doses of 8 to
40 mg per kg on gestational days 9, 10 or 11. Gibson (1973)
used the compound orally (38.3 mg per kg) and
intraperitoneally (13.6 mg per kg) on days 10 through 12 in
the mouse and found no teratogenic action.

Gibson, J.E.: Teratology studies in mice with 2-sec-butyl-
-4,6-dinitrophenol (dinoseb). Food Cosmet. Toxicol. 11:
31-43, 1973.

478

Goldman, A.S. and Yakovac, W.C.: Salicylate intoxication and congenital anomalies. Arch. Environ. Health 8: 648-656, 1964.

479 Dioctyl Sodium Sulfosuccinate and 1,8-dihydroxy anthraquinone (Solven, Danthron)

Ichikawa and Yamamoto (1980) fed this laxative combination to rats on days 7-17 in doses of up to 800 mg per kg. At the highest dose viability of the fetuses was decreased. No other ill effects were found.

Ichikawa, Y.; Yamamoto, Y.: Teratology study of solven in rats. Gendai Iryo 12:819-831, 1980.

480 Dinoseb (2-sec-butyl-4,6-dinobrophenol)

This herbicide was administered orally, subcutaneously or intraperitoneally to mice in doses of up to 20 mg per kg per day. Doses over 17.7 to 20 mg per kg were toxic to the mother. Several time schedules during organogenesis were employed. At 17.7 mg per kg doses by the intraperitoneal and subcutaneous route, malfomations were found. These included skeletal defects, cleft palate, hydrocephalus and adrenal agenis. Oral administration produced no gross or soft tissue defects but some skeletal defects were seen at maternally toxic levels.

Gibson and Rao (1973) have studied the herbicides distribution in the pregnant mouse.

McCormack et al (1980) studied postnatal renal function in rats exposed on days 10-12 of gestation by maternal intraperitoneal injection of 16 mg per kg. The dilated tubules and pelves seen in the neonatal period were not found or reduced by 42 days postnatally and renal function was normal. Beaudoin and Fisher (1981) administered 10 mg per kg intraperitoneally on day 9 of rat pregnancy and studied the embryos in vitro after day 10. Little or no effect was observed on growth and development of the embryos.

Beaudoin, A.R.; Fisher, D.L.: An in vivo - in vitro evaluation of teratogenic action. Teratology 23:57-61, 1981.

Gibson, J.E.: Teratology studies in mice with 2-sec-butyl-4, 6-dinitrophenol (dinoseb). Fd. Cosmet. Toxicol. 11:31-34, 1973.

Gibson, J.E.; Rao, K.S.: Disposition of 2-sec-b3tyl-4, dinitro- phenol (dinoseb), Fd. Cosmet. Toxicol. 11:45-52, 1973.

McCormack, K.M.; Abuelgasim, A.; Sanger, V.L.; Hook, J.B.: Postnatal morphology and functional capacity of the kidney following prenatal treatment with dinoseb in rats. J. Toxicol. Environ. Health 6:633-643, 1980.

481   Dioxin (see 2,3,7,8-Tetrachlorodibenzo-p-dioxin)

482   1,2-bis(3,5-dioxopiperazine-1-yl)propane (1CRF-159)

Duke (1975) reported studies of this chemotherapeutic agent
in mice, rats and rabbits. At these doses some malformations occurred in the rat offspring and these included eye,
brain and skeletal defects as well as cleft palate. The
most sensitive time of administration was the period of day
6 through 8. The offspring of the mice were retarded in
growth.

Duke, D.I.: Prenatal effects of the cancer chemotherapeutic
drug 1CRF159 in mice, rats and rabbits. Teratology 11:
119-126, 1975.

483   Diphenylamine

Crocker and Vernier (1970) fed a diet of 2.5 percent
diphenylamine to rats during the last 6 days of pregnancy
and produced cystic dilitation of the renal collecting ducts
and degeneration of the proximal tubules in the fetuses.
Tube feeding of 2 ml of a 1 percent solution also produced
the fetal kidney changes.

Crocker, J.F.S. and Vernier, R.L.: Chemically induced
polycystic disease in the newborn. (abstract) Pediatr.
Res. 4: 448, only, 1970.

484   4,5 Diphenyl-2-bis-(2-hydroxyethyl)aminooxazol (see Ditazol)

485   Diphenylhydantoin

The offspring of epileptic mothers treated with
diphenylhydantoin have been reported to have about twice the
expected rate of congenital defects (Janz and Fuchs, 1964;
Speidel and Meadow, 1972; Fedrick, 1973; Monson, et al,
1973). The type of defect encountered has included cleft
lip and palate, congenital heart disease and microcephaly.
Czeizel studied medications ingested by mothers of babies
with cleft lip and-or palate and found 11 out of 413 (2.7
percent) had taken phenytoins. Hypoplasia of the nails and
distal phalanges may represent a specific malformation in as
many as 18 percent of pregnancies associated with this drug.
(Barr et al, 1974; Hill, et al, 1974). This type of defect
tends to become less noticeable with age and it could be
easily overlooked in the newborn (Hanson and Smith, 1975).
Hanson, et al (1976) drawing on a Seattle study and the
records of the Collaborative Perinatal Project of the
National Institute of Neurological and Communication
Disorders and Stroke, emphasize that while only 11 percent
of exposed offspring have the hydantoin syndrome, three
times as many have impairment of performance, especially
intellectual.

Some reports have indicated no increase in malformation
after dilantin exposure and these studies tended to be more

prospective rather than retrospective in nature. Goujard et al (1974) in a study of their own and a review of five prospective studies could find no increase in malformations. Meyer (1973) studied retrospectively 199 children born of mothers treated with antiepileptics and could not establish any proof of teratogenic activity. Livingston et al (1973) also had negative findings. Other factors associated with chronic seizure conditions may contribute to a slight increase in malformations. Many malformations probably have a multifactorial etiology; the role of folic acid deficiency and genetic predisposition need to be more thoroughly studied here. Shapiro et al (1976) drawing on the Collaborative Perinatal Project in the United States and a large Finnish registry, recorded an increase in malformations in the offspring when either the mother or father was epileptic and suggested that the increased rate was not due only to drug exposure. Based on 701 at-risk parents, the defect rate was 10.5 percent when the mother was epileptic as compared to 8.3 when the father was affected and 6.4 when neither parent was affected. The Committee on Drugs of the American Academy of Pediatrics (1979) in a recent review gives sound recommendations useful to those advising pregnant women with epilepsy.

Mirkin (1971) has shown that diphenylhydantoin equilibrates across the human placenta at term and when the fetus is 8 to 10 cm in crown-rump length.

Cancers derived from neural crest cells appear to be more common than expected in children exposed to diphenylhydantoin. At least 4 cases are reported in the literature (Ehrenbard and Chaganti, 1981.

Harbinson and Becker (1969) used 75 to 150 mg per kg in mice on days 8 through 13 and produced cleft lip and palate, ectrodactyly and minor skeletal defects. Hydronephrosis and internal hydrocephalus was found in those fetuses treated on day 9. Open eye was common in fetuses exposed on day 8. Elshove (1969) produced cleft palate in mice also and wondered if the mechanism of action was through folic acid deficiency induced by the drug. Schardein, et al (1973) could not prevent cleft palate in diphenylhydantoin-treated mice by giving folinic acid to 100 mg per kg. Khera found embryolethality in the rat given 2 mg per kg.

Finnell (1981) studied several strains of mice including one type with seizures (quaker) and found that the malformation rate correlated with both the dose and blood level of the drug. In the rabbit doses of 75 and 100 mg per kg per day were teratogenic (McClain and Langhoff, 1980). Cleft palate and limb defects were found.

Barr, M.; Pozanski, A.K. and Schmickel, R.D.: Digital hypoplasia and anticonvulsants during gestation, a teratogenic syndrome. J. Pediat. 4: 254-256, 1974.

Committee on Drugs: American Academy of Pediatrics: Anticonvulsants and pregnancy. Pediatrics 63: 331-333, 1979.

Czeizel, A.: Diazepam, phenytoin and etiology of cleft lip and-or palate. Lancet 1: 81, only, 1976.

Ehrenbard, L.T.; Chaganti, R.S.K.: Cancer in the fetal hydantoin syndrome. Lancet 2:97, only, 1981.

Elshove, J.: Cleft palate in the offspring of female mice treated with phenytoin. Lancet 2: 1074, only, 1969.

Fedrick, J.: Epilepsy and pregnancy: A report from Oxford record linkage study. Brit. Med. J. 2: 442-448, 1973.

Finnell, R.H.: Phenytoin-induced teratogenesis: A mouse model. Science 211:483-484, 1981.

Goujard, J.; Huel, G. and Rumeau-Rouquette, C.: Antiepileptiques et malformations congenitales. J. Gyn. Obst. Biol. Repr. 8: 831-842, 1974.

Hanson, J.W. and Smith, D.W.: The fetal hydantoin syndrome. J. Pediat. 87: 285-290, 1975.

Hanson, J.W.; Myrianthopoulos, N.C.; Harvey, M.A.S. and Smith,D.W.: Risks to the offspring of women treted with hydantoin anticonvulsants, with emphasis on the fetal hydantoin syndrome. J. Pediat. 89: 662-668, 1976.

Harbinson, R.D. and Becker, B.A.: Relation of dosage and time of administration of diphenylhydantoin to its terato-genic effect in mice. Teratology 2: 305-312, 1969.

Hill, R.M.; Verniaud, W.M.; Horning, M.G.; McCulley, L.B. and Morgan, N.F.: Infants exposed in utero to antiepileptic drugs. Am. J. Dis. Child. 127: 645-653, 1974.

Janz, D. and Fuchs, U.: Sind Antiepileptische Medikamente wahrend der Schwangerschaft Schadlich. Dtsch. Med. Wochenschr. 89: 241-243, 1964.

Khera, K.S.: Teratogenicity study of hydroxyurea and diphenylhydantoin in the rat. Teratology 20:447-452, 1970.

Livingston, S.; Berman, W. and Pauli, L.: Maternal epilepsy and abnormalities of the fetus and newborn. Lancet 2: 1265 (only), 1973.

McClain, R.M.; Langhoff, L.: Teratogenicity of diphenylhydantoin in the New Zealand white rabbit. Teratology 21:371-379, 1980.

Meadow, S.R.: Congenital abnormalities and anticonvulsant drugs. Proc. R. Soc. Med. 63: 48-49, 1970.

Meyer, J.G.: The teratological effects of anticonvulsants and the effects on pregnancy and birth. Europ. Neurol. 10: 179-190, 1973.

Mirkin, B.L.: Diphenylhydantóin: Placental transport, fetal localization, neonatal metabolism and possible teratogenic effects. J. Pediatr. 78: 329-337, 1971.

Monson, R.R.; Rosenberg, L.; Hartz, S.C.; Shapiro, S.; Heinonen, O.P. and Slone, D.: Diphenylhydantoin and selected malformations. New Eng. J. Med. 289: 1049-1052,

485

1973.

Schardein, J.L.; Dresher, A.J.; Hentz, D.L.; Petrere, J.A.; Fitzgerald, J.E. and Kurtz, S.M.: The modifying effect of folinic acid on diphenylhydantoin-induced teratogenicity in mice. Toxicol. Appl. Pharm. 24: 150-158, 1973.

Shapiro, S.; Hartz, S.C.; Siskind, V.; Mitchell, A.A.; Slone, D.; Rosenberg, L.; Monson, R.R.; Heinonen, O.P.; Idanpaan-Heikkila, J.; Haro, S. and Saxen, L.: Anticonvulsants and parental epilepsy in the development of birth defects. Lancet 1:272-275, 1976.

Speidel, B.D. and Meadow, S.R.: Maternal epilepsy and abnormalities of the fetus and newborn. Lancet 2: 839-843, 1972.

486 Diphenhydramine HCl

Heinonen et al (1977) reported no significant increase in congenital defects among the offspring of 595 women who used the drug in the first 4 lunar months of their gestation.

This antihistamine was given to rats and rabbits and no defects were produced (Schardein et al.; 1971). The compound was given orally in amounts of 15 to 20 mg per kg during active organogenesis. Saxen (1975) reported that a concentration of 1 microgm per ml delayed fusion of explanted mouse palatal shelves.

Heinonen, O.P.; Slone, D.; Shapiro, S.: Birth Defects and Drugs in Pregnancy. Publishing Sciences Group, Inc., 1977.

Saxen, I.: Etiological variables in oral clefts. Proceedings of the Finnish Dental Society. 71: Suppl. 3, 3-40, 1975.

Schardein, J.L.; Hentz, D.L.; Petrere, J.A. andd Kurtz, S.M.: Teratogenesis studies with diphenhydramine HCl. Toxicol. Appl. Pharmacol. 18: 971-976, 1971.

487 Dipropylacetate, Sodium (DPA)

Esaki et al (1975) administered orally 200 and 400 mg per kg to pregnant monkeys on days 23 through 35. Two of the three pregnancies treated at 400 mg terminated with dead fetuses while the three pregnancies at 200 mg were not altered.

Esaki, K.; Tanioka, Y.; Ogata, T. and Koizumi, H.: Influence of sodium dipropylacetate (DPA) on the fetuses of the Rhesus monkey. (Japanese) CIEA Preclin. Rpt. 1:157-164, 1975.

488 Dipterex (0,0-Dimethyl-1-hydroxy-2,2,2- trichloroethyl-phosphonate)

This organophosphate insecticide was given by gavage or in the diet to rats on days 6 through 15 (Staples et al, 1976).

488

With gavage at 145 mg per kg per day, malformations of the skull and brain occurred in the fetus as well as skeletal and palate defects. In the diet experiment, 75 mg per kg did not cause malformations. Martson and Voronina (1976) gave 80 mg per kg on day 9 and produced open eye and exencephaly in the rat fetus. Eight mg per kg throughout gestation caused no malformation increase.

Martson, L.V. and Voronina, V.M.: Experimental study of the effect of a series of phosphoroorganic pesticides (dipterex and imidan) on embryogenesis. Envir. Health Persp. 13: 121-125, 1976.

Staples, R.E.; Kellam, R.G. and Haseman, J.K.: Developmental toxicity in the rat after ingestion or gavage of organophosphate pesticides (dipterex, imidan) during pregnancy. Envir. Health Persp. 13: 133-140, 1976.

489 2,2 Dipyridyl

This chelator for ferrous iron was given intraperitoneally to rats on days 11.5 through 14.5 in doses of 60 to 75 mg per kg. (Oohira and Nogami, 1978). Skeletal defects especially of the limbs were found.

Oohira, A. and Nogami, H.: Limb anomalies produced by 2,2 dipyridyl in rats. Teratology 18: 63-70, 1978.

490 Diquat [1,1-Ethylene-2,2-dipyridilium Dibromide]

Khera et al. (1970) reported studies on this herbecide. Pregnant rats were injected with 7 or 14 mg per kg on one of several days during organogenesis. Maternal death occurred often with the higher dose. Skeletal defect of the sternum and lack of ossification or absence of one of the auditory occicles were detected in some fetuses. Using repeated intraperitoneal injections of 0.5 mg per kg daily no terato-genic effects were found.

Khera, K.S.; Whitta, L.L. and Clegg, D.J.: Embryopathic effects of diquat and paraquat in rats. In, Pesticides Symposia. Inter-American Conference on Toxicology and Occupational Medicine, 1970. pp 257-261.

491 Disodium Etidronate

Nolen and Buehler (1971) tested this material in pregnant rats and rabbits and found no evidence of teratogenicity. The rats were given 500 mg per kg per day.

Nolen, G.A. and Buehler, E.U.: The effects of disodium etidronate on the reproductive functions and embryology of albino rats and New Zealand rabbits. Toxicol. Appl. Pharmacol. 18: 548-561, 1971.

492 Disopyramide phosphate

This drug was given intravenously to rats before, during or at the end of pregnancy in doses of up to 30 mg per kg and no adverse effects were observed (Umemura et al, 1981). In the rabbit intravenous doses of up to 11 mg per kg had no adverse effect during organogenesis. (Esaki and Yanagita, 1981).

Esaki, K.; Yanagita, T.: Effects of intravenous administration of disopyramide phosphate on the rabbit fetus. Preclin. Rep. Cent Inst. Exp. Animal. 7:189-198, 1981.

Umemura, T.; Sasa, H.; Esaki, K.; Suzuki, S.; Unagami, S.; Yanagita, T.: Effects of disopyramide phosphate on reproduction in rats. Preclin. Rept. Cent. Inst. Exp. Animal 7:157-173, 1981.

493 Disulfiram [Antabuse-R]

Rats fed 100 mg daily from day 3 were found to have 88 percent resorptions on day 13 (Salgo and Oster 1974). Surviving fetuses had no gross malformations as also reported by Robens (1969). The mechanism of embryotoxicity is believed to be via copper chelation but excess dietary copper was not used to reverse the resorption effect. Veghelyi et al (1978) found that ethanol (4 ml) followed by disulfiram (150 mg per kg) in the pregnant rat on day 4 through day 13 was associated with a 65 percent resorption rate, reduced fetal weight and skeletal retardation. No comment on defects in the offspring was given. Based upon one patient with elevated acetaldehyde they postulated that the fetal alcohol syndrome might occur in women with acetaldehyde levels over 30 micromolar.

Favre-Tissot and Delatour (1965) reported that among 5 women treated with disulfiram and tranquilizers during pregnancy there were two offspring with club foot and one spontaneous miscarriage. They also administered up to 400 mg per kg to rats on days 5 through 10 and produced no increase in fetal anomalies.

Favre-Tissot, M. and Delatour, P.: Psycopharmacologie et teratogenese a propos du sulfirame: Essai experimental. (French) Annales Medico-psychogiques 1:735-740, 1965.

Robens, J.F.: Teratologic studies of carbaryl diazionin, norea, disulfiram and thiram in small laboratory animals. Toxicol. Appl. Pharmacol. 15: 152-163, 1969.

Salgo, M.P. and Oster, G.: Fetal resorption induced by disulfiram in rats. J. Reprod. Fert. 39: 375-377, 1974.

Veghelyi, P.V.; Osztovics, M.; Kardos, G.; Leisztner, L.; Szaszovszky, S.I.; Imprei, J.: The fetal alcohol syndrome: symptoms and pathogenesis. Acta Paed. Acad. Scient. Hung. 19:171-189, 1978.

494 Ditazol (4,5-Diphenyl-2-bis(2-hydroxy-ethyl)aminoxazol)

494

Caprino et al (1973) gave this antiinflammatory compound to
pregnant mice, rats and rabbits during active organogenesis
and except for mild growth failure in the rat, found no
fetal changes.

Caprino, L.; Borrelli, F. and Falchetti, R.: Toxicological
investigation of 4,5-diphenyl-2-bis (2-hydroxyethyl)-amino-
xazol (Ditazol or S222). Arzneim Forsch 23:1287-1291, 1973.

495 2,2-Dithio-bis-(pyridine-1-oxide)   (see Magnesium Sulfate
Adduct)

496 Dithiocarbamate [Maneb-R] [Zineb-R]

This fungicide in its manganese or zinc form was given
orally to rats in doses of 2 to 4 gm per kg on days 11 or 13
and a high incidence of neural tube closure defects, cleft
lip and palate and skeletal defects resulted. These dose
levels are at least one-half the LD-50 maternal dose. Below
0.5 gm per kg no defects occurred. They also studied the
effect of inhalation of 100 mg of zineb per cubic meter for
4 hours per day after implantation through the end of
gestation and found no adverse fetal effects. Larsson et al
found teratogenic effects in the rat treated by gavage with
770 mg per kg on day 11 but in the mouse treated on day 9 or
13 with up to 1420 mg per kg, no fetal changes occurred.
They studied two other related pesticides, mancozeb and
propineb, in mice and rats. No teratogenicity was found in
mice but at 1320 mg per kg for mancozeb and 230 mg per kg
for propineb, teratogenic activity was found.

Larsson, K.S.; Arnander, C.; Cvekanova, E. and Kjellberg,
M.: Studies of teratogenic effects of the dithiocarbamates
maneb, mancozeb and propineb. Teratology 14:171-184, 1976.

Petrova-Vergieva, T. and Ivanova-Tchemishanska, L.:
Assessment of the teratogenic activity of dithiocarbamate
fungicides. Food Cosmet. Toxicol. 11: 239-244, 1973.

497 Doca (see Deoxycorticosterone Acetate)

498 Dobutamine Hydrochloride

Nagaoka et al (1979) gave rats up to 50 mg per kg daily
intravenously before mating and during the first 7 days of
gestation. During organogenesis up to 70 mg per kg was
given and perinatally 50 mg per kg was used. At 70 mg per
kg there was some delay in ossification of the fetus. In
the perinatal studies growth retardation of the offspring
occurred to 35 days of age. In the rabbit intravenous doses
of up to 30 mg per kg produced no fetal ill effects.

Nagaoka, T.; Fuchigami, K.; Shigemura, T.; Takatouka, K.;
Osuga, F.; Hatano, M.: Reproductive studies on S-1000
(dobutamine hydrochloride) Yakuri to Chiryo 7:1691-1706,
1707-1730, 1731-1741, 1742-1763, 1979.

499

499 Dodecylethoxysulphate, Sodium (see Surfactants)

500 Domperidone

Hara et al (1980) gave this antiemetic orally to mice, rats and rabbits in maximum doses of 120, 200 and 120 mg per kg respectively. The percent of successful mating was decreased at 1 mg per kg. Maternal and fetal weight was reduced and fetal survival was lower at 70 and 200 mg per kg treatment during organogenesis. Displacement of the subclavian artery, skeletal defects and eye defects occurred at 200 mg per kg. No postnatal effects were found except for retarded genital development at doses over 70 mg per kg. The same authors studied the effects of intravenous and intraperitoneal dosing at up to 25 and 30 mg per kg respectively. Fertility was reduced when the dose exceeded 0.2 mg per kg. Following treatment with 15 or 30 mg per kg during organogenesis, growth retardation and skeletal delay were found. Postnatal studies were not remarkable except for growth retardation. Rabbits treated during organogenesis had fetuses with reduced survival (25 mg per kg) but no significant increase in defects.

Hara, T.; Nishikawa, S.; Miyazaki, E.; Ogura, T.: Toxicologic studies on KW-5338 reproductive studies. Yakuri to Chiryo 8: 4045- 4060, 4125-4136, 1980.

501 Don (see 6-Diazo-5-oxo-1-norleucine)

502 L-Dopa [3-(3,4-Dihydroxyphenyl)-1-alanine]

Staples and Mattis (1973) gave this medication by intubation to rabbits in doses up to 250 mg per kg per day from days 8 through 15 of gestation. At doses of 125 and 250 mg per kg malformations of the circulatory system were found. In mice treated with up to 500 mg per kg per day on days 6 through 15 only fetal stunting was significant.

Samojlik et al (1969) administered 10 mg per kg daily or for 5 days from day 10 or 15 of the pregnancy of the rat. Many of the offspring died during suckling. Of 216 fetuses exposed during the entire gestation period there were two with cataracts, 17 with suppurative inflammation of the eyes and one with polydactyly.

Samojlik, E.; Khing, O.J. and Chang, M.C.: Effects of dopamine on reproductive processes and fetal development in rats. Am. J. Obstet. Gynecol. 104: 578-585, 1969.

Staples, R.E. and Mattis, P.A.: Teratology of L-dopa (abstract) Teratology 8: 238 (only), 1973.

503 Doxapram

Imai (1974a) studied this respiratory stimulant in pregnant mice using an intraperitoneal maximum dose of 144 mg per kg per day of major organogenesis. At the highest dose some fetal death and growth retardation occurred but no gross defects. One treated pregnancy gave fetuses with minor skeletal defects. Post-natal studies for 6 weeks did not show any differences between the treated and control group. No teratogenicity was found in rats (Imai 1974b).

Imai, K.: Effect of doxapram hydrochloride administered to pregnant mice on pre- and post-natal development of their offsprings. (Japanese) Oyo Yakuri 8: 229-236, 1974a.

Imai, K.: Effect of doxapram hydrochloride administered to pregnant rats on pre- and post-natal development of their offsprings. Oyo Yakuri 8: 237-243, 1974b.

504   Doxepin   HCl   [N,N-Dimethyldibenz[b,e]oxepin-delta-11   (6H) gamma-propylamine HCl]

Owaki et al (1971, a and b) treated rabbits and rats during pregnancy with this psychotherapeutic agent. In rabbits doses up to 100 mg per kg during organogenesis produced some increase in neonatal death but no increase in gross malformations. The rats were treated with maximal doses of 270 mg per kg per day. At the highest levels postnatal survival was decreased but no congenital defects were found.

Owaki, Y.; Momiyama, H. and Onodera, N.: Effects of doxepin hydrochloride administered to pregnant rabbits upon the fetuses. Oyo Yakuri 5: 905-912, 1971a.

Owaki, Y.; Momiyama, H. and Onodera, N.: Effects of doxepin hydrochloride administered to pregnant rats upon the fetuses and their postnatal development. Oyo Yakuri 5: 913-924, 1971b.

505   Doxycycline (see Vibramicin-R)

506   Doxylamine Succinate [Decapryn-R]

Gibson et al. (1968) using 100 mg per kg per day in the rabbit and 100 mg per kg per day in the rat during periods of organogenesis produced no increase in congenital defects as compared to controls. At the highest doses which were toxic to the mother a reduction in fetal weight occurred.

Gibson, J.P.; Staples, R.E.; Larson, E.J.; Kuhn, W.L.; Holtkamp, D.E. and Newberne, J.W.: Teratology and reproduction studies with an antinauseant. Toxicol. Appl. Pharmacol. 13: 439-447,1966.

507   Duazomycin

Thiersch (1971) gave rats 4 to 10 mg per kg on day 7 of gestation and found increased resorptions and fetal stunting with minor unspecified malformations.

Thiersch, J.B.: Investigations into the differential effect of compounds on rat litter and mother. In,

507

Tuchmann-Duplessis, H. (ed.): Malformations Congenitales Des Mammiferes. Paris: Masson et Cie, 1971. pp 95-113.

508 Ebstein-Barr Virus (Infectious Mononucleosis)

Ebstein-Barr infection of the mother has been associated with at least three newborns with congenital defects (summarized by Brown and Stenchever, 1978). No pattern of defects has been identified; cleft lip and palate, microphthalmus, cardiovascular defects and cataracts were included in the case reports.

Brown, Z.A.; Stenchever, M.A.: Infectious mononucleosis and congenital malformations. Am. J. Obstet. Gynecol. 131:108-109, 1978.

509 Econazole

This antimycotic agent was given to mice and rabbits subcutaneously in maximum daily doses of 100 and 75 mg per kg respectively. Although no teratologic changes occurred, the mice at 100 mg per kg had prolonged gestation and increased fetal deaths. The rabbits had maternal deaths at 75 mg and some increase in fetal deaths at 25 mg per kg. (Maruoka et al, 1978).

Maruoka, H.; Kadota, Y.; Ueshima, M.; Uesako, T.; Takemoto, Y. and Sato, H.: Toxicological studies on econazole nitrate 4 Teratological studies in mice and rabbits. Iyakuhin Kenkyu 9:955-970, 1978.

510 E.D.T.A. (Ethylenediaminetetracetic Acid)

Tuchmann-Duplessis and Mercier-Parot (1956) reported that 20 to 40 mg E.D.T.A. Injected during embryogenesis caused tail defects and polydactyly in rat fetuses. Swenerton and Hurley (1971) produced cleft palate, brain and eye defects and skeletal anomalies in rat fetuses exposed to 2 or 3 percent E.D.T.A. in the diet after day 6 of gestation. By adding 1000 PPM of zinc to their experimental diet they were able to prevent the defects. Schardein et al (1981) gave up to 1000 mg per kg by gavage pm days 7 through 14 of the rat gestation. Neither EDTA nor its sodium and calcium salts produced adverse fetal changes. Congeital defects in the quail were produced with E.D.T.A. by Craig et al. (1968).

Craig, R.M.; Kratzer, F.H. and Vohra, P.: Growth and reproductive performance of coturnix fed several levels of E.D.T.A. (abstract) Poultr. Sci. 47: 1664-1665, 1968.

Swenerton, H. and Hurley, L.S.: Teratogenic effects of a chelating agent and their prevention by zinc. Science 173: 62-64, 1971.

Schardein, J.L.; Sakowski, R.; Petreve, J.; Humphrey, R.R.: Teratogenesis studies with EDTA and its salts in rats. Toxicol. Appl. Pharm. 61:423-428, 1981.

Tuchmann-Duplessis, H. and Mercier-Parot, L.: Influence d'un corps de chelation, l'acide ethlenediaminetetraacetique sur la gestation et le developpment foetal du rat. C. R. Acad. Sci. (Paris) 243: 1064-1066, 1956.

511 Elymoclavine

Witters et al, 1975 injected 3, 30 or 40 mg per kg on the 10th day and produced rib and vertebral defects in the offspring mouse fetuses.

Witters, W.L.; Wilms R.A.; Hood, R.D.: Prenatal effects of elymoclavine administration and temperature stress. J. Animal Science 41:1700-1705, 1975.

512 EM-12 (2-(2,6-dioxopiperiden-3-Yl)phthalimidine)

This analogue of thalidomide is teratogenic in monkeys and rabbits (Schumacher et al, 1972). In the rat oral doses of 250 mg per kg or intravenous doses of 10 mg per kg for three days failed to produce typical thalidomide malformations. Jackson and Schumacher (1979) administered 150 mg per kg intraperitoneally to rats maintained on a low zinc diet and produced phocomelia in over 50 percent of the fetuses. EM-12 treatment was on days 8-10 of pregnancy.

Jackson, A.J.; Schumacher, H.J.: The teratogenic activity of thalidomide analogus EM-12 in rats on a low-zinc diet. Teratoloogy 19:341-344, 1979.

Schumacher, H.J.; Terapane, J.J.; Jordan, R.L.; Wilson, J.G.: The teratogenic activity of a thalidomide analogue, EM-12 in rabbits, rats and monkeys. Teratology 5:233-240, 1972.

513 Emorfazone
(4-Ethoxy-2-methyl-5-morpholino-3(2H)-pyridazinone)

This antiflammatory agent was given to rabbits orally in doses of up to 300 mg per day on days 6 to 18 of gestation. Tanigawa et al (1979) gave rats up to 600 mg per kg orally before and during early pregnancy or in the late gestational period and observed no ill effects in the offspring.

Tanigawa, H.; Obori, R.; Tanaka, H.; Yoshida, J.; Kosazuma, E.: Reproductive study of 4-ethoxy-2-methyl 5-morpholino-3(2H)-pyridazinone (M 73101) on rabbits administration of M73101 during the period of major organogenesis. J. Toxicol. Sci. 4:162-174, 1979A.

Tanigawa, H.; Yoshida, J.; Tanaka, H.; Obori, R.; Kosazuma, T.: Reproductive study of 4ethoxy-2-methyl-5-morpholino-3(2H)-pyridazone (M73101) in rats. Oyo Yakuri 18:417-447, 1979B.

514 Emotional Stress

514

Rosenzweig (1966) has reviewed the experimental literature on psychologic stress and production of cleft palates. A number of stress techniques have caused an increase in cleft palate in the naturally susceptible AJAX strain of mice. Warkany and Kalter (1962) exposed two strains of mice to audiogenic stimuli and observed no increase in cleft palate in the offspring. Besides handling, restraint and avoidance, an effect of air transportation has been shown (Brown et al.; 1972).

Hartel and Hartel (1960) subjected pregnant rats to 6 hour periods of intermittent ringing of bells and flashing of light on the 9th through the 12th day and found no defects in 13 litters. Ishii and Yokobori (1960) exposed mice to noise for six hours daily on days 11 through 14 of gestation and produced seven defects among 130 survivors. The fetal weight was reduced and the stillbirth rate increased by the treatment. Kimmel et al (1976) in a carefully controlled exposure of mice and rats to noise stress (100 DB), found no teratogenicity but in mice maternal weight was reduced and also resorption rates were increased. Nawrot et al (1980) studied various types of noise stimuli in mice (126 dBA for 4 hours daily) and found that the extremely high frequency (jet type) had an embryo lethal effect on days 1-6 and that very high frequency (110 dBA) had the same effect on days 6-15. No malformations were produced. Maternal corticosterone levels were not elevated. Hamburgh et al (1974) produced a 9.5 percent incidence of malformations in the offspring of mice which were stressed by over crowding.

Stott (1973) made a study of 153 pregnancies and found no increase in physical defects in 14 where personal tension existed during gestation.

Brown, K.S.; Johnston, M.C. and Niswander, J.D.: Isolated cleft palate in mice after transportation during gestation. Teratology 5: 119-124, 1972.

Hamburgh, M.; Mendoza, L.A.; Rader, M.; Lang, A.; Silverstein, H. and Hoffman, K.: Malformations induced in offspring of crowded and parabiotically stressed mice. Teratology 10: 31-38, 1974.

Hartel, A. and Hartel, G.: Experimental study of teratogenic effect of emotional stress in rats. Science 132: 1483-1484, 1960.

Ishii, H. and Yokobori, K.: Experimental studies on teratogenic activity of noise stimulation. Gunma J. Med. Sci. 9: 153-167, 1960.

Kimmel, C.A.; Cook, R.O. and Staples, R.E.: Teratogenic potential of noise in mice and rats. Toxicol. Appl. Pharm. 36:239-245, 1976.

Nawrot, P.S.; Cook, R.O.; Staples, R.E.: Embryotoxicity of various noise stimuli in the mouse. Teratology 22:279-289, 1980.

Rosenzweig, S.: Psychological stress in cleft palate etiology. J. Dent. Res. 45: 1585-1593, 1966.

514

Stott, D.H.: Follow-up study from birth of the effects of prenatal stress. Develop. Med. Child Neurol. 15: 770-787, 1973.

Warkany, J. and Kalter, H.: Maternal impressisons and congenital malformation. Plastic and Reconstructive Surgery 30: 628-637, 1962.

515   3-(1,4-Endomethylene-cyclohexane-2,3-endo-cis-dicarboximido-)-pipe ridine2,6-dione

This hypnotic drug structurally similar to thalidomide was tested in the pregnant rabbit and found to be non-teratogenic (Stockinger and Koch, 1969). It was given orally from day 7 through 12 in amounts of 150 mg per kg. The authors suggest that their findings give evidence that aromatic phthalidimide moiety of thalidomide is responsible for the embryotoxic activity.

Stockinger, L. and Koch, H.: Teratologische Untersuchvng einer neuen, dem Thalidomid Stuckturell Nahestehenden Sedativ-hypnotisch wirksamen Verbindung (K-2004). Arzneim. Forsch. 19: 167-169, 1969.

516   Endosulfan

This insecticide was given orally on days 6 through 14 in doses of 5 and 10 mg per kg to rats and no soft tissue defects were found. Some delayed ossification occurred with treatment (Gupta et al, 1978)

Gupta, P.K.; Chandra, S.V. and Saxena, D.K.: Teratogenic and embryotoxic effects of endosulfan on rats. Acta Pharmacol. et Toxicol. 42:150-152, 1978.

517   Endotoxin

Ornoy and Altshuler (1976) treated pregnant rats with E. coli endotoxin intraperitoneally. When the treatment was given on days 10, 13 an 16, or on days 11, 14 and 17, hydrocephalus and or neuronal necrosis was increased in the fetus. Kanoh and Ema (1980) gave up to 1000 micrograms intravenously to rats on days 7, 12 or 17 and produced resorptions and dead fetuses but no congenital defect increase.

Kanoh, S.; Ema, M.: Effects of bacterial endotoxin on pregnant rats and their offspring. Cong. Anom. 20:151-155, 1980.

Ornoy, A. and Altshuler, G.: Maternal endotoxemia, fetal anomalies, and central nervous system damag: a rat model of a human problem. Am. J. Obstet. Gynecol. 124:196-204, 1976.

518
     3-(1,4-Endoxo-cyclohexane-2-exo-3-exo-dicarboximido)-piperidine-2

518

-6-dione

This sedative chemically related to thalidomide was
non-teratogenic in the offspring of rabbits receiving 150 mg
per kg orally from day 7 through 13 (Koch and Stockinger,
1971).

Koch, H. and Stockinger, L.: Teratologische Untersuchung
des 3-(1,4-endoxocyclohexan-2-exo-3-dicarboximido)-piper-
idin-2,6-dion

N, einer weiteren dem Thalidomide stuckturell Nahestehenden,
Sedativ-hypnotisch Wirksamen Verbindung. Arzneim. Forsch.
21: 2022-2025, 1971.

519   Endrin-R

Noda et al (1972) gave rat and mice 0.58 mg per kg four
times weekly for a month and then after a week or more
without treatment the animals were allowed to become
pregnant. A reduced survival rate was found in both
species. Nine mouse fetuses with club foot were found in
the treated group of 177 and only one in the control group
of 303.

Noda, K.; Hirabayashi, M.; Yonemura, I.; Maruyama, M. and
Endo, I.: Influence of pesticides on embryos 2. On the
influence of organochloric pesticides (Japanese) Oyo Yakuri
6: 673-679, 1972.

520   Enflurane   [2-Chloro-1,1,2-trifluoro Ethyl Diethyl Methyl
Ether]

Saito et al (1974) exposed pregnant rats and mice to one
hour of this anesthetic daily during major organogenesis.
Concentrations for the rat were 1.25 percent and for the
mouse 0.75 percent. No teratogenicity was found. No
post-natal changes were found in a 6 week study. Wharton et
al (1979) confirmed this work using 4 hour daily exposures.

Saito, N.; Urakawa, M. and Ito, R.: Influence of
enflurance on fetus and growth after birth in mice and rats.
(Japanese) Oyo Yakuri 8: 1269-1276, 1974.

Wharton, R.S.; Wilson, A.I.; Rice, S.A. and Mazze, R.I.:
Teratogenicity of enflurane in Swiss- ICR mice. (abs)
Teratology 19:53A only, 1979.

521   Enovid-R

This oral progestin which contains 9.85 mg 17-alpha-
-ethinyl-17-OH-5(10) estren-3-one and 0.15 mg
ethynylestradiol 3 methyl ether per 10 mg tablet has been
given in 10 mg daily doses to a mother who produced a girl
with labio-scrotal fusion and clitoromegaly (Grumbach et
al.; 1959).

Grumbach, M.M.; Ducharme, J.R. and Moloshok, R.E.: On the

fetal masculinizing action of certain oral progestins. J.
Clin. Endocrinol. Metab. 19: 1396-1380, 1959.

522 Enteroviruses

Brown and Karunas (1972) collected sera from 22,935 women
early in pregnancy and again at delivery. Among 82 mothers
who gave birth to children with urogenital malformation a
significantly higher number (37) were found to have had
infections with one of the 5 coxsackie B viruses (B2 and B4
mainly). Among a group of 77 infants with cleft lip or
palate, pyloric stenosis or other gastrointestinal tract a-
nomalies, there was an increase in the number of women with
serologic evidence of enterovirus A-9. A significant
increase in the number of maternal titers against coxsackie
B3 and B4 was found in pregnancies associated with congenital heart conditions.

Brown, G.C. and Karunas, R.S.: Relationship of congenital
anomalies and maternal infection with selected
enteroviruses. Am. J. Epidem. 95: 207-217, 1972.

523 Ephedrine (see Epinephrine)

524 Epidermal Growth Factor

Bedrick and Ladda (1978) injected pregnant mice on days
11-15 with 40 microgram per gm of animal and produced no
defects. Epidermal growth factor did cause an increase in
cortisone-induced cleft palates.

Bedrick, A.D. and Ladda, R.L.: Epidermal growth factor
potentiates cortisone-induced cleft palate in the mouse.
Teratology 17:13-18, 1978.

525 Epidihydrocholestrin

This steroid precursor was given subcutaneously in doses of
up to 200 mg per kg to mice and no fetal alterations were
detected. Treatment was on days 6 through 15. (Matumoto et
al, 1978).

Matumoto, H.; Tujitani, N.; Ouchi, S.; Jida, T.; Tomizawa,
S. and Kamata, J.: Teratogenicity test of epidihydro-
cholesterine in mice (Japanese). Clinical Report
12:479-492, 1978.

526 Epinephrine [Adrenalin]

Jost et al. (1969) have summarized their experiments with
adrenalin-induced limb defects in the rabbit. They injected
5 to 50 microgms of adrenalin directly into rabbit fetuses
at 18 to 22 days of gestational age and noted hemorrhages,
edema and necrosis of the distal extremities. A recessively
inherited syndrome (br) in the rabbit produces similar types
of defects, and they showed that the concentration of

adrenalin is elevated in the adrenal medulla of these affected fetuses; this raised the possibility of excess endogenous adrenalin leading to the genetic limb defect.

Jost, in his original work (1953), produced limb defects in rat fetuses injected directly with 1 to 50 microgm of adrenalin on the 17th day.

Gatling (1962) dropped 20 to 200 microgm of this material on the chorio-allantoic membrane of the chick once on the 10th, 11th or 12th day and produced hemorrhages of the head, skin and extremities. Similar findings occurred when norepinephrine and Neosynephrine-R were used. Ephedrine and serotonin gave negative results.

Hodach et al (1974) administered 5 micrograms of epinephrine to chick embryos at intervals between 24 and 190 hours of incubation. Treatment between 96 and 124 hours produced over 50 percent aortic arch anomalies in the surviving embryos.

Gatling, R.R.: The effect of sympathomimetic agents on the chick embryo. Am. J. Pathol. 40: 113-127, 1962.

Hodach, R.J.; Gilbert, E.F. and Fallon, J.F.: Aortic arch anomalies associated with administration of epihephrine in chick embryos. Teratology 9: 203-210, 1974.

Jost, A.: Degenerescence des extremites du foetus de rat provoquee par l'adrenaline. C. R. Acad. Sci. (Paris) 236: 1510-1512, 1953.

Jost, A.; Roffi, J. and Cowitat, M.: Congenital amputations determined by the br gene and those induced by adrenalin injection in the rabbit fetus. In, Swinyard, C.A. (ed.): Limb Development and Deformity: Problems of Evaluation and Rehabilitation. Springfield: C.C. Thomas, 1969. pp 187-199.

527 Eptazocine (L-1,4-Dimethyl-10-hydroxy-2,3,4,5,6,7-hexahydro-1,6-methano-1H-4-benzazonine hydrobromide)

Matsuda et al (1980) in a series of papers reported reproductive studies in the mouse and rabbit. Using up to 125 mg per kg subcutaneously during organogenesis and 100 mg per kg subcutaneously before mating and the first 7 days of gestation or during days 15 through 21, they observed no ill effects except for a decrease in fetal weight and delayed ossification at the higher doses. Transient behavioral alterations were observed. In rabbits 100 mg per kg was given on days 6 through 18 and no adverse fetal effects were found.

Matsuda, M.; Minami, Y.; Kawakami, T.; Nogami, M.; Ikeda, M.; Kumada, S.; Urata, M.; Kihara, T.: Reproductive studies of 1-1,4-dimethyl-10-hydroxy-2,3,4,5,6,7-hexahydro-1,6-methano-1H-4-benzazonine hydrobromide (Eptazocine HBr, 1-ST-2121) Oyo Yakuri 20: 501-526, 703-714, 803-811, 1980.

528   2 Alpha, 3-alpha-epithio-5-alpha-androstan-17-beta-01

This long-acting antiestrogenic compound was given to mice
and rats during pregnancy and at doses of 10 and 40 mg per
kg per day delayed parturition and maternal death occurred.
Administration late in pregnancy of 2.5 mg per kg caused no
effect on the reproductive ability of the male offspring but
none of the female offspring showed reproductive ability.
Deformities of the female mice sex organs were seen with
doses of 10 mg per kg per day (Minesita, et al, 1973).

Minesita, T.; Hasegawa, Y.; Yoshida, T.; Kozen, T.;
Sakaguchi, I.; Okamoto, A. and Ohara, T.: Teratological
and reproductive studies on 2-alpha,3-alpha-epithio-5-alpha
androstan-17-beta-01 in mice and rats. (Japanese). Oyo
Yakuri 7: 723-752, 1973.

529   Ergotamine

David (1972) reported that among 10 newborns with Poland's
syndrome five were adopted and of the remaining 5, 3
attempted abortion.   One of these mothers took ergonovine.
Wainscott et al (1978) studied the outcome of women treated
during pregnancy for migraine and reported no adverse
effects. Graham et al (1983) reported jejunal atresia in a
mother who took cafergot.

Grauwiler and Schon (1973) studied the effect of this drug
on pregnant mice, rats and rabbits and found no specific
defects but compression effects on the fetus (reduced fetal
weight and skeletal retardation) were found at oral doses of
100 mg per kg in mice and 10 mg per kg in rats. The rodents
were treated on day 6 through 15 and the rabbits on day 6
through 18.

David, T.J.: Nature and etiology of Poland anomaly. New
Eng. J. Med. 238:487-489, 1972.

Graham, J.M.; Marin-Padilla, M.; Hoefnagel, D.: Jejunal
atresia associated with cafergot ingestion during pregnancy.
Clinical Pediatrics (in press)

Grauwiler, J. and Schon, H.: Teratological experiments
with ergotamine in mice, rats and rabbits. Teratology 7:
227-236, 1973.

Wainscott, G.; Sullivan, F.M.; Volans, G.N.; Wilkinson, M.:
The outcome of pregnancy in women suffering from migrane.
Postgraduate Med. J. 54:98, 1978.

530   Estradiol

Using 0.8 to 35 mg estradiol during the 12th to 19th
gestational days of the rat, Greene et al. (1939, 1940)
produced complete feminization of the external genitalia of
male fetuses with testes retained in the female position and
reduction or absence of epididymus, vas, seminal vesicles
and prostate. A rudimentary vagina was present in the
males.   In the female fetus there was enlargement of the

uterus and a paradoxical retention of the wolffian bodies.
In both sexes the number of nipples was increased. At high
dose levels fetal loss was common.

Burns (1955) was able to produce ovo testes by treating
premature opossum embryos with topical estradiol
diproprionate (0.1 to 5 microgm per day).

Nishihara (1958) produced 14 percent cleft palates in the
mouse fetus by injecting the mother with 1 mg on the 11th
through the 16th day. Closure of the fetal mouse eye lids
has also been delayed by the use of estradiol on the 17th
gestational day (Raynaud, 1942).

Burns, R.K.: Experimental reversal of sex in the gonads of
the opossum Didelphis virginiana. Proc. Nat. Acad. Sci.
USA 41: 669-676, 1955.

Greene, R.R.; Burrill, M.W. and Ivy, A.C.: Experimental
intersexuality: the paradoxicol effects of estrogens on the
sexual development of the female rat. Anat. Rec. 74:
429-438, 1939.

Greene, R.R.; Burrill, M.W. and Ivy, A.C.: Experimental
intersexuality: the effects of estrogens on the antenatal
sexual development of the rat. Am. J. Anat. 67: 305-345,
1940.

Nishihara, G.: Influences of female sex hormones in
experimental teratogenesis. Proc. Soc. Exp. Biol. Med.
97: 809-812, 1958.

531   Estramustine phosphate disodium

This chemical combination of estradiol and nitrogen mustard
was tested in rats and rabbits by Nomura et al (1980 and
1981). Rats received orally up to 4.0 mg per kg before
mating on days 7-17 or on day 17-21. Dosing prenatally and
during the first 7 days of gestation was not associated with
any adverse effects. Treatment with 4.0 mg per kg during
organogenesis was followed by an increase in ectopic kidneys
and skeletal defects. Late treatment with 4.0 mg per kg was
associated with increased abnormalities of the external
genitalia and decreased fertility in the female offspring.
Both males and females had increased exploratory behavior at
55-58 postnatal days. Rabbits treated on days 6-18 had
interruption of pregnancy at 0.2 mg per kg and at 0.1 mg
resorptions were increased. At 0.1 mg per kg no increase in
defects was found.

Nomura, A.; Watanabe, M.; Ninomiya, H.; Enomoto, H.:
Reproductive studies of estramustine phosphate disodium
(EMP). Oyo Yakuri 20:1211- 1236, 21:41-65, 1980 and 1981.

532   Estrone

Nishihara produced 12.4 percent cleft palate in mouse
fetuses whose mothers were injected with 1 mg estrone on the
11th through the 16th gestational days. Among

injection-control fetuses, the incidence of cleft palate was 0.7 percent.

Nishihara, G.: Influence of female sex hormones in experimental teratogenesis. Proc. Soc. Exp. Biol. Med. 97: 809-812, 1958.

533 Ethambutol

Bobrowitz (1974) studied 42 pregnancies in which 15 to 25 mg per kg was given. There was neither intrauterine growth retardation no increase in prematurity. Although there were some minor malformations observed, there was no increase in the rate. Lewit et al (1974) could find no abnormalities in aborted embryos exposed to the drug.

Bobrowitz, I.D.: Ethambutol in pregnancy. Chest 66:20-24, 1974.

Lewit, T.; Nebel, L.; Terracina, S. and Karman, S.: Ethambutol in pregnancy: observations on embryogenesis. Chest 66:25-26, 1974.

534 Ethamoxytriphetol [MER-25] [1-(P-2-Diethylamino-ethoxyphenyl)-1-phenyl-2-p-methoxyphenyl Ethanol]

Heller and Jones (1964) produced ovarian dysgenesis in rat fetuses by administering this anti-estrogenic compound in oral doses of 25 mg per kg on day 13 through 19. The fetal ovaries were necrotic and hemorrhagic in about half of the female fetuses. Although the number of fetuses per litter and fetal weight were reduced in the treated group, no other effects were noted. The fetal testes were histologically normal but increased in weight.

Heller, R.H. and Jones, H.W.: The production of ovarian dysgenesis in the rat by ethamoxytriphetol (MER-25). Am. J. Obstet. Gynecol. 90: 264-270, 1964.

535 Ethane-1-hydroxy 1,1-diphosphonate

Eguchi et al (1982) administered this calcification inhibitor subcutaneously to mice on days 11-17 of gestation in doses of 200 mg per kg daily. Decrease in mineralization and angulations of fetal long bones were produced.

Eguchi, M.; Yamaguchi, R.; Shiota, E.; Handa, S.: Fault of ossification and calcification and angular deformities of long bones in the mouse fetuses caused by high doses of ethane-1-hydroxy-1,1- diphosphonate (EHDP) during pregnancy. Cong. Anomal. 22:47-52, 1982.

536 Ethanol (see alcohol)

537 Ethidine (2,6 - Dimethyl-3,5-dicarbethoxy-1,4-dihydropirine)

537

Maganova and Zaitsev (1978) studied the effect of this compound in pregnant rats (100 and 500 mg per kg) and mice (1000 mg per kg) and found no mutagenic, embryotoxic or any adverse postnatal effect.

Maganova, N.B. and Zaitsev, A.N.: A study of mutagenic and embryotoxic action produced by ethidine. Vopr. pitaniya (USSR) 4:70-74, 1978.

538 17-Alpha-ethinyl-19-nor-testosterone [Norlutin-R]

This oral progestin can produce masculinization of the external genitalia in the female fetus. Details appear under 17-Alpha-ethinyl testosterone.

539 17-Alpha-ethinyl-testosterone   [Pranone-R]   [Lutocylol-R]
[Pregneninolone]

Although 17-hydroxyprogesterone is not teratogenic (Johnston and Franklin, 1964; Suchowsky and Junkmann, 1961), certain derivatives can cause virilizing effects in animals and man. Wilkins et al. (1958) and Wilkins (1960) reported that 17-alpha-ethinyl-testosterone in daily doses of 20 to 200 mg used during the 1st trimester of pregnancy caused masculinization of the external genitalia of female offspring. Jacobson (1962) with daily doses of 10 to 20 mg of 17-alpha-ethinyl-19-nor-testosterone reported 15 percent of female newborns to be masculinized. Grumbach et al. (1959) pointed out that labio-scrotal fusion was produced only in fetuses exposed prior to the 13th gestational week, but clitoromegaly could still be produced after this period. Serment and Ruf (1968) give a good general summary of the types of progestins that cause masculinization. They cite four incidences where normethandrone was implicated.

There is a fairly extensive experimental literature on the effect of progestins on masculinization of the female fetus. Courrier and Jost (1942) first warned that this compound could masculinize the fetus. Johnstone and Franklin (1964) used the mouse, Revesz et al. (1960) and Suchowsky et al. (1961) the rat and Jost (1946) the rabbit. Some of these fetuses also had blind vaginas or absence of portions of the uterus.

Courrier, R. and Jost, A.: Intersexualite foetale provoqvee par pregneninolone au cours de la grossesse. C. R. Soc. Biol. (Paris) 136: 395-396, 1942.

Grumbach, M.M.; Ducharme, J.R. and Moloshok, R.E.: On the fetal masculinizing action of certain oral progestins. J. Clin. Endocrinol. Metab. 19: 1369-1380, 1959.

Jacobson, B.D.: Hazards of norethindrone therapy during pregnancy. Am. J. Obstet. Gynecol. 84: 962-968, 1962.

Johnstone, E.E. and Franklin, R.R.: Assay of progestins for fetal virilizing properties using the mouse. Obstet. Gynecol. 23: 359-362, 1964.

Jost, A.: Recherches sur la differenciation sexuelle de l'embryon de lapin. Action des androgenes de synthese sur l'histogenese genitale. Arch. Anat. Microsc. Morphol. Exp. 36: 242-270, 1946.

Revesz, C.; Chappel, C.I. and Gaudry, R.: Masculinization of the female fetuses in the rat by progestational compounds. Endocrinology 66: 140-144, 1960.

Serment, H. and Ruf, H.: Therapeutiques hormonales. Bull. Fed. Soc. Gynecol. Obstet. Lang. Fr. 20: 69-76, 1968.

Suchowsky, G.K. and Junkmann, K.: A study of the virilizing effect of progestogens on the female rat fetus. Endocrinol. 68: 341-349, 1961.

Wilkins, L.: Masculinization due to orally given progestins. J.A.M.A. 172: 1028-1032, 1960.

Wilkins, L.; Jones, H.W.; Holman, G.H. and Stempfel, R.S.: Masculinization of the female fetus associated with administration of oral and intramuscular progestins during gestation: non-adrenal female pseudohermaphrodism. J. Clin. Endocrinol. Metab. 18: 559-585, 1958.

540 Ethionamide

Fujimori et al. (1965) gave rats by mouth 200 mg per kg from the 6th through the 14th gestational day and found a low incidence of omphalocele (5.2 percent), exencephaly (2.7 percent) and cleft palate (1.4 percent). Takekoshi (1965) gave mice 75 mg orally during days 6 through 13 of gestation and found no defects. When hydroxymethylpyrimidine (0.75 mg) was added to 7.5 mg of ethionamide, 23 percent defects occurred (exencephaly and facial clefts).

Potworowski et al (1966) found seven deformities among 23 exposed infants but two of these were Down's syndrome. No pattern of malformation was apparent and they included congenital heart, spina bifida and atresia of the gastrointestinal tract.

Fujimori, H.; Yamada, F.; Shibukawa, N.; Goda, S. and Itani, I.: The effect of tuberculostatics on the fetus: An experimental production of congenital anomaly in rats by ethionamide. (abstract) Proceedings of the Congenital Anomalies Research Association of Japan 5: 34-35, 1965.

Potworowski, M.; Sianozecka, E. and Szufladowicz, R.: Ethionamide treatment and pregnancy. Pol. Med. J. 5:1152-1158, 1966.

Takekoshi, S.: Effects of hydroxymethylpyrimidine on isoniazid- and ethionamide-induced teratosis. Gunma J. of Med. Sc. 14:233-244, 1965.

541 Ethionine

Feldman and Waddington (1955) injected approximately 1 mg of

541

this substance into chick eggs before incubation and found
after 42 hours incubation that neurulation was defective.
Methionine given concommitantly resulted in normal development. Proffit and Edwards (1962) injected 200 mg of D-L
ethionine during the 2nd week of the rats' gestation and
produced no congenital defects. Landauer and Salam (1974)
produced beak abnormalities, muscle hypoplasia and malformations of the cervical vertebrae in chicks by injecting 4.5
mg at 96 hours of incubation.

Feldman, M. and Waddington, C.H.: The uptake of
methionine-S(35) by the chick embryo and its inhibition by
ethioninee. J. Embryol. Exp. Morphol. 3: 44-58, 1955.

Landauer, W. and Salam, N.: Experimental production in
chicken embryos of muscular hypoplasia and associated
defects of beak and cervical vertebrae. Acta Embryol.
Experimentalis 1: 51-66, 1974.

Proffit, W.R. and Edwards, L.E.: Effects of ethionine administration during pregnancy in the rat. J. Exp. Zool.
150: 135-142, 1962.

542 Ethnodiol diacetate

Saunders and Elton (1967) treated rats and rabbits buccally
and subcutaneously with the compound and found neither
defects nor infertility in the offspring. The treatment
periods were for various periods of gestation as well as the
entire period. The highest dose during the entire period
was 2 mg per kg per day for rats and 0.05 mg per kg per day
for rabbits. In mice Andrew et al (1972) found 30 percent
malformations when 1.0 mg per kg was given on days 7 through
9.

The effect of oral contraceptives on pregnant women is
discussed under oral contraceptives.

Andrew, F.D.; Williams, T.L.; Gidley, J.T. and Wall, M.E.:
Teratogenicity of contraceptive steroids in mice. (abs)
Teratology 5:249 (only) 1972.

Saunders, F.J. and Elton, R.L.: Effects of ethnodiol
diacetate and mestranol in rats and rabbits, on conception,
on the outcome of pregnancy and on the offspring. Toxicol.
Appl. Pharm. 11:229-244, 1967.

543 Ethosuximide (Zarotin-R)

The suxinimides (ethosuximide, methsuximide and
phensuximide) appear to have much less teratogenic potential
than the oxazolidine-2,4-diones (trimethadione and
parmethadione) (Fabro and Brown, 1979). These authors
summarized a large number of case histories and found only 6
percent (5 per 89) malformations in the suxinimide group
while the other group had 36 percent (5 per 14). Kao et al
(1979) have shown in mice that the suxinimides are less
teratogenic than the oxazolidine-2,4-diones.

page 184

Fabro, S. and Brown, N.A.: The teratogenic potential of anticonvulsants. New Eng. J. Med. 300:1280-1281, 1979.

Kao, J.; Brown, N.A.; Shull, G. and Fabro, S.: Chemical structure and teratogenicity of anticonvulsants (abs). Fed. Proc. 38:438 (only), 1979.

544 2-Ethoxyethanol (see Ethylene glycol monoethyl ether)

545 Ethoxzolamide

Wilson et al. (1968) fed this carbonic anhydrase inhibitor to rats as 0.3 or 0.6 percent of their diet throughout pregnancy. The acetazolamide syndrome consisting of localized post-axial forelimb defects was observed in about 10 percent of the fetuses. Occasionally other organ systems were involved also.

Wilson, J.G.; Maren, T.H.; Takano, K. and Ellison, A.C.: Teratogenic action of carbonic anhydrase inhibitors in the rat. Teratology 1: 51-60, 1968.

546 1-Ethyl-2-acetylhydrazine (see 1-methyl-formylhydrazine)

547 2-Ethylamino-1,3,4 Thiadiazole (also see Acetazolamide) [Thiadiazole]

Murphy et al. (1957) using one-quarter to one-half the maternal LD-50 (200 mg per kg) produced skeletal defects in rat fetuses with treatment on the 11th day. On the 12th day cleft lips and palates and encephaloceles were seen. But the most distinctive feature was absence of the tail. Ellison and Maren (1972) confirmed the work of Murphy et al. (1957).

Maren, T.H. and Ellison, A.C.: The teratological effect of certain thiadiazoles related to acetazolamide with a note on sulfanilamide and thiazide diuretics. Johns Hopkins Med. J. 130: 95-104, 1972.

Murphy, M.L.; Dagg, C.P. and Karnofsky, D.A.: Comparison of teratogenic chemicals in the rat and chick embryos. Pediatrics 19: 701-714, 1957.

548 Ethyl Acrylate

Murray et al (1981) exposed rats for 6 hours daily on days 6-15 to 50 or 150 ppm. Maternal toxicity occurred at the highest dose but no adverse fetal effects were found.

Murray, J.S., Miller, R.R., Deacon, M.M., Hanley, T.R., Hayes, W.C., Rao, K.S., John, J.A.: Teratological evaluation of inhaled ethyl acrylate in rats. Toxicol. Appl. Pharm. 60:106-111, 1981.

549 Ethyl Carbamate (see Urethan)

550 Ethylene Chloride (see 1,2-dichoroethane)

551 Ethylenediaminetetraacetic Acid (see E.D.T.A.)

552 Ethylene dibromide

Haar (1980) reviewed the existing human epidemiologic data and concluded there was no reproductive adverse effect among workers.

Haar, T.G.: An investigation of possible sterility and health effects from exposure to ethylene dibromide. Bambury Report No. 5 Ethylene dichloride edited by B. Ames, P. Infante and R. Reitz, Cold Spring Harbor Laboratory, 1980, 149-161.

553 Ethylene glycol-monoethyl Ether (2-Ethoxyethanol, Cellosolve-R)

Stenger et al. (1971) tested this material by mouth and injection in pregnant mice, rats and rabbits. Some fetal skeletal defects were found in rats with doses over 100 microliters per kg per day but no other defects were described in the three species. The type of skeletal defects was not mentioned. Hardin et al (in press) applied 0.25 ml two times daily to the skin of pregnant rats on days 6-15. Maternal and fetal weight were reduced as were fetal survivors. Five of 35 survivors had cardiovascular defects and 13 had enlarged cerebral ventricles. Hardin et al (1981) exposed rats and rabbits to 200-765 or 160-615 PPM for 7 hours daily during most of gestation. In rabbits the higher concentration was lethal to the embryos but at the lower concentration 10 of 167 had cardiovascular defects and some increase in vertebral defects was found. Cardiovascular and skeletal defects were increased in the rat fetuses exposed to the lower dose at which maternal toxicity did not occur. Postnatal behavior effects have been reported (Nelson et al (1981).

Hardin, B.D.; Bond, G.P.; Sikov, M.R.; Andrew, F.D.; Beliles, R.P.; Niemeier, R.W.: Testing of selected workplace chemicals for teratogenic potential. Scand. J. Work Envir. ₊Heath 7:Suppl 4, 66-75, 1981.

Hardin, B.D.; Niemier, R.W.; Smith, R.J.; Kuczuk, M.H.; Mathinos, P.R.; Weaver, T.F.: Teratogenicity of 2 ethoxyethanol by dermal application. Drug and Chemical Toxicol. (in press)

Nelson, B.K.; Brightwell, W.S.; Setzer, J.V.; Taylor, B.J.; Hornung, R.W.; O'Donohue, T.L.: Ethoxyethanol behavioral teratology in rats. Neurotoxicology 2:231-249, 1981.

Stenger, E.G.; Aeppli, L.; Muller, D.; Peheim, E. and Thomann, P.E.: Zur Toxikologie des

A+hylenglykol-monoathylathers.   Arzneim.   Forsch.   21:
880-885, 1971.

554 Ethylene Oxide

Kimmel and Laborde (1979) injected this material intravenously on several days during organogenesis in the mouse.
Skeletal malformations occurred in fetuses whose mothers
received 150 mg per kg which produced maternal toxicity.
Doses of 75 mg per kg caused no defects. Shellings et al
(1982) exposed rats on days 6-15 of gestation for 6 hours
daily to 10 to 100 PPM. At the highest dose fetal growth
retardation occurred but there was no increase in congenital
defects.

Hemminki et al (1982) studied the abortion rate in 1443
hospital workers exposed during pregnancy to sterilizing
procedures by ethylene oxide. The frequency was 16.7 as
compared to appropriate hospital controls with 5.6%

Hemminki, K.; Mutanen, P.; Saloniemi, I.; Niemi, M-L.;
Vainio, H.: Spontaneous abortions in hospital staff engaged
in sterilising instruments with chemical agents. Brit.
Med. J. 285:1461-1463, 1982.

Kimmel, C.A. and Laborde, J.B.: Teratogenic potential of
ethylene oxide (abs) Teratology 19:34A-35 , 1979.

Shellings, W.M.; Maronpot, R.R.; Zdenak, J.P.; Laffoon,
C.P.: Teratology study in Fischer 344 rats exposed to
ethylene oxide by inhalation. ʿToxicol. Appl. Pharm.
64:478-481, 1982.

555 Ethylenethiourea

Ruddick and Khera (1975) studied this fungicide degradation
product in rats during several periods of organogenesis at
10 to 80 mg per kg per day. Above 10 mg per kg, neural tube
closure defects, hydrocephalus and other malformations of
the brain were found along with kinky tails and limb
defects. In the rabbit at 80 mg per kg, decreased brain
weight was found. Ruddick et al (1976) have studied the
distribution and metabolism of the compound in pregnant
rats. Lu and Staples (1978) produced defects in the rat
even following thyroparathyroidectomy and suggested the mode
of action was not via a maternal thyroid effect. Khera and
Iverson (1981) gavaged (200 mg per kg) or gave
intraperitoneally (400 mg per kg) of a similar antithyroid
N-methyl-2-thioimidazole and found no adverse effects in rat
fetuses.

Ruddick et al (1976) studied the correlation of teratogenicity with molecular structure of 16 related chemicals. The
only chemical which was teratogenic was 4-methylethyl-
ene-thiourea at a dose of 240 mg per kg on day 12 or 13 in
the rat. The following chemicals were not teratogenic
(although minor skeletal changes were present): allylthiourea (240), allylisothiocyanate (60), ethyl-
ene-bis-isothiocyanate (25), ethylenethiuram monosulfide

(60), ethyleneurea (240), N,N-dimethyl- thiourea (240), imidazole (240), 3-(2-imidazoline-2- yl)-2-imida zo-lidinethione (Jaffe's base, 200), 2- mercaptobenzimidazole (120), 2-mercapto-1-methyl- imidazole (240), 2-mercaptothiazoline (240), N-methylethylenethiourea (240), 3,4,5,6-tetrahydro- 2-pyrimidinethiol (240), 1,1,3,3-tetra-methyl-2-thiourea (240). The figure in parenthesis following the drug is the dosage used in mg per kg on day 12 or 13. A sulfur in the 2 position and the imidazolidine ring appeared to be necessary in producing the teratogenic activity of ethylenethiourea.

Khera, K.S.; Iverson, F.: Effects of pretreatment with SKF-525A, N-methyl-2-thioimidazole sodium phenobarbital or methyl cholanthrene on ethylenethiourea-induced teratogenicity. in rats. Teratology 24: 131-137, 1981.

Lu, M.H. and Staples, R.E.: Teratogenicity of ethyl-enethiourea and thyroid function in the rat. Teratology 17:171-178, 1978.

Ruddick, J.A. and Khera, K.S.: Pattern of anomalies following single oral doses of ethylene- thiourea to pregnant rats. Teratology 12:277-282, 1975.

Ruddick, J.A.; Newsome, W.H.; and Nash, L.: Correlation of teratogenicity and molecular structure. Ethylenethiourea and related compounds. Teratology 13:263-266, 1976.

Ruddick, J.A.; Williams, D.T.; Hierlihy, L. and Khera, K.S.: [14-C]ethylenethiourea: distribution, excretion and metabolism in pregnant rats. Teratology 13:35-39, 1976.

556 Ethylenebisisothiocyanate (see Ethylenethiourea)

557 Ethylene Chlorhydrin (2-chlorethanol)

This breakdown product of ethylene oxide was given by gavage to mice during organogenesis (Courtney et al, 1982). Doses of up to 227 mg per kg in the water or 100 mg per kg by gavage produced no malformations. With the gavage dosing, both maternal and fetal weights were reduced. Shellings et al (1979) have reported no teratogenicity after treating rats.

Courtney, K.D.; Andrews, J.E.; Grady, M.: Teratogenic evaluation of ethylene chlorhydrin. J. Envir. Sc. Health B17 381-391, 1982.

Shellings, W.M.; Pringle, J.L.; Dorke, J.D.; Kintigh, W.J.: Teratology and reproduction studies with rats exposed to 10, 33 or 100 ppm of ethylene oxide (abs). Toxicol. Appl. Pharmacol 48:A84, 1979.

558 Ethylenethiuram Monosulfide (see Ethylenethiourea)

559 Ethyleneurea (see Ethylenethiourea)

560 Ethyl P-(6-guanidinohexanoyloxy) Benzoate Methansulfonate

Fujita et al (1975) studied this chemical in pregnant mice and rats giving up to 100 mg per kg to mice and 30 mg per kg to rats during organogenesis. No teratogenic activity was detected.

Fujita, T.; Suzuki, Y.; Yamamoto, Y.; Yokohama, H.; Yonezawa, H.; Ozeki, Y.; Mori, T. and Matsuoka, Y.: Toxicities and teratogenicity of ethyl P-(6-guanidinohexanyloxy) benzoate methanesulfate (FOY). (Japanese) Oyo Yakuri 9: 743-760, 1975.

561 N-2-Ethylhexyl-beta-oxybutyramide Semisuccinate

Kuraishi et al (1974) gave this compound orally to pregnant mice from days 7 through 11 of gestation in maximum doses of 1,000 mg per kg per day and found no teratogenic effect.

Kuraishi, K.; Nabeshima, J.; Haresaku, M. and Inoue, S.: Teratologic study with N-2-ethylhexyl-beta-oxybutyramide semisuccinate (M-2H) in mice. Oyo Yakuri 8: 1413-1421, 1974.

562 2-Ethyl-5-methylbenzimidazole (see Benzimidazole)

563 N-Ethylnicotinamide

Landauer and Wakasugi (1967) injected 2.5 to 10 mg of this compound into the yolk sac at 24 or 96 hours of incubation and observed shortening of the legs, abnormal upper beaks and a low incidence of rumplessness in the 17 day survivors. Supplementation with ADP tended to protect the embryos.

Landauer, W. and Wakasugi, N.: Problems of acetazolamide and N-ethylnicotinamide as teratogens. J. Exp. Zool. 164: 499-516, 1967.

564 Ethylnitrosourea

Druckrey et al. (1966) injected 80 mg per kg on the 15th day and found abnormalities of the paws of the rat offspring. Three of five surviving fetuses subsequently developed brain tumors. Subsequent work (Ivankovic and Druckrey, 1968) indicated that a single dose of only 5 mg per kg on the 15th day was sufficient to produce postnatal tumors. Druckery, et al (1972) found that ethylnitrosabiuret produced postnatal neurogenic tumors. Druckrey(1973) and Druckrey et al(1972) have recently summarized the role of this compound and other indirect alkylating compounds.

Alexandrov and Janisch (1970) fed pregnant rats a combination of ethyl urea and nitrite on the 9th and 10th gestational days and produced hydrocephalus, anencephalus and absence of the eye. These defects were felt to be due to absorption of ethyl nitroso-urea which was formed in the gastrointestinal tract. The dosage used was 0.3 to 1

564

percent nitrite in the feed and 0.5 percent ethyl urea in the water with tube feeding of ethyl urea 100 or 200 mg per kg per day. Alexandrov (1976) has reviewed the extensive Russian experimental work on transplacental carcinogenesis of the compound and related chemicals. He reported that when 15 mg per kg was given intravenously on the 21st day, 78 percent of the rat offspring had postnatal tumors of the central nervous system.

Alexandrov, V.A. and Janisch, W.: Die Teratogene wirkung von Athylharnstoff und Nitrit bei Ratten. Experienta 27: 538-539, 1971.

Alexandrov, V.A.: Some results and prospects of transplacental carcinogenesis studies. Neoplasia 23:285-299, 1976.

Druckrey, H.; Ivankovic, S. and Preussmann, R.: Teratogenic and carcinogenic effects in the offspring after single injection of ethylnitrosourea to pregnant rats. Nature 210: 1378-1379, 1966.

Druckrey, H.; Ivankovic, S.; Preussmann, R.; Zulch, K. and Mennel, H.D.: Selective induction of malignant tumors of the nervous system by resorptive carcinogens, In Kirsch, W.M.; Paoletti, E.G. and Paoletti, P. (eds): The Experimental Biology of Brain Tumors. Springfield: C.C. Thomas, 1972, pp 107-108.

Druckrey, H.: Specific carcinogenic and teratogenic effects of indirect alkylating methyl and ethyl compounds, and their dependency on stages of ontogenic developments. Xenobiotica 3: 271-303, 1973.

Ivankovic, S. and Druckrey, H.: Transplacentare Erzeugnung Maligner Tumoren des Nervensystems: Athyl-Nitroso-Harnstoff (ANH) an BD IX-Ratten. Z. Krebsforsch. 71: 320-360, 1968.

565 Ethylparathion

Noda et al (1972) applied this pesticide percutaneously once a day to rats for 7 days starting on day zero or the 7th day of gestation. No effects were seen in the group treated starting on the 7th day but a decrease in implantations was found in the group started on day zero.

Noda, K.; Numata, H.; Hirabayashi, M. and Endo, I.: Influence of pesticides on embryos. 1. On influence of organophosphoric pesticides. Oyo Yakuri 6: 667-672, 1972.

566 Ethylpyrimidine (see 2,4-Diamino-5-(p-chlorophenyl)-6-ethyl-pyrimidine)

567 Ethyndiol (see Ethnodiol Diacetate)

568 2-Ethoxyethanol (see ethylene glycol monoethyl ether)

569 Etizolam   (6-(o-Chlorophenyl)8-ethyl-1-methyl-4H-S-triazolo
(3,4-C)thieno(2,3-e)(1,4)-diazepine)

Hamada et al (1979) studied this anti-anxiety drug in
pregnant rats, mice and rabbits at maximum oral doses of
100, 500 and 25 mg per kg respectively. In rats and rabbits
there were no increases in congenital defects. Some
decrease in fetal weight gain occurred in all species at the
highest doses. In mice at 500 mg per kg six exencephalic
fetuses were found from 167 exposed while only one occurred
in the control group of 229. No adverse effects on
reproduction in rats was found when 25 mg per kg was given
63 days before mating and for 7 days after fertilization
(Hamada and Imanishi, 1979). No adverse perinatal or
postnatal effects were observed in rats after 100 mg per kg
from day 17 through 21 (Hamada and Imanishi, 1979).

Hamada, Y.; Imanishi, M.: Fertility study of etizolam in
rats. Oyo Yakuri 17:781-785, 1979.

Hamada, Y.; Imanishi, M.: Perinatal and postnatal study of
etizolam in rats. Oyo Yakuri 17:787-797, 1979.

Hamada, Y.; Imanishi, M.; Onishi, K.; Hashiguchi, M.:
Teratogenicity study of etizolam (P-INN) in mice, rats and
rabbits. Oyo Yakuri 17: 763-779, 1979.

570 Etofenamate

Terada et al (1982) studied the effect of this non-steroidal
antiinflammatory agent on reproduction in the rat. Using
doses of up to 80 mg per kg daily in males and females no
loss of reproductive capacity was found. The pregnant
females were treated on days 7-17 subcutaneously with the
same dose and no adverse fetal effects were found. At 80 mg
per kg a significant number of the mothers had intestinal
ulcers.

Terada, Y.; Nishimura, K.; Shigematsu, K.; Imura, Y.;
Sasaki, H.; Yoshioka, M.; Tasumi, H.; Hashimoto, M.;
Yoshida, K.: Reproductive study of etofenamate: Fertility
and teratogenicity studies in the rat. Ikakuhin Kenkyu
13:886-909, 1982.

571 Etoperidone

Barcellona et al (1977) gave oral doses of up to 300 mg per
kg in the rat and 50 mg per kg in the rabbit during
organogenesis and found no increase in fetal malformations.

Barcellona, P.S.; Fanelli, O. and Campana, A.:
Teratological study of etoperidone in the rat and rabbit.
Toxicology 8:87-94, 1977.

572 Etretinate   (ethyl
(all-E)-9(4-methoxy-2,3,6-trimethyl-phenyl)-3,
7-dimethyl-2,4,6,8-nonatetracnoate)

572

Aikawa et al (1982) gave this vitamin A analog to rats
orally in doses of 2-8 mg per kg daily on days 7-17. The
defect rate was higher after 4 and 8 mg dosage schedules.
Exencephaly, craniofacial defects, cleft palate and skeletal
defects were found. Using 40 mg per kg on a single day on
days 8-13 they found increases in defects in each study
group.

Aikawa, M.; Sato, M.; Noda, A.; Udaka, K.: Toxicity study
of etretinate. III Reproductive segment 2 study in rats.
Yakuri to Chiryo 9:5095-5108, 5117-5143, 1982.

573 Evans blue

Wilson (1955) reported that injection of 10 mg on day 7, 8
and 9 produced brain defects and also occasional eye and
heart anomalies in the rat fetus. This azo dye probably
affects yolk sac nutrition in a way similar to the action of
trypan blue. A review on the subject of teratogenicity of
azo dyes was wriitten by Beck and Lloyd (1966).

Beck, F. and Lloyd, J.B.: Teratogenic effects of azo dyes.
In, Woollam, D.H.M. (ed.): Advances in Teratology, Vol.
1. London: Logos Press, 1966. pp 131-193.

Wilson, J.G.: Teratogenic activity of several azo dyes
chemically related to trypan blue. Anat. Rec. 123:
313-334, 1955.

574 Fasting (Including Starvation)

The mouse appears to be the animal most susceptible to
fasting teratogenesis (see Kalter and Warkany (1959) for a
concise review). A 24 to 30 hr fast in the mouse during the
7th to 10th gestational day produced vertebral and rib
defects and occasionally exencephaly (Miller, 1962).
Fasting on the 8th or 9th day produced the highest incidence
of defects. Interruption of the fast with glucose or
various aminoacids prevented the defects (Runner and Miller,
1956). Kalter (1950) has reported that cortisone has a
synergetic effect with fasting on teratogenesis in the
mouse.

Miller (1973) made a study of the effect of fasting in the
mouse and found that cleft palate incidence was increased
especially when fasting occurred on day 13. Fasting on days
11 through 13 produced 58 percent clefts. Administration of
succinate or glucose reduced the number of clefts.

A comprehensive paper on protein malnutrition and the growth
of the rat central nervous system is available (Morgane et
al, 1978).

The effect of starvation in the human has been carefully
reported in a book by Stein et al (1975). During the war
famine of 1945-46 in the Netherlands the head circumference
of newborns was decreased but no measurable intellectual
deficit was found in adult survivors. For infants exposed
to famine during early gestation there was a significant

increase   in   the   incidence   of   hydrocephalus   and
meningomyelocele.

Evidence that nutritional deprivation in early childhood may
lead to congenital nervous system defects in the subsequent
offspring of those deprived has been summarized by Emanuel
and Sever (1973).

Emanuel, I. and Sever, L.E.: Questions concerning the
possible association of potatoes and neural-tube defects,
and an alternative hypothesis relating to maternal growth
and development. Teratology 8: 325-332, 1973.

Kalter, H.: Teratogenic action of a hypocaloric diet and
small doses of cortisone. Proc. Soc. Exp. Biol. Med.
104: 518-520, 1950.

Kalter, H. and Warkany, J.: Experimental production of
congenital malformations in mammals by metabolic procedure.
Physiol. Rev. 39: 69-115, 1959.

Miller, J.R.: A strain difference in response to the teratogenic effect of maternal fasting in the mouse. Can. J.
Genet. Cytol. 4: 69-78, 1962.

Miller, T.J.: Cleft palate formation: The effects of
fasting and iodoacetic acid on mice. Teratology 7: 177-182,
1973.

Morgane, P.J.; Miller, M.; Kemper, T.; Stern, W.; Forbes,
W.; Hall, R.; Bronzino, J.; Kissane, J.; Hawrylewicz, E.
and Resnick, O.: Effects of protein malnutrition on the
developing central nervous system in the rat. Neuroscience
and Behavioral Reviews 2:137-230, 1978.

Runner, M.N. and Miller, J.R.: Congenital deformity in the
mouse as a consequence of fasting. (abstract) Anat. Rec.
124: 437-438, 1956.

Stein, Z.A.; Susser, M.; Saenger, G. and Marolla, F.:
Famine and Human Development, the Dutch Hunger Winter of
1944-45. New York: Oxford University Press, 1975.

575 Fatty Acids

Martinet (1952) reported that rats maintained on a bread,
sucrose, caseine and oat diet with added vitamins A and D
produced fetal hemorrhages in 20 percent of the offspring.
By supplementing this diet with various dietary substances,
he concluded that even small amounts of cottonseed oil, rich
in linoleic acid, prevented the hemorrhages. No other
defects were described.

Martinet, M.: Hemorragies embryonnaires par deficience en
acid linoleique. Ann. Med. Interne 53: 286-333, 1952.

576 Feline Panleucopenia Virus

This virus can cross the placenta and by interfering with

576

proliferating cerebellar cells result in ataxia in offspring
of the cat (Johnson et al.; 1967). Kalter (1968) has
summarized this subject.

Johnson, R.H.; Margolis, G. and Kilham, L.: Identity of
feline ataxia virus with feline panleucopenia virus. Nature
214: 175-177, 1967.

Kalter, H.: Teratology of the central nervous system.
Chicago: University of Chicago Press, 1968. p. 263 only.

577 Fenfluramine

Gilbert et al (1971) reported negative teratologic testing
in rats, rabbits and mice. Doses of up to 45 mg per kg were
given subcutaneously to rats on days 5 through 14 of
gestation. Postnatal studies of rats whose mothers received
20 mg per kg daily during most of gestation were reported to
be different from controls. Locomotor tests (pivoting) were
the most altered. Brain weight, but not DNA, was
significantly reduced in the pups at 70 days of postnatal
life.

Gilbert, D.L.; Franko, B.V.; Ward, J.W.; Woodard, G. and
Courtney, K.D.: Toxicologic studies of fenfluramine.
Toxicol. Appl. Pharm. 19: 707-711, 1971.

Vorhees, R.C.; Brunner, R.L. and Butcher, R.E.:
Psychotropic drugs as behavioral teratogens. Science
205:1220-1225, 1979.

578 Fenoprofen (B-L-2-(3-phenoxy-phenyl)proprionic Acid)

No teratologic effects were found in the rat or rabbit given
up to 100 mg per kg orally (Emmerson et al, 1973). Powell
and Cochrane (1975) administered 50 mg per kg to the rat
orally starting on the 18th day and produced premature
closure of the ductus arteriosus in 4 to 10 percent of the
offspring treated for 3.5 to 5 days.

Emmerson, J.L.; Gibson, W.R.; Pierce, E.C. and Todd, G.C.:
Preclinical toxicology of fenoprofen (abs) Toxicol. Appl.
Pharm. 25:44 (only), 1973.

Powell, J.G. and Cochrane, R.L.: The effects of the administration of fenoprofen or indomethacin to rat dams during
late pregnancy with special reference to the ductus
arteriosus of the fetuses and neonates. Toxicol. Appl.
Pharmacol. 45:783-796, 1978.

579 Fenoterol (1-(3,5-dihydroxyphenyl)-2-{[1-(4-hydroxy-benzyl)
ethyl]-amino}-ethanol hydrobromide)

Nishimura et al (1981) tested this beta-adrenoreceptor
stimulant orally in rats and rabbits during organogenesis at
maximum doses of 25 (rats) and 100 mg per kg (rabbits) per
day. No teratogenic effects were found. Early
embryogenesis and postnatal function was also studied. No

ill effects were found except for some delay in partuition.

Nishimura, M.; Kast, A.; Tsunenari, Y.: Reproduction studies of fenoterol (Th 1165a) in rats and rabbits (Japanese). Iyakuhin Kenkyu 12:742-761, 1981.

580 Fentiazac (4-(p-chlorophenyl)-2-phenyl-5-thiazoleacetic acid)

Shimazu et al (1979) gave this non-steroidal antiinflammatory agent to rats and rabbits by mouth. They gave up to 50 mg in rats and 100 mg per kg in rabbits. An increase in stillbirths was found at 50 mg per kg in the rat. No adverse fetal effects were found in either species.

Shimazu, H.; Ichibana, T.; Matsuura, M.; Kojima, N.: Reproductive studies on 4(p-chlorophenyl)-2-phenyl-5-thiazoleacetic acid. Kiso to Rinsho 13:1929-1945, 1979.

581 Fenthion-R

This organophosphorus insecticide was given to mice intraperitoneally on single or in 3 day periods during organogenesis in doses up to 80 mg per kg. Some reduction in fetal weight occurred but no defects were found. (Budreau and Singh, 1973).

Budreau, C.H. and Singh, R.P.: Teratogenicity and embryotoxicity of demeton and fenthion in CF No. 1 Mouse Embryos. Toxicol. Appl. Pharm. 24: 324-332, 1973.

582 Feprazone (4-prenyl-1,2-diphenyl-3,5-pyrazolidinedione)

Kato et al (1979) in a series of papers studied reproduction in the rat and rabbit using oral doses of up to 480 mg and 240 mg per kg respectively. At the highest dose in the rat preimplantation losses were increased and in the rabbits at doses above 120 mg per kg fetal lethality was increased. In neither species was any increase in defects found. Behavioral studies in the rat offspring exposed up to 120 mg per day were not different from controls.

Kato, M.; Matsuzawa, K.; Enjo, H.; Makita, T. and Hashimoto, Y.: Reproductive studies of feprazone 1-3 Ikakuhin Kenkyu 10:142-175, 1979.

583 Fern

Yasuda et al (1974) fed a diet containing 33 percent dried bracken fern to pregnant mice. The offspring had an increase in cervical and lumbar ribs and a delay in ossification as well as growth retardation. The treated group did not have an increase in other types of malformations.

Yasuda, Y.; Kihara, T. and Nishimura, H.: Embryotoxic

583

effects of feeding bracken fern (Pteridium aquilinum) to
pregnant mice. Toxicol. Appl. Pharm. 28: 264-268, 1974.

584 Fertilization, Delayed (see Delayed Fertilization)

585 Alpha-fetoprotein Antibodies

In a preliminary report Smith (1972) has produced abnormalities including neural tube closure defects in chick and rat
embryos given species-specific anti-alpha-fetoprotein
antiserum.

Smith, J.A.: Alpha-fetoprotein: A possible factor necessary
for normal development of the embryo. Lancet 1: 851 only,
1972.

586 Flagyl-R (see Metronidazole)

587 Fluocortolone

Ezumi et al (1976 and 1977) treated mice and rabbits with
this steroid. At 20 mg per kg injected subcutaneously or
given orally on day 13, the mouse fetuses had increased
cleft palate. Rabbit dams injected with 2.5 mg per kg
produced fetuses with cleft palates and exencephaly.

Ezumi, Y.; Tomoyama, J. and Kodama, N.: Teratogenicity
(cleft palate formation) in mouse embryos of fluocortolone
by a single injection. (Japanese). Yakabutsu Ryoho 9:
1623-1632, 1976.

Ezumi, Y.; Tomoyama, J.; Kodama, N. and Tanaka, M.:
Effects of subcutaneous injection of flucortolone to rabbit
embryos. Yakabutsu Ryoho 10;151-156, 1977.

588 N-2-Fluorenylacetamide

Izumi (1966) injected a single dose of 0.1 mg per gm into
mice (D-D strain) on the 8th to the 15th gestational day and
found mainly skeletal defects, but some cleft lips and
palates and cerebral hernias occurred.

Izumi, T.: Developmental anomalies in offspring of mice
induced by administration of 2-acetylaminofluorene during
pregnancy. Acta Anat. Nippon 37: 239-249, 1966.

589 Fluorine

Mottled dental enamel has been found in the deciduous teeth
of children whose mothers used well water containing 12 to
18 parts of fluorine per million (Smith and Smith, 1935).
This fluorine level is over 20 times higher than usually
found. The rat has been used for experimental study of this
subject (Schour and Smith, 1935).

The lack of association between Down's syndrome and fluoridation has been well studied and discussed (Needleman et al, 1974). Erickson (1980) has added further evidence for lack of association between fluoridation and Down's syndrome.

In explanted chick embryos both Spratt (1950) and Duffy and Ebert (1957) have reported a differential inhibition of cardiac development. Concentrations over 5 x 10(-3)m had less effect on heart development; pyruvate in concentrations of 2 x 10(-2)m prevented the effect of fluoride.

Flemming and Greenfield (1954) found decalcification and histologic changes in the teeth of mouse fetuses when the mothers received 600 microgm of CAF(2) or 1,000 microgm of NAF.

Duffy, L.M. and Ebert, J.D.: Metabolic characteristics of the heart-forming areas of the early chick embryo. J. Embryol. Exp. Morphol. 5: 324-339, 1957.

Erickson, J.D.: Down Syndrome, water fluoridation and maternal age. Teratology 21:177-180, 1980.

Flemming, H.S. and Greenfield, V.S.: Changes in the teeth and jaws of neonatal Webster mice after administration of NAF and CAF(2) to the female parent during gestation. J. Dent. Res. 33: 780-788, 1954.

Needleman, H.J.; Pueschel, S.M. and Rothman, K.J.: Fluoridation and the occurrence of Down's syndrome. N. Eng. J. Med. 291: 821-823, 1974.

Schour, I. and Smith, M.C.: Mottled teeth: An experimental and histologic analysis. J. Am. Dent. Assoc. 22: 796-813, 1935.

Smith, C.M. and Smith, H.V.: The occurrence of mottled enamel on the temporary teeth. J. Am. Dent. Assoc. 22: 814-817, 1935.

Spratt, N.T.: Nutritional requirements of the early chick embryo. III The metabolic basis of morphogenesis and differentiation as revealed by the use of inhibitors. Biol. Bull. 98: 120-135, 1950.

590 Fluoroacetate

This inhibitor of citrate oxidation via the Krebs cycle was given to rats on day 9, 10 or 11 in a dose of 1 mg per kg and no malformations detected (Spielmann et al, 1973). These same authors noted a reduction in the Q O2 of rat embryos studied in the presence of fluoroacetate.

Spielmann, H.; Meyer-Wendecker, R. and Spielmann, F.: Influence of 2-deoxy-O-glucose and sodium fluoroacetate on respiratory metabolism of rat embryos during organogenesis. Teratology 7:127-143, 1973.

591

591   5-Fluorocytosine

Chaube and Murphy (1969) produced defects in the offspring
of rats receiving 700 to 1000 mg per kg on day 11 or 12 of
gestation. The defects included cleft lip and palate,
micrognathia and other skeletal defects. They comment that
this compound was considerably less effective as a teratogen
than 5-fluorodeoxycytidine.

Takeuchi et al (1976 A and B) studied the agent in rats and
mice and found teratogenicity at doses over 10 mg per kg.
Vertebral fusions were found at 40 mg per kg given orally.
At 400 mg per kg, the mouse fetuses were reduced in size and
a small number had cleft palate.

Chaube, S. and Murphy, M.L.: The teratogenic effects of
5-fluorocytosine in the rat. Cancer Res. 29: 554-557,
1969.

Takeuchi, I.; Takagaki, T.; Yoshino, T.; Noda, A.; Shimizu,
M. and Udaka, K.: Toxicological studies on flucytosine
(5-FC) 4. Teratology study in rats. (Japanese) Basic
Pharmacology and Therapeutics 4: 59-80, 1976.

Takeuchi, I.; Shimizu, M.; Tamitani, S.; Noda, A. and
Udaka, K.: Toxicologic studies on flucytosone (5-FC) 5.
Embryotoxicity study in mice (Japanese) Basic Pharmacology
and Therapeutics 4: 101-123, 1976.

592   5-Fluoro-2-deoxycytidine

Chaube and Murphy (1968) in their general review of
fluoropyrimidines report that this compound is 200 times
more lethal in the rat fetus than in the mother. A dose of
0.15 to 2.5 mg per kg on the 11th or 12th day of gestation
causes defects of the central nervous system, palate and
skeleton. In the rat this is by weight the most potent
teratogen of the fluoropyrimidine group. Chaube and Murphy
(1968) were unable to prevent teratogenicity by thymidine
administration. Degenhardt et al. (1968) have published
detailed studies of the effect of timed dosages on incidence
and type of congenital defect produced.

Chaube, S. and Murphy, M.L.: The teratogenic effects of
the recent drugs active in cancer chemotherapy. In,
Woollam, D.H.M. (ed.): Advances in Teratology, Vol. 3.
London: Logos Press, 1968. pp 181-237.

Degenhardt, K.H.; Franz, J. and Yamamura, H.: A model in
comparative teratogenesis: dose response to
5-fluoro-2-deoxycytidine (FCDR, RO5-1090) in organogenesis
of mice strains C57Bl-6JHANFFM and C57Bl-10JFM. Teratology
1: 311-334, 1968.

593   5-Fluoro-2-deoxyuridine   [2-Deoxy-5-fluorouridine]
      [Floxuridine]

This pyrimidine analogue used in cancer chemotherapy is
teratogenic in chicks, mice and rats (see Review by Chaube

and Murphy, 1968). In the rat the fetal LD-100 is 8 times greater than the maternal LD-100. Given on the 11th or 12th day 75 to 150 mg per kg causes defects of the central nervous system, palate and skeleton. Bro-Rasmussen et al. (1971) have described embryonic hemorrhages which they believe contribute to production of the defects. Ferguson (1977;1978) has presented data that the mechanism producing cleft palate is related to lack of water binding by mucopolysaccharides and elevation of the shelves. By injecting into the yolk sac of the alligator embryo Ferguson (1981) was able to produce facial clefts.

Bro-Rasmussen, F.; Jensen, B.; Hansen, O.M. and Ostergaard, A.H.: Fluorodeoxyuridine-induced malformations in mice. Studies of early embryogenesis. Acta Pathol. Microbiol. Scand. (a) 79: 55-60, 1971.

Chaube, S. and Murphy, M.L.: The teratogenic effects of the recent drugs active in cancer chemotherapy. In, Woollam, D.H.M. (ed.): Advances in Teratology, Vol. 3. New York: Academic Press, 1968. pp 181-237.

Ferguson, M.W.J.: The mechanism of palatal shelf elevation and the pathogenesis of left palate. Virchows Arch. A. Path. Anat. and Histol. 375:97-113, 1977.

Ferguson, M.W.J.: The teratogenic effects of 5-fluoro-2-desoxyuridine (FUDR) on the Wistar rat fetus, with particular reference to cleft palate. J. Anat. 126:37-49, 1978.

Ferguson, M.W.J.: Review: The value of the American alligator as a model for research in craniofacial development. J. Craniofacial Genetics and Developmental Biology 1:123-144, 1981.

594 9-Fluoro-11-beta-21-dihydroxy-16-alpha-methylpregna-1, 4-diene-3, 20-dione

This antiinflammatory agent was tested in pregnant rats and mice (Miyamoto et al, 1975). Cleft palate was found at 1,600 microgm per kg per day when given to mice during organogenesis.

Miyamoto, M.; Ohtsu, M.; Sugisaki, T. and Sakaguchi, T.: Teratogenic effect of 9-fluoro-11-beta,21-dihydroxy-16-alpha-methylpregna-1, 4-diene-3,20-dione (A41304) a new antiinflammatory agent, and of dexamethasone in rats and mice. (Japanese) Folia Pharmacol. Japon 71: 367-378, 1975.

595 M-Fluorodimethylaminoazobenzine (see Aminoazobenzine)

596 5-Fluoro-n-(4)-methyl-2-deoxycytidine

This fluoropyrimidine is teratogenic in the mouse at doses of 5 to 300 mg per kg. Defects of the palate, central nervous system and skeleton have been reported (Chaube and Murphy, 1968).

596

Chaube, S. and Murphy, M.L.: The teratogenic effects of the recent drugs active in cancer chemotherapy. In, Woollam, D.H.M. (ed.): Advances in Teratology, Vol. 3. New York: Academic Press, 1968. pp 181-237.

597 Flurazepam (Dalmane-R)

In doses up to 80 mg per kg during various periods of gestation in the rat, neither teratogenic nor postnatal changes were produced in the offspring. In the rabbit, doses of 20 mg per kg per day from day 6 through 18 produced no observable adverse fetal effects (Hoffmann-LaRoche, 1979).

Hoffmann-LaRoche: personal communication to the author, 1979.

598 Flutofrazepam (7-chloro-1-cyclopropylmethyl-1,3-dihydro-5-(2H-1,4-benzodiazepin-2-one)

Yokoi et al (1981) gave this tranquilizer to rats before mating (700 mg per kg) during organogenesis (1000 mg per kg) and on days 17-21 (700 mg per kg). No adverse effects were noted following the first two treatments but in the perinatal test doses of 100 mg per kg or more were associated with increased death of the offspring. Learning ability and reproduction were not altered.

Yokoi, Y.; Yoshida, H.; Nagano, M.; Sagara, J.; Mitsumori, T.; Hirano, K.; Tsunawaki, M.; Nose, T.: Reproductive studies of 7- chloro-1-cyclopropylmethyl-1,3-dihydro-5-(2-fluorphenyl) 2H-1,4-benzodiazepin-2-one (KB-509). Oyo Yakuri 21:1-40, 1981.

599 5-Fluoroorotic Acid

Chaube and Murphy (1968) report that 150 to 200 mg per kg on the 11th or 12th gestational day produced deformities of the skeleton in the rat.

Chaube, S. and Murphy, M.L.: The teratogenic effects of the recent drugs active in cancer chemotherapy. In, Woollam, D.H.M. (ed.): Advances in Teratology, Vol. 3. New York: Academic Press, 1968. pp 181-237.

600 P-Fluoro-phenylalanine

Waddington and Perry (1958) produced growth inhibition with large blisters on each side of the embryonic axis in chick embryos explanted to media containing 0.2 to 0.4 mg per ml. Equimolar concentrations of phenylalanine prevented the effect.

Waddington, C.H. and Perry, M.M.: Effects of some amino--acid and purine antagonists on chick embryos. J. Embryol. Exp. Morphol. 6: 365-372, 1958.

1-(Bis(4-Fluorophenyl)methyl)4-(3-phenyl-2-propenyl)piperizine Dihydrochloride)

This drug increased cerebral blood flow. Miyazaki et al (1982) gave it orally to pregnant rats and rabbits in amounts of up to 30 or 36 mg per kg respectively. Some growth retardation and increase in embryo lethality was found in the rat. In neither species was there an increase in congenital defects. After postnatal studies in rats there was decreased nursing rates among the offspring.

Miyazaki, E.; Haro, T.; Nishikawa, S.; Oguro, T.: Toxicologic studies of K-W-3149. Kiso to Rinsho 16:1832-1839, 1840-1859, 1860-1871, 1982.

602 5-Fluorouracil

This pyrimidine analogue given on the 11th or 12th day in doses of 12 to 37 mg per kg produces defects of the central nervous system, palate and skeleton in the rat (Chaube and Murphy, 1968). Defects in the mouse fetus have been studied by Dagg (1960). The mechanism of action for the 5-fluoropyrimidines is through interference with RNA and DNA synthesis. They inhibit thymidylate synthetase producing thymidine deficiency and a syndrome termed thymidineless death. The general subject is reviewed by Chaube and Murphy (1968). Puchkov (1967) studied the effect of this compound on 4 to 23 somite chick embryos.

Stephens et al (1980) have reported a human pregnancy during which the mother received 600 mg intravenously five times weekly at 11 to 12 fetal weeks. Radial aplasia, imperforate anus, esophageal aplasia and hypoplasia o the duodenum, lung and aorta were present.

Chaube, S. and Murphy, M.L.: The teratogenic effects of the recent drugs active in cancer chemotherapy. In, Woollam, D.H.M. (ed.): Advances in Teratology, Vol. 3. New York: Academic Press, 1968. pp 181-237.

Dagg, C.P.: Sensitive stages for the production of developmental abnormalities in mice with 5-fluorouracil. Am. J. Anat. 106: 89-96, 1960.

Puchkov, V.F.: Teratogenic action of aminopterin and 5-fluorouracil on 4-23 somite chick embryos after application in ovo. Bull. Exptl. Biol. (Russian) 7: 99-102, 1967.

Stephens, T.D.; Golbus, M.S.; Miller, J.R.; Wilber, R.R.; Epstein, C.J.: Multiple congenital anomalies in a fetus exposed to 5-fluorouracil during the first trimester. Am. J. Obst. Gyn. 137:747-749, 1980.

603 5-Fluorouridine

This fluoropyrimidine produces defects of the central nervous system, palate and skeleton in rat fetuses when the

603

mother rats are treated with 25 to 50 mg per kg on the 11th or 12th gestational day (Chaube and Murphy, 1968). The maternal LD-50 is 400 to 800 mg per kg. Chaube and Murphy have reviewed this general subject (1968).

Chaube, S. and Murphy, M.L.: The teratogenic effects of the recent drugs active in cancer chemotherapy. In, Woollam, D. H.M. (ed.): Advances in Teratology, Vol. 3. New York: Academic Press, 1968. pp 181-237.

604   Flutazolam

Sato et al (1978) administered this benzodiazepin derivative orally to rats on days 8 through 15. The maximum dose of 1000 mg per kg per day did not alter fetal development.

Sato, R.; Sato, H. and Kashima, M.: Studies on the possible teratogenicity of flutazolam 3. Teratogenicity test in rats. (Japanese) Basic Pharmacology and Therapeutics 6:1692-1738, 1978.

605   Flutoprazepam

Fukunishi et al (1982) gave rabbits orally up to 50 mg per kg during organogenesis and produced no adverse fetal effects.

Fukunishi, K.; Yoshida, H.; Hirano, K.; Yokoi, Y.; Nagano, M.; Mitsumori, T.; Terasaki, M.; Nose, T.: Teratological studies on flutoprazepam in rabbits. Kiso to Rinsho 16:658-666, 1982.

606   Folic Acid Deficiency [Pteroylglutamic Acid deficiency]

Deficiency of this substance has been used widely to experimentally produce a wide variety of congenital defects. The general literature is reviewed by Kalter and Warkany (1959) and by Giroud and Tuchmann-Duplessis (1962). By altering the timing and period of the deficiency regimen, the incidence of particular anomalies can be altered (Nelson et al.; 1955). During days 7 through 8 before major organogenesis, the deficiency state had no effect. In most animal models the deficient diet is supplemented by a folic acid antagonist such as X-methyl-pteroylglutamic acid or its more purified component 9-methyl-pteroylglutamic acid. Aminopterin, another antimetabolite, produces defects in animals and man and is covered under its separate heading.

Although the mouse can be used, the rat has been the most common test subject. Cardiovascular defects were produced by Baird et al. (1954) in 57 percent of rat fetuses exposed to a deficient diet along with X-methyl-pteroylglutamic acid and succinylsulfathiazole on days 7 through 9 of gestation. No cardiovascular defects were produced when the diet was started on day 11. Genito-urinary tract defects produced by a deficiency diet on days 10 through 13 were described by Monie et al. (1957) and included renal hypoplasia, renal ectopia, absence of kidney, hydronephrosis and hydroureter.

Asling et al (1955) made detailed studies of the skeletal defects.

Johnson (1964) by careful studies of early deficient embryos suggested that mitotic arrest at metaphase might play a role in the mechanism of action of this teratogen. Further studies by Chepenik et al (1970) have shown that the embryonic deficiency is associated with decreased levels of adenosine triphosphate.

Pritchard et al. (1970) have reported that among women with folate deficiency during pregnancy no increase in malformations of their offspring was found. Pritchard et al. (1971) studied women with anticonvulsant-induced lowered serum folate and found no increase in fetal complications.

There has been evidence presented that neural tube closure defects in the human may be related to folic acid deficiency (or some other nutritional supplement). Smithells et al (1981) supplemented the diet of 202 mothers who had given birth to infants with neural tube defects. Only two recurrences of the defect were found as compared to a group of 198 controls with 10 recurrences. The controls consisted of women who entered the study after becoming pregnant. The supplement used included vitamins, calcium phosphate and iron. The folic acid content was 0.36 mg. Laurence et al (1981) gave a daily supplement of 4 mg of folic acid to 44 mothers who had had previous pregnancies with neural tube defects and had no recurrences. There were 6 recurrences among the 77 controls or non-compliers.

Asling, C.W.; Nelson, M.M.; Wright, H.V. and Evans, H.M.: Congenital skeletal abnormalities in fetal rats resulting from maternal pteroylglutamic acid deficiency during gestation. Anat. Rec. 121: 775-800, 1955.

Baird, C.D.C.; Nelson, M.M.; Monie, I.W. and Evans, H.M.: Congenital cardiovascular anomalies induced by pteroylglutamic acid deficiency during gestation in the rat. Circ. Res. 2: 544-554, 1954.

Chepenik, K.; Johnson, E.M. and Kaplan, S.: Effects of transitory maternal pteroylgluutamic acid (PGA) deficiency on levels of adenosine phosphates in developing rat embryos. Teratology 3: 229-236, 1970.

Giroud, A. and Tuchmann-Duplessis, H.: Malformations congenitales role des facteurs exogenes. Pathol. Biol. 10: 119-151, 1962.

Johnson, E.M.: Effects of maternal folic acid deficiency on cytologic phenomena in the rat embryo. Anat. Rec. 149: 49-56, 1964.

Kalter, H. and Warkany, J.: Experimental production of congenital malformations in mammals by metabolic procedure. Physiol. Rev. 39: 69-115, 1959.

Laurence, K.M.; James, N.; Miller, M.H.; Tennant, G.B. and Campbell, H.: Double-blind randomized controlled trial of folate treatment before conception to prevent recurrence of neural tube defects. Brit. Med. J. 282:1509-1511, 1981.

Monie, I.W.; Nelson, M.M. and Evans, H.M.: Abnormalities of the urinary system of rat embryos resulting from transitory deficiency of pteroylglutamic acid during gestation. Anat. Rec. 127: 711-724, 1957.

Nelson, M.M.; Wright, H.V.; Asling, C.W. and Evans, H.M.: Multiple congenital abnormalities resulting from transitory deficiency of pteroylglutamic acid during gestation in the rat. J. Nutr. 56: 349-370, 1955.

Pritchard, J.A.; Scott, D.E.; Whalley, P.J. and Haling, R.F.: Infants of mothers with megaloblastic anemia due to folate deficiency. J.A.M.A. 211: 1982-1984, 1970.

Pritchard, J.A.; Scott, D.E. and Whalley, P.J.: Maternal folate deficiency and pregnancy wastage. IV. Effects of folic acid supplements, anticonvulsants and oral contraceptives. Am. J. Obstet. Gynecol. 109: 341-346, 1971.

Smithells, R.W.; Sheppard, S.; Schorah, C.J.; Seller, M.J.; Nevin, N.C.; Harris, R.; Read, A.P.; Fielding, D.W.; Walker, S.: Vitamin supplementation and neural tube defects. Lancet 1:425 (only) 1981.

607 Folpet [N-Trichloromethylthiophthalamide]

Verrett et al. (1969) injected the chick egg via the air cell or yolk sac with 3 to 20 mg before incubation and found 8.2 percent defects. Abnormalities of the eye and central nervous system with skeletal defects were present. Amelia and phocomelia were the most noteworthy. Doses of 75 mg per kg in rabbits and 500 mg per kg in rats given at critical stages of organogenesis were non-teratogenic (Kennedy et al.; 1968).

Kennedy, G.L.; Fancher, O.E. and Calandra, J.C.: An investigation of the teratogenic potential of captan, folpet, and difolatan. Toxicol. Appl. Pharmacol. 13: 420-430, 1968.

Verrett, M.J.; Mutchler, M.K.; Scott, W.F.; Reynaldo, E.F. and McLaughlin, J.: Teratogenic effects of captan and related compounds in the developing chicken embryo. Ann. N. Y. Acad. Sci. 160: 334-343, 1969.

608 Fominoben (PB 89Cl)

This antitussive was studied by Iida et al (1978) in rats. No teratogenicity was found at oral doses of 1,500 mg per kg during organogenesis. Maternal weight was reduced at 1,000 and 1,500 mg levels, and sucklings had reduced weight gain at 1,000 mg per kg given to the mother. Postnatal reproduction was not modified.

Iida, H.; Matsuo, A.; Kast, A.; Tsunenari, Y.: Reproductive studies with fominoben hydrochloride (PB 89Cl) in rats.

Iyakuhin Kenkyu 9:724-735, 1978.

609 Food Dye Red. No. 102

This dye was fed in amounts of 1 percent of the diet to pregnant rats and no teratogenic or postnatal alterations were found. (Kihara et al, 1977)

Kihara, T.; Yasuda, Y.; Tanimura, T.: Effects on pre- and postnatal offspring of pregnant rats fed Food Dye No. 102 (abs) Teratology 16:111-112, 1977.

610 Food Dye Red No. 105

Kanoh and Hori (1982) fed a diet of 2.5% dye to rats on days 8-21 of gestation. Slight fetal weight decrease occurred and four of 55 fetuses had dilated lateral cerbral ventricles.

Kanoh, S.; Hori, Y.: Fetal toxicity of food red no. 105. Oyo Yakuri 24:391-397, 1982.

611 Food Dye Yellow No. 4

Kanoh et al (1982) fed rats up to 5% dye in the diet on days 7-14 and observed no increase in defects but the neonatal death rate was increased.

Kanoh, S.; Ema, M.; Kawasaki, H.: Fetal toxicity of food yellow No. 4. Oyo Yakuri 24:399-404, 1982.

612 Formaldehyde

Pushkina et al. (1968) exposed rats continuously during pregnancy to formaldehyde vapors (1 mg per cubic meter) and found no visible fetal malformations. The ascorbic acid content of the treated fetuses was lower than controls but the body weight was increased. The fetal DNA content was decreased and the RNA content was increased. Gofmekler (1968) found a 14-15 percent increase in the duration of rat gestation with exposure of 1 mg per cu. meter. Hurni and Ohder (1973) fed Beagles 125 and 375 PPM in the diet from 4 through 56 days of gestation and found no reproductive or fetal changes. Marks et al (1981) gave mice formaldehyde or potentiated glutaraldehyde (Sonacide-R) by gavage on days 6-15 of gestation. Maximum doses of formaldehyde (185 mg per kg) and glutaraldehyde (5.0 ml of a 2% solution per kg) did not produce increased malformations except in the group receiving the highest dose of glutaraldehyde which was lethal to a number of pregnant mice.

Gofmekler, V.A.: Effect on embryonic development of benzene and formaldehyde in inhalation experiments. Gig. Sanit. 33:12-16, 1968.

Hurni, H.; Ohder, H.: Reproductive study of formaldehyde and hexamethylene tetramine in beagle dogs. Fd. Cosmet.

Toxicol. 11: 459-462, 1973.

Marks, T.A.; Worthy, W.C.; Staples, R.E.: Influence of formaldehyde and Sonacide-R (Potentiated acid glutaraldehyde) on embryo and fetal development in mice. Teratology 22:51-58, 1981.

Pushkina, N.N.; Gofmekler, V.A. and Klertsova, G.N.: Changes in content of ascorbic acid and nucleic acids produced by benzene and formaldehyde. Bull. Exp. Biol. Med. (Russian) 66: 868-869, 1968.

613 Formamide

Thiersch (1971) gave 1 ml intraperitoneally to rats on gestational days 11 through 16 and found 36 percent resorption and, of the survivors, 46 percent were stunted. Defects of the palate and extremities also occurred.

Thiersch, J.B.: Investigations into the differential effect of compounds on rat litter and mother. In, Tuchmann-Duplessis, H. (ed.): Malformations Congenitales Des Mammiferes. Paris: Masson, 1971. pp 95-113.

614 Fosfomycin

Koeda and Moriguchi (1979 and 1980) gave this antibiotic intraperitoneally during organogenesis to rats and rabbits at maximum daily doses of up to 150 mg and 800 mg per kg respectively. Maternal and fetal toxicity was seen at the highest doses but no increase in defects or decrease in postnatal performance was found. Male and female rats treated before mating and during the first 7 days of gestation with up to 1500 mg per kg were found to have normal fertility. Perinatal studies were also done and no differences from controls were found. Similar studies were done using fosfomycin-calcium orally. The rats received up to 14,000 mg per kg and the rabbits 420 mg per kg daily during organogenesis. No adverse fetal effects were found. Fertility and perinatal and postnatal studies were carried out without finding any adverse effects except for a reduction of fetal weight and survival at the 2,800 mg per kg dose level.

Koeda, T.; Moriguchi, M.: Effects of fosfomycin-Na on reproduction of rats and rabbits. Japanese J. Antibiotics 32:155-163, 164-170, 171- 179, 1979.

Koeda, K.; Moriguchi, M.: Effect of fosfomycin-calcium on reproduction of the rat and rabbit. Japanese J. Antibiotics 32: 546-554, 1979; 33:613-617, 733-737, 478-486, 1980.

615 Fumagillin

This antibiotic produced complete litter destruction in the rat when given on the 7th gestational day in amounts of 25 mg per kg (Thiersch, 1971). Treatment on the 11th day caused 68 percent of the survivors to be stunted.

Thiersch, J.B.: Investigations into the differential effect of compounds on rat litter and mother. In. Tuchmann-Duplessis, H. (ed.): Malformations Congenitales Des Mammiferes. Paris: Masson, 1971. pp 95-113.

616 Furbiprofen (2-(2-Fluoro-4-biphenylyl)proprionic Acid)

Yoshinaka et al (1976) studied the teratogenicity of this compound in rats and rabbits giving oral doses on days 9 through 14 (rat) and 8 through 17 (rabbit). The maximum daily dose per kg was 10 mg in the rat and 25.5 mg in the rabbit. The only positive finding was an increase in skeletal variation (hypoplasia of sternebrae) in the rat fetuses.

Yoshinaka, I.; Saito, K.; Hikida, S.; Komori, S.; Okuda, T.; Matubara, T.; Moriji, H. and Saito, H.: Studies on toxicity of FP-70 2. Teratogenicity test in rats and rabbits. (Japanese) Clinical Report 10:1890- 1915, 1976.

617 Furosemide

This diuretic was given twice daily in amounts of 37.5 to 300 mg per kg to rats on days 6-17 of gestation (Robertson et al, 1981). Decreased fetal weight was seen at 150 and 300 mg levels. Wavy ribs and some skeletal defects were found at these levels. These defects were not seen when KCl was given concurrently.

Robertson, R.T.; Minsker, D.H.; Bokelman, D.L.; Durand, G.; Conquet, P.: Potassium loss as a causative factor for skeletal malformations in rats produced by indacrinone: a new investigational loop diuretic. Toxicol. Appl. Pharm. 60:142-150, 1981.

618 Furylfuramide

Miyaji (1971) fed pregnant mice a diet containing 0.2 percent of this compound after the 7th day of mating and observed no increase in malformations. The fertility of males was diminished in a 3-generation test using a diet with 0.0125 percent furylfuramide.

Miyaji, T.: Effect of furylfuramide on reproduction and malformation. Tohoku J. Exp. Med. 103: 381-388, 1971.

619 Fusaric Acid-Ca

Matsuzaki et al (1976 and 1977) did teratologic studies in mice, rats and rabbits. In the mouse and rat, a maximum daily dose of 125 mg per kg orally caused no defects but delay in ossification and growth of the mouse fetuses was found. At the same dose, no effects were found in the rabbit.

Matsuzaki, A.; Akutsu, S.; Mukaikawa, H. and Shimamura, T.:
Studies on the possible teratogenicity of fusaric acid–Ca 3.
Effects on the mouse and rat embryo. (Japanese) Japanese J.
of Antibiotics 5: 543–551, 1976.

Matsuzaki, A.; Akutsu, S.; Shimamura, T. and Nakatani, H.:
Studies on the possible teratogenicity of fusaric acid–Ca 3.
Effects on the embryos of oral administration to pregnant
rabbits. (Japanese) Japanese J. of Antibiotics 30:321–333,
1977.

620   Galactoflavin (also see Riboflavin Deficiency)

This analogue of riboflavin has been used to augment the
riboflavin-deficient state in experimental animal models
(Nelson et al.; 1956). The usual dose of galactoflavin is
60 mg per kg of riboflavin-deficient diet, and this
combination given during the entire gestation produces in
the rat fetus a syndrome characterized by growth
retardation, hypoplasia of mandible and reduction defects of
the extremities. Hydronephrosis (26 percent), cleft palate
(34 percent) and subcutaneous edema (30 percent) are
frequently observed also (Shepard et al.; 1968). The exact
mechanism by which galactoflavin and riboflavin deficiency
interfere with the development of the terminal electron
transport system is not known (Aksu et al.; 1968); however,
if 600 mg of riboflavin is added to the deficient diet with
galactoflavin, the anomalies are prevented.

Aksu, O.; Mackler, B.; Shepard, T.H. and Lemire, R.J.:
Studies of the development of congenital anomalies in
embryos of riboflavin-deficient galactoflavin fed rats. II.
Role of the terminal electron transport systems. Teratology
1: 93–102, 1968.

Nelson, M.M.; Baird, C.D.C.; Wright, H.V. and Evans, H.M.:
Multiple congenital abnormalities in the rat resulting from
riboflavin deficiency induced by the antimetabolite
galactoflavin. J. Nutr. 58: 125–134, 1956.

Shepard, T.H.; Lemire, R.J.; Aksu, O. and Mackler, B.:
Studies of the development of congenital anomalies in
embryos of riboflavin-deficient galactoflavin fed rats. I.
Growth and embryonic pathology. Teratology 1: 75–92, 1968.

621   Galactose

Bannon et al. (1945) fed a 25 percent galactose diet to
rats and found cataracts starting on day 15 of gestation.
Demeyer (1959) fed rats 55 percent galactose diets and
produced anophthalmia and lens abnormalities in the fetuses.
The most sensitive period was the 8th, 9th and 10th day of
gestation. Segal and Bernstein (1963) demonstrated that
galactose crosses the placenta of the rat.

Evidence that galactose toxicity reduces the weight and the
content of protein and DNA of the fetal brain has been given
by Haworth and Ford (1973).

Bannon, S.L.; Higginbottom, R.M.; McConnell, J.M. and Kaan, H.W.: Development of the galactose cataract in the albino rat. Arch. Ophthalmol. 33: 224-228, 1945.

Demeyer, R.: Action teratogene du galactose administre a la rate gravide. Ann. Endocrinol. (Paris) 20: 203-211, 1959.

Haworth, J.C. and Ford, J.D.: Effect of galactose toxicity on incorporation of tritiated thymidine into fetal brain. Brain Res. 63: 470-473, 1973.

Segal, S. and Bernstein, H.: Observations on cataract formation in the newborn offspring of rats fed a high galactose diet. J. Pediatr. 62: 363-370, 1963.

622 Gallamine Triethiodide

Jacobs using 8 to 64 mg per kg on day 15.3 of gestation was able to produce flaccid paralysis in the rat fetus but no cleft palates resulted.

Jacobs, R.M.: Failure of muscle relaxants to produce cleft palate in mice. Teratology 4: 25-30, 1971.

623 Gallium

Ferm and Carpenter (1970) injected 40 mg per kg intravenously into hamsters on day 8 of gestation and found no increase in malformation rate in 237 fetuses.

Ferm, V.H. and Carpenter, S.J.: Teratogenic and embryopathic effects of indium, gallium and germanium. Toxicol. Appl. Pharmacol. 16: 166-170, 1970.

624 Gas Fuel (see Methane)

625 German Measles (see Rubella)

626 Germanium

Ferm and Carpenter (1970) injected hamsters intravenously on day 8 of pregnancy with 40 or 100 mg per kg and reported no increase in congenital defects.

Ferm, V.H. and Carpenter, S.J.: Teratogenic and embryopathic effects of indium, gallium, and germanium. Toxicol. Appl. Pharmacol. 16: 166-170, 1970.

627 Germine [Protoverine]

This alkaloid of Veratrum californicum has been tested in pregnant ewes with negative results.

Keeler, R.F. and Binns, W.: Teratogenic compounds of Veratrum californicum (Durand). V. comparison of cyclopian effects of steroidal alkaloids from plant and structurally related compounds from other sources. Teratology 1: 5-10, 1968.

628 Gliclazide (Sulfonylurea Gliclazide)

Kawanishi et al (1981) administered this new antidiabetic to rats and rabbits orally in maximum doses of 800 and 120 mg per kg respectively. No adverse fetal effects were found except for fetal weight reduction in the rat at 400 and 800 mg per kg. Maternal weight was also reduced. Learning ability and reproductive function of rat offspring was not affected after dosing on days 17 of gestation through day 21 poostnatally.

Kawanishi, H.; Takeshima, T.; Igarashi, N.; Tauchi, K.: Reproductive studies of gliclazide a new sulfonylurea antidiabetic agent. Yakuri to Chiryo 9:3551-3571, 1981.

629 Glossypol

This product of the cotton plant used for birth control in China reduced the weight and hatchability of cotton leaf worm larvae (El- Sebae et al, 1981).

El-Sebae, A.H.; Sherby, S.I.; Manscrit, N.A.: Glossypol as inducer and inhibitor in Spodoptera littoralis larvae. J. Environ. Sci. Health B. 16:167-178, 1981.

630 Glucagon

Scaglione (1960) reported production of fetal cataracts after daily administration of 20 or 200 microgm of glucagon to pregnant rats. Tuchmann-Duplessis and Mercier-Parot (1962) produced glaucoma in fetal rats by injecting 300 microgm on the 7th, 8th and 9th days. When the dosage was increased to 400 or 500 microgm, microphthalmia and defects of the skeleton were found.

Scaglione, S.: Recherches sur l'action du cortisone de l' acth, du glucagone et de l'iode (131) sur les embryons des rates pleines. Folia Hered. Pathol. 9: 143-150, 1960.

Tuchmann-Duplessis, H. and Mercier-Parot, L.: Production de malformations congenitales chez le rat traite par le glucagon. C. R. Acad. Sci. (Paris) 254: 2655-2657, 1962.

631 Glucose

Cockroft and Coppola (1977) studied the effect of 1200 and 1500 mg of D-glucose per ml on explanted rat embryos and found fusion of the anterior to the posterior neural folds in many of the specimens. L-glucose retarded growth and did not produce abnormalities.

Cockroft, D.L. and Coppola, P.T.: Teratogenic effects of

excess glucose on head-fold rat embryos in culture.
Teratology 16:141-146, 1977.

632 Glutamate (see Monosodium Glutamate)

633 Beta-L-Glutamyl-amino Propionitrile (also see Lathyrism)

This compound is an active principle of lathyrus odoratus
seeds (Schilling and Strong, 1954) and produces the lathyrus
syndrome in mammalian fetuses (see Lathyrism).

Schilling, E.D. and Strong, F.M.: Isolation, structure and
synthesis of a lathyrus factor from 1. Odoratus. J. Am.
Chem. Soc. 76: 2848 only, 1954.

634 Glutaraldehyde

Marks et al (1980) using Sonacide-R a potentiated acid
glutaraldehyde gave mice the equivalent of 100 mg per kg on
days 6-15. Although this dose was lethal in 19 of 35 dams
no evidence of teratogenicity was detected.

Marks, T.A.; Worthy, W.C.; Staples, R.E.: Influence of
formaldehyde and Sonacide-R (potentiated acid
glutaraldehyde) on embryo and fetal development of mice.
Teratology 22:51-58, 1980.

635 Glutethimide

McColl et al. (1963) reported that a diet coontaining 0.4
percent glutethimide fed during pregnancy failed to produce
defects in the rat fetus. Double vertebral centra which
occurred in 4 of 17 fetuses represent probably only a delay
in ossification. Tuchmann-Duplessis and Mercier-Parot
(1963) produced resorptions but no congenital defects in the
rabbit, mouse and rat.

Kotin and Ignatyeva (1982) injected pregnant rats (with
200-400 mg per kg on days 14 and 15) and observed some
behavioural abnormalities in the first progeny of animals
under test.

Kotin, A.M. and Ignatyeva: Variation in rat behavior after
exposure to glutethimide during antenatal neurogenesis.
Farmakol. Toksikol. (USSR) 4:73-78, 1982.

McColl, J.D.; Globus, M. and Robinson, S.: Drug induced
skeletal malformations in the rat. Experientia 19: 183-184,
1963.

Tuchmann-Duplessis, H. and Mercier-Parot, L.: Repercussion
d'un somnifere, le glutethimide, sur la gestation et le
developpement foetal du rat, de la souris et du lapin. C.
R. Acad. Sci. (Paris) 256: 1841-1843, 1963.

636 Glycopyrrolate

Kagiwada et al (1973) gave this anticholinergic agent orally
to pregnant mice and rats during active organogenesis. The
maximum dose in the rat was 150 mg per kg per day and in the
mouse it was 100 mg. No increase in defects was found and
postnatal studies for 3 weeks were negative.

Kagiwada, K.; Ishizaki, O. and Saito, G.: Effects of
glycopyrrolate on pre- and post-natal developments of the
offsprings in pregnant mice and rats. (Japanese) Oyo Yakuri
7: 617-626, 1973.

637 L-Goitrin

This thioamide present as its glycoside in vegetables such
as turnips and cabbage can inhibit the metabolism of the
thyroid gland in the developing chick. A total dose of 1.0
mg given during the 7th to 15th days of incubation caused
thyroid hypertrophy and reduction of radioiodine uptake in
the chick embryo on the 17th day (Shepard, 1960).

Shepard, T.H.: Unpublished data, 1960.

638 Gold

Ridgway and Karnofsky (1952) using $AuCl(3)$ determined that
the LD-50 for chick embryos was less than 20 mg per egg. No
congenital defects were noted.

Kidston et al (1971) reported a 25 percent malformation rate
in rats exposed to somewhat higher than human serum levels
of gold (aurothiomalate). These malformations included
hydronephrosis, hydrocephalus with some eye, heart and
palate defects. Gold accumulated in the yolk sac lyosomes.
Szabo et al (1978A and B) studied two oral forms and a
thiomalate subcutaneous compound in rats and rabbits treated
during day 6-15 and 6-18, respectively. At the higher dose
levels (6-44 mg gold per kg per day), they found a small
increase in defects. Hydrocephalus, eye defects and rib
fusion were the most frequent defects in rats while
gastroschisis and umbilical hernia were most common in
rabbits.

Transfer of gold across the placenta of a 20 week human
pregnancy has been documented (Rocker and Henderson, 1976)
but Hollander (1972) documents a series where several women
received gold without untoward effects on their fetuses.
Miayamoto et al (1974) in a survey found 26 patients who
received gold during pregnancy and all of these offspring
were normal. Another 93 patients took gold during only the
first part of their pregnancy and among these offspring
there was one with dislocated hip and one with a flattened
acetabulum.

Hollander, J.L.: Arthritis and Allied Conditions edited by
J.C. Hollander and D. J. McCarthy, Philadelphia, 1972, p.
479.

Kidston, M.E.; Beck, F. and Lloyd, J.B.: Effects of
myocrisin injection in rats. J. Anat. 108:590-591, 1971.

Miyamoto, T.; Miyaji, S. and Horiuchi, Y.: Gold therapy in bronchial asthma - special emphasis upon blood level of gold and its teratogenicity (Japanese) J. of Japanese Soc. of Int. Med. 63: 1190-1197, 1974.

Ridgway, L.P. and Karnofsky, D.A.: The effects of metals on the chick embryo: Toxicity and production of abnormalities in development. Ann. N. Y. Acad. Sci. 55: 203-215, 1952.

Rocker, I. and Henderson, W.J.: Transfer of gold from mother to fetus. Lancet 2:1246 only, 1976.

Szabo, K.T.; Guerriero, F.J. and Kang, Y.J.: Effects of gold-containing compounds on pregnant rats and their fetuses. Vet. Path. 15 (suppl. 5) 89-96, 1978A.

Szabo, K.T.; DiFebbo, M.E. and Phelan, D.G.: The effects of gold-containing compounds on pregnant rabbits and their fetuses. Vet. Path. 15 (suppl. 5) 97-102, 1978B.

639 Gonadotropin, Human Chorionic

Hultquist and Engfeldt (1949) gave human chorionic gonadotropin injections in the rat and produced some increase in weight of the newborn fetuses. Whether this size increase was due to delay in parturition or reduction in number of fetuses per litter was not evident. No defects were found.

Hultquist, G.T. and Engfeldt, B.: Growth of rat fetuses produced experimentally by means of administration of hormones to the mother during pregnancy. Acta Endocrinol. (KBH) 3: 365-376, 1949.

640 Griseofulvin

Solonitskaya (1969) injected 50 to 500 mg per kg into pregnant rats on the 11th through the 14th day. WWith the largest dose 22 percent of the fetuses were abnormal. A wide range of defects was seen including the eye, skeleton, urogenital tract and central nervous system. Injection during the first four days of pregnancy did not cause defects or embryonic death. Chronic injection on each day of pregnancy was less toxic to the embryo than acute administration during the critical periods of organogenesis.

Klein and Beall (1972) using doses of 1250 to 1500 mg per kg daily from the 6th through the 15th day of gestation in the rat produced an 8 to 10 percent incidence of tail defects in the offspring. Occasionally exencephaly was found. These dosages are 60 to 75 times those used therapeutically in man.

Klein, M.F. and Beall, J.R.: Griseofulvin; a teratogenic study. Science 175: 1483-1484, 1972.

Slonitskaya, N.N.: Teratogenic effect of grisofulvin-forte on rat fetus (Russian). Antibiotiki 14: 44-48, 1969.

641 Guanfacine   (N-Amidino-2(2,6-dichlorophenyl)   acetamide
hydrochloride)

Esaki and Nakayama (1979A) gave 0.5 to 2 mg per kg daily to
pregnant rabbits from the 6th to 18th day of gestation.
Even though the weight gain of the mothers was reduced at
the 1 mg level and above, no increase in defects was found.
In another series of papers using similar dosing in the
mouse no evidence of teratogenicity or reproductive
dysfunction was observed (Esaki and Hirayama, 1979).
Postnatal studies were also negative although some neonatal
mortality increase was found at 1.0 mg per kg (Esaki et al,
1980).

Esaki, K.; Nakayama, T.: Effects of oral administration of
BS 100-1441 on;the rabbit fetus. Preclin. Rept. Cent.
Inst. Exp. Animal 5:129-136, 1979.

Esaki, K.; Hirayama, M.: Effect of oral administration of
BS-100- 141 on reprodu;tion in th; mouse. Preclin. Rept.
Cent. Exp. Animal 5:107-128, 1979.

Esaki, K.; Oshio, K.; Yamaguchi, K.: Effects of oral
administration of BS-100-141 on reproduction in mice:
observations on behavior. Preclin. Rep. Cent. Exp.
Animal 6:117-122, 1980.

642 Guanine (also see 2-Deoxyguanosine)

This substance was injected by Karnofsky and Lacon (1961)
into 4-day chick eggs and no abnormalities were found. The
LD-50 for the embryo on the 4th day was 8 mg per egg.

Karnofsky, D.A. and Lacon, C.R.: Effects of physiological
purines on the development of the chick embryo. Biochem.
Pharmacol. 7: 154-158, 1961.

643 Guanosine (also see 2-Deoxyguanosine)

Karnofsky and Lacon (1961) found that the LD-50 for 4-day
chick embryos was 8 mg per egg. Using 2 to 12 mg they
reported that 12 percent of the embryos were abnormal. The
type of defects was not specified.

Karnofsky, D.A. and Lacon, C.R.: Effects of physiological
purines on the development of the chick embryo. Biochem.
Pharmacol. 7: 154-158, 1961.

644 Hadacidin [N-Formyl-N-hydroglycine]

Chaube and Murphy (1963) reported that rats receiving 1 to 5
mg per kg on days 9 through 12 or single injections on day
10, 11 or 12 produced fetuses with exencephaly, cleft palate
or other skeletal defects. Two analogues of hadacidin,
N-acetyl hydroxyaminoacetic acid and hydroxyaminoacetic acid
at the same dose ranges were toxic to the fetuses but did
not produce malformations. Lejour-Jeanty (1966) has studied
the pathoembryogenesis of the cleft lip deformity and found

that cell death played a prominent role in preventing the lateral nasal process to fuse with the medial nasal and maxillary processes. Milaire (1971) made a study of the pathogenesis of the syndactyly which occurrs and found an associated reduction in proliferation of the limb blastema along with some hyperplasia of the apical ectodermal ridge.

Chaube, S. and Murphy, M.L.: Teratogenic effect of hadacidin (a new growth inhiibitory chemical) on the rat fetus. J. Exp. Zool. 152: 67-73, 1963.

Lejour-Jeanty, M.: Becs-de-lievre provoques chez le rat par un derive de penicilline, l'hadacidine. J. Embryol. Exp. Morphol. 15: 193-211, 1966.

Milaire, J.: Etude morphogenetique de la syndactylie postaxiale provoquee chez le rat par l'hadacidine: 2 les bourgeous de membres chez les embryons de 12 a 14 jours. Arch. Biol. (Liege) 82: 253-322, 1971.

645 Hair Dyes

A composite of a series of commercially available semipermanent hair colorings (mostly phenylendiamines) was added to the diet of rats in the maximal amount of 7800 ppm from day 6 through 15 and no fetal effects were found. Rabbits were also tested by gavage on days 6-18 of gestation with doses up to 97.5 mg per kg per day and no teratogenicity was found (Wernick et al, 1975). Marks et al (1981) studied the effects of 2-nitro-p- phenylenediamine (2-NPPD), 4-nitro-0-phenyldiamine (4-NOPD) and 2,5-toluenediamine sulfate (2,5TDS) by subcutaneous injection on days 6-15 in the pregnant mouse. At doses which were toxic to the mother defects were prouced with 2-NPPD and 4-NOPD (160 mg and 256 mg per kg per day respectively). Cleft palate was the most common defect but mineralization of the myocardium also was observed. 2,5-TDS was not teratogenic at 64 mg per kg.

Marks, T.A.; Gupta, B.N.; Ledoux, T.A.; Staples, R.E.: Teratogenic evaluation of 2-nitro-p-phenylenediamine, 4-nitro-0- phenylenediamine and 2,5-toluenediamine sulfate in the mouse. Teratology 24:253-265, 1981.

Wernick, T.; Lanman, B.M. and Fraux, J.L.: Chronic toxicity, teratologic and reproductive studies with hair dyes. Toxicol. Appl. Pharm. 32: 450-460, 1975.

646 Haloperidol

Tuchmann-Duplessis and Mercier-Parot (1971) have shown that this tranquilizer has a remarkable delaying effect on time of implantation in the mouse and rat. In the rat treated immediately after mating with 2 to 10 mg per kg daily about 50 percent of the fetuses on day 20 were the size of 14-day embryos. If delivery was allowed to occur, normal fetuses appeared 2 to 8 days later than in the controls. No defects were associated with this delay in growth. Yamamura et al (1982) found a delay in the first three cleavages of the

646

mouse morula when 3.5 mg per kg was administered subcutaneously.

Van Waes and Van De Velde studied 100 pregnancies in which 0.6 mg was administered twice daily for varying periods. Not a single malformation was found in 94 newborns examined and no adverse effects on pregnancy were observed.

Tuchmann-Duplessis, H. and Mercier-Parot, L.: Influence of neuraleptics on prenatal development in mammals. In, Tuchmann-Duplessis, H.; Fanconi, G. and Burgio, G.R. (eds.): Malformations, Tumors and Mental Defects, Pathogenetic Correlations. Milan: Carlo Erba Foundation, 1971.

Van Waes, A.; Van De Velde, W.: Safety evaluation of haloperidol in the treatment of hyperemesis gravidarum. J. of Clinical Pharmacy 9:224-227, 1969.

Yamamura, H.; Kukui, K.; Fukui, Y.; Inamoto, M.: Effects of haloperidol, an antipsychotic agent, on preimplantation development in the mouse. Cong. Anom. 22:145-160, 1982.

647 Halothane

Basford and Fink (1968) reported that when rats were exposed to 0.8 percent halothane for 24 hours on day 9 a significant increase in defects of the ribs and vertebrae were found in the offspring as compared to controls exposed to air and also starved during day 9.

Basford, A.B. and Fink, B.R.: The teratogenicity of halothane in the rat. Anesthesiology 29: 1167-1173, 1968.

648 Hb 419 [N-4-[2-(5-Chlor-2-methoxybenzamido)-ethyl-]phenylsulfonyl-N-cyclo hexylurea]

This oral antidiabetic drug was tested in mice, rats and rabbits with negative results (Baeder and Sakaguchi, 1969). Doses up to 350 mg per kg per day were used.

Baeder, C. and Sakaguchi, T.: Teratologische untersuchungen mit HB 419. Arzneim. Forsch. 19: 1419-1420, 1969.

649 Heliotrine

This pyrrolizidine alkaloid occurring in several plant families can cause liver disease in animals and man. Green and Christie (1961) injected 150 or 200 mg per kg into the rat. Vertebral and rib defects occurred when the rats were treated after the 11th day. Mandibular hypoplasia and cleft palate were seen when the higher dose was used.

Green, C.R. and Christie, G.S.: Malformations in foetal rats induced by the pyrrolizidine alkaloid heliotrine. Br. J. Exp. Pathol. 42: 369-378, 1961.

650 Hemlock

Edmonds et al. (1972) reported an outbreak of congenital defects in the offspring of sows who ingested poison hemlock (Conium maculatum). Seven of 55 newborn piglets had defects of the hind legs and 34 had classic signs of hemlock poisoning including trembling and ataxia. Sows from the same farm pastured in an area where poison hemlock did not grow gave birth to normal offspring.

Edmonds, L.D.; Selby, L.A. and Case, A.A.: Poisoning and congenital malformations associated with consumption of poison hemlock by sows. J. Am. Vet. Med. Ass. 160: 1319-1324, 1972.

651 Heparin

With a molecular weight of 20,000, heparin apparently does not cross the placenta. The author has found no studies of this drug in pregnant animals. Complications of pregnancy are common and may include the central nervous system (Pauli and Hall, 1982).

Pauli, R.M.; Hall, J.G.: Warfarin embryopathy. Am. J. Med. 68:122-144, 1980.

652 Hepatitis

Siegel and Fuerst (1966) in a prospective study of the offspring of 60 mothers with hepatitis found no increase in congenital defect rate. Low birth rate was found in 37 percent of mothers having the infection after 20 weeks of gestation. Adams and Combes (1965) found no fetal wastage in 34 patients.

Schweitzer et al (1973) followed 31 infants whose mothers had hepatitis B during or shortly after pregnancy. Neonatal infection occurred in only one out of 10 women infected in the first 2 trimesters but in 16 out of 21 infants exposed in the 3rd trimester. Of the infected babies, 35 percent were less than 2,500 gm at birth. Hieber et al (1977) in a study of 50 pregnancies confirmed these findings by observing no congenital defects. They found a higher incidence of low birth weight and some asymptomatic carriers among infants whose mothers were infected in the last trimester. Drew et al (1978) found that when either parent was HBS Ag positive, there was a very high sex ratio in their offspring (60 males and 24 females). Beasley et al (1981) were able to significantly reduce the carrier rate in offspring of HBsAg carrier mothers by immunizing from birth with hepatitis B immune globulin.

Adams, R.H. and Combes, B.: Viral hepatitis during pregnancy. J.A.M.A. 192: 195-198, 1965.

Beasley, R.P.; Lin, C-C; Wang, K-Y; Hsieh, F-S.; Hwang, L-Y; Stevens, C.E.; Sun T.S.; Szmuness, W.: Hepatitis B immune globulin (HBIG) efficiency in the interruption of perinatal transmission of Hepatitis B virus carrier state. Lancet

2:388-393, 1981.

Drew, J.S.; London, W.T.; Lustbader, E.D.; Hesser, J.E.; and Blumberg, B.S.: Hepatitis B virus and sex ratio of off-spring. Science 201:687-692, 1978.

Heiber, J.P.; Dalton, D.; Shorey, J. and Combes, B.: Hepatitis in pregnancy. J. Pediatr. 91:545-549, 1977.

Schweitzer, I.L.; Dunn, A.E.G.; Peters, R.L. and Spears, R.L.: Viral hepatitis B in neonates and infants. Am. J. Med. 55: 762-771, 1973.

Siegel, M. and Fuerst, H.T.: Low birth weight and maternal virus diseases. A prospective study of rubella, measles, mumps, chicken pox and hepatitis. J.A.M.A. 197: 680-684, 1966.

653 Heptabarbital (see Barbituric Acid)

654 2-hepta-5-methylbenzimidazole (see Benzimidazole)

655 Heroin (diacetylmorphine)

Teausch et al (1973) injected 3 to 12 mg of uncut heroin intravenously to the rabbit on days 24 through 26 of gestation. The fetal body weight was reduced but lung maturation was accelerated. Naeye et al (1973) have reported that newborns from addicted mothers have diminished numbers of cells in most of their tissues. Except for a higher rate of infection, no other disorders were increased in these 39 infants. Heinonen et al (1976) found no increase in defects among 11 exposed infants.

Heinonen, O.P.; Slone, D. and Shapiro, S.: Birth Defects and Drugs in Pregnancy. Publishing Sciences Group, Inc.; Littleton, Mass.; 1977.

Naeye, R.L.; Blanc, W.; LeBlanc, W. and Khatamee, M.A.: Fetal complications of maternal heroin addiction. J. Pediatr. 83:1055-1061, 1973.

Taeusch, H.W.; Carson, S.H.; Wang, N.S. and Avery, M.E.: Heroin induction of lung maturation and growth retardation in fetal rabbits. J. Pediat. 82: 869-875, 1973.

656 Herpes Virus

South et al. (1969) report a newborn infant with microcephaly, intracranial calcifications, eye defects and vescicular skin lesions. Type 2 herpes virus was recovered from the child and the mother reported genital blisters and vaginal discharge in the early weeks of pregnancy. Schaffer (1965) reported a similar patient with herpes virus isolated. Florman et al (1973) report an infant infected with herpes 1 who had microcephaly, intracranial calcifications and owl eye inclusion bodies in the urine.

They summarize 5 reported cases of herpes 2 infection. Eye and retinal disease are associated with the brain damage. All of the 5 cases reported have been suspected because of a vesicular rash in the newborn period.

Heath et al (1956) have produced microcephaly and flexion deformities in chick embryos receiving herpes simplex at 48 hours of incubation.

Heath, H.D.; Shear, H.H.; Imagawa, D.T.; Jones, M.H. and Adams, J.M.: Teratogenic effects of herpes simplex vaccinia, influenza-A (NWS) and distemper virus infections on early chick embryos. Proc. Soc. Exp. Biol. Med. 92: 675-682, 1956.

Florman, A.L.; Gershon, A.A.; Blackett, P.R. and Nahmias, A.J.: Intrauterine infection with herpes simplex virus. Resultant congenital anomalies. J.A.M.A. 225: 129-132, 1973.

Schaffer, A.J.: Diseases of the newborn. Philadelphia: W.B. Saunders Co. (2nd ed.), 1965. pp 733-734.

South, M.A.; Thompkins, W.A.F.; Morris, C.R. and Rawls, W.E.: Congenital malformation of the central nervous system associated with genital type (type 2) herpes virus.. J. Pediatr. 75: 13-18, 1969.

657 Hexachlorobenzene

Khera (1974) gave single oral doses to rats during several periods of organogenesis and until day 21 of gestation. The doses varied from 10 to 120 mg per kg per day. At the higher doses extra 14th ribs were found but this was associated in the maternal toxicity. The fetal weights and survival rates did not differ from controls and no other defects were found. Dominant lethal studies were negative. Courtney et al (1975) used 100 mg per kg in the mouse and found no significant fetal changes.

The transplacental passage of the chemical has been found in the rat and mouse (Svendsgaard et al, 1979); swine, (Hansen et al, 1979); rat (Villeneuve and Hierlihy, 1975); rabbit, (Villeneuve et al, 1974) and human (Astolfi et al, 1974).

Astolfi, E.; Alonso, A.H.; Mendizabal, A.; Zubizarreta, E.: Pesticides chlores de l'accorichee et du cordin ombilical des nouveau-nes. J. European Toxicol. 1:330-338, 1974.

Courtney, K.D.; Copeland, M.F.; Robbins, A.: The effects of pentochloronitrobenzene, hexachlorobenzene and related compounds on fetal development. Toxicol. Appl. Pharmacol. 35:239-256, 1976.

Hansen, L.G.; Simon, J.; Dorn, S.B.; Teske, R.H.: Hexachlorobenzene distribution in tissues of swine. Toxicol. Appl. Pharmacol. 51:1-7, 1979.

Khera, K.S.: Teratogenicity and dominant lethal studies of hexachlorobenzene in rats. Fd. Cosmet. Toxicol.

657

12:471-477, 1974.

Svendsgaard, D.J.; Courtney, K.D.; Andrews, J.E.: Hexachlorobenze (HCB) deposition in maternal and fetal tissues of rat and mouse. Environ. Res. 20:267-281, 1979.

Villeneuve, D.C.; Hierlihy, S.L.: Placental transfer of hexachlorobenzene in the rat. Bull Environ. Contamin. Toxicol. 13: 489-491, 1975.

Villeneuve, D.C.; Panopio, L.G.; Grant, D.L.: Placental transfer of hexachlorobenzene in the rabbit. Envir. Physiol. Biochem. 4:112- 115, 1974.

658 3,3',4,4',5,5'-Hexachlorobiphenyl

Marks et al (1981) gavaged mice on days 6-15 of gestation with 0.1 to 16 mg per kg per day. At 8 mg per kg the dams had a decrease in weight gain. Cleft palate and hydronephrosis were found to be increased beginning at 2 and 4 mg dose levels respectively.

Marks, T.A.; Kimmel, G.L.; Staples, R.E.: Influence of symmetrical polychlorinated biphenyl isomers on embryo and fetal development in mice. Toxicol. Appl. Pharm. 61:269-276, 1981.

659 Hexachloropentadiene

John et al (1979) gavaged pregnant mice and rabbits with up to 75 mg per kg per day during active organogenesis and observed no teratogenic effect.

John, J.A.; Murray, F.J.; Murray, J.S.; Schwetz, B.A. and Staples, R.E.: Evaluation of environmental contaminants tetrachloroacetone, hexochlorocyclopentadiene and sulfuric acid aerosol for teratogenic potential in mice and rabbits. (abs) Teratology 19:32A-33A, 1979.

660 Hexachlorophene

Levels of 100 to 500 PPM fed to rats have not produced gross changes in the fetal brain; but at the highest levels which were toxic to the mothers 3 of 44 fetuses had cleft palate (Oakley and Shepard, 1972). Kimbrough and Gaines (1971) reported cystic changes in the white matter of the brain of rats fed 500 PPM (25 mg per kg per day) hexachlorophene for two weeks. Kimmel et al. (1972) administered hexachloro- phene to rats by intravaginal application on days 7, 8, 9 and 10. The approximate dosage was 300 mg per kg daily. Microphthalmia, hydrocephalus and wavy ribs were produced in the fetuses. only two cleft palates were produced out of 82 surviving fetuses. Kennedy et al (1975) using 6 mg per kg on days 6 through 18 in the pregnant rabbit produced no soft tissue anomalies and only 3 out of 175 had rib malforma- tions. Transplacental studies of the material in mice have been reported (Brandt et al, 1979).

Brandt, I.; Dencker, L. and Larsson, Y.: Transplacental passage and embryonic-fetal accumulation of hexachlorophene in mice. Toxicol. Appl. Pharmacol. (in press), 1979.

Kennedy, G.L.; Smith, S.H.; Keplinger, M.L. and Calandra, J.C.: Evaluation of the teratological potential of hexachlorophene in rabbits and rats. Teratology 12: 83-88, 1975.

Kimbrough, R.D. and Gaines, T.B.: Hexachlorophene effects on the rat brain. Arch. Environ. Health 23: 114-118, 1971.

Kimmel, C.A.; Moore, W. and Stara, J.F.: Hexachlorophene teratogenicity in rats. Lancet 2: 765 only, 1972.

Oakley, G.P. and Shepard, T.H.: Possible teratogenicity of hexachlorophene in rats. (abstract) Teratology 4: 264 only, 1972.

661 N-hexane (and metabolites)

N-hexane can be metabolically activated to methyl n-butyl ketone (MBK) and 2,5-hexanedione (2,5-HD). Pregnant rats were exposed 6 hours per day to 1000 ppm N-hexane on days 8-12, 12-16, or 8-16 of gestation (Bus et al, 1979). No increase in resorptions, fetal deaths or malfomations were observed in the fetus. Concentrations in the fetuses of N-hexame, MBK and 2,5-HD were approximately equal that in the maternal blood.

Bus, J.J.; White, E.L.; Tyl, R.W.; Barrow, C.S.: Perinatal toxicity and metabolism of n-hexane in Fischer 344 rats after inhalation exposure during gestation. Toxicol. Appl. Pharmacol. 51:295-302, 1979.

662 Hexafluoroacetone

Brittelli et al (1979) applied this organic solvent to the skin of pregnant rats on days 6 through 16 and at absorbed doses of 5 and 25 mg per kg found hematomas, hydronephrosis, hydrocephalus and other defects. Some hydronephrosis increase was found at a dose of 1 mg per kg.

Brittelli, M.R.; Culik, R.; Dascheill, O.L. and Fayerweather, W.E.: Skin absorption of hexafluoroacetone: Teratogenic and lethal effects in the rat fetus. Toxicol. Appl. Pharmacol. 47:35-39, 1979.

663 Hexobarbital (also see Barbitaric Acid)

Persaud (1965) treated 10 pregnant rats with 50 to 100 mg injections on the 4th, 8th and 18th day and observed no defective offspring.

Persaud, T.V.N.: Tierexperimentelle Untersuchungen zur Frage der Teratogenen wirkung von Barbituraten. Acta Biol. Med. Ger. 14: 89-90, 1965.

664 1-Hexylcarbamoyl-5-fluorouracil

Sato et al (1980) gave this antimetabolite orally to pregnant rats and rabbits. No ill effects on fertility were found using up to 50 mg per kg in both rat sexes. Administration of the same dose during organogenesis was associated with a few skeletal variations in the fetuses. At a dose of 100 mg per kg there was increased fetal death. No adverse postnatal findings were detected. In the rabbit they used 50 mg per kg and no adverse fetal effects occurred.

Sato, T.; Nagaoka, T.; Kaneko, Y.; Osuga, F.; Naramo, I.; Sejima, Y.: Reproductive studies of 1-hexylcarbamoyl-5-fluorouracil. Kiso to Rinsho 14:1373-1402, 1980.

665 Histamine

Gatling (1962) dropped 50 microgm of histamine on the chorio-allantoic membrane of the 11-day chick embryo and found no defects.

Gatling, R.R.: The effect of sympathomimetic agents on the chick embryo. Am. J. Pathol. 40: 113-127, 1962.

666 Hog Cholera Vaccine

Sautter et al. (1953) injected this vaccine on the 14th to 16th gestational day and produced a syndrome in pigs consisting of generalized edema, ascites, mottling of the liver and skeletal defects. Small lungs and pitted kidneys were found in other effected fetuses (Young et al.; 1955).

Cerebellar hypoplasia with congenital tremors and hypomyelinogenesis has been associated with vaccination against hog cholera when given from the 20th to 97th gestational day (Emerson and Delez, 1965). Macrocephaly, contraction of tendons, edema and hemorrhages were also found in the pig fetuses.

Emerson, J.L. and Delez, A.L.: Cerebellar hypoplasia, hypomyelinogenesis and congenital tremors of pigs, associated with prenatal hog cholera vaccination of sows. J. Am. Vet. Med. Assoc. 147: 47-54, 1965.

Sautter, J.H.; Young, G.A.; Luedke, A.J. and Kitchell, R.L.: The experimental production of malformations and other abnormalities in fetal pigs by means of attenuated hog cholera virus. J. Am. Vet. Med. Assoc. 90: 146-150, 1953.

Young, G.A.; Kitchell, R.L.; Luedke, A.J. and Sautter, J.H.: The effect of viral and other infections of the dam on fetal development in swine. I. Modified live hog cholera viruses, immunological, virological and gross pathologic studies. J. Am. Vet. Med. Assoc. 126: 165-171, 1955.

667   Homopantothenic Acid

Nishizawa et al. (1969) found no evidence of teratogenicity in the rat and mouse. They gave 2 gm per kg to both species during active organogenesis.

Nishizawa, Y.; Kodama, T.; Noguchi, Y.; Nakayama, Y.; Hori, M. and Kowa, Y.: Chronic toxicity and teratogenic effect of homopantothenic acid. J. Vitaminol. 15: 26-32, 1969.

668   HVJ Virus [Hemagglutinating Virus of Japan]

Ohba (1958) administered chorio-allantoic fluid containing this virus intranasally or intravenously to mice on the 8th day of pregnancy and some abnormalities of the central nervous system were observed in the embryos. The author found 20.9 percent abnormal embryos in the treated group and only 4.4 percent in the controls, but he was cautious in ascribing the cause to the viral agent itself.

Ohba, N.: Formation of embryonic abnormalities of the mouse by a viral injection of mother animals. Acta Pathol. Jap. 9: 149-157, 1959.

669   Hycanthone Methane Sulfate

Moore (1972) administered intramuscularly either 35 or 50 mg per kg to mice on the 7th gestational day. There was a high incidence of congenital defects which were mainly exencephaly, hydrocephaly, microphthalmia or skeletal. At a dose level of 10 mg per kg there was no increase in fetal defects. Human therapeutic doses are 3 to 4 mg per kg.

Moore, J.A.: Teratogenicity of hycanthone in mice. Nature 239: 107-109, 1972.

670   Hydralazine (1-Hydrazinephthalazine)

This compound which inhibits hydroxylation steps in collagen syntheis has been used to produce skeletal defects which are similar to those produced by manganese deficiency. (Rapaka et al, 1978).

Rapaka, R.S.; Parr, R.W.; Lin, T-Z and Bhatnagar, R.S.: Biochemical basis of skeletal defects induced by hydralazine. Teratology 15:185-194, 1977.

671   Hydrazine

Stoll et al. (1967) using doses close to the LD-50 produced a low incidence of skeletal defects in chicks receiving 30 to 200 microgm on the 3rd day of incubation. Several derivatives of hydrazine have been found to be embryotoxic, but only in the early embryo (Poulson and Robson, 1963).

Poulson, E. and Robson, J.M.: The effect of amine oxidase inhibitors on pregnancy. J. Endocrin. 27:147-152, 1963.

671

Stoll, R.; Bodit, F. and Maraud, R.: Sur l'action teratogene de hydrazine et de substances voisines chez l'embryon de poulet. C. R. Soc. Biol. (Paris) 161: 1680-1684, 1967.

672 P-Hydrazinobenzoic Acid (see Semicarbazide)

673 Hydrochlorthiazide

Maren and Ellison using 250 mg per kg on gestational days 9, 10, 11 and 12 produced no defects in the rat fetus.

Heinonen et al (1977) reported no significant increase in defect rate among 107 women exposed during the first 4 months.

Heinonen, O.P.; Slone, D.; Shapiro, S.: Birth Defects and Drugs in Pregnancy. Publishing Sciences Group, Inc., 1977.

Maren, T.H. and Ellison, A.C.: The teratological effect of certain thiadiazoles related to acetazolamide, with a note on sulfanilamide and thiazide diuretics. Johns Hopkins Med. J. 130: 95-104, 1972.

674 Hydrocortisone [Cortisol] (also see Cortisone)

Kalter and Fraser (1952) observed that when hydrocortisone was given to mice in doses of 2.5 mg on the 110th or 11th day many offspring had cleft palates.

Pinsky and Digeorge (1965) have compared the cleft palate producing effect of this compound with several other corticoids.

Using the AJAX mouse they found that injections of 4 mg on days 11 through 18 produced 18 percent cleft palate. Aoyama et al (1974) studied the effect of hydrocortisone-17-alpha butyrate in pregnant mice and rats. Doses were given subcutaneously up to 1.0 mg per kg per day in mice and 9 mg per kg per day in rats. No increase in congenital malformations was found.

Hydrocortisone 17-butylate 21-propionate was studied by subcutaneous route in rats and rabbits by Yamada and Coworkers (1981A). In the male and female rat doses of up to 0.4 mg per kg per day subcutaneously did not interfere with reproduction. During organogenesis doses of 10 and 50 mg per kg increased congenital defects (omphaloceles, cleft palate and edema). Doses of 1 mg perinatally had no adverse effect on postnatal behavior. In the rabbit at 0.5 mg per kg during organogenesis cleft palate and open neural tube defects were increased over controls. Using single daily doses subcutaneously of up to 200 mg per kg Yamada et al (1981B) resorption, fetal growth retardation and an increase in umbilical hernias occurred at the highest dose. Some fetal weight decrease and lethality was found with percutaneous doses of 0.5 percent cream or ointment (Yamada et al, 1981C).

Aoyama, T.; Furuoka, R.; Hasegawa, N. and Terabayashi, M.: Teratological studies on hydrocortisone-17-alpha-butyrate (H-17B) in mice and rats. Oyo Yakuri 8: 1035-1047, 1974.

Kalter, H. and Fraser, F.C.: Production of congenital defects in the offspring of pregnant mice treated with compound f. Nature 169: 665 only, 1952.

Pinsky, L. and DiGeorge, A.M.: Cleft palate in the mouse: A teratogenic index of glucocorticoid potency. Science 147: 402-403, 1965.

Yamada, T.; Suzuki, H.; Matsumoto, S.; Nakane, S.; Sasajima, M.; Ohzeki, M.: Reproductive studies of hydrocortisone 17-butyrate 21- propionate in rats and rabbits. Oyo Yakuri 21:427-482, 1981A.

Yamada, T.; Nogariya, T.; Ichikawa, A.; Nakane, S.; Sasajima, M.; Ohzeki, M.: Teratogenicity study in rats by a single injection. Yakuri to chiryo 9:3083-3104, 1981B.

Yamada, T.; Nogariya, R.; Ichikawa, A.; Nakane, S.; Sasajima, M.; Ohzoki, M.: Hydrocortisone 17-butyrate 21-propionate teratogenicity study in rats by percutaneous administration. Yakuri to Chiryo 9: 3045-3082, 1981C.

675 Hydrogen Peroxide

Moriyama et al (1982) fed pregnant rats a diet containing up to 10 percent hydrogen peroxide. Maternal and fetal weights were reduced but no significant malformations were reported.

Moriyama, I.; Fuyita, M.; Hiraoka, K.; Ichija, M.; Kanoh, S.: Effects of food additive hydrogen peroxide on fetal development (abstract) Teratology 26:28A, 1982.

676 N-Hydroxyethylpromethazine Chloride [Aprobit-R]

West (1962) reported that this antihistamine which accumulates in the placenta without crossing was toxic to the rat fetus at doses of 0.25 mg per kg. Other antihistamines cyproheptadine and promethazine produced fetal death at a much higher dose (25 mg per kg). Details, including the presence or absence of fetal defects, were not included in this report.

West, G.B.: Drugs and rat pregnancy. J. Pharm. Pharmacol. 14: 828-830, 1962.

677 6-Hydroxylaminopurine

Chaube and Murphy (1969) injected this adenine antagonist into pregnant rats on day 11 or 12 of gestation and produced malformations with doses of 200 to 900 mg per kg. The defects included cleft palate, micrognathia and deformed appendages. Inosine provided complete protection against this teratogen.

677

Chaube, S. and Murphy, M.L.: Teratogenic effects of 6-hydroxylaminopurine in the rat: Protection by inosine. Biochem. Pharmacol. 18: 1147-1156, 1969.

678 7-Hydroxymethyl-12-methylbenz-(a)-anthracene [7-OHM-12-MBA]

Bird et al. (1970) injected intravenously 25 mg per kg on day 17 of gestation and produced adrenal necrosis in rat fetuses.

Bird, C.C.; Crawford, A.M. and Currie, A.R.: Foetal adrenal necrosis induced by 7-hydroxymethyl-12-methyl-benz(a)-anthracene and its prevention. Nature 228: 72-73, 1970.

679 4-Hydroxy-N-dimethylbutyramide 4-chlorophenoxy-isobutyrate

Da Lage et al (1972) fed this cholesterol reducing agent to mice orally during the entire gestation in doses up to 400 mg per kg and no malformations resulted.

Da Lage, C.; Labie, Ch.; Loiseau, G.; Lohier, G.; Marquet, J.P. and Trichaud, M.: Etude toxicologique et teratologique d'un hypocholesterolemiant (mg 46). Europ. J. Toxicol. 4: 239-253, 1972.

680 17-Hydroxymethyl-12-methylbenz-(a)-anthracene (see 7-12-Di-methylbenz-(a)-anthracene)

681 Hydroxymethylpyrimidine (see Ethionamide)

682 P-Hydroxyphenyl Lactic Acid

Zharova et al (1979) injected CC-57BR and C-57BL mice with 5 mg of this substance either on days 1 through 10 or during the last week of pregnancy and found no teratogenic effect. Malignant and benign neoplasms in the progeny of CC-57BR and C-57BL mouse strains occurred in 88 and 78% of cases respectively.

Zharova, E.I.; Sergeeva, T.I.; Malakhova, N.V.; Romanenko, V.I.; Chitoridi, N.G. and Raushenbakh, M.O.: Transplacental blastomogenic action of p-hydroxyphenyl lactic acid. Byull. Eksper. Biol. Med. (USSR) 87:46-48, 1979.

683 17-Hydroxyprogesterone

Suchowsky and Junkmann (1961) found that this compound had no masculinizing effect on the female rat fetus.

The rare occurrence of masculinization of the female human fetus has been summarized by Serment and Ruf (1968) who state that in more than 1,500 treated cases only two cases of clitoral hypertrophy were found.

Serment, H. and Ruf, H.: Therapeutiques hormonales. Bull.
Fed. Soc. Gynecol. Obstet. Lang. Fr. 20: 69-76, 1968.

Suchowsky, G.K. and Junkmann, K.: A study of the
virilizing effect of the progestogens on the female rat
fetus. Endocrinology 68: 341-349, 1961.

684 4-Hydroxypyrazolo-(3,4-d)-pyrimidine

Chaube and Murphy (1968) gave 50 to 500 mg per kg to
pregnant rats on the 11th or 12th gestational day and found
no defects in fetuses surviving to the 21st day.

Chaube, SS. and Murphy, M.L.: The teratogenic effects of
the recent drugs active in cancer chemotherapy. In,
Woollam, D.H.M. (ed.): Advances in Teratology, Vol. 3.
New York: Academic Press, 1968. pp 181-237.

685 Hydroxystreptomycin (see Streptomycin)

686 5-Hydroxytryptamine (see Serotonin)

687 Hydroxyurea

Chaube and Murphy (1966) injected pregnant rats with 185 to
1000 mg per kg on the 9th, 10th, 11th or 12th gestational
day and produced defects of the central nervous system,
palate and skeleton. Large doses of hydroxylamine or
urethan did not cause fetal abnormalities. Scott et al.
(1971) have shown that DNA synthesis is depressed by the
presence of hydroxyurea in the embryo. Extensive cell death
in the limb buds and central nervous system was noted 5
hours after maternal administration of 750 mg per kg.
Soukup et al. (1967) found no chromosome changes in embryos
after the rat was treated with 750 mg per kg on the 13th
day. Murphy and Chaube (1964) have shown that this
substance produced a low incidence of beak defects in the
chick embryo. Khera (1979) found teratogenicity in the cat
given 50 or 100 mg per kg daily orally during organogenesis.
Wilson et al (1975) have studied the teratogenicity in
monkeys.

Adlard and Dobbing (1975) studied the post natal maze
learning after administering 1 or 2 gm per kg to the mother
rat on the 14th day. A decrease in performance was found
along with body and brain growth reduction. Pigmentation
was also less in the treated offspring. In another study
using 150 mg per kg on days 6, 9, 12 15 and 18 of rat
gestation, Brunner et al (1978) were not able to show
alterations in postnatal behavioral tests. The authors
point out that in this case behavioral changes were less
sensitive than morphological measures.

Adlard, B.P.F. and Dobbing, J.: Maze learning by adult
rats after inhibition of neuronal multiplication in utero.
Pediat. Res. 9: 139-142, 1975.

Brunner, R.L.; McLean, M.; Vorhees, C.V. and Butcher, R.E.:
A comparison of behavioral and anatomic measures of hydroxyurea induced abnormalities. Teratology 18:379-384, 1978.

Chaube, S. and Murphy, M.L.: The effects of hydroxyurea
and related compounds on the rat fetus. Cancer Res. 26:
1448-1457, 1966.

Khera, K.S.: Teratogenicity study on hydroxyurea and
diphenylhydantoin in cats. Teratology 20:447-452, 1970.

Murphy, M.L. and Chaube, S.: Hydroxyurea (NSC-32065) as a
teratogen. Cancer Chemother. Rep. 40: 1-7, 1964.

Scott, W.J.; Ritter, E.J. and Wilson, J.G.: DNA synthesis
inhibition and cell death associated with hydroxyurea teratogenesis in rat embryos. Dev. Biol. 26: 306-315, 1971.

Soukup, S.; Takas, E. and Warkany, J.: Chromosome changes
in embryos treated with various teratogens. J. Embryol.
Exp. Morphol. 18: 215-226, 1967.

Wilson, J.G.; Scott, W.J.; Ritter, E.J.; Fradkin, R.:
Comparative distribution and embryotoxicity of hydroxyurea
in pregnant rats and Rhesus monkeys. Teratology 11:169-178,
1975.

688 Hydroxyurethane

Chaube and Murphy (1966) injected 225 to 700 mg per kg into
rats on the 9th, 10th, 11th or 12th day of gestation and
produced defects of the central nervous system, palate or
skeleton. Tail defects were especially common after
treatment on the 11th or 12th day.

Chaube, S. and Murphy, M.L.: The effects of hydroxyurea
and related compounds on the rat fetus. Cancer Res. 26:
1448-1457, 1966.

689 Hydroxyzine (also see Meclizine)

This antihistamine belongs to the benzhydrylpiperazine
series of compounds. It has been used as a teratogen in the
rat. The details are discussed under meclizine.

690 Hyperbaric Air

Bolton and Alamo (1981) exposed gravid rats to 6 atmospheres
of air during several periods of organogenesis and found no
adverse changes in their fetuses.

Bolton, M.E.; Alamo, A.L.: Lack of teratogenic effects of
air at high ambient pressure in rats. Teratology
24:181-185, 1981.

691 Hypercalcemia (also see Vitamin D)

The association of hypercalcemia with congenital heart disease (supravalvular aortic stenosis) has been suggested (Black and Bonham-Carter, 1963). The subject is covered more fully under vitamin D.

Black, J.A. and Bonham-Carter, R.E.: Association between aortic stenosis and facies of severe infantile hypercalcemia. Lancet 2: 745-749, 1963.

692 Hyperglycemia

Sadler (1980) exposed mouse embryos to 5 and 8 times the normal blood glucose level in vitro and produced a high frequency of exencephaly.

Sadler, T.W.: Effects of maternal diabetes on early rat embryogenesis: 2. Hyperglycemia-induced exencephaly. Teratology 21:349-356, 1980.

693 Hyperoxia

Ferm produced umbilical hernias, exencephaly, spina bifida and limb defects in a small but significant number of hamster fetuses by exposing the mother to 3.0 to 4.0 atmospheres of oxygen for periods of 2 to 3 hours on the 6th, 7th or 8th day of gestation.

Grote (1965) exposed rabbits to 70 to 96 percent oxygen and produced no vertebral or other fetal defects.

Ferm, V.H.: Teratogenic effects of hyperbaric oxygen. Proc. Soc. Exp. Biol. Med. 116: 975-976, 1964.

Grote, W.: Storung der Embryonalentwicklung bie Erhohtem CO_2 und O_2-Partialdruck und bie Unterdruck. Z. Morphol. Anthropol. 56: 165-194, 1965.

694 Hypertension (preclampsia, eclampsia)

Brazy et al (1982) studied the offspring of 28 women with severe hypertension before the 36th week of pregnancy. All the mothers had diastolic pressures above 110 mm Hg and 4 had hypertension prior to pregnancy. Most were treated with intravenous magnesium sulfate and other antihypertensive agents. Growth retardation, microcephaly, thrombocytopenia, leukopenia, patent ductus arteriosus and hypotonia of the skeletal and gut musculature were significantly increased over controls with similar gestational ages. Eight of the infants had head circumferences below the 10th percentile.

Preclampsia and eclampsia are often associated with placental insufficiency which can lead to intrauterine growth retardation. The evidence for this has been summarized by Dancis (1975).

Brazy, J.E.; Grimm, J.K.; Little, V.A.: Neonatal manifestations of severe maternal hypertension occurring before the thirty-sixth week of pregnancy. J. Pediat.

694

100:265-271, 1982.

Dancis,   J.:   Fetomaternal   interaction   in   Avery,   G.B.
Neonatology, J.B. Lippincott, Philadelphia, 1975, p.   44.

695   Hyperthermia

Smith   et   al   (1978) in a retrospective study of 13 infants
exposed to hyperthermia during the first trimester, reported
that   all had nervous system complications with microcephaly
in 3 and hypotonia in 9. Microopthalmia occurred   in   five.
Miller   et   al   (1978)   studied 63 mothers who gave birth to
anencephalics   and   found   5   with   temperatures   from   38.9
degrees   C   to   40.0 degrees   C and   two who had possible
hyperthermia related to sauna bathing (see   Sauna   Bathing).
Of   special   note,   all   the   mothers had their hyperthermia
during the period the anterior   neural   tube   closes   (14-28
days).   In another study, Fraser and Skelton (1978) randomly
reviewed records of children with congenital defects to
determine whether or not any particular type of defect was
associated with maternal fever.   In a group of 55 they found
six with microophthalmia and this number was significantly
higher than in controls.   Chance and Smith (1978) studied
the   pregnancy history of 43 women who gave birth to infants
with meningomyeloceles, and in three, fevers of over 102
degrees F (38.9 degrees C) occurred between the 25th to 28th
day of gestation.   None of the 63 controls had fever at this
time.   Layde   et   al (1980) found a significant increase in
fever among mothers who delivered infants with spina bifida.
In   a   prospective   study   of 165 women with first trimester
fever from 55,000 pregnancies, no significant differences in
defect rate or intelligence of the offspring were identified
as compared to matched controls.   (Clarren   et   al,   1979).
Most   of   these fevers were for brief episodes. Pleet et al
(1981) have reviewed the clinical syndromes associated with
hyperthermia.   Kleinbrecht et al (1979) found no significant
increase in neural tube or eye defects among   the   offspring
of women having fever in the first 12 weeks.

Shiota (1982) made a study of the histories from   113   women
who donated embryos with neural tube defects to the Kyoto
University embryo collection of Professor Nishimura.   The
histories   were   supplied   at   the   time the therapeutically
aborted   specimen   was   sent   to   the   collection.   The
obstetrician did not know the condition of the embryo.
Maternal fever was mentioned in 18 percent of   the   50   with
anterior neural tube defects, significantly higher than the
matched controls of 4.9 percent.   Among the 63 embryos with
myeloschisis 11.1 percent had a histoy of fever.

A moderately large literature exists on hyperthermia   as   an
experimental agent for producing congenital defects.   Kalter
(1968) has reviewed this literature.   In   the   rabbit
Brinsmade and Rubsaamen (1957) produced fever by injecting
milk   on   the   7th   and 8th gestational days and   found
microcephaly or encephalocele in 3 of 65 embryos.   Skreb and
Frank (1963) immersed one uterine horn in water of 40 to 41
degrees C for 40 to 60 minutes on the 8th to 16th day of
pregnancy of the rat and produced closure defects or   severe

histological effects of the central nervous system. Defects
of the eye, extremity or palate occurred also. A high
resorption rate was found on each day. Diathermy has been
used to produce defects of the central nervous system in rat
fetuses (Hofmann and Dietzel, 1966). Exencephaly has been
produced by hyperthermia in the hamster (Kilham and Ferm,
1976).

Lecyk (1966) subjected mice to 40 to 41 degrees C for
20-hour periods on gestational days 7 through 12 and
observed a 25 percent incidence of rib or vertebral defects
in the survivors. About one-third of the mothers died, and
strict controls to exclude the teratogenic effect of fasting
were not performed. Edwards (1969) studied the effect of a
one hour daily exposure of guinea pigs to 43 degree external
temperature. When exposed from the 18th to the 25th day 86
percent of the fetuses had multiple anomalies which included
microcephaly, reduction defects of the extremities,
exomphalos and renal agenesis. An unusual form of
amyoplasia was found also. Fetal death and resorptions were
common when treatment was carried out before the 18th day.
Postnatal studied of this model indicated persistent
impairment of learning (Johnson et al, 1976).

Cockroft and New (1978) isolated the rat embryo from the
mother by embryo culture from the egg cylinder stage to the
25 somite stage. Temperature exposure of 40.5 C retarded
whole embryo growth: at 40 degrees C both the size and
protein content of the brain were reduced.

Hartley et al (1974) exposed ewes to increased temperature
for 9 hours daily during the last one-third or two-thirds of
pregnancy and produced a high incidence of brain cavitation
and microcephaly in a large proportion of the lambs. The
ewes body temperatures ranged from 40 to 41 degrees
centigrade after treatment. Poswillo et al (1974) in a
preliminary study exposed marmosets to an incubator
temperature of 42 degrees C for one hour daily from days 25
through 50 of gestation and the offspring were small and had
a higher incidence of skeletal changes resembling rickets
than did the controls.

Edwards and Wanner (1977) have reviewed the animal
teratogenicity of hyperthermia.

Brinsmade, A.B. and Rubsaamen, H.: Zur Teratogenetischen
Wirkung von Unspezifischem Fieber auf den sich Entwickelnden
Kaninchenembryo. Beitr. Pathol. Anat. 117: 154-164,
1957.

Chance, P.F.; Smith D.W.: Hyperthermia and meningomyelocele
and anencephaly. Lancet 1:769-770, 1978.

Clarren, S.K.; Smith, D.W.; Harvey, M.A.S.; Ward, R.H.; and
Myrianthopoulos, N.C.: Hyperthermia - a prospective
evaluation of a possible teratogenic agent in man. J.
Pediatr. 95: 81-83, 1979.

Cockroft, D.L. and New, D.A.T.: Abnormalities induced in
rat embryos by hyperthermia. Teratology 17:277-284, 1978.

695

Edwards, M.J.: Congenital defects in guinea pigs: fetal resorptions, abortions and malformations following induced hyperthermia during early gestation. Teratology 2: 313-328, 1969.

Edwards, M.J.; Wanner, R.A.: Extremes of temperature in Handbook of Teratology, Vol. I, edited by Wilson, J.G. and Fraser, F.C., Plenum Press, Chicago, 1977, p. 421-444.

Fraser, F.C. and Skelton, J.: Possible teratogenicity of maternal fever. Lancet 2:634 (only), 1978.

Hartley, W.J.; Alexander, G. and Edwards, M.J.: Brain cavitation and microcephaly in lambs exposed to prenatal hyperthermia. Teratology 9: 299-304, 1974.

Hofmann, D. and Dietzel, F.: Abort und Missbildungen nach Kurzwellendurchflutung in der Schwangerschaft. Geburts. Frauenheilk 26: 378-390, 1966.

Jonson, K.M.; Lyle, J.G.; Edwards, M.J. and Penny, R.H.C.: Effect of prenatal heat stress on brain growth and serial discrimination reversal learning in the guinea pig. Brain Research Bulletin 1:133-150, 1976.

Kalter, H.: Teratology of central nervous system. Chicago: University of Chicago Press, 1968. pp 180-181.

Kilham, L. and Ferm, V.H.: Exencephaly in fetal hamsters exposed to hyperthermia. Teratology 14: 323-326, 1976.

Kleinbrecht, J.; Michaelis, H.; Michaelis, J.; Koller, S.: Fever in pregnancy and congenital defects. Lancet 1:1403, 1979.

Layde, P.M.; Edmonds, L.D.; Erickson, J.D.: Maternal fever and neural tube defects. Teratology 21:105-108, 1980.

Lecyk, M.: The effect of hyperthermia applied in the given stages of pregnancy on the number and form of vertebrae in the offspring of white mice. Experientia 22: 254-255, 1966.

Miller, P.; Smith, D.W. and Shepard, T.H.: Hyperthermia as one possible etiology of anencephaly. Lancet 1:519-521, 1978.

Pleet, H.B.; Graham, J.M.; Smith, D.W.: Central nervous system and facial defects associated with maternal hyperthermia at four to 14 weeks gestation. Pediat. 67:785-795, 1981.

Poswillo, D.E.; Nunnerly, H.; Sopher, D.; Keith, J.: Hyperthermia as a teratogenic agent. Ann. Roy. College of Surg. of England 55:171-174, 1974.

Shiota, K.: Neural tube defects and maternal hyperthermia in early pregnancy: Epidemiology in a human embryo population. Am. J. Med. Genetics 12: 281-288, 1982.

Skreb, N. and Frank, Z.: Developmental abnormalities in the rat induced by heat shock. J. Embryol. Exp. Morphol.

11: 445-457, 1963.

Smith, D.W.; Clarren, S.K. and Harvey, M.A.S.: Hyperthermia as a possible teratogenic agent. J. Pediatr. 92:877-883, 1978.

696 Hypervitaminosis A (also see Retinoic Acid)

Since the discovery by Cohlan (1954) that large doses of vitamin A given by mouth could produce congenital defects this experimental model has been used widely (see Summary by Kalter, 1968). Cohlan tube-fed rats 35,000 I.U. of vitamin A from the 2nd, 3rd or 4th to the 16th day of gestation and found 52 percent of the offspring to be abnormal. All the defective fetuses had exencephaly which was associated with an increased amount of bloody amniotic fluid. Thirty-eight percent had cleft palate and eye defects were found also. Giroud and Martinet (1956) studied the effect of time of administration of vitamin A to the rat and type of malformation. The peak effect on neural tube closure was seen when treatment was started on day 8 and the highest incidence of cleft palate and skeletal defects was noted when treatment commenced on day 11. Giroud et al. (1956) demonstrated a small increase in vitamin A content of the treated fetuses. Giroud and Martinet (1957) showed that the exencephaly was associated with failure of the anterior portion of the neural tube to close and externalization of the choriod plexuses occurred. Kalter and Warkany (1961) have produced defects in the mouse. A number of the fetuses with genitourinary abnormalities had absence of the umbilical artery and a compensatory retention of the vitelline (superior mesenteric) artery. Marin-Padilla and Ferm (1965) and Marin-Padilla (1966) studied the syndrome in hamsters and noted that cell necrosis in the somites and notochord was an early effect of treatment. A comprehensive review of the animal studies on vitamin A teratogenesis was made by Geelen, (1979)

Postnatal studies of rats receiving 60,000 units of vitamin A on days 14 and 15 or 17 and 18 revealed learning and fine motor changes respectively (Hutchings et al, 1973 and Hutchings and Gaston, 1973). Vorhees et al (1979) have confirmed this. Newman et al (1982) found that vitamin A administration on days 15-19 was associated with decreased 0-2 consumption in the neonates.

Bernhardt and Dorsey (1974) report that the offspring of a mother taking 25,000 IU daily during the 1st 3 months of gestation was found to have an aberrant ureter which was dilated and entered the vagina. Fantel et al (1977) reported cleft palate, craniofacial, skeletal and urogenital anomalies in pigtail monkeys treated with 10 mg of retinoic acid per kg from day 20 through 44. These authors cite another case with urogenital anomaly in a mother who ingested large amounts of vitamin A. A third report (Mounoud et al, 1975) gives a description of an infant with Goldenhar's syndrome following inadvertent ingestion of the

696

vitamin.

Bernhardt, I.B. and Dorsey, D.J.: Hypervitaminosis A and congenital renal anomalies in a human infant. Obstet. Gynecol. 43: 750-755, 1974.

Cohlan, S.Q.: Congenital anomalies in the rat produced by the excessive intake of vitamin A during pregnancy. Pediatrics 13: 556-569, 1954.

Fantel, A.G.; Shepard, T.H.; Newell-Morris, L.L.; and Moffett, B.C.: Teratogenic effects of retinoic acid in pigtail monkeys (Macaca nemistrina). Teratology 15:65-72, 1977.

Geelen, J.A.G.: Hypervitaminosis A induced teratogenesis. CRC Critical Reviews in Toxicology. 6:351-376, 1979.

Giroud, A.; Gounelle, H. and Martinet, M.: Concentration de la vitamine a chez la mere et le foetus au cours de la teratogenese par hypervitaminose A. C. R. Soc. Biol. 150: 2064-2065, 1956.

Giroud, A. and Martinet, M.: Teratogenese par hautes doses de vitamin A en fonction des stades du developpement. Arch. Anat. Micr. Morph. Exp. 45: 77-98, 1956.

Giroud, A. and Martinet, M.: Morphogenese de l'anencephalie. Arch. Anat. Micr. Morph. Exp. 46: 247-264, 1957.

Hutchings, D.E.; Gibbon, J.; Kaufman, M.A.: Maternal vitamin A excess during the early fetal period: Effects on learning and development in the offspring. Developmental Psychology 6:445-457, 1973.

Hutchings, D.E.; Gaston, J.: The effects of vitamin A excess administered during mid-fetal period on learning and development in rat offspring. Developmental Psychology 7:225-233, 1973.

Kalter, H.: Teratology of the central nervous system. Chicago: University of Chicago Press, 1968. pp 45-56.

Kalter, H. and Warkany, J.: Experimental production of congenital malformations in strains of inbred mice by maternal treatment with hypervitaminosis A. Am. J. Pathol. 38: 1-20, 1961.

Marin-Padilla, M.: Mesodermal alterations induced by hypervitaminosis A. J. Embryol. Exp. Morphol. 15: 261-269, 1966.

Marin-Padilla, M. and Ferm, V.H.: Somite necrosis and developmental malformations induced by vitamin A in the golden hamster. J. Embryol. Exp. Morphol. 13: 1-8, 1965.

Mounoud, R.L.; Klein, D. and Weber, F.: A propos d'un case de syndrome de Goldenhar intoxication aique a la vitamin A chez la mere pendent la grossesse. J. Genet Hum.

23:135-154, 1975.

Newman, L.M.; Johnson, E.M.; Cadogan, A.S.A.: Predictability of postnatal survival in prenatally hypervitamin A exposed rat pups based on 0-2 consumption values on day of delivery (abstract) Teratology 25: 64A, 1982.

Vorhees, C.V.; Brunner, R.L.; Butcher, R.E.: Psychotropic drugs as behavioral teratogens. Science 205:1220-1225, 1979.

697 Hypoglycemia (also see Fasting)

Although hypoglycemia was not studied specifically, Runner and Miller (1956) were able to prevent defects in fasted mice by administration of glucose (see Also insulin, carbutamide and tolbutamide).

Runner, M.N. and Miller, J.R.: Congenital deformity in the mouse as a consequence of fasting. (abstract) Anat. Rec. 124: 437-438, 1956.

698 Hypoglycin A

This analogue of leucine present in the fruit Blighia sapida was administered by Persaud and Kaplan (1970) to rats intraperitoneally on the 1st through the 6th gestational day in amounts of 30 mg per kg. Ninety-two percent of the off-spring were defective; gastroschisis, stunting, encephalocele and syndactyly were found. Chick embryos were not effected by the substance, and this result was thought to be related to the large leucine pools present in the egg. Persaud (1972) has reviewed the subject.

Persaud, T.V.N.: Teratogenic effect of hypoglycin-A. In, Woollam, D.H.M. (ed.): Advances in Teratology, Vol. 5. New York: Academic Press, 1972. pp 78-95.

Persaud, T.V.N. and Kaplan, S.: The effects of hypoglycin-A, a leucine analogue, on the development of the rat and chick embryos. Life Sci. 9: 1305-1313, 1970.

699 Hypothermia

Kalter (1968) has reviewed this subject. Generally, studies at low temperature have resulted in reduction of litter size. Smith (1957) maintained pregnant hamsters for 30 minutes in baths at minus 5 degrees C. The pregnancies were uneffected except for uterine hemorrhage followed by resorption when treatment was on day 9, 10 or 11. When cooling was extended to 45 minutes on days 6, 7 and 8, defects of the neural tube, palate and extremities occurred. Lecyk (1965) subjected mice to 24 hours at 20 degrees C on day 7.5 or 8.5 and produced defects of the vertebral column in over one-half of the offspring. The control animals also receiving chloropromazine were placed in an incubator and produced only 9 skeletal defects among 175 offspring.

Unfortunately, this author did not perform controls to exclude the effect of fasting which can produce similar defects in the mouse fetus.

Kalter, H.: Teratology of the central nervous system. Chicago: University of Chicago Press, 1968. pp 181-182.

Lecyk, M.: The effect of hypothermia applied in the given stages of pregnancy on the number and form of vertebrae in the offspring of white mice. Experientia 21: 452-453, 1965.

Smith, A.U.: The effects on foetal development of freezing pregnant hamsters (Mesocricetus auratus). J. Embryol. Exp. Morphol. 5: 311-323, 1957.

700 Hypothyroidism (also see Thyroidectomy)

Lu and Staples (1978) parathyroidectomized rats and 20 days later mated them. Decrease in implantations and a 10 percent malformation rate was found. Hydrocephalus and convoluted retinae were the most common type of defect.

Lu, M.H. and Staples, R.E.: Teratogenicity of ethyl-enethiourea and thyroid function in the rat. Teratology 17: 171-178, 1978.

701 Hypoxanthine (also see 2-Deoxyinosine)

Karnofsky and Lacon (1961) injected 2 to 8 mg into the chick yolk sac on the 4th day and produced no defects. Inosine and 2-deoxyinosine were teratogenic under these conditions.

Karnofsky, D.A. aand Lacon, C.R.: Effects of physiological purines on the development of the chick embryo. Biochem. Pharmacol. 7: 154-158, 1961.

702 Hypoxia

This experimental tool has been used extensively by teratologists and is reviewed critically by Kalter and Warkany (1959). In general, lowered atmospheric pressure has been used.

In the mouse exposed for 5 hours to 260 to 280 mm Hg on the 9th, 10th or 15th gestational day Ingalls et al. (1952) and Ingalls and Curley (1957) produced hemivertebra, fused ribs, cleft palate and cranioschisis. Curley and Ingalls (1957) using a mixture of 6 percent oxygen and nitrogen produced similar defects in mice. The rat and hamster (Ferm, 1965) appear to be resistant to the teratogenic effect of hypoxia, but Degenhardt and Knoche (1959) have produced vertebral and rib defects in the rabbit and observed that the most effective day of treatment was the 9th. Murakami and Kameyama (1963) have described in detail the vertebral defects produced in the mouse.

Petter et al. (1971) have produced a syndrome of generalized edema followed by hemorrhages in the extremities of fetuses after maternal exposure to a variety of hypoxia-producing conditions at 16.5 days of gestation. These conditions included vascular occlusion of maternal blood supply, reduced respiratory oxygen, fuel gas and potassium ferric cynide.

Pregnant mice (C57 BL x CBA) were exposed by Udalova (1978) to low atmosphere pressure (230 mm Hg) for 3 hours on 7 - 10th days of pregnancy. No damage to embryonic development or effect on sex ratio of embryos was found in the treated animals. Khokhlova et al (1979) have reported that rats subjected on the 15th day of pregnancy to 2-hour hypoxia corresponding to 8,000 m altitude delivered offspring with delay of differentiation and maturation of the brain cortex neurons.

in a study of children born at high altitude, Lichty et al. (1957) found their birth weight reduced but no increase in the rate of congenital defects. Penaloza et al. (1964) summarize data suggesting that the frequency of patent ductus is increased at high altitudes and rises to 1 percent of newborns at altitudes over 4500 meters. Warkany (1971) has discussed critically the reports dealing with hypoxia and congenital heart disease.

Curley, F.J. and Ingalls, T.H.: Hypoxia at normal atmospheric pressure as a cause of congenital malformations in mice. Proc. Soc. Exp. Biol. Med. 94: 87-88, 1957.

Degenhardt, K.H. and Knoche, E.: Analysis of intrauterine malformations of vertebral column induced by oxygen deficiency. Can. Med. Assoc. J. 80: 441-445, 1959.

Ferm, V.H.: Teratogenic effects of hyperbaric oxygen. Proc. Soc. Exp. Biol. Med. 116: 975-976, 1964.

Ingalls, T.H. and Curley, F.J.: Principles governing the genesis of congenital malformations induced in mice by hypoxia. N. Engl. J. Med. 257: 1121-1127, 1957.

Ingalls, T.H.; Curley, F.J. and Prindle, R.A.: Experimental production of congenital abnormalities: Timing and degree of anoxia as factors causing fetal deaths and congenital abnormalities in the mouse. N. Engl. J. Med. 247: 758-768, 1952.

Kalter, H. and Warkany, J.: Experimental production of congenital malformations in mammals by metabolic procedure. Physiol. Rev. 39: 69-115, 1959.

Khokhlova, V.A. and Kazakova, P.B.: Effect of maternal hypoxia on neurogenesis of the brain cortex in rat progeny (autoradiographic study). Byull, Eksper. Biol. Med. (USSR) 87,5: 485-487, 1979.

Lichty, J.A.; Ting, R.Y.; Bruns, P.D. and Dyar, E.: Studies of babies born at high altitude. I. Relation of altitude to birth weight. A.M.A. J. Dis. Child. 93: 666-669, 1957.

Murakami, U. and Kameyama, Y.: Vertebral malformations in

702

the mouse foetus caused by maternal hypoxia during early
stages of pregnancy. J. Embryol. Exp. Morphol. 11:
107-118, 1963.

Penaloza, D.; Arias-Stella, J.; Sime, F.; Recavarren, S.
and Marticorena, E.: The heart and pulmonary circulation in
children at high altitudes; physiological, anatomical and
clinical observations. Pediatrics 34: 568-582, 1964.

Petter, C.; Bourbon, J.; Maltier, J. and Jost, A.:
Production d'hemorragies des extremites chez le foetus de
rat soumis a une hypoxie in utero. C. R. Acad. Sci. (D)
(Paris) 272: 2488-2490, 1971.

Udalova, L.D.: The influence of acute hypoxia on adult and
embryonic mortality and sex ratio of the embryos. Byull.
Eksper. Biol. Med. (USSR) 86,7:88-89, 1978.

Warkany, J.: Congenital Malformations: Notes and Comments.
Chicago: Year Book Medical Publishers, 1971. P. 465 only.

703 Ibuprofen [2-(4-Isobutylphenyl)-proprionic Acid]

This anti-inflammatory antipyretic was tested in rabbits and
rats by Adams et al. (1969) and no evidence for teratogenicity was found. The rabbits received oral doses of up to
60 mg per kg, and the rats received up to 180 mg per kg.
The treatments were given throughout pregnancy.

Ono et al (1982) administered up to 100 mg per kg rectally
before and for 7 days following fertilization and found a
reduction in the number of implants. At 200 mg per kg
rectally during organogenesis no adverse fetal effects were
found. Administration of 100 mg rectally on days 17-21
produced no significant postnatal changes in the offspring.

Ono, M.; Ogawa, Y.; Ogihara, K.; Nagase, M.; Asimi, K.:
Reproductive studies of ibuprofen by rectal administration.
Oyo Yakuri 24:467-473, 539-547, 1982.

Adams, S.S.; Bough, R.G.; Cliffe, E.E.; Lessel, B. and
Mills, R.F.N.: Absorption, distribution and toxicity of
ibuprofen. Toxicol. Appl. Pharmacol. 15: 310-330, 1969.

704 Ifenprodil

This alphaa receptor blocker was given intraperitoneally to
the rat and mouse in maximum daily doses of 40 mg per kg
during organogenesis. Maternal weight gain in the rat was
found at 40 mg per kg. No effects were observed in the
fetus of either species.

Kihara, J.; Sugisawa, A.; Kumura, I.; Fukui, Y. and
Sakaokibara, E.: The effect of Ifenprodil (FX-505 on rat
and mice embryos. Yakubutsu Ryoho 9:45-65, 1979.

705 Ifosfamide

This structural analogue of cyclophosphamide when injected intraperitoneally into pregnant mice on day 11 at a dose of 20 mg per kg produced skeletal and renal malformations and hydrocephalus in the offspring (Bus and Gibson, 1973.

Ifosfamide was tested intravenously by Nagaoka et al (1982) in rats and rabbits. Treating rats of both sexes before mating and during the first 7 days of gestation with 2.5 or 5.0 mg per kg they found decreased viability at term. In perinatal studies using up to 10 mg per kg an increase in stillbirths and hydrocephalus was found. Studies during organogenesis were followed by an increase in defects mostly involving the central nervous system when 5.0 mg per kg was used. In rabbits ectrodactylia was produced when 20 mg per kg was given during organogenesis.

Bus, J.S. and Gibson, J.E.: Teratogenicity and neonatal toxicity of ifosfamide in mice. Proc. Soc. Exp. Biol. Med. 143:965-970, 1973.

Nagaoka, T.; Oishi, M.; Narama, I.: Reproductive studies of ifosfamide. Kiso to Rinsho 16:508-516, 517-541, 542-552, 553-568, 1982.

706 Imidan [0,0-Dimethyl S-phthalidomethyl Phosphorodithioate]

Fabro et al. (1966) fed 35 mg per kg daily to rabbits on gestational days 7 through 12 and found no congenital defects in the offspring. Martson and Voronina (1976) found hydrocephalus in rat fetuses whose mothers received 30 mg per kg on day 14 of gestation. Staples et al (1976) gavage fed rats up to 30 mg per kg from day 6 through 15 and produced only an increase in minor skeletal fetal anomalies.

Fabro, S.; Smith, R.L. and Williams, R.T.: Embryotoxic activity of some pesticides and drugs related to phthalimide. Food Cosmet. Toxicol. 3: 587-590, 1966.

Martson, L.V. and Voronina, V.M.: Experimental study of the effect of a series of phosphoroorganic pesticides (dipterex and imidan) on embryogenesis. Envir. Health Prosp. 13:121:125, 1976.

Staples, R.E.; Kellam, R.G. and Hasseman, J.K.: Developmental toxicity in the rat after ingestion or gavage of organophosphate pesticides (dipterex, imidan) during pregnancy. Envir. Health Prosp. 13:133-140, 1976.

707 Imidazole (see Ethylenethiourea)

708 3-(2-Imidazoline-2-yl)-2-imidazolidinethione (Jaffe's Base) (see Ethylenethiourea)

709 Beta, Beta-Iminodipropionitrile

Miike and Chou (1981) gave approximately 40-70 mg per kg daily during gestation to rats. Hind limb paresis was found

in 7 of 137 offspring and about 50 percent of the newborns
died. The paresis appeared 3-6 weeks after birth and was
associated with subluxation and A-D angulation of the
thoracic vertebrae. The effects were considered to be due
to the monomer of the chemical beta-aminopropionitrile.

Miike, T.; Chou, S.M.: Lordosis of thoracic vertebrae
column and following paraparesis of hind-limbs induced by
maternal administration of beta, beta-iminodipropionitrile
(IDPN) during pregnancy in rats. Cong. Anom. 21:407-413,
1981.

710 Imipramine   [5-(3-Dimethylaminopropyl)-10,11-dihydro-
-5-H-dibenz(b,f)-azepine hydrochloride]

Robson and Sullivan (1963) injected rabbits with about 15 mg
per kg starting on the 1st day and until the 13th to 20th
day of gestation. From 12 mothers they observed one fetus
with encephalocele and another with incomplete palatal
development and spina bifida occulta. Some of the other
fetuses had hemorrhages of the cranium and abnormal limb
flexion. Larsen (1963) using another strain of rabbit and
conditions quite similar to the above found only one
abnormal fetus (single kidney) out of 53 examined. Harper
et al. (1965) using rabbits found no defective fetuses
among 46 whose mothers were given by injection 15 mg per kg
from day 6 through day 16. Administration by the injection
route was associated with some increased fetal loss. At a
dosage range of 30 mg per kg which was toxic to the mother,
four of 29 surviving fetuses were abnormal. Harper et al.
(1965) produced no fetal defects in the mouse or rat exposed
to 150 and 15 mg per kg respectively. These negative
results with the rabbit and rat were further supported by
Stenger et al (1965) and Hendrickx (1975) found no teratogenicity in monkeys given up to 1000 mg per kg per day
during 20 day periods of early gestation. In a Finnish
study of 2,784 congenital malformations, 3 mothers had taken
this drug as compared to one in a matched control.
(Idanpaan-Heikkila and Saxen, 1973).

Although a possible association between this drug and human
defects has appeared from Australia (McBride, 1972),
surveillance groups in the United States and Canada reviewed
histories of hundreds of mothers who gave birth to children
with limb reduction defects and found no supporting evidence
of an association (Rachelefsky et al.; 1972; Banister et
al.; 1972).

Banister, P.; DaFoe, C.; Smith, E.S.O. and Miller, J.:
Possible teratogenicity of tricyclic antidepressants.
Lancet 1: 838-839, 1972.

Harper, K.H.; Palmer, A.K. and Davies, R.E.: Effect of
imipramine upon the pregnancy of laboratory animals.
Arzneim. Forsch. 15: 1218-1221, 1965.

Hendrickx, A.G.: Teratologic evaluation of imiprimine
hydrochloride in bonnet (Macaca mulatta). Teratology 11:
219-222, 1975.

Idanpaan-Heikkila, J. and Saxen, L.: Possible teratogenicity of imipraminechloropyramine. Lancet 2: 281-283, 1973.

Larsen, V.: Teratogenic effects of thalidomide, imipramine HCl and imipramine N-oxide HCl on white Danish rabbits. Acta Pharmacol. Toxicol. 20: 186-200, 1963.

McBride, W.G.: Limb deformities associated with iminodibenzyl hydrochloride. Med. J. Aust. 1: 492 only, 1972.

Rachelefsky, G.S.; Flynt, J.W.; Ebbin, A.J. and Wilson, M.G.: Possible teratogenicity of tricyclic antidepressants. Lancet 1: 838 only, 1972.

Robson, J.M. and Sullivan, F.M.: The production of foetal abnormalities in rabbits with imipramine. Lancet 1: 638-639, 1963.

Stenger, E.G.; Aeppli, L. and Fratta, I.: Zur frage der Keimschadigenden Wirkung von N-(gamma-dimethylaminopropyl-)-iminodibenzyl-HCl am Tier. Arzneim Mittelforschung 15: 1222-1224, 1965.

711 Immobilization

Immobilization of the mouse fetus by muscle relaxants at the time of palate closure failed to produce cleft palate (Jacobs, 1971). Drachman and Coulombre (1962) produced arthrogryposis and clubfoot in chick embryos immobilized by D-tubocurarine.

Hartel and Hartel (1960) produced 36.7 percent cleft palates in rat fetuses when the vitamin-A-treated mother was immobilized for 3 to 4 hours on the 9th through the 12th day of gestation. The vitamin A alone (15,000 I.U. daily on the 8th through 12th day) produced only 4.5 percent cleft palates and immobilization alone produced no defects.

Drachman, D.B. and Coulombre, A.J.: Experimental clubfoot and arthrogryposis multiplex congenita. Lancet 2: 523-526, 1962.

Hartel, A. and Hartel, G.: Experimental study of teratogenic effect of emotional stress on rats. Science 132: 1483-1484, 1960.

Jacobs, R.M.: Failure of muscle relaxants to produce cleft palate in mice. Teratology 4: 25-30, 1971.

712 Imuran-R (see Azathioprine)

713 Indacrinone

Robertson et al using this diuretic at 40-120 mg per kg on days 6-17 of rat gestation produced wavy ribs and skeletal abnormalities in the fetus. This finding was reversed by coadministration of extra potassium chloride.

713

Robertson, R.T.; Minsker, D.H.; Bokelman, D.L.; Durand, G.;
Conquet, P.: Potassium loss as a causative factor for
skeletal malformations in rats produced by indacrinone: A
new investigational loop diuretic. Toxicol. Appl. Pharm.
60: 142-150, 1981.

714 Indapamide

Seki et al (1982) administered this antihypertensive orally
to rats and rabbits in maximum doses of 1000 and 80 mg per
kg daily. Ferrtility was unaffected in the rat. Studies
during organogenesis and on days 17-21 were done and no
adverse effects were found in the rat fetuses or in the
behavior of the offspring. Some growth retardation was seen
in rat fetuses at the highest dose schedule. No adverse
fetal effects were found in the rabbit.

Seki, T.; Fujitani, M.; Osumi, S.; Yamamoto, T.; Eguchi, K.;
Inoue, N.; Sakka, N.; Suzuki, M.R.: Reproductive studies of
indapamide. Yakuri to Chiryo 10:1325-1335, 1337-1353,
1355-1362, 1363-1314, 1982.

715 Inderal-R (see Propanolol)

716 Indiogofera Extract

The extract of Indiogofera spicata, a hardy pasture plant,
has been fed to the rat and cleft palate was produced in
about 60 percent of the offspring (Pearn, 1967).

Pearn, J.H.: Report of a new site-specific cleft palate
teratogen. Nature 215: 980-981, 1967.

717 Indium

Ferm and Carpenter (1970) injected indium nitrate (0.5 to
1.0 mg per kg intravenously) on day 8 of gestation of the
hamster and observed digital defects in over one-half of the
surviving fetuses. Dosage over 1 mg per kg caused
intrauterine death.

Ferm, V.H. and Carpenter, S.J.: Teratogenic and
embryopathic effects of indium, gallium and germanium.
Toxicol. Appl. Pharmacol. 16: 166-170, 1970.

718 Indoleacetic Acid

Ruddick et al (1974) gave pregnant rats up to 100 mg per kg
by gavage on days 6 through 15 and found no fetal changes.

Ruddick, J.A.; Harwig, J. and Scott, P.M.: Nonteratogenicity in rats of blighted potatoes and compounds contained
in them. Teratology 9: 165-168, 1974.

719 Indole-3-acetic Acid

John et al (1979) gavaged mice and rats on days 7-15 of gestation with 50 to 500 mg per kg per day. At the highest dose fetuses from both species had increased numbers of cleft palate. The mouse fetuses also had increased rates of exencephaly, dilated cerebral ventricles and crooked tails.

John, J.A.; Blogg, C.D.; Murray, F.J.; Schwetz, B.A.; Gehring, P.J.: Teratogenic effects of the plant hormone indole-3-acetic acid in mice and rats. Teratology 19:321-326, 1979.

720 Indomethacin

Kalter (1973) administered this antipyretic agent to mice on the 9th through the 15th day by oral, subcutaneous and intramuscular route. Dosage up to the maternal lethal dose (7.5 mg per kg) did not produce teratogenic activity. Kusang et al (1977) using 7.5 mg per kg orally on days 7-15 produced fused ribs, vertebral abnormalities and other skeletal defects in mouse fetuses. Similar negative findings in the rat using 4 mg per kg during organogenesis were reported by Klein et al (1981). Powell and and Cochrane (1978) used 1.6 mg per kg orally starting on day 18 in the rat and caused premature closure of the ductus arteriosus in 1 to 3 percent of the offspring whose mothers were treated for 3.5 to 5 days.

Levin et al (1978) have reported an infant with pulmonary artery changes following short term prenatal exposure (25 mg daily) to the mother.

Kalter, H.: Nonteratogenicity of indomethacin in mice. (abstract) Teratology 7: A-19, 1973.

Klein, K.L.; Scott, W.J.; Clark, K.E.; Wilson, J.G.: Indomethacin- placental transfer, cytotoxicity and teratology in the rat. Am. J. Obst. and Gyn. 141:448-452, 1981.

Kusanag, T.; Ihara, T. and Mizutani, M.: Teratogenic effects of non-steroid anti-inflammatory agents in mice (Japanese) Cong. Anom. 17:177-185, 1977.

Levin, D.L.; Fixler, D.E.; Morriss, F.C.; Tyson, J.:Morphologic analysis of pulmonary vascular bed in infants exposed in utero to prostoglandin synthetase inhibitors. J. Pediat. 92:478-483, 1978.

Powell, J.G. and Cochrane, R.L.: The effects of the administration of fenoprofen or indomethacin to rat dams during late pregnancy with special reference to the ductus arteriosus of the fetuses and neonates. Toxicol. Appl. Pharmacol. 45:783-796, 1978.

721 Influenza Viruses

There is a major body of literature on the role that influenza viruses might play in production of congenital defects (see review by Brown, 1966). Some epidemiologic

721

studies report a small non-specific increase in defects
(Hardy et al.; 1961; Saxen et al.; 1960; Coffey and Jessop,
1963); an almost equal number of studies have reported none
(Wilson et al.; 1959; Ingalls, 1960; Walker and Mckee, 1959;
Doll et al.; 1960; Korones et al.; 1970). Hardy et al.
(1961) reported an increase in fetal wastage associated with
an influenza outbreak. Leck (1963) noted that the incidence
of esophageal atresia was especially high; and Doll et al.
(1960), Coffey and Jessop (1963) and Hakosalo and Saxen
(1971) found anencephaly to be more frequent following
epidemics of Asian influenza. The data from many of these
reports are difficult to assess because of the following
factors: lack of serologic proof of the infection, unknown
attack rates in the control population, restricted numbers
of congenital defects or inadequate controls. A number of
investigators have suggested that the small increase in
attack rates during epidemics may be caused by fever,
medications or other non-viral associated factors. Saxen
(1975) analyzed the effect of non-viral components of
influenza attacks.

Studies of the effect of influenza virus on chicks (Adams et
al.; 1956) and mice (Siem et al.; 1960) have induced some
decrease in number of offspring but no clear-cut congenital
defects were produced. In the study by Siem et al. (1960),
the virus did not cross the mouse placenta until late in the
gestation period.

Adams, J.M.; Heath, H.D.; Imagawa, D.T.; Jones, M.H. and
Shear, H.H.: Viral infections in the embryo. Am. J. Dis.
Child. 92: 109-114, 1956.

Brown, G.C.: Recent advances in the viral aetiology of congenital anomalies. In, Woollam, D.H.M. (ed.): Advances in
Teratology, Vol. 1. London: Logos Press, 1966. pp.
55-80.

Doll, R.; Hill, A.B. and Sukula, J.: Asian influenza in
pregnancy and congenital defects. Br. J. Prev. Soc.
Med. 14: 167-172, 1960.

Hakosalo, J. and Saxen, L.: Influenza epidemic and congenital defects. Lancet 2: 1346-1347, 1971.

Hardy, J.B.; Azarowicz, E.N.; Mannini, A.; Medearis, D.N.
and Cooke, R.E.: The effect of Asian influenza on the
outcome of pregnancy, Baltimore, 1957-1958. Am. J. Public
Health 51: 1182-1188, 1961.

Ingalls, T.H.: Prenatal human ecology. Am. J. Public
Health 50: 50-54, 1960.

Korones, S.B.; Todaro, J.; Roane, J.A. and Sever, J.L.:
Maternal virus infection after the first trimester of pregnancy and status of offspring to 4 years of age in a
predominantly Negro population. J. Pediatr. 77: 245-251,
1970.

Leck, I.: Incidence of malformations following influenza
epidemics. Br. J. Prev. Soc. Med. 17: 70-80, 1963.

Saxen, L.: Newborn monitoring. In, Shepard, T.H.; Miller, J.R. and Marois, M. (eds.): Methods for Detection of Environmental Agents Which Produce Congenital Defects, Amsterdam: North-Holland American Elsevier, 1975, pp. 205-216.

Saxen, L.; Hjelt, L.; Sjostedt, J.E.; Hakosalo, J. and Hakosalo, H.: Asian influenza during pregnancy and congenital malformations. Acta Pathol. Microbiol. Scand. 49: 114-126, 1960.

Siem, R.A.; Ly, H.; Imagawa, D.T. and Adams, J.M.: Influenza virus infections in pregnant mice. J. Neuropathol. Exp. Neurol. 19: 125-129, 1960.

Walker, W.M. and McKee, A.P.: Asian influenza in pregnancy relationship to fetal anomalies. Obstet. Gynecol. 13: 394-398, 1959.

Wilson, M.G.; Heins, H.L.; Imagawa, D.T. and Adams, J.M.: Teratogenic effects of Asian influenza. J.A.M.A. 171: 116-119, 1959.

722 Influenza Vaccine

Heinonen et al (1973 and 1977) studied 3,051 pregnancies where influenza immunization was given and found no increase in defect rate or postnatal malignancies. Sarnat et al (1979) report one infant with cerebral malformation after the mother received swine influenza vaccine 6 weeks post conception.

Heinonen, O.P.; Slone, D.; Shapiro, S.: Birth Defects and Drugs in Pregnancy. Publishing Sciences Group, Inc., 1977.

Heinonen, O.P.; Shapiro, S.; Monson, R.R.; Hartz, S.C.; Rosenberg, L.; Slone, D.: Immunization during pregnancy agains poliomyelitis and influenza in relation to childhood malignancy. Int. J. Epid. 2:229-235, 1973.

Sarnat, H.B.; Rybak, G.; Kotagal, S.; Blair, J.D.: Cerebral embryopathy in late first trimester: Possible association with swine influenza vaccine. Teratology 20:93-100, 1979.

723 Inosine (also see 2-Deoxyinosine)

Karnofsky and Lacon (1961) injected 2 to 8 mg into 4-day-old chick yolk sacs and found a 9 percent incidence of unspecified defects. The LD-50 under these conditions was 4 to 8 mg.

Mercier-Parot and Tuchmann-Duplessis (1973) gave 500 mg per kg on the 12th day of rat gestation intraperitoneally and found no abnormal fetuses.

Karnofsky, D.A. and Lacon, C.R.: Effects of physiological purines on the development of the chick embryo. Biochem. Pharmacol. 7: 154-158, 1961.

Mercier-Parot, L. and Tuchmann-Duplessis, H.: Malformations squelettiques chez le rat produites par la 6-hydroxyl-aminopurine. Essais de Prevention. Compt. R. S. Soc. Biol. 167: 5-10, 1973.

724 Insulin

Kalter (1968) and Kalter and Warkany (1959) have reviewed this subject. A number of negative reports using the rat have appeared (see Kalter, 1968). Ferrill (1943) using 20 to 40 units per kg from weaning could find no defects in the rat offspring that were produced during five generations. Love et al. (1964) giving 0.5 units every 12 hours during the last two weeks of pregnancy produced no defects in the rat.

The mouse has been used by Smithberg et al. (1956) and Smithberg and Runner (1963) who injected 0.1 units of protamine zinc insulin 8.5 days post coitum and found a high incidence of exencephaly, rib and vertebral defects. The teratogenic effects of insulin or tolbutamide alone or in conjunction with nicotinamide were compared by Smithberg and Runner (1963) in three strains of mice. The primary role of insulin is hard to judge when the mouse is sensitive also to fasting teratogenesis.

In the rabbit Chomette (1955) and Brinsmade et al. (1956) have produced microcephaly and other central nervous system defects. Landauer (1947) produced rumplessness, micromelia and other skeletal defects in chicks by injecting 2 units of insulin into the yolk sac at 24 or 120 hours of incubation. Riboflavin given with the insulin caused an increase in the number of deformities (Landauer, 1952), but nicotinamide reduced the incidence (Landauer and Rhodes, 1952). Landauer (1972) has reviewed the evidence that insulin alone is teratogenic.

Sobel (1960) was able to identify 17 incidences where the mother was treated with insulin shock; four fetal deaths and two fetuses with multiple congenital anomalies were reported.

Brinsmade, A.B.; Buchner, F. and Rubsaamen, H.: Missbildungen am Kaninchenembryo durch Insulininjektion beim Muttertier. Naturwissenschaften 43: 259, only, 1956.

Chomette, G.: Entwichlungsstorungen nach Insulinschock beim Trachtigen Kaninchen. Beitr. Pathol. Anat. 115: 439-451, 1955.

Ferrill, H.W.: Effect of chronic insulin injections on reproduction in white rats. Endocrinology 32: 449-450, 1943.

Kalter, H.: Teratology of the central nervous system. Chicago: University of Chicago Press, 1968.

Kalter, H. and Warkany, J.: Experimental production of congenital malformations in mammals by metabolic procedure. Physiol. Rev. 39: 69-115, 1959.

Landauer, W.: Insulin-induced abnormalities of the beak, extremities and eyes in chickens. J. Exp. Zool. 105: 145-172, 1947.

Landauer, W.: Malformations of chicken embryos produced by boric acid and the probable role of riboflavin in their origin. J. Exp. Zool. 120: 469-508, 1952.

Landauer, W.: Is insulin a teratogen? Teratology 5: 129-135, 1972.

Landauer, W. and Rhodes, M.B.: Further observations on the teratogenic nature of insulin and its modification by supplementary treatment. J. Exp. Zool. 119: 221-261, 1952.

Smithberg, M. and Runner, M.N.: Teratogenic effects of hypoglycemic treatment in inbred strains of mice. Am. J. Anat. 113: 479-489, 1963.

Smithberg, M.; Sanchez, H.W. and Runner, M.N.: Congenital deformity in the mouse induced by insulin. (abstract) Anat. Rec. 124: 441, only, 1956.

Sobel, D.E.: Fetal damage due to ECT, insulin coma, chlorpromazine, or reserpine. A.M.A. Gen. Psych. 2: 606-611, 1960.

725 Iodide

Protracted ingestion of iodide containing medications (expectorants) by the mother may result in fetal thyroid enlargement which can lead in some cases to tracheal compression and choking in the newborn (Parmelee et al.; 1940; Galina et al.; 1962). These goiters are due to fetal thyroid inhibition with secondary compensatory hypertrophy. Klevit (1969) has reviewed this subject. Pharoah et al (1971) were able to prevent endemic cretinism and the associated mental retardation by injection of iodised oil before conception.

Galina, M.P.; Avnet, N.L. and Einhorn, A.: Iodides during pregnancy. An apparent cause of death. N. Engl. J. Med. 267: 1124-1127, 1962.

Klevit, H.D.: Iatrogenic thyroid disease. In, Gardner, L.I. (ed.): Endocrine and Genetic Diseases of Childhood. Philadelphia: W.B. Saunders, 1969. pp. 246-247.

Parmelee, A.H.; Allen, E.; Stein, I.F. and Buxbaum, H.: Three cases of congenital goiter. Am. J. Obstet. Gynecol. 40: 145-147, 1940.

Pharoah, P.O.D.; Buttfield, I.H.; Hetzel, B.S.: Neurological damage to the fetus from severe iodine deficiency during pregnancy. Lancet 1:308-310, 1971.

726 Iodine-131

726

This isotope of iodine if given in millicurie doses can damage or ablate the developing thyroid of the human fetus. Hypothyroidism, either congenital or of late onset, has been reported in at least five children whose mothers were treated with I(131) during pregnancy (Russel et al.; 1957; Hammill et al.; 1961; Fisher et al.; 1963; Green et al.; 1971). The risk of fetal radiochemical thyroidectomy increases with the onset of the iodide concentrating ability of the fetal thyroid at around the 74th gestational day (Shepard, 1968).

Stoffer and Hamburger (1976) surveyed 517 physicians and obtained information on 182 pregnancies. The general complication rate was not increased. However, 6 infants had hypothyroidism and of these, 4 were mentally retarded.

Speert et al. (1951) first studied the thyroid damaging effect of I(131) in the mouse fetus whose mother was given 200 microcuries after the 15th gestational day.

Fisher, W.D.; Voorhess, M.L. and Gardner, L.I.: Congenital hypothyroidism in infant following maternal I(131) therapy. J. Pediatr. 62: 132-146, 1963.

Green, H.G.; Gareis, F.J.; Shepard, T.H. and Kelley, V.C.: Cretinism associated with maternal sodium iodide I(131) therapy during pregnancy. Am. J. Dis. Child. 122: 247-249, 1971.

Hammill, G.C.; Jarman, J.A.; Wynne, M.D.: Fetal effects of radioactive iodine therapy in a pregnant woman with thyroid cancer. Am. J. Obstet. Gynecol. 81: 1018-1023, 1961.

Russel, K.P.; Rose, H. and Starr, P.: The effects of radioactive iodide on maternal and fetal thyroid function during pregnancy. Surg. Gynecol. Obstet. 104: 560-564, 1957.

Shepard, T.H.: Onset of function in the human fetal thyroid: Biochemical and radioautographic studies from organ culture. J. Clin. Endocrinol. Metab. 27: 945-958, 1967.

Speert, H.; Quimby, E.H. and Werner, S.C.: Radioiodine uptake by the fetal mouse thyroid and resultant effects in later life. Surg. Gynecol. Obstet. 93: 230-242, 1951.

Stoffer, S.S. and Hamburger, J.I.: Inadvertent I-131 therapy for hyperthyroidism in the first trimester of pregnancy. J. Nucl. Med. 17:146-149, 1976.

727 Iodine Deficiency

Warkany (1971) has comprehensively reviewed the role that iodine deficiency played in production of endemic and congenital goiters. Before the introduction of modern transportation of iodinated foods isolated communities drawing their food and water supply from glaciated terrain were the source of most cases of endemic goiter.

Warkany, J.: Congenital Malformations: Notes and Comments.

Chicago: Year Book Medical Publishers, 1971. pp. 106-107.

728 Iodoacetate

Runner and Dagg (1960) injected 1 mg of iodoacetate intraperitoneally into mice on day 8 of gestation and found deformed ribs and vertebrae in 62 percent of the offspring. Miller (1973) injected 0.5 mg intramuscularly on days 12 through 14 and produced 14 percent cleft palates in the mouse and was able to lower the incidence by giving succinate concurrently.

Miller, T.J.: Cleft palate formation: The effects of fasting and iodoacetic acid on mice. Teratology 7: 177-182, 1973.

Runner, M.N. and Dagg, C.P.: Metabolic mechanisms of teratogenic agents during morphogenesis. Natl. Cancer Inst. Monogr. 2: 41-54, 1960.

729 5-Iododeoxyuridine

Skalko and Packard (1973) administered this compound on single days intraperitoneally to mice from day 7 through 11. Doses of 300 and 500 mg per kg were highly embryolethal and teratogenic while at 100 mg per kg fewer defects and resorptions were found. Exencephaly, polydactyly, skeletal reduction defects and cleft palate were found.

Percy (1975) treating pregnant rats and mice for 3 days toward the end of gestation produced cerebellar dysplasia, microcystic kidneys and rare retinal changes. The changes could be produced by doses of 50 mg per kg. Itoi et al (1975) applied a 0.1 percent solution to rabbit eyes four times daily for 12 days during organogenesis and found exophthalmos and clubbing of the forefeet in the fetuses. Trifluorothymidine (1 percent) did not produce abnormalities when applied in a similar manner.

Itoi, M.; Gefter, J.W.; Kaneko, N.; Ishii, Y.; Ramer, R.M. and Gasset, A.R.: Teratogenicities of ophthalmic drugs 2. Antiviral ophthalmic drugs. Arch. Ophth. 93: 46-49, 1975.

Percy, D.H.: Teratogenicity effects of pyrimidine analogues 5-iododeoxyuridine and cytosine arabinoside in late fetal mice and rats. Teratology 11: 103-108, 1975.

Skalko, R.G. and Packard, D.S.: The teratogenic response of the mouse embryo to 5-iododeoxyuridine. Experientia 29: 198-200, 1973.

730 Ionizing Radiation (see Radiation, Ionizing)

731 Ipratropium Bromide (Sch 1000)

Nishimura et al (1978) gavage fed rats and rabbits with maximum daily doses of 500 and 125 mg per kg during

organogenesis. The only positive finding was a slight
reduction in weight of the rat fetuses at the highest dose.

Nishimura, M.; Kast, A. and Tsunenari, Y.: Reproduction
studies of ipratropium bromide (Sch 1000) on rats and
rabbits. Iyakuhin Kenkyu 9:393-416, 1978.

732 Iproniazid

This compound which inhibits the breakdown of 5-hydroxy-
tryptamine was used by Poulson et al. (1960) to produce
hemorrhages in rat placentas. They gave 5 to 10 mg per day
and reported a reduction in fertility when it was administered during the first half of pregnancy. Teratogenic
results were not reported.

Poulson, E.; Botros, M. and Robson, J.M.: Effect of 5-
hydroxytryptamine and iproniazid on pregnancy. Science 131:
1101-1102, 1960.

733 Irradiation (see Radiation)

734 Isofluorophate (DFP, diisopropyl phosphorofluoridate)

This organophosphate cholinesterase inhibitor was tested by
Fish (1966) in rats which received doses on days 7 through
12 of gestation. At doses up to 4 mg per kg, no adverse
effects on reproduction were found.

Fish, S.A.: Organophosphorus cholinesterase inhibitors and
fetal development. Am. J. Obst. & Gynecol.
96:1148-1154, 1966.

735 Isoniazid [Isonicotinic Acid Hydrazide]

There are a number of reports on the effect of treating
pregnant women with antituberculous drugs including
isoniazid. Lowe (1964) examined 74 exposed infants and
Marcus (1967) 19 children and found no increase in congenital defects. Varpela (1964) reported 12 anomalies in 123
children exposed in utero to various antituberculous drugs.
Heinonen et al (1977) reported 10 malformed children from 85
mothers exposed during the first 4 months of pregnancy. The
types of defects were not given. Monnet (1967) studied 5
children with severe encephalopathies after their mohers
were treated with INH. Warkany (1975) has published a
complete review of the effects of antituberculosis drugs in
human pregnancy.

Heinonen, O.P.; Slone, D. and Shapio, S.: Birth Defects
and Drugs in Pregnancy. Publishing Sciences Group Inc.;
Littleton, Mass.; 1977.

Lowe, C.R.: Congenital defects among children born to women
under supervision or treatment for pulmonary tuberculosis.
Br. J. Prev. Soc. Med. 18: 14-16, 1964.

Marcus, J.C.: Non-teratogenicity of antituberculous drugs.
S. Afr. Med. J. 41: 758-759, 1967.

Monnet, P.; Kalb, J.C.; Pujol, M.: Doit-on craindre une
influence teratogene eventuelle de l'isoniazide. Rev.
Tubercul. (Paris) 31: 845-848, 1967.

Varpela, E.: On the effect exerted by first-line
tuberculosis medicines on the fetus. Acta Tuberculosea et
Pneumologica Scandinavica 35: 53-69, 1964.

Warkany, J.: Antituberculous drugs. Teratology 20:133-138,
1979.

736 Isonicotinic Acid-2-isopropylhydrazide (see 1-Methyl-
-formylhydrazine)

737 Iproniazid (see 1-Methyl-formylhydrazine)

738 P-IsooctylPolyoxyethylphenol polymer (see Triton W-R 1339)

739 Isopropyl Alcohol

Antonova and Salmina (1978) reported that this compound
induced death in 31% of embryos and malformations in 14% of
embryos. The substance was given to pregnant rats
0.018-1008 mg per kg. Behaviour abnormalities in progeny of
treated females were also found.

Antonova, V.I. and Salmina, Z.A.: The maximum permissible
concentration of isopropyl alcohol in water bodied with due
regard for its action on the gonads and the progeny.
Gigiena i Sanitariya (USSR) 1:8-11, 1978.

740 N-Isopropyl-P-(2-methylhydrazinomethyl)benzamide [Natulan-R]

Von kreybig et al (1973) gave this compound to rats on the
13th gestational day and at levels of 250 mg per kg found a
teratogenic effect. They found deformed skulls and defects
of the brain and extremities.

Von Kreybig, T.; Preussmann, R. and Von Kreybig, I.:
Chemische Konstitution und teratogene Wirkung bei der Ratte.
3. N-alkylcarbonhydrazide, weitere Hydrazinderivate.
Arzneim-Forsch 20: 363-367, 1970.

741 Isoproterenol

Vogin et al. (1970) administered isoproterenol to rats and
rabbits by aerosol spray and produced no congenital defects.

The rats received 150 or 450 microgm per kg per day from day
5 through day 16. The rabbits received 36.5 microgm per kg
daily from day 6 through day 16. Hodach et al (1975) administered 0.4 micromoles in 5 microliters directly to the

chick embryo and produced cardiovascular anomalies.
Increased heart rates in explanted rat embryos have been
found at exposure doses of 500 nanograms per ml of medium
(Robkin et al, 1976).

Hodach, R.J.; Hodach, A.E.; Fallon, J.F.; Folts, J.D.;
Bruyere, H.J. and Gilbert, E.F.: The role of Beta-
adrenergic activiy in the production of cardiac and aortic
arch anomalies in chick embryos. Teratology 12:33-49, 1975.

Robkin, M.A.; Shepard, T.H. and Dyer, D.C.:

Autonomic receptors of the early rat embryo heart: Growth
and development. Proc. Soc. Exp. Biol. Med.
151:799-803, 1976.

Vogin, E.E.; Goldhamer, R.E.; Scheimberg, J.; Carson, S.
and Boxill, G.C.: Teratology studies in rats and rabbits
exposed to an isoproterenol aerosol. Toxicol. Appl.
Pharmacol. 16: 374-381, 1970.

742 Isoprothiolane

This fungicide was given orally to mice on days 6 through 12
in doses to 600 mg per kg and only reduced fetal weight and
ossification centers were found. (Sukurai and Kasai, 1976).

Sukurai, K. and Kasai, T.: Teratological studies of
isoprothiolane in mice (abs) Teratology 14:251, only, 1976.

743 Isouracil

Kosmachevskaya and Tichodeeva (1968) produced malformations
in 18 percent of chick embryos injected with 0.5 to 4 mg of
isouracil at 24 hours of incubation. Microphthalmia,
rumplessness, beak and axial skeletal defects and
sirenomelia were found. Embryonic mortality was
insignificant.

Kosmachevskaya, E.A. and Tichodeeva, I.I.: Relation
between embryotoxic activity of some pyrimidine derivatives
and their chemical structure. Chick Embryo Test.
Pharmacol. Toxicol. (Russian) No. 5: 618-620, 1968.

744 Janus Green B

Braun (1954) inoculated chicken eggs at the beginning of
incubation or once during the first three days of incubation
with 65 to 300 microgm of Janus green. Over 90 percent of
the embryos receiving the dosage schedule of 100 microgm
were defective. The defects included hydrocephalus,
microphthalmia, cerebral dysplasia, phocomelia and
hemorrhages in various places. The author postulated that
the dye reduced the oxygen consumption of the cells which
led to the defective development.

Braun, S.: Janus green B teratological action in
embryonated hen's eggs and embryogenetic and carcinogenic

bearings of its mechanism of action. Acta Morphologica 4: 61-79, 1954.

745 Japanese B Encephalitis Virus

Burns (1950) isolated Japanese B encephalitis virus from newborn pigs with encephalomalacia or internal hydro-cephalus. At the time there was a large epidemic of this infection in both man and pigs, and the fetal morbidity in swine was 60 to 70 percent. Shimizu et al. (1954) injected the virus intravenously into susceptible pigs and produced hydrocephalus in some, but virus recovery was successful from the fetuses only during early gestation.

Burns, K.F.: Congenital Japanese encephalitis infection of swine. Proc. Soc. Exp. Biol. Med. 75: 621-625, 1950.

Shimizu, T.; Kawakami, Y.; Fukuhara, S. and Matumoto, M.: Experimental stillbirth in pregnant swine infected with Japanese encephalitis virus. Jap. J. Exp. Med. 24: 363-375, 1954.

746 Japanese Equinine Encephalitis

A high incidence of hydrocephalus in newborn calves was reported by Tabuchi et al. (1953) during an epidemic of Japanese equinine encephalitis. Isolation of the virus from the fetuses was unsuccessful.

Tabuchi, A.; Narita, R.; Ebi, Y. and Hosoda, T.: Studies on hydrocephalus of newborn calves in Aomori, Akita and Iwate prefectures. Experimental Report of the Government Experimental Station of Animal Hygiene (Tokyo) 26: 21-26, 1953.

747 Jervine (also see Cyclopamine)

The alkaloid prepared from Veratrum californicum has been administered (0.9 to 2.4 gm) to ewes on the 14th gestational day and produced cyclopian fetuses (Keeler and Binns, 1968).

Keeler, R.F. and Binns, W.: Teratogenic compounds of Veratrum californicum (Durand) 5 comparisons of cyclopian effects of steroidal alkaloids from plant and structurally related compounds from other sources. Teratology 1: 5-10, 1968.

748 Josamycin Proprionate

Oshima and Iwadare (1973) administered this compound orally to pregnant mice and rats in doses up to 2000 mg per kg during 7 days of their organogenesis and found no significant fetal effects.

Oshima, T. and Iwadare, M.: Studies of josamycin proprionate. Jap. J. Antibiotics 26: 148-153, 1973.

749   Kanamycin

Bevelander and Cohlan (1962) injected rats with 100 mg per
kg from the 8th through 16th day and produced no fetal
changes.

Akiyoshi et al (1977) studied the effect of 100-200 mg per
kg given intramuscularly on the guinea pig fetuses from day
7 through day 56. At both doses cochlear hair cell damage
was found and hearing impairment using the pinna reflex test
was reduced at higher frequencies in some offspring.   Tests
with amikacin at the same dose showed no hearing impairment
but some hair cell damage occurred.

Akiyoshi, M.; Yano, S.; Tajima, T.; Matsuzaki, M.; Akutsu,
S.; Nishimoto, K. and Maeda, M.: Ototoxic effect of BB-K-8
administered to pregnant guinea pigs on development of inner
ear of intrauterine litters. (Japanese) Japanese J.
Antibiotics 196:53-64, 1977.

Bevelander, G.; Cohlan, S.Q.: The effect on the rat of
transplacentally acquired tetracycline. Biol.   Neonate
4:365-370, 1962.

750   Kanechlor

This polychlorinated biphenyl was administered orally to
pregnant rats from days 8 to 14 or from day 15 through 21 in
amounts of 20 or 100 mg per kg per day (Shiota et al,
1976A).   At the highest dose some fetal and maternal
toxicity occurred but no congenital defect increase was
found.   Post-natal function was measured and maze learning
was slower in the offspring exposed in utero.   At dietary
levels of 500 PPM Kanechlor 300 and Kanechlor 500 were
associated with fetal weight decrease but there was no
increase in defects (Shiota, 1976B).

Shiota, K.:   Embryotoxic effects of polychlorinated
biphenyls (Kanechlors 300 and 500) in rats. Okijimas Fol.
Anat. 53:93-104, 1976A.

Shiota, K.:   Postnatal behavioral effects of prenatal
treatment with PCBs (Polychlorinated biphenyls) in rats.
Okajimas Fol. Anat. 53:105-114, 1976B.

751   Kepone   (Decachlorooctahydro-
      -1-3-4-metheno-2h-cyclobuta(6d)pentalen-2-one) (chlordecone)

This polychlorinated organic insecticide and fungicide was
fed to mice in amounts of 40 PPM (Huber, 1965).
Reproduction failure related to constant   estrus was
observed.   The average young per litter was reduced by 30
PPM. Although the material was detected in fetuses, no congenital defects were reported. Cannon and Kimbrough (1979)
feeding rats 25 ppm for 3 months completely inhibited
reproduction.   Chernoff and Rogers (1976) reported enlarged
cerebral ventricles and dilated renal pelves in rat fetuses
exposed by gavage to 10 and 6 mg per kg on days 7-16. In
the mouse, clubfeet were increased over controls at 12 mg

per kg.

Cannon, S.B. and Kimbrough, R.D.: Short-term chlordecone toxicity in rats including effects on reproduction, pathological organ changes, and their reversibility. Toxicol. Appl. Pharmacol. 47:469-476, 1979. reversibility.

Chernoff, N. and Rogers, E.H..: Fetal toxicity of kepone in rats and mice. Toxicol. Appl. Pharmacol. 38:189-194, 1976.

Huber, J.J.: Some physiologic effects of the insecticide kepone in the laboratory mouse. Toxicol. Appl. Pharmacol. 7: 516-524, 1965.

752 Ketamine

This general anesthetic agent related to phencyclidine was tested in pregnant rats by El-Karim and Benny (1976). They gave 120 mg per kg intramuscularly from the ninth through the thirteenth day. No adverse fetal effects were noted.

El-Karim, A.H.B. and Benny, R.: Embryotoxic and teratogenic action of ketamine hydrochloride in rats. Ain Shavis Med. J. 27:459-463, 1976.

753 4-Ketocyclophosphamide (see Cyclophosphamide)

754 Ketoprofen (M-Benzoylhyratropic Acid)

This antiinflammatory analgesic has been tested in mice, rats and monkeys (Esaki et al, 1975A and B, Tanioka and Koizumi, 1975 and Tanioka et al, 1975). Mice and rats were treated on days 7 through 13 and 9 through 15 respectively. The maximum daily subcutaneous doses were 100 mg and 5 mg and orally 10 and 3 mg respectively in the mouse and rat. There were no ill effects to the fetuses, but in several groups in both species the treated fetuses were heavier than controls. In monkeys intramuscular (30 mg) and oral doses (150 mg) were given from day 23 through 35 without detectable effect on the fetuses at day 60.

Esaki, K.; Tsukada, M.; Izumiyama, K. and Oshio, K.: Teratogenicity of sodium ketoprofen (19583RP-Na) tested by subcutaneous administration in mice and rats 1:101-109, 1975.

Esaki, K.; Tsukada, M.; Izumiyama, K. and Ohshio, K.: Teratogenicity of ketoprofen (19583RP) tested by oral administration in mice and rats. (Japaanese) CIEA Preclinical Reports 1:91-100, 1975.

Tanioka, Y. and Koizumi, H.: Teratogenicity test by intramuscular administration of ketoprofen-Na (19583 RP-Na) in Rhesus monkeys. CIEA Preclinical Report 3:87-96, 1977.

Tanioka, Y.; Koizumi, H.; Ogata, T. and Esaki, K.: Terato-

754

genicity of ketoprofen (19583RP) in the Rhesus monkey. CIEA
Preclinical Report 1:67-73, 1975.

755 Ketotifen

Nakajima et al (1979) studied this antiallergic agent in
pregnant rats using 30 mg per kg daily by mouth. Dosing was
in both sexes before mating and during the first 7 days,
during days 7-17 or on days 17-21. No adverse fertility
effects were found and the fetuses were similar to controls.
Some decrease in postnatal survival and weight was found.

Nakajima, T.; Ishizaka, K.; Hamada, M.; Matsuda, M.:
Reproductive studies of HC-20-511 in rats. Kiso to Rinsho
13:4096-4114, 1979.

756 Kwell-R (see Lindane)

757 Labetalol Hydrochloride

Nagaoka et al (1981) studied this beta blocker in rats and
rabbits using oral routes of up to 300 mg and 200 mg per kg
respectively. The copulation rate was decreased in rats at
the 300 mg level. No defects were found after treatment.
In the perinatal studies (days 17-21) decreased viability
and size was found with the 300 mg and 150 mg doses. Only a
slight decrease in survival was found in rabbit fetuses at
the 200 mg per kg level.

Nagaoka, T.; Shigemura, T.; Narama, I.:   Reproductive
studies on labetalol hydrochloride. Yakuri to Chiryo
9:839-850, 851-867, 869- 877, 879-893, 1981.

758 Laetrile (D,L-Amygdalin)

Oral D,L-amygdalin, the main constituent of laetrile
administered orally in amounts of 250 mg per kg or more to
hamsters was associated with neural tube defects (Willhite,
1982). Intravenous administration was not teratogenic.
D-prunasin at oral doses of 177 mg per kg was associated
with neural tube defects also. Since thiocyanide blocked
the teratogenicity of amygdalin it was suggested that
cyanide was the teratogenic metabolite.

Willhite, C.C.: Congenital malformations induced by
laetrile. Science 215:1513-1515, 1982.

759 Lampren [3-(P-Chloranilino)-10-(p-chlorphenyl)-2,10-dihydro-
     -2-(isopropylimino)-phenazine]

Stenger et al. (1970) gave this antibiotic orally to mice,
rats and rabbits during their gestational periods and found
no evidence of teratogenic activity. The rats and mice
received up to 50 mg per kg and rabbits 15 mg per kg daily.

Stenger, E.G.; Aeppli, L.; Peheim, E. and Thomann, P.E.:

Zur   Toxikologie   des   Leprostaticums
3-(P-chloranilino)-10-(P-chlorphenyl)-2-10-dihydro-2-(iso-
propylim ino)phenazin(G-30320).   Arzneim.   Forsch.   20:
794-799, 1970.

760   Laporotomy

Johnson   (1971)   laporotomized   rabbits on the 7th, 8th, 9th
and 10th post-coital days.   Pentobarbital   (40   mg   per   kg)
which   was   used   as   an anesthetic did not cause congenital
defects, but on the 9th and 10th day the resorption rate was
increased.   Laporotomy   with   uterine   exposure   to   the
atmosphere caused an increase in resorptions   on   all   days,
but no congenital defects were produced.   Brent and Franklin
(1960)   laporotomized   rats   on   the   9th   day   and   in   the
non-traumatized   horns   found   significant   increases   in
resorption rates.

Brent, R.L.   and Franklin, J.B.:   Uterine vascular clamping:
New procedure for the   study   of   congenital   malformations.
Science 132: 89-91, 1960.

Johnson, W.E.:   Fetal   loss   from   anesthesia   and   surgical
trauma   in   the   rabbit.   Toxicol.   Appl.   Pharmacol.   18:
773-779, 1971.

761   Lathyrism

Stamler (1955) fed   a   diet   containing   50   percent   ground
lathyrus odoratus peas and found that after the 17th day the
lathyrism syndrome could be produced in the rat fetus.   This
syndrome   consisted   of   poorly   developed   muscles   and
connective tissue with scanty collagen formation, dissecting
aneurisms   of   the   aorta   and   severe   spinal   deformities.
Beta-aminopropionitrile   bis-(beta-cyanoethyl)amine   and
aminoacetonitrile   produced similar findings when fed in the
diet at 0.01 to 0.05 percent levels.   These   compounds   had
little   effect on fetuses when fed to the rat during the 1st
16 days of gestation.   Tris(beta-cyanoethyl)amine and   beta-
-dimethylaminopropionitrile   had   no effect when given after
the 17th day.   Steffek et al.   (1972) produced cleft palates
in   rat   fetuses   by   feeding the mothers sweet pea seeds or
giving single 500 mg doses of beta-aminopropionitrile.   The
most   effective   time   of   administration   was   on   day   15.
Rosenberg   (1957)   has   produced   the   syndrome   in   chicks.
Barrow et al (1974) have reviewed the subject.

Barrow, M.V.; Simpson, C.F.   and Miller, E.J.:   Lathyrism: a
review.   Quart.   Rev.   Biol.   49: 101-128, 1974.

Rosenberg,   E.E.:   Teratogenic   effects   of   beta-aminopropionitrile   in   the   chick   embryo.   Nature 180: 706-707,
1957.

Stamler,   F.W.:   Reproduction   in rats fed lathyrus peas or
aminonitriles.   Proc.   Soc.   Exp.   Biol.   Med.   90: 294-298,
1955.

Steffek, A.J.; Verrusio, A.C.   and   Watkins,   C.A.:   Cleft

761

palate in rodents after maternal treatment with various lathyrogenic agents. Teratology 5: 33-40, 1972.

762 Latomoxef

This oxacephalosporin was given intraperitoneally by Kobayashi and Hara (1980) to rats of both sexes before pregnancy and during the first 7 days of gestation. Up to 200 mg per kg per day had no adverse effect on reproduction. Using the intravenous route and same dose rats were treated on days 7-17 or 17-21 and no adverse effects were found in the fetuses or in postnatal development of the offspring (Kobayashi and Audo, 1980 and Hasegawa and Yoshida, 1980).

Hasegawa, Y.; Yoshida, T.: Teratology study of 6059-S on rats. Chemotherapy 28:1119-1141, 1980.

Kobayashi, F.; Ando, M.: Perinatal-postnatal study on 6059-S in rats. Chemotherapy 28:1142-1157, 1980.

Kobayashi, F.; Hara, K.: Fertility study of 6059-S in rats. Chemotherapy 28:1108-1118, 1980.

763 Lead

Ridgway and Karnofsky (1952) reported brain hemorrhage and damage followed by hydrocephalus in chick embryos exposed to 0.10 mg of lead nitrate on the 4th day. Murakami et al. (1954) give examples of nervous system defects in mice receiving unspecified amounts of lead carbonate on the 7th and 8th days of gestation. In hamsters, Ferm and Carpenter (1967) injected 50 mg per kg of various lead salts on day 8 and found a high incidence of tail and sacral defects in the offspring. Later they studied the genesis of these caudal defects and found that edematous blebs and hemorrhage led to the production of the malformations (Carpenter and Ferm, 1977). McClain and Becker (1975) administered lead nitrate intravenously to rats and on the 9th day using 35 to 70 mg per kg a teratogenic effect was observed. The malformation consisted of urorectalcaudal syndrome which included a decrease in vertebral bodies, often associated with sirenomelia, absence of the rectum or external genitalia and tail defects. Treatment on the 16th day resulted in hydrocephalus and brain hemorrhage. Gerber and Maes using diets containing 0.25, 0.5 and 1.0 percent lead acetate showed reduced iron uptake and weight in fetal mice. Carson et al (1974) found learning defects in lambs exposed in utero to maternal blood levels of 34 micrograms per 100 ml.

Angle and McIntyre (1964) and Cantarow and Trumper (1944) have summarized the evidence that lead poisoning increases the incidence of abortion and stillbirths in humans. The evidence that lead affects the development of the central nervous system of the human fetus is not complete. Beattie et al (1975) have suggested that lead from water pipes might produce mental retardation. Moore et al (1977) have found some increase in blood lead among newborns who subsequently were found to be mentally retarded. Minsker et al (1979) exposed rat fetuses during late gestation and-or lactation to 5 or 25 mg per kg of lead nitrate intravenously (maternal) by mouth and found no behavioral or neurohistologic alterations. Hackett et al (1979) studied the kinetics of lead exposure in the rat and reported only small amounts in the fetus.

Wide (1978) found that intravenously administered lead did not interfere with blastocyst attachment or growth in the rat but in vitro exposure did cause changes. Gerber et al (1980) have summarized the data from animal experiments and humans. Rom (1976) has reviewed the ancient and modern literature on reproduction in lead exposed women.

Angle, C.R. and McIntyre, M.S.: Lead poisoning during pregnancy: fetal tolerance of calcium disodium edetate. Am. J. Dis. Child. 108: 436-439, 1964.

Beattie, A.D.; Moore, M.R.; Goldberg, A.; Finlayson, M.J.W.; Mackie, E.M.; Graham, J.F.; Main, J.C.; McLaren, D.A.; Murdock, R.M. and Stewart, G.T.: Role of chronic low-level lead exposure in the aetioloy of mental retardation. Lancet 1:589-592, 1975.

Cantarow, A. and Trumper, M.: Lead poisoning. Baltimore: Williams and Wilkins, 1944. pp. 84-86, 142-144.

Carpenter, S.J. and Ferm, V.H.: Embryopathic effects of lead in the hamster. Lab. Invest. 37:369-385, 1977.

Carson, T.L.; Vangelder, G.A.; Karas, G.G.; Buck, W.B.: Development of behavioral tests for the assessment of neurologic effects of lead in sheep. Environ. Health Perspect., May, 233-237, 1974.

Ferm, V.H. and Carpenter, S.J.: Developmental malformations resulting from administration of lead salts. Exp. Mol. Pathol. 7: 208-213, 1967.

Gerber, G.B.; Maes, J.: Heme synthesis in the lead-intoxicated mouse embryo. Toxicology 9:173-179, 1978.

Gerber, G.B.; Leonard, A.; Jacquet, P.: Toxicity, mutagenicity and teratogenicity of lead. Mutation Research 76:115-141, 1980.

Hackett, P.L.; Hess, J.O. and Sikov, M.R.: Cross-placental transfer and distribution or inhaled or ingested lead nitrate in rats (abs) Teratology 19:28A, 1979.

McClain, R.M. and Becker, B.A.: Teratogenicity, fetal toxicity, and placental transfer of lead nitrate in rats. Toxic. Appl. Pharmacol. 31: 72-82, 1975.

Minsker, D.H.; Moskalski, N.; Peter, C.P.; Robertson, R.T. and Bokelman, D.L.: Effects of lead exposure in utero or postpartum on brain histomorphology and behavior in rat offspring (abs) Teratology 19: 40A (only), 1979.

Moore, M.R.; Meredith, P.A. and Goldberg, A.: A retrospective analysis of blood-lead in mentally retarded children. Lancet 1:717-719, 1977.

763

Murakami, U.; Kameyama, Y. and Kato, T.: Basic processes seen in disturbance of early development of the central nervous system. Nagoya J. Med. Sci. 17: 74-88, 1954.

Ridgway, L.P. and Karnofsky, D.A.: The effects of metal on the chick embryo: Toxicity and production of abnormalities in development. Ann. N. Y. Acad. Sci. 55: 203-215, 1952.

Rom, W.N.: Effects of lead on the female and reproduction: A review. Mount Sinai J. of Med. 43:542-552, 1976.

Wide, M.: Effect of inorganic lead on the mouse blastocyst in vitro. Teratology 17:165-170, 1978.

764 Lecitin (see Concanavalin A)

765 Leucine

Persaud (1969) injected pregnant rats intraperitoneally with 15 mg per kg on days 1 through 6 or days 6 through 9. In each group about 45 percent of the fetuses were defective. The defects included microphthalmia, anophthalmia, encephalocele, skeletal defects and eventration of the abdominal wall. Bergstrom et al. (1967) reported inward flexion of the toes in chicks treated with leucine on the 9th day.

Bergstrom, R.M.; Erila, T. and Pirskanen, R.: Teratogenic effects of the amino acid leucine in the chicken. Experientia 23: 767-768, 1967.

Persaud, T.V.N.: Developmental abnormalities in the rat induced by the amino acid leucine. Naturwissenschaften 56: 37-39, 1969.

766 Levamisole Hydrochloride

Ohguro et al (1982) gave rats and rabbits orally up to 240 and 90 mg per kg daily respectively. Fertility and perinatal studies in the rat indicated some decrease in implantation at 120 and 240 mg levels and some decrease in viability over 60 mg per kg. No defect increases were found in either species but some growth retardation was found at 120 mg per kg in the rat.

Ohguro, Y.; Imamura, T.; Hara, T.; Nishikawa, S.; Miyazaki, E.: Study on safety of KW-2-LE-T (Levamisole Hcl) Reproductive studies. Yakuri to Chiryo 10:3155-3167, 1982.

767 D-Limonene [D-P-Mentha-1,8-diene]

The gallstone solubilizer was given to pregnant rats in doses of up to 2,869 mg per kg during organogenesis. Although maternal toxicity and fetal growth reduction occurred no teratogenicity was found (Tsuji et al, 1975).

Tsuji, M.; Fujisaki, Y.; Okubo, A.; Arikawa, Y.; Noda, K.;
Hiroyuki, I. and Ikeda, T.: Studies on D-limonene as a
gallstone solubilizer 5. Effects on development of rat
fetuses and offsprings. Oyo Yakuri 10: 179-186, 1975.

768 Lindane (benzene hexachloride, Kwell-R)

Palmer et al (1978A) studied three generations of rats
exposed to up to 100 ppm and found no adverse effects on the
reproduction or fetuses. Administration of up to 15 mg per
kg in the rat and rabbit during organogenesis produced no
teratogenic effect (Palmer et al, 1978B).

The International Agency for Research on Cancer (1979) has
reviewed the embryotoxicity and teratogenicity.

Anonymous: Hexachlorocyclohexane (technical HCH and
Lindane). IARC Monographs an Evaluation of Carcinogenic
Risk of Chemicals to Humans. 20:217-218, 1979.

Palmer, A.K.; Cozens, D.D.; Spicer, E.J.F. and Worden,
A.N.: Effects of lindane upon reproduction function in a
3-generation study of rats. Toxicology 11: 45-54, 1978A.

Palmer, A.K.; Bottomley, A.M.; Worden, A.N.; Frohberg, H.
and Bauer, A.: Effect of lindane on pregnancy in the rabbit
and rat. Toxicology 9:239- 247, 1978B.

769 Linoleic acid

Cutler and Schneider (1973) fed rats and mice a diet
containing 10 percent oxidized linoleic acid. Although
there was no change in survival rate, a significant increase
in urogenital malformations was found only in the rat
fetuses. These defects included agenesis of uterine horn
and ovary, pelvic kidneys and cysts of the kidneys.

Cutler, M.G. and Schneider, R.: Malformations produced in
mice and rats by oxidized lineolate. Food Cosmet. Toxicol.
11: 935-942, 1973.

770 Linuron

Khera et al (1978) gavage fed pregnant rats on days 6
through 15 of gestation with 100 or 200 mg per kg.
Formulation from one supplier was teratogenic at 200 mg per
kg. Wavy ribs were the most common defect.

Khera, K.S.; Whalen, C. and Trivett, G.: Teratogenicity
studies on linuron, malathion, and methoxychlor in rats.
Toxicol. Appl. Pharm. 45:435-444, 1978.

771 Lipase AP

This fat solubility agent extracted from mold was given
orally to rats and mice on days 7-13 of gestation by
Tsutsumi et al (1981). Maximum doses in both species of

4,500 mg per kg produced no adverse fetal effects.

Tsutsumi, S.; Kawaguchi, M.; Yoshida, H.; Simomura, H.;
Sakuma, N.: Teratological study of lipase AP in mice and
rats. Kiso to Rinsho 15: 2577-2524, 1981.

772 Lisuride Hydrogen Maleate

Kodama et al (1981) fed mice up to 30 mg per kg daily before
mating and during the first 6 days of gestation and found no
changes in fertility. Similar doses did not increase
malformations and postnatal function was not altered.
Rabbits were given up to 10 mg per kg orally during
organogenesis without producing an increase in congenital
defects.

Kodama, N.; Tsubota, K.; Ezumi, Y.: Reproductive studies of
lisuride hydrogen maleate. Kiso to Rinsho 15:2299-2310,
2311-2377, 2338-2345, 2346-2371, 1981.

773 Lithium

Wright et al (1971) gave rats 50 mg LiCl intraperitoneally
on the 1st, 4th, 7th and 9th day followed by 20 mg per day
until the 17th day and produced defects of the palate, eye
and external ear. Szabo (1970) produced cleft palates in
mouse fetuses whose mothers were gavaged with 300 to 465 mg
of lithium carbonate per kg daily from day 6 to day 15 of
gestation. Smithberg and Dixit (1982) found defects in mice
receiving intraperitoneal doses of 200 mg per kg. The
recommended human therapeutic dose is 90 to 1,800 mg per
day. Johansen (1971) using a different strain of rat found
only one defect in 42 animals injected with 212 mg LiCl(2)
per kg on day 4, 7 or 9 and followed until day 19 by a daily
dose of 85 mg per kg. Gralla and McIlhenny (1972) found no
teratogenicity testing rats, rabbits and monkeys dduring
organogenesis. The rats received 27 mg, the rabbits 7 mg,
and the monkeys 4 mg per kg per day.

Schou and Amidsen (1971) found three malformations in 60
children born of mothers receiving lithium. They point out
that although the number studied is small, the incidence of
anomalies was not increased over that of the general
population. Nora et al (1974) first observed an increase in
Ebstein's anomaly among the offspring of women taking
lithium. Weinstein (1979) found 17 cardiovascular defects
among 212 offspring exposed in utero to lithium therapy.
Six of these children had a rare cardiac defect, Ebstein's
anomaly. A registry of lithium treated pregnancies is
maintained by the Langley Porter Neuropsychiatric Clinic in
San Francisco.

Gralla, E.J.; McIlhenny, H.M.: Studies in pregnant rats,
rabbits and monkeys with lithium carbonate. Toxicol. &
Appl. Pharmacol 21: 428-433, 1972.

Johansen, K.T.: Lithium teratogenicity. Lancet 1:
1026-1027, 1971.

Nora, J.J.; Nora, A.H. and Toews, W.H.: Lithium, Ebstein's anomaly and other congenital heart defects. Lancet 2:594-595, 1974.

Schou, M. and Amidsen, A.: Lithium teratogenicity. Lancet 1: 1132 only, 1971.

Smithberg, M.; Dixit, P.K.: Teratogenic effects of lithium in mice. Teratology 26:239-246, 1982.

Szabo, K.T.: Teratogenic effect of lithium carbonate in the foetal mouse. Nature 225: 73-75, 1970.

Weinstein, M.R.: Lithium teratogenesis in Lithium, Controversies and Unresolved Issues, edited by Cooper, T.B., Gershon, S., Kline, N.S., Schou, M., Excerpta Medica, Amsterdam, 1979, pp. 432-446.

Wright, T.L.; Hoffman, L.H. and Davies, J.: Teratogenic effects of lithium in rats. Teratology 4: 151-156, 1971.

774 Lividomycin

Mori et al (1972) gave pregnant mice up to 400 mg per kg per day from the 7th through the 14th days and found no defects. The treated fetuses on the 18th day had a delay in ossification but no postnatal differences were observed in groups allowed to suckle. Studies in the pregnant rabbit showed no teratogenicity using 100 mg per kg intramuscularly during organogenesis (Mori et al, 1973).

Mori, H.; Kakishita, T. and Kato, Y.: The safety test of lividomycin 2. The effect of lividomycin on development of fetuses and newborns of mouse. (Japanese) Oyo Yakuri 6: 813-820, 1972.

Mori, H.; Saito, N. and Kato, Y.: The safety test of lividomycin 5. Effect of lividomycin on development of fetuses and newborn rabbits. Oyo Yakuri 7: 1241-1250, 1973.

775 Locoweed

Locoweed, Astragalus pubentissimus, was fed to pregnant sheep at various periods during the 1st 120 days of gestation, and many of the lambs exhibited weakness and contractures of the joints of the legs (James et al.; 1969). The sheep ate 400 to 680 gm of the dried material daily. The authors postulated a lathyrogenic mechanism of terato-genesis.

James, L.F.; Keeler, R.F. and Binns, W.: Sequence in the abortive and teratogenic effects of locoweed fed to sheep. Am. J. Vet. Res. 30: 377-380, 1969.

776 Lofepramine (N-Methyl-N-(4-chlorophenacyl)-3- [10,11-di-hydro-5H-dibenz(b,f)-azepin-5-yl]-propylamine Hydrochloride

Suzuki et al (1976) treated mice and rats orally with up to

200 and 100 mg per kg respectively during active organogenesis. At the higher doses, maternal weight was reduced in both species and fetal weight in the rat fetus.

Suzuki, K.; Watanabe, T.; Oura, K.; Matuhashi,K.; Kouchi, T.; Morita, T. and Akimoto, K.: Effects of a new antidepressant lofepramine on the reproduction of small laboratory animals. Clinical Report 10:2186- 2205, 1976.

777 Lorazepam

Esaki et al (1975) gave up to 4.0 mg per kg daily during organogenesis to the mouse and rat. Some reduction in fetal weight was observed in both species. No malformation increase occurred.

Esaki, K.; Tanioka, Y.; Tsukada, M. and Izumiyama, K.: Teratogenicity of lorazepam (WY-4036) in mice and rats. CIEA Preclinical Reports 1:25-34, 1975.

778 LSD (see Lysergic Acid Diethylamide)

779 Lymphocytic Choriomeningitis

Kreschover and Hancock (1956) studied the effect of this virus in mice and found that fetal infection and resorption was much more common following inoculation during the 1st 7 days of gestation. Dental abnormalities which were relatively infrequent in the young were characterized by disturbed amelogenesis.

Kreschover, S.J. and Hancock, J.A., Jr.: Effect of lymphocytic choriomeningitis on pregnancy and dental tissues in mice. J. Dent. Res. 35: 467-478, 1956.

780 Lupus Erythematosis (see Rheumatic Disease of the Mother)

781 Luteinizing Hormone-releasing Hormone [LH-RH]

Tanabe et al (1974) injected this synthetic neuroendocrine compound intraperitoneally into mice in doses of 0.04 mg to 4 mg per kg (days 6 through 15) and produced delayed parturition but there was no growth inhibition or increase in congenital defects. Postnatal studies to 8 weeks revealed no differences.

Ishihara et al (1980) gave 0.002 to 2.0 mg per kg per day intraperitoneally to male and female rats for 63 days before mating and during the first 7 days of gestation. Mating performance in both sexes was decreased at all dose levels. No teratogenic effects were noted.

Ishihara, H.; Asano, Y.; Nito, S.; Higaki, K.: Fertility study of rats intraperitoneally treated with synthetic luteinizing hormone- releasing hormone. Oyo Yakuri 20: 149-161, 1980.

Tanabe, Y.; Ariyuki, F. and Higaki, K.: Effects of synthetic LH-RH administration to pregnant mice on pre- and post-natal development of their offsprings. Oyo Yakuri 8: 685-695, 1974.

782 Lysergic Acid Diethylamide (LSD)

A good deal of controversy exists about whether or not lysergic acid diethylamide is teratogenic in either animals or man. Although sporadic case reports of defective infants born to mothers taking LSD have appeared, no specific pattern or clear evidence has been produced (Zellweger et al; 1967; Aase et al; 1970; Assemany et al.; 1970). McGlothlin et al. (1970) carried out a study of 121 pregnancies and found no increase in defects but a possible increase in spontaneous abortions in the mothers who took LSD as compared to pregnancies where only the father took it.

A critical analysis of the experimental teratologic work is beyond the scope of this catalog; accordingly, the references showing teratogenicity will be mentioned and in a following paragraph the published negative experiments will be given. Auerbach and Rugowski (1967) reported central nervous system abnormalities in day -11 mouse embryos after injecting 0.05 to 1.0 microgm on day 7. No dose response effect was seen. They used inbred mouse lines. Hanaway (1969) injected Swiss-Webster mice on days 6,7, 8 or 9 of pregnancy with 5 microgm of LSD-25 and found a high incidence of histologic abnormalities of the lens. No mention of gross defects was made. In the Wistar-O'Grady rat, Alexander et al. (1970) produced fetal loss by administering LSD by mouth or subcutaneously (20 microgm and 5 microgm respectively) between the 1st and 4th day of gestation. No specific congenital defects were reported. Geber (1967) in the hamster using 0.08 to 410 microgm per kg on the 8th day found a small increase in defects of the central nervous system in 12-day embryos. No dose response effect was found. Dipaolo et al. (1968) could not produce defects in the hamster, but in one of two mouse strains (A-CUM) an increase in congenital defects was found when 30 microgm was injected during organogenesis.

Warkany and Takacs (1968) gave total doses of 1.5 to 300 microgm to Wistar rats on the 7th through 12th gestational days and found no increases in congenital defects. They also gave 1 to 100 microgm on the 4th or 5th day and did not confirm the fetal loss effect found by Alexander et al. (1970). Roux et al. (1970) injected rats with 5 to 100 microgm on the 4th through the 7th day or the 7th through the 13th day and found no increase in fetal death or deformity. They injected Swiss mice with 5 to 500 microgm per kg between the 4th and 14th day of gestation and found no increased fetal mortality or defects. In their experiments with hamsters, they injected 50 to 500 microgm per kg during the 7th to 13th days and found no fetal changes. Including all three species, a total of 1,723 fetuses were examined. Fabro and Sieber (1968) reported no teratogenicity in rabbits injected with 100 microgm per kg on the 7th, 8th and 9th days of pregnancy. Long (1972) has recently critically reviewed the literature.

Aase, J.M.; Laestadius, N. and Smith, D.W.: Children of mothers who took L.S.D. in Pregnancy. Lancet 1:100-101, 1970.

Alexander, G.J.; Gold, G.M.; Miles, B.E. and Alexander, R.B.: Lysergic acid diethylamide intake in pregnancy: Fetal damage in rats. J. Pharmacol. Expt. Ther. 173:48-59, 1970.

Assemany, S.R.; Neu, R.L. and Gardner, L.I.: Deformities in a child whose mother took L.S.D. Lancet 1: 1290 only, 1970.

Auerbach, R. and Rugowski, J.A.: Lysergic acid diethylamide: Effects on embryos. Science 157:1325-1326, 1967.

Dipaolo, J.A.; Givelber, H.M. and Erwin, H.: Evaluation of teratogenicity of lysergic acid diethylamide. Nature 220:490-491, 1968.

Fabro, S. and Sieber, S.M.: Is lysergic acid a teratogen? Lancet 1:639 only, 1968.

Hanaway, J.K.: Lysergic acid diethylamide: effects on the developing mouse lens. Science 164:574-575, 1969.

Long, S.Y.: Does LSD induce chromosomal damage and malformation? A review of the literature. Teratology 6:75-90, 1972.

McGlothlin, W.H.; Sparkes, R.S. and Arnold, D.O.: Effect of LSD on human pregnancy. J.A.M.A. 212:1483-1487, 1970. mice and hamsters. Science 169:588-589, 1970.

Roux, C.; Dupuis, R. and Aubry, M.: LSD: no teratogenic action in rats, mice and hamsters. Science 169:588-589, 1970.

Warkany, J. and Takacs, E.: Lysergic acid diethylamide (LSD): No teratogenicity in rats. Science 159: 731-732, 1968.

Zellweger, H.; McDonald, J.S. and Abbo, G.: Is lysergic-acid diethylamide a teratogen? Lancet 2:1066-1068, 1967.

783 Lysine

Bergstrom et al. (1970) injected a 1 percent solution of lysine into the chick amniotic sac at 7 to 9 days of incubation and found anomalies of the legs with muscle spasticity and weakness. The total amount of lysine was not stated.

Bergstrom, R.M.; Erila, T. and Pirskanen, R.: Teratogenic effects of lysine in the chicken. Naturwissenschaften 57: 134 only, 1970.

784 Mafenide Acetate

This antibacterial agent was given by Tokunaga et al (1973) subcutaneously to mice and rats during active organogenesis. At the maximal dose (1.0 gm per kg per day), some decrease in implants was found but congenital defects were not increased.

Tokunaga, Y.; Kawada, K.; Nagano, A.; Kunimatu, H.; Miyakubo, H. and Miyagawa, E.: Influence of mafenide acetate on the offspring of rats and mice. Nichidai Igaku Zasshi 32: 973-995, 1973.

785 Magnesium Aluminosilicate

Sakai and Moriguchi (1975) administered up to 6000 mg per kg to mice from the 7th through the 12th day of gestation and found no fetal changes or postnatal effect.

Sakai, K. and Moriguchi, K.: Effect of magnesium aluminosilicate administered to pregnant mice on pre- and post-natal development of offsprings. (Japanese) Oyo Yakuri 9: 703-714, 1975.

786 Magnesium Deficiency

Gunther et al (1973) produced a very high resorption rate in rats placed on magnesium deficient diets for periods of their gestation. No significant increase in congenital defects was found.

Hurley (1971) reported studies in pregnant rats on a deficient diet (0.2 mg per 100 gm of diet.) When the diet was administered from day 6 through 12, 14 percent of the fetuses had defects and many others were resorbed. The defects included skeletal, cleft lip, hydrocephalus, heart, lung and urogenital anomalies. The author reviews the incomplete data on magnesium and human pregnancy.

Gunther, T.; Dorn, F. and Merker, H.J.: Embryo-toxic effects produced by magnesium deficiency in rats. Z. Klin. Chem. Klin. Biochem. 11: 87-92, 1973.

Hurley, L.S.: Magnesium deficiency in pregnancy and its effects on the offspring. In,Durlach, J. (ed) First Symposium International Sur Le Deficit Magnesique en Pathologie Humaine. 1 Volume des rapports (S.G.E.M.V.; Ed) Vittel. 1971, pp. 481-492.

787 Magnesium Sulfate Adduct of [2,2-dithio-bis-(pyridine-1-oxide)]

This antimicrobial antifungal chemical was applied dermally to pregnant swine to give a dose of 10, 30 and 100 mg per kg. Crooked tail occurred in some of the fetuses. In the rat receiving 30 or 100 mg per kg on days 6 through 15 of gestation, maternal toxicity, increased resorption sites and rib fusions were found (Wedig et al, 1977).

Wedig, J.H.; Kennedy, G.L.; Jenkins, D.H. and Keplinger, M.L.: Teratologic evaluation of magnesium sulfate adduct of [2,2-dithio-bis-(pyridine-1-oxide)] in swine and rats. Toxicol. Appl. Pharmacol. 42:561-570, 1977.

788 Malathion-R

This compound was given to rats in amounts of 240 mg per kg and no teratogenic activity was detected (Kalow and Marton, 1961). There was some increase in the mortality rate of the newborns from the treated mothers. Khera et al gavage fed pregnant rats with 300 mg per kg on days 6 through 15 and found no teratogenicity.

Kalow, W. and Marton, A.: Second-generation toxicity of malathion in rats. Nature 192: 464-465, 1961.

Khera, K.S.; Whalen, C. and Trivett,G.: Teratogenicity studies on linuron, malathion, and methoxychlor in rats. Toxicol. Appl. Phaarm. 45:435-444, 1978.

789 Malonate, Sodium

Spratt (1950) used 10(-3)m sodium malonate in the medium for explanted chick embryos and found that after 20 hr the central nervous system degenerated, while the heart continued to develop and function. Addition of succinate partially prevented the effect of malonate.

Spratt, N.T.: Nutritional requirements of the early chick embryo. III. Metabolic basis of morphogenesis and differentiation as revealed by the use of inhibitors. Biol. Bull. 98: 120-135, 1950.

790 Maltose

Maruoka and Kume (1973) gave this compound to rabbits intra-venously in maximum doses of 10 gm per kg per day and found no teratogenicity. This sugar was administered to rats and mice intravenously daily during organogenesis and no terato-genic effects were found. Up to 30 gm per kg were given to the rats and 10 gm per kg per day to the mice (Maruoka et al, 1972).

Maruoka, H.; Kume, M. and Horie, K.: Toxicological studies of maltose. 3 Teratological study 1. Influence of maltose on fetuses and suckling youngs of mouse and rat. (Japanese) Oyo Yakuri 6: 751-768, 1972.

Maruoka, H. and Kume, M.: Toxicological studies of maltose. 6 Teratological study. 2. Effect of maltose on growth and differentiation of fetuses and suckling youngs of rabbits. Oyo Yakuri 7: 1359-1369, 1973.

791 Manganese Deficiency

Hurley et al. (1958 and 1960) demonstrated that rats

maintained on a manganese-deficient diet gave birth to offspring with an ataxic condition secondary to defective
morphogenesis of the vestibular portion of the inner ear.
In a subsequent publication, Erway et al. (1966) showed
that in the mouse the defective morphogenesis was
characterized by absence of the vestibular otoliths. Their
diets were 1 and 3 PPM of manganese and the defect rate
increased from 4 to 100 percent during the course of three
consequent litters. A genetic condition in the mouse
(Pallid) also exhibits defective otolith formation (Lyons,
1955). Erway et al. (1966) in an interesting demonstration
treated the genetically defective (Pallid) mice with 1000
PPM of manganese and were able to completely inhibit the
genetic development of the otolithic defect.

Erway, L.C.; Hurley, L.S. and Fraser, A.: Neurological
defect: Manganese in phenocopy and prevention of a genetic
abnormality of the ear. Science 152: 1766-1767, 1966.

Hurley, L.S.; Everson, G.J. and Geiger, J.F.: Manganese
deficiency in rats: Congenital nature of ataxia. J. Nutr.
66: 309-319, 1958.

Hurley, L.S.; Wooten, E.; Everson, G.J. and Asling, C.W.:
Anomalous development in the inner ear of offspring of
manganese-deficient rats. J. Nutr. 71: 15-19, 1960.

Lyon, M.F.: The developmental origin of hereditary absence
of otoliths in mice. J. Embryol. Exp. Morphol. 3:
230-241, 1955.

792 Maprotiline

Esaki et al (1976) administered orally up to 30 mg per kg to
mice and rats during active organogeneis and observed no
fetal changes other than slight weight reduction at the
highest dose. Postnatal changes were not detected.

Esaki, K.; Tanioka, Y.; Tsukada, M. and Izumiyama, K.:
Teratogenicity of maprotiline tested by oral administration
to mice and rats. (Japanese) CIEA Preclinical Report
2:69-77, 1976.

793 Marihuana (Cannabis, delta-9-tetrahydrocannabinol)

In hamsters using to 500 mg per kg of D-9
tetrahydrocannabinol Joneja (1977) could not produce
malformations. Intragastric doses were given from day 7
through 13 of gestation. Joneja (1976) treated pregnant
mice intravenously, subcutaneously and by gavage with the
same material. Most dose levels gave no malformations but
200 mg per kg by mouth on day 8, 9 or 10 produced a low
increase in malformation rate over controls. Umbilical
hernias with occasional club foot, cleft palate and
exencephaly were found. The intravenous and subcutaneous
doses did not produce defects.

Geber and Schramm (1969) injected crude extract of marihuana
into rabbits and guinea pigs on gestational days 7 through

10 and 6 through 8 respectively. At doses over 150 mg per kg neural tube closure defects, phocomelia and other defects were reported. Persaud and Ellington (1968) gave resin (4.2 mg per kg) to pregnant rats and found 57 percent of the offspring had defects which included stunting, syndactyly, encephalocele and limb reductions. Banerjee et al (1975) injected up to 100 mg per kg of tetrahydrocannabinol in rats on day 7 through 16 of gestation and found no significant defects in the offspring. Sofia et al (1979) using synthetic delta-9-hydrocannabinol in rabbits subcutaneously at doses of up to 60 mg per kg per day on days 7-19 produced no teratogenicity. Gianutsos and Abbatiello (1972) injected 250 mg per kg of an extract of cannabis resin into rats on days 8 through 11 and then observed significant loss of maze learning in the offspring. No congenital defects were found in the fetuses after delivery. Borgen et al (1973) studied the offspring of rats injected subcutaneously with 10 mg per kg of tetrahydrocannabinol on days 10, 11 and 12 of gestation. Significant increases in open field activity and decreases in growth rate were found until weaning. Cross fostering techniques helped to exclude maternal effects on the post-natal activity. In the mouse Fleischman et al (1975) gave up to 150 mg of tetrahydrocannabinol per kg per day on day 6 through 15 of gestation and produced no fetal effects. Grilly et al (1974) exposed male and female chimpanzees to long term tetrahydrocannabinol (1.4 to 2.0 mg per kg per day) and then after discontinuing the drug mated the animals and found 7 normal offspring. Fleischman et al (1975) reviewed the animal literature.

In man only sporadic case reports have appeared and no pattern of malformation has emerged (Hecht et al, 1968; Neu et al, 1969).

Banerjee, B.N.; Galbreath, C. and Sofia, R.D.: Teratological evaluation of synthetic D-9-tetrahydrocannabinol. Teratology 11: 99-102, 1975.

Borgen, L.A.; Davis, W.M. and Pace, H.B.: Effects of prenatal delta-9tetrahydrocannabinol on development of rat offspring. Pharmacology Biochemistry and Behavior 1: 203-206, 1973.

Fleischman, R.W.; Hayden, D.W.; Rosenkrantz, H. and Braude, M.C.: Teratologic evaluation of delta-9-tetrahydrocannabinol in mice, including a review of the literature. Teratology 12: 47-50, 1975.

Geber, W.F. and Schramm, L.C.: Effect of marihuana extract on fetal hamsters and rabbits. Toxicol. Appl. Pharmacol. 14: 276-282, 1969.

Gianutsos, G. and Abbatiello, E.R.: The effect of prenatal cannabis sativa on maze learning ability in the rat. Psychopharmacologia (Berl) 27: 117-122, 1972.

Grilly, D.M.; Ferraro, D.P. and Braude, M.C.: Observations on the reproductive activity of chimpanzees following long-term exposure to marihuana. Pharmacology 11: 304-307, 1974.

Hecht, F.; Beals, R.K.; Lees, M.H.; Jolly, H. and Roberts, P.: Lysergic-acid-diethylamide and cannabis as possible teratogens in man. Lancet 2: 1087 (only), 1968.

Joneja, M.G.: Effects of delta-9-tetrahydrocannabinol on hamster fetuses. J. Tox. Envir. Health 2:1031-1040, 1977.

Joneja, M.G.: A study of teratological effects of intravenous, subcutaneous and intragastric administration of delta-9-tetrahydrocannabinol in mice. Toxicol. Appl. Pharm. 36:151-162, 1976.

Neu, R.L.; Powers, H.; Kings, S. and Gardner, L.I.: Cannabis and chromosomes. Lancet 1: 675 (only), 1969.

Persaud, T.V.N. and Ellington, A.C.: Teratogenic activity of cannabis resin. Lancet 2: 406-407, 1968.

Sofia, R.D.; Strasbaugh, J.E.; Banerjee, B.N.: Teratologic evaluation of synthetic delta-9-tetrahydrocannabinol. Teratology 19:361-266, 1979.

794 Maytansine

Sieber et al (1978) studied this plant extract using 0.1 to 0.25 mg per kg intraperitoneally on days 6, 7 or 8 and found numerous malformations including dextrocardia, axial skeleton defects and hydrocephalus.

Sieber, S.M.; Whang-Peng, J.; Botkin, C. and Knutsen, T.: Teratogenic and cytogenic effects of some plant-derived antitumor agents (vincristine, colchicine, maytansine, VP-16-213 and VM-26) in mice. Teratology 18:31-48, 1978.

795 Measles (see Rubeola)

796 Mebarol-R (see Mephobarbital)

797 Mebendazole   (Vermox-R,   Methyl   5-benzoylbenzimidazole-2-carbamate)

In doses up to 40 mg per kg on days 7 through 10 of rat gestation, no significant increases in defect rates were found and studies in the rabbit at the same dose were negative (Sargent, 1979). In 112 human pregnancies with exposure to the drug, only one malformation is known to have occurred and this was a digital reduction of one hand (Sargent, 1979)

Sargent, E.C.: Ortho Pharmaceutical Corporation, personal communication to the author, 1979.

798 Meclizine (1(P-Chloro-alpha phenyl benzyl)-4-(M-methyl benzyl)-piperazine)

Since Tuchmann-Duplessis and Mercier-Parot's original report (1963), the benzhydrylpiperazine series of compounds have been studied in the rat extensively (King et al.; 1965). The members of this series of drugs are buclizine, cyclizine, chlorcyclizine, hydroxyzine, meclizine and norchlorcyclizine. The syndrome in the rat fetus consists of cleft palate, micrognathia, microstomia and glossopalatine fusion (Posner and Darr, 1970). The drug (20 to 80 mg per kg) is usually given on the 13th through 16th days. Congenital defects have been found in the ferret (Steffek et al.; 1968) and mouse (King and Howell, 1966). The major tissue metabolite of these compounds, norchlorcyclizine, is teratogenic and produced cleft palate even when applied directly over the amniotic sac (Wilk, 1969). A number of antihistamines lacking the ethylamine as a ring structure were non-teratogenic (King et al.; 1965). Massive edema of the embryonic thorax may play a role in the mechanism which produces these defects (Posner and Darr, 1970). Chlorcyclizine, hydroxyzine and cyclizine produce a-bortions in the monkey (Steffek et al.; 1968). Tuchmann-Duplessis and Mercier-Parot (1963) have described eye defects resulting from treatment of the rat, rabbit and mouse with cyclizine.

In the wake of the thalidomide disaster, some of these compounds were suspected to be teratogens in the human (Watson, 1962), but on further analysis no association could be made (Carter and Wilson, 1962; David and Goodspeed, 1963). Lenz (1966) has summarized the reports on 3,333 infants exposed to meclizine during pregnancy and believes that the finding of 12 patients with cleft lip or palate in this group does not completely clear the drug of teratogenicity. Yerushalmy and Milkovich (1965) studied prospectively 8,090 births and did not observe an increased defect rate in the 330 fetuses exposed to meclizine early in pregnancy. The same series was enlarged to 613 offspring exposed during the first 84 days of pregnancy and no teratogenicity was detected (Milkovich and Van den Berg (1976).

Carter, M.P. and Wilson, F.W.: 'ancoloxin' and fetal abnormalities. Br. Med. J. 2: 1609 only, 1962).

David, A. and Goodspeed, A.H.: 'ancoloxin' and foetal abnormalities. Br. Med. J. 1: 121 only, 1963.

King, C.T.G.: Teratogenic effects of meclizine hydrochloride on the rat. Science 141: 353-355, 1963.

King, C.T.G. and Howell, J.: Teratogenic effect of buclizine and hydroxyzine on the rat and chlorcyclizine in the mouse. Am. J. Obstet. Gynecol. 95: 109-111, 1966.

King, C.T.G.; Weaver, S.A. and Narrod, S.A.: Antihistamines and teratogenicity in the rat. J. Pharmacol. Exp. Ther. 147: 391-398, 1965.

Lenz, W.: Malformations caused by drugs in pregnancy. Am. J. Dis. Child. 112: 99-106, 1966.

Milkovich, L. and Van den Berg, B.J.: An evaluation of the teratogenicity of certain antinauseant drugs. Am. J.

Obstet. Gyn. 125:244-248, 1976.

Posner, H.S. and Darr, A.: Fetal edema from benzhydro-
ylpiperizines as a possible cause of oral-facial malformations in the rat. Toxicol. Appl. Pharmacol. 17: 67-75,
1970.

Steffek, A.J.; King, C.T.G. and Wilk, A.L.: Abortive
effects and comparative metabolism of chlorcyclizine in
various mammalian species. Teratology 1: 399-406, 1968.

Tuchmann-Duplessis, H. and Mercier-Parot, L.: Action du
chlorhydrate de cyclizine sur la gestion et le developpement
embryonnaire du rat, de la souris et du lapin. C. R.
Acad. Sci. (Paris) 256: 3359-3362, 1963.

Watson, G.I.: Meclizine ('ancoloxin') and foetal abnormalities. Br. Med. J. 2: 1446 only, 1962.

Yerushalmy, J. and Milkovich, L.: Evaluation of the teratogenic effect of meclizine in man. Am. J. Obstet.
Gynecol. 93: 553-562, 1965.

799 Meclofenamate

Schardein et al. (1969) reported negative teratologic
studies of this anti-inflammatory drug in rats and rabbits.
Up to 3.5 mg per kg per day was given daily during the
period of active organogenesis.

Schardein, J.L.; Blatz, A.T.; Woosley, E.T. and Kaup, D.H.:
Reproductive studies on sodium meclofenamate in comparison
to aspirin and phenylbutazone. Toxicol. Appl. Pharmacol.
15: 46-55, 1969.

800 Medroxyprogesterone [Provera-R]

Burstein and Wasserman (1964) treated 172 women before the
12th menstrual week with 5 to 50 mg per day and observed
transient clitoral hypertrophy in only one newborn. The
mother had received 25 mg daily for 7 days during the 6th
menstrual week.

Although Aarskog (1979) reported that hypospadias could be
associated with synthetic progestins, Mau (1981) who studied
3,602 male newborns of whom 33 had hypospadias could not
confirm it. Of these 8 had been exposed giving a 1.4
percent rate which was not different from the controls at
0.8 percent. The type of hypospadias was correlated with
the time of ingestion in the study by Aarskog but not in
that of Mau.

Suchowsky and Junkmann (1961) produced masculinization of
the female rat fetus with this compound. Andrew and Staples
(1977) produced no malformations in rats and mice using up
to 3000 mg per kg during various days of organogenesis, but
in the rabbit with 0.3 to 30 mg per kg, cleft palates were
found. Eibs et al (1982A) using 30 mg per kg subcutaneously
early in the mouse gestation (days 1-12) were able to

800

produce defects of palate, urinary and respiratory tract. They point out that the drug has a long half-life. Eibs et al (1982B) have studied the toxicity of the compound on preimplantation stages of the rat in vitro. Prahalada and Hendrickx (1982) gave monkeys 300 mg per day from day 23 to day 41 of gestation. The fetuses removed at around day 100 had hypoplastic adrenals, thymus and thyroids and the females had masculinized external genitalia. The male monkey fetuses were hypospadic with micropenis.

Dickmann (1973) found that this compound when given on day 1 (12.5 mg) followed on day 3 by oestrone led to destruction of fertilized eggs.

Aarskog, D.: Maternal progestins as a possible cause of hypospadias. New Eng. J. Med. 300:75-78, 1979.

Andrew, F.D. and Staples, R.E.: Prenatal toxicity of medroxyprogesterone acetate in rabbits, rats and mice. Teratology 15:25-32, 1977.

Burstein, R. and Wasserman, H.C.: The effect of provera on the fetus. Obstet. Gynecol. 23: 931-934, 1964.

Dickmann, Z.: Postcoital contraceptive effects of medroxyprogesterone acetate and oestrone in rats. J. Reprod. Frt. 32: 65-69, 1973.

Eibs, H.G.; Spielmann, H.; Hagele, M.: Teratogenic effects of cyproterone acetate and medroxyprogesterone treatment during the pre- and post implantation period of the mouse. Teratology 25:27-36, 1982.

Eibs, H.G.; Spielmann, H.; Jacob-Muller, U.; Klose, J.: Cyproterone acetate and medroxyprogesterone acetate treatment before implantation in vivo and in vitro. Teratology 25:291-299, 1982.

Mau, G.: Progestins during pregnancy and hypospadias. Teratology 24:285-287, 1981.

Prahalada, S.; Hendrickx, A.G.: Teratogenicity of medroxyprogesterone acetate (MPA) in cynomolgus monkeys (abstract). Teratology 25:67A-68A, 1982.

Suchowsky, G.K. and Junkmann, K.: A study of the virilizing effect of the progestogens on the female rat fetus. Endocrinology 68: 341-349, 1961.

801 Meglumine Iotroxate

Koda et al (1980 and 1981) administered the contrast medium to rats and rabbits in doses of up to 1800 mg per kg daily. For the reproductive studies in rats an intraperitoneal route was used. For studies during organogenesis in both species intravenous routes were used. The perinatal studies were done by the intravenous route followed after birth by intraperitoneal administration to the dam. The only adverse effect was some postnatal growth retardation in rats exposed during organogenesis to 1800 and 360 mg per kg.

Kodama, N.; Tsubota, K.; Ezami, Y.: Effects of meglumine on reproduction in the rat and rabbit. Nichi-Doku Iho (Japanisch- Deutsche Medizinische Berichte). 25:398-405, 1980; 26:110-118, 119-135, 1981.

802 Mephobarbital (Mebaral-R)

Heinonen et al (1977) reported that among 8 women treated during the first 4 months of pregnancy no congenital defects occurred in their offspring.

Heinonen, O.P.; Slone, D.; Shapiro, S.: Birth Defects and Drugs in Pregnancy. Publishing Sciences Group, Inc. 1977.

803 Meprobamate (Miltown-R, Equinil-R)

Werboff and Kesher (1963) gave pregnant rats 60 mg per kg on days 5 through 8, 11 through 14 or 17 through 20 and then carried out several learning tests postnatally. Although they reported decreased scores in all treated groups, Kletzkin and Berger (1971) using similar conditions were unable to confirm their work. These later workers also reviewed the clinical literature and reported absence of teratogenic activity. Caldwell and Spille (1964) using up to 128 mg per kg in the rat's diet during the entire gestation period could not demonstrate learning impairment in the offspring. Nishikawa (1963) using near lethal doses (750 mg per kg) in the mouse produced some skeletal defects, but lower doses did not produce defects (Clavert, 1963; Brar, 1969).

Milkovich and Van Den Berg (1974) in a study of 19,044 births used a computer system of record linkage to study the association between prescriptions filled for women and serious congenital defects in their offspring. A four-fold increase in defect rate was found when mothers took meprobamate or chlordiazepoxide during the first 42 days of gestation. No pattern of malformations was identified but 5 infants from the 66 meprobamate takers had congenital heart disease. A group of women taking phenobarbital did not have an increased malformation rate in their offspring. Hartz et al (1975) in a follow-up of 50,282 pregnancies could not associate an increased defect rate with maternal ingestion of meprobamate or chlordiazepoxide. They had 1345 mothers in the meprobamate exposure group. Crombie et al (1975) reported four malformations among a group of 67 mothers who took meprobamate.

Brar, B.S.: The effect of meprobamate on fertility gestation and offspring viability and development of mice. Arch. Int. Pharmacodyn. 177: 416-422, 1969.

Caldwell, M.B. and Spille, D.F.: Effect on rat progeny of daily administration of meprobamate during pregnancy and lactation. Nature 202: 832-833, 1964.

Clavert, J.: Etude de l'action du meprobamate sur la formation de l'embryon. C. R. Soc. Biol. (Paris) 157: 1481-1482, 1963.

803

Crombie, D.L.; Pinsent, R.J.; Fleming, D.M.; Rumeau-Rouquette, C.; Goujard, J. and Huel, G.: Fetal effects of tranquilizers in pregnancy. New Eng. J. Med. 293:198-199, 1975.

Hartz, S.C.; Heinonen, O.P.; Shapiro, S.; Siskind, V. and Slone, D.: Antenatal exposure to meprobamate and chlordiazepoxide in relation to malformations, mental development and childhood mortality. New Eng. J. Med. 292: 726-728, 1975.

Kletzkin, M. and Berger, F.M.: Influence of mebrobamate on the fetus, fertility and post-natal development. In, Tuchmann-Duplessis, H. (ed.): Malformations Congenitales des Mammiferes. Paris: Masson, 1971. pp. 255-272.

Milkovich, L. and Van Den Berg, B.J.: Effects of prenatal meprobamate and chlordiazepoxide hydrochloride on human embryonic and fetal development. New Eng. J. Med. 291: 1268-1271, 1974.

Nishikawa, M.: Effect of meprobamate on the development of the fetus on pregnant mice. Acta Anat. Nippon 38: 258, , 1963.

Werboff, J. and Kesner, B.: Learning deficits of offspring after administration of tranquilizing drugs to the mothers. Nature 197: 106-107, 1963.

804 Mequitazine (10-(3-Quinuclidinylmethyl)phenothiazine)

Maeda et al (1981) gave oral doses of 1.25, 5 and 20 mg per kg to rats before pregnancy and during the entire gestation or on day 17-17. At the highest dose the maternal weight was decreased but no adverse fetal effects were found. Behavioral and fertility studies of the exposed offspring did not show significant differences from controls. Rabbits were given orally up to 125 mg per kg and no increase in malformations was found in the offspring.

Maeda, H.; Yoshifune, S.; Shimizu, Y.: Reproductive studies of 10-(3-quinclidinylmethyl)phenothiazine. Oyo Yakuri 21:855-898, 1982.

805 Mer-25 (see Ethamoxytriphetol)

806 Mercaptobenzimidazole (see Ethylenethiourea)

807 Mercapto-1-methyl-imidazole (see Ethylenethiourea)

808 6-Mercaptopurine (and Related Derivatives)

This SH-containing purine analogue and related derivatives are teratogenic in the chick, mouse, rabbit and rat. Chaube and Murphy (1968) reported results on 13 purine analogues and found the following teratogenic: 6-mercaptopurine,

6-mercaptopurine riboside, 6-mercaptopurine-3-N-oxide, 9-butyl-6-mercaptopurine, 9-ethyl-6-mercaptopurine, 6-chloropurine, 6-thioguanine, 6-thioguanosine and 6-hydroxylaminopurine. 6-mercaptopurine in doses of 31 to 125 mg per kg on the 11th or 12th day produced defects of the extremities and tail in rat fetuses. 6-mercaptopurine riboside and 6-mercaptopurine-3-N-oxide under similar conditions produced essentially the same syndrome except for inclusion of cleft palate. 9-butyl-6-mercaptopurine and 6-hydroxylaminopurine (in the mouse) and 9-ethyl-6-mercaptopurine and 6-chloropurine (in the rat) produced skeletal defects when the dosages were close to the LD-50 for the mother (400 to 900 mg per kg). 6-thioguanine and 6-thioguanosine produced skeletal defects in rats at dosage ranges of 12 to 50 mg per kg. Chaube and Murphy (1968) reported that 9-ethyl--6-mercaptopurine and 6-methyl-mercaptopurine riboside were non-teratogenic. In the chick Karnofsky (1960) used 400 microgm on the 4th day and produced some facial defects. Adams et al. (1961) injected 25 to 250 mg per kg into rabbits during ovulation and cleavage stages and found no morphologic changes in the embryos. Degeneration of the embryonic discs appear during the blastocyst stage and no conceptus survived after the mother received 75 mg per kg (Chaube and Murphy, 1968).

Experience with 6-mercaptopurine during human pregnancy has been reviewed by Sokal and Lessmann (1960). Five pregnant women treated during pregnancy produced five offspring without defects, but two were prematurely born.

Adams, C.E.; Hay, M.F. and Lutwak-Mann, C.: The action of various agents upon the rabbit embryo. J. Embryol. Exp. Morphol. 9: 468-491, 1961.

Chaube, S. and Murphy, M.L.: The teratogenic effects of the recent drugs active in cancer chemotherapy. In, Woollam, D.H.M. (ed.): Advances in Teratology, Vol. 3. New York: Logos and Academic Press, 1968. pp. 181-237.

Karnofsky, D.A.: Influences of antimetabolites inhibiting nucleic acid metabolism on embryonic development. Trans. Assoc. Am. Physicians 73: 334-347, 1960.

Sokal, J.E. and Lessmann, E.M.: Effects of cancer chemotherapeutic agents on the human fetus. J.A.M.A. 172: 1765-1771, 1960.

809   2-Mercaptothiazoline (see Ethylenethiourea)

810   Mercury

An epidemic of cerebral palsy with microcephaly occurred in Minimata, Japan, and the cause was felt to be maternal ingestion of fish contaminated with methyl mercury. Two autopsy reports with mercury analyses and detailed brain examination are given by Matsumoto et al. (1965). Murakami (1972) has reviewed the 25 cases of fetal Minimata disease and reports that cerebral palsy was the primary feature, but in 7 an association with microcephaly occurred. Subtle dental changes were observed also, but with the exception of one case of auricular deformity other congenital defects did not occur.

Snyder (1971) has reported severe central nervous system damage in an infant whose mother ate meat from a pig contaminated by a mercury-containing grain diet. The ingestion occurred during the third gestational month.

Wannag and Skjaerasen (1975) studied mothers exposed to elemental mercury through their dental work place and found significantly increased mercury content in their babies' placentae and membranes. Koos and Longo (1976) have summarized human experience with mercury poisoning giving exposure limits for women of childbearing age and levels at which toxicity might be expected. For the fetus and newborn, the toxic level is given as 3 micrograms Hg per gm.

Murakami (1972) has reviewed the work in experimental animals. Specific defects following inorganic mercury are uncommon. Inouye et al. (1972) injected methyl mercury chloride (30 mg per kg) into mice from day 6 to 13 of preg- nancy. Treatment after day 7 was associated with a high incidence of cleft palate and hydrocephalus. Spyker and Smithberg (1972) using methyl mercuric dicyandiamide and Khera and Nera (1971) using 1 mg of methyl mercuric chloride in mice found cleft palate and histopathologic and functional changes in neuronal development. Mottet (1974) studied the offspring of rats exposed to chronic low dose methylmercury hydroxide (total about 20 mg per kg) and could find no microscopic malformations or changes in behavior. MMurakami et al (1953) used a vaginal tablet containing 0.1 mg of phenylmercuric acetate on day 7 of the rat gestation and found tail and neural tube abnormalities. Inouye et al. (1972) have studied the rat fetus also. Harris et al (1972) have studied methyl mercuric chloride teratogenicity in the hamster.

Shtenberg and Safronova (1979) reported that in experiments on Wistar rats oral methyl mercuric iodide at doses of 0.85; 0.64; 0.42 and 0.21 mg per kg daily exerted no teratogenic or embryotoxic action. Administration at doses of 0.85 and 0.64 mg per kg produced in females a significant decrease in the SH- group content in renal and cerebral tissues, in the activity of acetylcholine esterase in the cerebellum (by 18-48%) and a rise in the activity of glucose - 6-phosphatase in the kidneys (by 48-70%). The doses of 0.42 and 0.21 mg per kg administered at various periods of pregnancy, did not exert any effect on the body of females under experimental conditions. The biochemical parameters of these animals did not differ from those of the control. Ignatyev (1980) treated male rats with inhalation of metallic mercury during 115 days. Alterations of spermatogenesis and DNA and RNA synthesis in the testis were found. Offspring of treated males (mated with intact females) had decreased weight and vitality. Exposure of rat females during the entire gestation with 6 and 1 mg per cubic millimeter produced slight embryotoxic and gonadotoxic effect.

Ramel and Magnusson (1969) have presented some evidence that organic mercury may produce meiotic nondisjunction in drosophila.

The disposition of organic mercury in the maternal-fetal system of the rat indicates a preferential concentration in the fetal brain (Yang et al, 1972; King et al, 1976).

Amin-Zaki et al (1974) reported studies on 15 infant-mother pairs poisoned in Iraq due to ingestion of home-made bread prepared from wheat treated with a methylmercury fungicide. In all cases but one the infants blood mercury level was higher than that of the mother. Six of the infants were severely impaired in their motor and mental development. Follow-up neurological examinations on 32 prenatally exposed children are given by Amin-Zaki et al(1979). Cerebral palsy occurred even when exposure was during the third trimester. Milder cases with developmental retardation in addition to exaggerated tendon reflexes and pathological extensor plantar reflexes were described.

Amin-Zaki, L.; Elhassani, S.; Majeed, M.A.; Clarkson, T.W.; Doherty, R.A. and Greenwood, M.R.: Intra-uterine methyl-mercury poisoning in Iraq. Pediat. 54: 587-595, 1974.

Amin-Zaki, L.; Majeed, M.A.; Elhassani, S.B.; Clarkson, T.W.; Greenwood, M.R. and Doherty, R.A.: Prenatal mercury poisoning, clinical observations over five years. A.M.A. Dis. Child 133:172-177, 1979.

Harris, S.B.; Wilson, J.G.; Printz, R.H.: Embryotoxicity of methyl mercuric chloride in golden hamsters. Teratology 6:139-142, 1972.

Ignatyev, V.M.: Gonadotoxic and embryotoxic effects of metallic mercury. Gigiena i. Sanit. 3:72-73, 1980.

Inouye, M.; Hoshino, K. and Murakami, U.: Effect of methyl mercuric chloride on embryonic and fetal development in rats and mice. Ann. Report Res. Inst. Environ. Med. Nagoya Univ. 19: 69-74, 1972.

Khera, K.S. and Nera, E.A.: Maternal exposure to methyl mercury and postnatal cerebellar development in mice. (abstract) Teratology 4: 233 only, 1971.

King, R.B.; Robkin, M.A. and Shepard, T.H.: Distribution of Hg-203 in the maternal and fetal rat. Teratology 13:275-290, 1976.

Koos, B.J. and Longo, L.D.: Mercury toxicity in the pregnant woman, fetus, and newborn infant. Am. J. Obstet. Gynecol. 126:390-409, 1976.

Matsumoto, H.; Koya, G. and Takeuchi, T.: Fetal Minimata disease: A neuropathological study of two cases of intrauterine intoxication by a methyl mercury compound. J. Neuropathol. Exp. Neurol. 24: 563-574, 1965.

Mottet, N.K.: Effects of chronic low-dose exposure of rat fetuses to methylmercury hydroxide. Teratology 10: 173-190,

810

1974.

Murakami, U.: Organic mercury problem affecting intrauterine life. In, Klingberg, M.A. (ed.): Proceedings of the International Symposium on the Effect of Prolonged Drug Usage on Fetal Development. Advances in Experimental Biology and Medicine, Vol. 27, New York: Plenum Publishing Corp.; 1972, pp. 301-336.

Murakami, U.; Kameyama, Y.; Kato, T.; Tsuji, S.; Imai, M. and Furakawa, E.: An Experiment by Mercury Compounds (preliminary report). Influences of The Contraceptive Agent upon Embryo and Mother Animal. Ann. Report Res. Inst. Environ. Med. Nagoya Univ. 5: 167-168, 1953.

Ramel, C. and Magnusson, J.: Genetic effects of organic mercury compounds. II. Chromosome segregation in drosophila melanogaster. Hereditas 61: 231-254, 1969.

Shtenberg, A.I. and Safronova, A.M.: Effect of minor quantities of methyl mercuric iodide on embryogenesis and some biochemical parameters. Vopr. pitaniya (USSR) 5:53-57, 1979.

Snyder, R.D.: Congenital mercury poisoning. New Eng. J. Med. 284: 1014-1016, 1971.

Spyker, J.M. and Smithberg, M.: Effects of methyl mercury on prenatal development in mice. Teratology 5: 181-190, 1972.

Wannag, A. and Skjaerasen, J.: Mercury accumulation in placenta and foetal membranes. A study of dental workers and their babies. Environ. Physiol. Biochem. 5:348-352, 1975.

Yang, M.G.; Krawford, K.S.; Garcia, J.D.; Wang, J.H.C. and Lei, K.Y.: Deposition of mercury in fetal and maternal brain. Proc. Soc. Biol. Med. 141: 1004-1007, 1972.

811 Mescaline [3,4,5-Trimethoxyphenethylamine]

Geber (1967) reported production of congenital defects in guinea pigs given a single intravenous dose of 0.45 to 3.25 mg per kg on the 8th day. The defects involved the central nervous system mainly. There was no correlation between dose and rate of congenital defects, but resorptions and runts increased with dose.

Geber, W.F.: Congenital malformations induced by mescaline, lysergic acid diethyamide and bromolysergic acid in the hamster. Science 158: 265-266, 1967.

812 Mestranol

The effect of oral contraceptives on women is discussed under oral contraceptives.

Saunders and Elton (1967) reported negative teratogenic
studies in the rat and rabbit. There was no fertility
problem in fetuses raised after intrauterine exposure. The
rabbits received up to 0.1 mg per kg buccally or 0.25 mg per
kg subcutaneously and the rats up to 0.1 mg per kg orally.
Anorectal distances in the rat fetuses were not changed.

Saunders, F.J. and Elton, R.L.: Effects of ethynodiol
diacetate and mestranol in rats and rabbits on conception,
on the outcome of pregnancy and on the offspring. Toxicol.
Appl. Pharm. 11:229-244, 1967.

813 Metahexamide

Bariliak (1968) gave 2000 mg per kg to rats on the 9th and
10th days of gestation and produced a high incidence of congenital defects which included hydrocephalus, microcephaly,
hydronephrosis and heart malformation.

Bariliak, I.R.: Comparison of antithyroidal and teratogenic
activity of some hypoglycemic sulphanylamides. Problems in
Endocrinology (Russian) 14: No. 6, 89-94, 1968.

814 Metepa [Tris-[1-2 2(methylaziridinyl)]-phosphine oxide]

Gaines and Kimbrough (1966) injected rats with 30 mg per kg
on the 12th day of pregnancy and found a high resorption
rate and malformations in the offspring. Ectrodactylia
occurred in 100 percent with some kinky tails and
meningoceles.

Gaines, T.B. and Kimbrough, R.D.: The sterilizing,
carcinogenic and teratogenic effects of Metepa on rats.
Bull. W.H.O. 34: 317-320, 1966.

815 Metformin (1,1-dimethylbiguanide)

Tuchmann-Duplessis and Mercier-Parot (1961) administered 500
to 1000 mg per kg to rats by tube and found anophthalmia and
anencephaly in a few fetuses. Major malformations occurred
in less than 0.5 percent of the fetuses suggesting that the
material was not strongly teratogenic.

Tuchmann-Duplessis, H. and Mercier-Parot, L.:
Reprocussions sur la gestation et le developpement foetal du
rat d'un hypoglycemiant, le chlorhydrate de N,N-dimethyl-
biguanide. C. R. Acad. Sci. (Paris) 253: 321-323, 1961.

816 Methacrylate Esters

Singh et al. (1972) administered six types of methacrylate
esters to pregnant rats on days 5, 10 and 15 of gestation in
doses up to one-third the acute intraperitoneal LD-50. The
maximum doses used were 0.44, 0.40, 0.78, 0.46 and 0.82 ml
per kg for the methyl, ethyl, n-butyl, isobutyl, isodecyl
methacrylate respectively. Hemangiomas were increased at
the highest doses as were resorptions. The fetal weight was

reduced by treatment. Acrylic acid was injected in volumes of up to 0.0075 ml per kg and this was associated with resorptions and hemangiomas. Fetal mortality and an incidence of up to 16 percent malformations were reported but only in an abstract. malformations were reported but only in an abstract.

Singh, A.R.; Lawrence, W.H. and Autian, J.: Embryo-fetal toxicity and teratogenic effects of a group of methacrylate esters in rats. J. Dent. Res. 51:1632-1638, 1972.

817 Methadone [D-1-6-dimethylamino-4,4-diphenyl-3-heptanone Hydrochloride]

Markham et al. (1971) gave pregnant rats and rabbits up to 40 mg per kg during days 6 through 15 and 6 through 18 respectively and detected no drug-related defects in the offspring. Geber and Schramm (1969) injecting guinea pigs on day 8 of gestation were able to find some defects in the embryos examined on the 12th day. Jurand (1973) injected subcutaneously 22 to 24 mg per kg into pregnant mice on the 9th day and produced exencephaly in 11 percent of the surviving 13 day embryos.

Geber and Schramm (1975) produced CNS defects in hamsters by giving 67 or more mg per kg subcutaneously on day 8. Nalorphine and other antagonists blocked the teratogenic action.

Geber, W.F. and Schramm, L.C.: Congenital malformations of the central nervous system produced by narcotic analgesics in the hamster. Am. J. Obstet. Gynecol. 123: 705-713, 1975.

Geber, W.F. and Schramm, L.C.: Comparative teratogenicity of morphine, heroin and methadone in the hamster.

(abstract) Pharmacologist 11: 248 only, 1969.

Jurand, A.: Teratogenic activity of methadone hydrochloride in mouse and chick embryos. J. Embryol. Exp. Morph. 30: 449-458, 1973.

Markham, J.K.; Emmerson, J.L. and Owen, N.V.: Teratogenicity studies of methadone HCl in rats and rabbits. Nature 233: 342-343, 1971.

818 Methallibure [1-Alpha-methyl-allyl-6-methyldithiobiurea]

King (1969) fed sows 100 mg daily for 20 days starting on the 29th or 30th day of gestation and found nearly all of the piglets to have contractures of the distal extremities with distorted mandibles and cranial bones. Treatment after the 49th day had no effect. Low (1972) has extensively reviewed the pharmacology of this compound including its teratogenicity. Schafer et al, (1973) in their studies found that this pituitary inhibitor when given to pigs between the 30th to 50th day of gestation in doses of 100 mg per day produced in the offspring alopecia, cranial bone thickening, dysplasia of the renal cortex and some musculo-skeletal defects.

King, G.J.: Deformities in piglets following administration of methallibure during specific stages of gestation. J. Reprod. Fertil. 20: 551-553, 1969.

Low, O.: Chemie, Pharmakologie und Anwendung des 1-methyl-thiocarbamoyl-2-(1-methylallyl) thiocarbamoylhydrazines. Arch. Exp. Veterinaermed. 58: 883-938, 1972.

Schafer, J.H.; Christensen, R.K.; Teaque, H.S.; Grifo, A.P.: Effects of methallibure on early pregnancy in the swine. J. Anim. Sci. 36: 722-725, 1973.

819 Methamphetamine (see Dextroamphetamine Sulfate)

820 Methampyrone [Sulpyrin]

Ungthavorn et al. (1970) injected this antipyretic into pregnant mice in doses up to 1000 mg per kg on days 8, 9 or 10. A low incidence of defects resulted and the incidence was not dose dependent. Six out of 68 fetuses receiving 750 mg per kg on day 9 had exencephaly or encephaloceles.

Ungthavorn, S.; Chiamsawatphan, S.; Chatsanga, C.; Tangsanga, K.; Limpongsanuruk, S. and Jeyasak, N.: Studies on sulpyrin-induced teratogenesis in mice. J. Med. Assoc. Thailand 53: 550-557, 1970.

821 Methane

Kato (1958) exposed pregnant mice on the 8th day for 1 hr to 5 to 8 percent concentration of fuel-gas. In addition to 85 percent methane most natural gases contain small amounts of ethane, propane and butane. Abnormalities of the fetal brains were found to result in brain hernia and hydrocephalus.

Kato, T.: Embryonic abnormalities of the central nervous system caused by fuel-gas inhilation of the mother animal. Folia Psychiatr. Neurol. Jap. 11: 301-307, 1958.

822 Methaqualone

McColl et al. (1963) fed rats a diet containing 0.8 percent methaqualone (a sedative) and found double vertebral centra and extra lumbar ribs in some of the offspring. Bough et al (1963) found no teratogenicity in rabbits given 200 mg per kg orally from day one through 29 and in rats given 100 mg per kg from day 1 through day 20.

Bough, R.G.; Gurd, M.R.; Hall, J.E. and Lessel, B.: Effect of methaqualone hydrochloride in pregnant rabbits and rats. Nature 200:656-657, 1963.

McColl, J.D.; Globus, M. and Robinson, S.: Drug induced

822

skeletal malformations in the rat. Experientia 19: 183-184, 1963.

823 Methazolamide (see Sulphonamides)

824 Methenamine

Among 299 exposed pregnancies Heinonen et al (1976) found 12 malformations which gave a rate that was not increased significantly.

Heinonen, O.P.; Slone, D.; Shapiro, S.: Birth Defects and Drugs in Pregnancy. Publishing Sciences Group, Inc., 1977.

825 Methimazole [Tapazole-R]

Milham and Elledge (1972) reported that ulcerlike midline defects of the scalp occurred in the offspring of 11 mothers and that two of these mothers were under treatment for hyperthyroidism with methimazole.

Milham, S. and Elledge, W.: Maternal methimazole and congenital defects in children. (letter) Teratology 5: 125 (only), 1972.

826 Methomyl (Methyl N-[[(methylamino)carbonyl]ethanimidothioate

Kaplan and Sherman (1977) fed rabbits 0, 50 and 100 ppm in the diet during days 8 through 16 of pregnancy and found no adverse effects in the fetuses on days 29 and 30.

Kaplan, M.A.; Sherman, H.: Toxicity studies with methyl N-[[methylamino)carbonyl]oxy]-ethanimidothioate. Toxicol. Appl. Pharmacol. 40:1-17, 1977.

827 Methophenazine (also see Chloropromazine, Prochlorperazine and Phenothiazine)

Horvath and Druga (1975) administered this tranquilizer to pregnant rats by mouth. With doses of 10 mg per kg per day from the 7th through the 14th day malformations were found which included micrognathia and micromelia of the hind limbs. With doses of 100 mg per kg given on the 8th, 9th, 10th or 11th days, a high fetal mortality was found. Single large doses on the 14th day produced cleft palate and hydronephrosis was common. These authors believe that the teratogenic action of phenothiazines is increased when the length of the N-alkyl side chain is lengthened.

Horvath, C. and Druga, A.: Action of the phenothiazine derivative methophenazine on prenatal development in rats. Teratology 11: 325-330, 1975.

828 Methotrexate [Amethopterin] [Methylaminopterin]

This methyl derivative of aminopterin is a folic acid antagonist. Milunsky et al. (1968) reported defects in a child whose mother ingested 2.5 mg daily for 5 days between the 8th to 10th week. The defects included absence of the frontal bones, premature craniosynostosis, rib defects and absence of digits (see aminopterin and folic acid deficiency).

Powell and Ekert (1971) report a similar child from the pregnancy of a mother who received 5 mg daily during the first two months for treatment of psoriasis. Adams et al. (1961) reported that 6.5 mg per kg in early pregnancy caused no visible effects on 6.5-day rabbit embryos. Berry (1971) used the compound in pregnant rats to study DNA inhibition in the fetus and embryo. Skalko and Gold (1974) have reported on the teratogenicity in mice and found no defects at 10 mg per kg but at 25 and 50 mg per kg exencephaly, omphalocele, ectrodactyly and cleft palate were found. Giving 30 mg per kg intravenously on days 29 through 32 in the monkey caused transitory embryonic growth retardation but was not teratogenic (Wilson et al, 1979).

Adams, C.E.; Hay, M.F. and Lutwak-Mann, C.: The action of various agents on the rabbit embryo. J. Embryol. Exp. Morphol. 9: 468-491, 1961.

Berry, C.L.: Transient inhibition of DNA synthesis by methotrexate in the rat embryo and fetus. J. Embryol. Exp. Morphol. 26: 469-474, 1971.

Milunsky, A.; Graef, J.W. and Gaynor, M.F.: Methotrexate-induced congenital malformations with a review of the literature. J. Pediatr. 72: 790-795, 1968.

Powell, H.R. and Ekert, H.: Methotrexate-induced congenital malformations. Med. J. Aust. 2: 1076-1077, 1971.

Skalko, R.G. and Gold, M.P.: Teratogenicity of methotrexate in mice. Teratology 9: 159-164, 1974.

Wilson, J.G.; Scott, W.J.; Ritter, E.J.; Fradkin, R.: Comparative distribution and embryotoxicity of methotrexate in pregnant rats and Rhesus monkeys. Teratology 19:71-80, 1979.

829 Methotrimeprazine (see Phenothiazines)

830 Methoxychlor

Khera et al (1978) gavage fed pregnant rats with 50 to 400 mg per kg on days 6 through 15. At 200 and 400 mg per kg, maternal and fetal toxicity occurred and many rat fetuses had wavy ribs.

Khera, K.S.; Whalen, C. and Trivett, G.: Teratogenicity studies on linoron, malathion, and methoxychlor in rats. Toxicol. Appl. Pharm. 45:435- 444, 1978.

831 2-Methoxyethanol

Nelson et al (1982) exposed rats to 50 or 100 ppm for 7 hours daly on days 7-15 of gestation. An increase in skeletal and cardiac malformations was reported. No embryotoxicity was found wih 2(2-ethoxy ethoxy) at 700 ppm. 2-butoxyethanol was toxic to the dams at 200 ppm but no increase in fetal defects was found.

Nelson, B.K.; Setzer, J.V.; Brightwell, W.S.; Mathinos, P.R.; Kuczuk, M.H.; Weaver, T.E.: Comparative inhalation teratogenicity of four industrial glycol ether solvents in rats. (abs) Teratology 25:64A (only) 1982.

832 L-3-Methoxy-omega-(1-hydroxy-1-phenyl-isopropylamino-)-propiopheno one-HCl [Oxyfedrin-R]

This compound was tested in mice, rabbits and rats and no evidence of teratogenicity was found (Habersang et al.; (1967). The rats were given up to 600 mg per kg daily, and the mice and rabbits received 50 mg per kg.

Habersang, S.; Leuschner, F. and Schlichtegroll, A.: Toxikologische antersuchungen uber eine neue myocard- und coronarwirksame verbindung aus der reihe der beta-amino-ketone. Arzneim. Forsch. 17: 1478-1491, 1967.

833 3-(0-Methoxyphenoxy)-2-hydroxypropyl Nicotinate (see Nicotinic Acid)

834 1-[2-[p[Alpha-(p-Methoxyphenyl)-beta-nitrostyryl] phenoxy]-ethyl]pyrrolidine monocitrate. [Ci628]

This estrogen antagonist was given to Beagle dogs orally during the first 15 days of gestation. At doses of 0.5 mg per kg pregnancy was prevented but at 0.125 and 0.25 mg per kg the offspring had malformations which included cleft palate, skeletal defects, persistent cloaca and diaphragmatic hernia.

Schardein, J.L.; Rentner, T.F.; Fitzgerald, J.E. and Kurtz, S.M.: Canine teratogenesis with an estrogen antagonist. Teratology 7: 199-204, 1973.

835 M-Methyl Acetamide (see Acetamide)

836 1-Methyl-acetylhydrazine (see 1-Methyl-formylhydrazine)

837 1-Methyl-2-P-allophanoyl-benzl-hydrazine

Mercier-Parot and Tuchmann-Duplessis (1968) gave the bromhydrate form of this compound orally to rats at various periods from the 8th through the 14th day. Daily doses of as low as 5 mg per kg resulted in fetal defects localized to the eye and extremities. Earlier treatment was associated

with microthalmia and anophthalmia while treatment after the
12th day produced limb defects. The same authors (1968)
extended this study by showing that the compound was teratogenic in mice and rabbits.

Mercier-Parot, L. and Tuchmann-Duplessis, H.: Action d'une
methyl-hydrazine, le bromhydrate D l-methyl-
-2-p-allophanoyl-benzl-hydrazine sur la morphogenese du rat.
C. R. Acad. Sci. (d) (Paris) 267: 444-447, 1968.

Mercier-Parot, L. and Tuchmann-Duplessis, H.: Mise en
evidence chez deux autres rongeurs: la souris et le lapin,
de l'action teratogene du bromhydrate de l-methyl-
-2-p-allophanoyl-benzyl-hydrazine. C. R. Acad. Sci. (d)
(Paris) 268: 1088-1091, 1969.

838   Methylamphetamine (see Amphetamine)

839   Methyl Arsenate

Ancel (1946) used 1.0 mg of the disodium salt dropped onto
the developing 26 hour chick to produce spina bifida.

Ancel, P.: Reserche experimentale sur le spina bifida.
Arch. Anat. Microscop. Morphol. Exp. 36: 45-68, 1946.

840   Methylazoxymethanol [Cycasin]

This chemical is the glycone of cycasin which occurs in the
seeds of the tropical plants Cycas circinalis and C.
revoluta. Spatz et al. (1967) injected 25 mg per kg into
guinea pigs on the 8th gestational day and produced fetal
defects including exencephaly, spina bifida,
craniorachischisis and oligodactyly. This compound is also
mutagenic and carcinogenic. Spatz (1969) found neoplasms of
the jejunum and brain in the offspring of mothers fed 3
percent cycasin.

Haddad et al (1975) have reported post-natal studies of rats
which were treated with this compound.

Haddad, R.; Rabe, A. and Dumas, R.: Functional
consequences of chemically induced cerebellar dysplasia in
the rat. (abstract) Teratology 11: 20A (only), 1975.

Spatz, M.: Toxic and carcinogenic alkylating agents from
cycads. Ann. N.Y. Acad. Sci. 163:848-855, 1969.

Spatz, M.; Dougherty, W.J. and Smith, D.W.E.: Teratogenic
effects of methylazoxymethanol. Proc. Soc. Exp. Biol.
Med. 124: 467-478, 1967.

841   l-Methyl-2-benzyl-hydrazine (see 1,2-Diethylhydrazine)

842   0-Methyl-0-(4-bromo-2,5-dichlorophenyl)phenyl
       thiophosphonate (Phosrel-R)

Kanoh et al (1981) fed 125, 50 and 12.5 ppm in the diet of rats on days 8-20. Some fetal growth retardation was found at 12.5 and 125 mg dose levels. There was some delay in ossification and 5 out of 150 fetuses had dilated renal pelves.

Kanoh, S.; Ema, M.; Hori, Y.: Fetal toxicity of 0-methyl-0-(4-bromo-2,5-dichlorophenyl) phenyl thiophosphonate. Oyo Yakuri 22:373-380, 1981.

843 1-Methyl-5-chloroindoline Methylbromide

Irikura et al (1973) studied this parasympathomimetic drug in mice and rabbits using the oral and subcutaneous routes during active organoggenesis. No teratogenic effects were seen with oral maximum doses of 30 mg per kg per day and subcutaneous maximal doses of 10 mg.

Irikura, T.; Suzuki, H. and Sugimoto, T.: Teratological study of 1-methyl-5-chloroindole methylbromide. (Japanese) Oyo Yakuri 7: 1171-1180, 1973.

844 2-Methyl-4-Chlorophenoxyacetic Acid

Buslovich et al (1979) observed single administration one-half LD-50 on the 9th and 10th day of pregnancy induced teratogenic and embryotoxic effects in rat embryos. Phenobarbital (80 mg per kg) administered to pregnant rats before the agent decreased the embryotoxic action.

Buslovich, S.Yu.; Aleksashina, Z.A. and Kolosovskaya, V.M.: Effect of phenobarbital on the embryotoxic action of 2-methyl-4- chlorophenoxyacetic acid. Farmakol. i Toksicol. (USSR) 42, 2:167-170, 1979.

845 Methylcholanthrene

Savkur et al. (1961) injected 2.5 microgm into each embryonic site of the pregnant mouse on the 10th day and found a high incidence of tail defects and subcutaneous hemorrhages. The limited extent and description of the defects casts some doubt about the teratogenicity of this compound. The incidence of the defects did not increase with dose and a persistence of defects in subsequent untreated litters was noted.

Tomatis et al. (1971) administered orally 8.4 mg of 3-methylcholanthrene to mice during their last week of pregnancy. They found that the treatment group had a three fold increase in the incidence of tumors. The most common type was lymphoma and lung tumor. Khera and Iverson (1981) injected intraperitoneally 20 mg per kg on days 11, 12 and 13 of the gravid rat and produced no adverse effects in the fetuses.

Khera, K.S.; Iverson, F.: Effects of pretreatment with SKF-525A, N-methyl-1-2-thioimidazole, sodium phenobarbital, or methyl cholanthrene on ethylenethiourea-induced teratogenicity in rats. Teratology 24:131-137, 1981.

Khera, K.S.; Iverson, F.: Effects of pretreatment with SKF-525A, N-methyl-2-thioimidazole, sodium phenobarbital, or methyl cholanthrene on ethylenethiourea-induced teratogenicity in rats. Teratology 24:131-137, 1981.

Savkur, L.D.; Batra, B.K. and Sridharan, B.N.: Effect of 20-methylcholanthrene on mouse embryos. II Strain C3-H (JAX). J. Reprod. Fertil. 2: 374-380, 1961.

Tomatis, L.; Turusov, V.; Guibbert, D.; Duperray, B.; Malaveille, C. and Pacheco, H.: Transplacental carcinogenic effect of 3-methylcholanthrene in mice and its quantitation in fetal tissues. J. Natl. Cancer Inst. 47: 645-651, 1971.

846 Methyldigoxin (see Digoxin)

847 Methyldopa (Aldomet-R)

Redman et al (1976) carried out a controlled study in which 122 women with hypertension were treated with this drug. Only one malformation occurred (absent kidney with 2 umbilical vessels). A better pregnany outcome was associated with the treatment.

Redman, C.W.G.; Beilin, L.J.; Bonnar, J. and Ounsted, M.K.: Fetal outcome in trial of antihypertensive treatment in pregnancy. Lancet 2:753-756, 1976.

848 Methylene Blue

Gillman et al. (1951) reported that this dye was not tera-togenic in the rat.

Gillman, J.; Gilbert, C.; Spence, I. and Gillman, T.: A further report on congenital anomalies in the rat produced by trypan blue. S. Afr. J. Med. Sci. 16: 125-135, 1951.

849 Methylene Chloride

Schwetz et al (1975) exposed pregnant mice and rats to this vapor in concentrations which were twice the maximal allowable limit for human industrial exposure (1225 ppm). Both species were exposed for 7 hour daily periods on days 6 through 15 of gestation. No fetal toxicity or teratogen-icity was found.

Schwetz, B.A.; Leong, B.K.J. and Gehring, P.J.: The effect of maternally inhaled trichorethylene, perchloroethylene, methyl chloroform and methylene chloride on embryonal and fetal development in mice and rats. Toxicol. Appl. Pharmacol. 32: 84-96, 1975.

850   Methylethylenethiourea (see Methylenethiourea)

851   Methyl ethyl ketone

Schwetz et al (1974) exposed rats for 7 hours a day on days 6 through 15 of gestation to 1000 and 3000 ppm. At the highest dose mandibular hypoplasia and tail defects were increased among the fetuses.

Schwetz, B.A.; Leong, B.K.J.; Gehring, P.J.: Embryo- and fetotoxicity of inhaled carbon tetrachloride, 1,1-dichoroethane and methyl ethyl ketone in rats. Toxicol. Appl. Pharmacol. 28:452-464, 1974.

852   1-Methyl-formylhydrazine

Von Kreybig et al (1970) reported that this compound given at 100 mg per kg on day 13 to rats produced congenital malformations. They found misshaped skulls with hypoplasia of the telencephalon and skeletal defects of mandible and extremities. 1-methyl-acetylhydrazine and 1-ethyl-2-acetyl hydrazine were not teratogenic. Podophyllinic acid ethylhydrazide and isonicotinic acid 2-isopropylhydrazide and isonicotinic acid 2-isopropylhydrazide phosphate (Iproniazid-R) were toxic at high levels but not teratogenic.

Von Kreybig, T.; Preussmann, R. and Von Kreybig, I.: Chemische Konstitution und teratogene Wirkung bei der Ratte. 3. N-alkylcarbonhydrazide Weitere Hydrazinderivate. Arzneim-Forsch 20: 363-367, 1970.

853   Methylhydrazine   [1-Methyl-2-P-(isopropyl-carbamoyl)benzyl-hydrazine Chlorhydrate]

Mercier-Parot and Tuchmann-Duplessis (1969) extended their initial observations on rats to the mouse and rabbit. With oral doses of 20 mg per kg when administered on days 8 through 12 of the mouse pregnancy, they found 36 percent of the offspring malformed. A dose of 200 mg per kg in the rabbit on the 14th day produced an equal number of defective offspring. The anomalies consisted of anencephaly, eye defects and complex facial bone deformities.

Mercier-Parot, L. and Tuchmann-Duplessis, H.: Action embryotoxique et teratogene d'une methylhydrazine chez la souris et le lapin. C. R. Soc. Biol. (Paris) 163: 16-20, 1969.

854   Methyl 0-(4-hydroxy-3-methoxycinnamoly)reserpate

Shimazu et al (1979) gave this raumalfia alkaloid to pregnant rats and rabbits in maximum oral doses of 200 and 30 mg per kg respectively. Delayed implantation was found in rats receiving 100 mg per kg. At 200 mg per kg during organogenesis an increase in dead fetuses and resorptions was found. Perinatal administration of 100 mg per kg was associated with decreased suckling and weight gain. General behavior was not altered. No effect was seen following treatment of rabbits during organogenesis.

Shimazu, H.; Ikka, T.; Matsura, M.; Tamada, T.; Fujimoto, Y.: Teratological and reproductive studies of methyl 0-(4-hydroxy-3- methoxycinnamoly)reserpate in rats and rabbits. Oyo Yakuri 18:105-124, 1979.

855 N-Methyl-N-(1 naphthyl)-fluoroacetamide

This pesticide was given to mice orally from day 1 through day 12 of gestation in maximum doses of 20 mg per kg. Some growth retardation occurred with the highest dose but no malformation increase was found (Makita et al, 1970).

Makita, T.; Hashimoto, Y. and Noguchi, T.: Teratological studies of N-methyl-N-(1-naphthyl)-fluoroacetamide in mice. Oyo Yakuri 4: 463-468, 1970.

856 2-Methyl-4-nitro-1-(4-nitrophenyl)imidazole   [Imidazole Derivative]

Bauer et al (1972) reported that this chemical given orally to rats, mice and dogs was non-teratogenic. The multiple oral doses given were 200 mg per kg for rats, 100 mg per kg for mice and 50 mg per kg for rabbits.

Bauer, A.; Froberg, H.; Jochmann, G. and Schilling, B.V.: Reproduction and mutagenicity trials of 2-methyl--4-nitro-1-(4-nitrophenyl)imidiazole. (abstract) Naunyn Schmiedebergs Arch. Pharmakol. Suppl. 274: R-15 (only), 1972.

857 N-Methyl-N-nitro-N-nitrosoguanidine

Inouye and Murakami (1975) studied this potent mutagen and carcinogen in pregnant mice at dose levels of 40 to 80 mg per kg given as a single intraperitoneal injection on day 7, 8, 9, 10, 11 or 12. Hydrocephalus, cleft palate, micrognathia and reduction defects of the extremities were found in the fetus. The highest incidence of hydrocephalus was found in the group treated on day 10 with 60 mg per kg. At 80 mg per kg approximately one-third of the mothers died.

Inouye, M. and Murakami, U.: Teratogenic effect of N-methyl-N-nitro-N-nitrosoguanidine in mice. Teratology 18: 263-268, 1978.

858 Methylnitrosourea (also see Ethylnitrosourea)

Napalkov and Alexandrov (1968) found a 80 percent malformation rate in rat fetuses whose mothers received injections of 20 mg per kg on the 9th day. Koyama et al (1970) using 10 mg of methylnitrosourea per kg in the rat on single gestational days from the 8th through the 15th day produced hydrocephalus, exencephaly, hypoplasia of the pallium or

858

microcephaly. The exencephaly occurred in the earlier
treated group with hydrocephalus on the 9th and 10th days
and microcephalus after the 11th day. Alexandrov (1976) has
reviewed the extensive Russian experimental work on
transplacental carcinogenesis of this and related compounds.

Alexandrov and Schreiber (1978) and Alexandrov (1979)
studied brain blastomogenesis against the background of the
developmental deformities induced by the combined
transplacental effect of methylnitrosourea (MNU) and
ethylnitrosourea (ESU). To induce brain defects such as
microcephaly MNU was injected on the 15th day, whereas to
induce cerebellar defects - on the 21st day of
embryogenesis. Moreover, at the 13th or 17th day ENU was
additionally injected which is found to be highly effective
for inducing brain tumors. It was found that in MNU
exposure (at the 15th day) until ENU exposure (at the 17th
day of embryogenesis) no reliable decrease in brain tumor
occurrence was noted, compared to when only ENU was
employed. In the reverse sequence, i.e., first the exposure
to ENU on the 13th day and then to MNU on the 15th day the
occurrence of tumors located in cerebral hemispheres was 3
times less. It is assumed that cytotoxic effect of NMU
leading to microcephaly is likely to cause the death of a
considerable amount of the cell population previously
transformed. Dimant and Beniashvili (1978) reported the
results of exposure wth a number of carcinogenic agents in
rabbits. They remarked that NEU had the greatest
carcinogenic and neurotropic effects.

Alexandrov, V.A.: Some results and prospects of
transplacental carcinogenesis studies. Neoplasia 23:
285-299, 1976.

Alexandrov, V.A. and Schreiber, D.: Combined
transplacental carcinogenic action of N-nitrosomethylurea
(NMU) and N-nitrosoethylurea in rats. Vopr. Onkol. (USSR)
24.4: 38-43, 1978.

Alexandrov, V.A.: The pattern of N-nitrosoethylurea action
in rats during embryogenesis. Vopr. Onkol. (USSR) 25.6:
60-65, 1979.

Dimant, I.N. and Beniashvili, D.Sh.: Some aspects of the
transplacental blastomogenesis in rabbits. Byull. Eksper.
Biol. Med. (USSR) 85:3:343, 1978.

Koyama, T.; Handa, J.; Handa, H. and Matsumoto, S.: M-
ethylnitrosourea-induced malformations of brain in SD-JCL
rat. Arch. Neurol. 22: 342-347, 1970.

Napalkov, N.P. and Alexandrov, V.A.: On the effects of
blastomogenic substances on the organism during
embryogenesis, z. Krebsforsch. 71: 32-50, 1968.

859   4-Methyl 5-Oxyuracil

Kosmachevskaya and Tichodeeva (1968)

produced death (28 percent) injecting 4 mg per chick egg at 24 hours. Twenty-seven percent of the survivors had abnormalities of the extremities, ventral body wall or tail. UUsing 3000 mg per kg of body weight on the 9th and 10th day in immobilized rats Kosmachevskaya and Chebotar (1968) produced hydronephrosis or unilateral renal agenesis in 60 percent of the fetuses. Renal defects were the sole type found.

Kosmachevskaya, E.A. and Tichodeeva, I.I.: Relation between embryotoxic activity of some pyrimidine derivatives and their chemical structure. Chick embryo test. Pharmacol. Toxicol. (Russian) No. 5: 618-620, 1968.

Kosmachevskaya, E.A. and Chebotar, N.A.: The damaging effect of 4-methyl-5-oxyuracil on rat embryogenesis in conditions of maternal stress. Bull. Exptl. Biol. (Russian) No. 12: 89-91, 1968.

860   O-Methylpantothenic Acid (see Pantothenic Acid deficiency)

861   X-Methyl Pantothenic Acid (see Pantothenic Acid Deficiency)

862   Methyl Parathion [Dimethyl-0-4-mitrophenyl Phosphorothioate]

This cholinesterase inhibitor was given to rats in amounts of 24 mg per kg on days 9 or 15 of gestation, and no defects were seen in the offspring (Fish, 1966). Some perinatal mortality increase was seen, and the growth rate after birth was reduced. Cerebral cortical cholinesterase was reduced in the fetuses.

Tanimura et al (1967) found no teratogenicity with doses of 15 mg per kg on day 12 in the rat. In the mouse, cleft palate occurred at 60 mg per kg on day 10. The material was given intraperitoneally.

Fish, S.A.: Organophosphorus cholinesterase inhibitor and fetal development. Am. J. Obstet. Gynecol. 96: 1148-1154, 1966.

Tanimura, T.; Katsuya, T.; and Nishimura, H.: Embryotoxicity of acute exposure to methyl parathion in rats and mice. Arch. Envir. Health 15: 609-613, 1967.

863   Methylphenidate (Ritalin-R)

Heinonen et al (1977) included 11 mothers who took this drug in the first 4 lunar months of gestation among a group of 96 in which there was no significant increase in defect rate among the offspring.

Heinonen, O.P.; Slone, D.; Shapiro, S.: Birth Defects and Drugs in Pregnancy. Publishing Sciences Group, Inc., 1977.

864   Methylprednisolone

Walker using the mouse (AJAX) produced cleft palate using 0.5 mg daily on day 11 through 14. Doses of up to 8.0 mg daily in the rat did not produce cleft palates.

Walker, B.: Induction of cleft palate with anti-inflammatory drugs. Teratology 4:39-42, 1971.

865 9-Methyl-pteroylglutamic Acid (also see Folic Acid Deficiency)

This analogue of folic acid is used to potentiate the folic acid deficiency state in experimental models.

866 X-Methyl-pteroylglutamic Acid (also see Folic Acid Deficiency)

This is an unpurified substance which was used to potentiate the folic acid deficiency state in experimental models. It contains 9-methyl-pteroylglutamic acid.

867 Methylsalicylate (see Salicylate)

868 Methyltestosterone

This androgen is capable of masculinizing the human female fetus (Grumbach and Ducharme, 1960) as well as female fetuses of experimental animals (Jost, 1955). (see Testosterone for a more complete coverage)

Golubeva et al (1978) reported that this drug applied directly to the skin of pregnant rats (0.01-0.05 mg per kg from day 1 through 15) induced in the offspring some behavior abnormalities and slight disturbances in the function of cardio-vascular system.

Golubeva, M.I.; Shashkina, L.F.: Starkov, M.V. and Fedorova, Z.A.: Development of the progeny of rats after application of androgens to the skin throughout the entire pregnancy. Gigiena Tr. Prof. Zabol. (USSR) 6:25-28, 1978.

Grumbach, M.M. and Ducharme, J.R.: The effects of androgens on fetal sexual development androgen-induced female pseudohermaphroditism. Fertil. Steril. 11: 157-180, 1960.

Jost, A.: Biologie des androgenes chez l'embryon. In, Reunion Des Endocrinologists De Langue Francaise (third). Paris: Masson, 1955. pp. 160-180.

869 N-Methyl-2-thioimidazole (see ethylenethiourea)

870 Methylthiouracil

Freiesleben and Kjerulf-Jensen (1947) reported a 5-month old fetus with thyroid hypertrophy following maternal treatment during pregnancy. In pregnant rats fed 0.25 mg per 10 gm diet they demonstrated fetal thyroid changes histologically.

Toriumi (1959) fed rabbits 50 mg per kg and observed histologic changes in the fetal thyroid after the 18th day. By the 21st day grossly enlarged fetal thyroids occurred. Klosouskii (1963) gave chinchillas 300 mg per kg and produced cretinism, hypoplastic brains and some dextrocardia and transposition of the great vessels.

Freiesleben, E. and Kjerulf-Jensen, K.: The effect of thiouracil derivatives on fetuses and infants. J. Clin. Endocrinol. 7: 47-51, 1947.

Klosovskii, B.N.: The development of the brain and its disturbance by harmful factors. Translated from Russian and edited By B. Haigh. New York: MacMillian, 1963. pp. 161-167.

Toriumi, K.: Embryological studies on the experimental congenital goiter due to methylthiouracil in rabbits. Journal of the Osaka City Medical Center 8: 1281-1293, 1959.

871 1-Methyl-5-p-toluoylpyrrole-2-acetate dihydrate, Sodium (Tolmetin Sodium)

This non-steroid antiinflammatory was given orally by Nishimura et al (1977) to pregnant rabbits on days 6 through 18 in amounts of up to 100 mg per kg daily. At 100 mg per kg, the dam's weight gain was reduced and fetal mortality was increased. No teratogenic effect was found.

Nishimura, K.; Fukagawa, S.; Shigematsu, K.; Makumoto, K.; Terada, Y.; Sasaki, H.; Nanto, T. and Tatsumi, H.: Teratogenicity study of tolmetin sodium in rabbits. (Japanese) Iyakuhin Kenkyu 8:158-164, 1977.

872 Alpha-methyltyrosine

Kvist and Rubin (1975) reported studies in the chick egg with this tyrosine analogue. Twenty mg were injected at 20-22 hours of incubation and 30 percent of the survivors had defects including anencephaly and spina bifida.

Kvist, T.N. and Rubin, C.: The role of catecholamines in neural tube closure and head flexure formation in the chick embryo (abstract). Teratology 11: 26A-27A, 1975.

873 4-Methyl Uracil

Kosmachevskaya and Tichodeeva (1968) injected chick eggs with 4 mg of this substance and produced abnormalities of the brain or eye in 24 percent. No defects were produced in rat fetuses when the mother received 3000 mg per kg of body weight on the 9th and 10th day of gestation (Kosmachevskaya and Chebotar, 1968).

873

Kosmachevskaya, E.A. and Tichodeeva, I.I.: Relation
between embryotoxic activity of some pyrimidine derivatives
and their chemical structure. Chick Embryo Test.
Pharmacol. Toxicol. (Russian) No. 5: 618-620, 1968.

Kosmachevskaya, E.A. and Chebotar, N.A.: The damaging
effect of 4-methyl uracil on rat embryogenesis in conditions
of maternal stress. Bull. Exptl. Biol. (Russian) No.
12: 89-91, 1968.

874 4-Methylumbelliferyl-beta-D-xyloside (see Beta-D-xyloside)

875 Methylurea

Von Kreybig et al. (1969) showed that the dimethyl, tri-
methyl and tetramethyl form of this compound was teratogenic
in rats. Reduction defects of the skeletal system were
produced by administration of 500 to 1000 mg per kg on the
13th or 14th day of gestation. Cros et al (1972) give
detailed studies of the teratogenicity of tetramethylurea in
mice. They found exencephaly and reduction defects of the
extremities.

Cros, S.B.; Moisand, C. and Tollon, Y.: Influence de la
tetramethyluree sur le developpement embryonnaire de la
souris. Ann. Pharm. Franc. 9: 585-593, 1972.

Von Kreybig, T.; Preussmann, R. and Von Kreybig, I.:
Chemische Konstitution und teratogene Wirkung bei der Ratte.
II. N-alkylharnstoffe, N-alkylsulfonamide,
N,N-dialkylacetamide, N-methylthioacetamid, Chloracetamid.
Arzneim. Forsch. 19: 1073-1076, 1969.

876 Metiapine

Gibson and Newberne (1973) gave up to 30 mg per kg orally to
pregnant rats and rabbits during organogenesis and produced
no defects. At the highest doses postnatal survival was
reduced in the rats.

Gibson, J.P. and Newberne, J.W.: Teratology and
reproductive studies with metiapine. Toxicol. and Appl.
Pharm. 25: 212-219, 1973.

877 Metiazinic Acid [10-Methyl-2-phenothiazinyl Acetic Acid]

Julou et al. (1969) found no teratogenicity in mice, rats
and rabbits when they used up to 60 mg per kg per day during
active organogenesis. This antiinflammatory agent was
tested orally in pregnant rats by Nakamura et al, (1974).
Doses up to 80 mg per kg per day were given from the 8th
through the 14th day of gestation. No teratogenicity or
postnatal effects of treatment were found.

Julou, L.; Ducrot, R.; Fournel, J.; Ganter, P.; Populaire,
P.; Durel, J.; Myon, J.; Pascal, S. and Pasquet, J.: Etude
toxicologique de l'acide metiazinique (16091 R.P.).

877

Arzneim. Forsch. 19: 1207-1214, 1969.

Nakamura, E.; Kimura, M.; Kato, R.; Honma, K.; Tsuruta, M.;
Uchida, S.; Kaneka, K. and Sato, H.: Teratogenic studies
on metiazinic acid. Oyo Yakuri 8: 1587-1631, 1974.

878 Metolazone (7-Chloro 1,2,3,4 tetrahydro-2-methyl-4-
oxo-3-0-tolyl-6-quinazolinesulfonamide)

Nakajima et al (1978 A and B) studied the effect of this
diuretic on pregnant rats and rabbits. The dose range was 2
to 250 mg per kg daily orally during active organogenesis.
Fetal hydronephrosis was increased in the rat fetuses
exposed to 2 mg per kg but not at higher doses. Ureteric
dilitation was found in fetuses exposed to 2,10 and 50 mg
per kg. No limb changes were detected. In the rabbit the
only fetal change was a weight reduction at 10 mg per kg.

Nakajima, T.; Ishisaka, K.; Taylor, P. and Matuda, S.:
Effects of metolazone on the reproduction function of rats.
2 Teratogenicity test.(Japanese) Clinical Report
12:3394-3406, 1978A.

Nakajima, T.; Ishisaka, K.; Taylor, P. and Matuda, S.:
Effects of metolazone on reproduction of rabbits Teratogenicity test (Japanese) Clinical Report 12:3417-3421, 1978B.

879 Metoprolol Tartrate

Fukuhara et al (1979) studied the adrenergic blocker in rats
and rabbits. The rabbits received 64 mg and the rats 500 mg
per kg. In the rat implantation was inhibited at 500 mg per
kg. No adverse fetal effects were noted in either species
except for slight growth retardation in the rat. Neonatal
mortality was increased among fetuses exposed on days 17-21
of gestation. Some increase in embryolethality was noted in
the rabbit fetuses exposed to 64 mg per kg.

Fukuhara, Y.; Fujii, T.; Emi, Y.; Kado, Y.; Watanabe, N.:
Reproductive studies of metoprolol tartrate. Kiso to Rinsho
13: 3216-3224, 1979.

880 Metrizamide

Kodama et al (1979) administered up to 1800 mg per kg of
this contrast media to rats before mating and during the
first 7 days, on days 7-17 or on days 17-21. The fertility
studies were done by intraperitoneal route and the
teratological and perinatal by intravenous route.
Implantations were reduced in the treated group and a
borderline decrease in viability was reported. Other
adverse fetal effects were not reported.

Kodama, N.; Tsubota, K.; Ezumi, Y.: Effects of metrizamide
on rat reproduction. Nichi-doku Iho (Japanisch-Deutsche
Medizinische Berichte 24:277-285, 287-302, 303-318, 1979.

881

881 Metronidazole (Flagyl-R)

Gauter et al used 100 mg per kg during the entire rat pregnancy and observed neither change in number of viable offspring nor any malformations.

Monitoring of the offspring of treated pregnant women has
been carried out for 20 years, and several large studies are
summarized by Berget and Weber (1972). Their review
included 1,469 pregnant women, of whom 206 were treated in
the first trimester. No increase in the incidence of malformation, abortion, or stillbirth was found. Postnatal
followup was done in some of the patients.

Legator et al (1975) found evidence of mutagenic activity
using a salmonella typhimurium test when urine from patients
taking metronidazole was assayed. The importance of this
test is still unresolved. We have determined that about
half of the chemicals found to be mutagenic in these
bacterial tests are teratogenic in animal tests. Positive
animal teratogenicity tests do not by any means imply that
the drug is embryo- or fetotoxic in the human.

Berget, A.; Weber, T.: Metronidazole and pregnancy.
Ugeskr. Laeger 134:2085-2089, 1972.

Gauter, P.; Jolou, L.; Cosar, C.: Study of the action of
metronidazole (No. 8832RP.) on the genital system of the
rat. Gynecol. Obstet. 59:609-620, 1960.

Legator, M.S.; Conner, T.H. and Stoeckel, M.: Detection of
mutagenic activity of metronidazole and niradazole in body
fluids of humans and mice. Science 188:1118-1119, 1975.

882 Mevinolinic Acid

Robertson et al (1981) fed 800 mg per kg to the gravid rat
on days 6-17 and produced fetal malformations of the
vertebrae and ribs.

Robertson, R.T.; Minsker, D.H.; MacDonald, J.S.; Bokelman,
D.L.; Christian, M.S.: Mevalonic acid antagonism of the
teratogenic effects of mevinolic acid, a potent inhibitor of
hydroxymethylglutaryl-coenzyme A reductase (abstract)
Teratology 23:58A, 1981.

883 Mezlocillin

Hamada and Imanishi (1978) gave intravenously up to 1000 mg
per kg on days 7 through 17 and found no fetal changes in
rats. Tanioka and Koizumi (1978) found no evidence of teratogenicity in monkeys given up to 100 mg per kg from days 23
through 47 of gestation.

Hamada, Y. and Imanishi, M.: Reproduction study of
mezlocillin in rats. 2 Teratogenicity study (Japanese)
Iyakuhin Kenkyu 9:986-996, 1978.

Tanioka, Y. and Koizumi, H.: Influence of sodium

mezlocillin on fetuses of Rhesus monkeys. (Japanese) CIEA
Preclin. Rpt. 4:11-22, 1978.

884 Miconazole

Ito et al (1976A and B) tested this antimycotic in rats and
rabbits during active organogenesis. At the maximum dose of
100 mg per kg both species had an increase in fetal
mortality. In the rat, difficult labor occurred. No malformation rate increase was found.

Ito, C.; Shibutani, Y.; Inoue, K.; Nakano, K. and Ohnishi,
H.: Toxicological studies of miconazole 2. Teratological
studies of miconazole in rats. Iyakuhin Kenkyu 7:367-376,
1976.

Ito, C.; Shibutani, Y.; Taya, K. and Ohnishi, H.:
Toxicological studies of miconazole 3. Teratological
studies of miconazole in rabbits. Iyakuhin Kenkyu
7:377-381, 1976.

885 Microwave Radiations (Diathermy, Shortwave, Ultrasound)

The effects of microwave and shortwave radiation have been
studied extensively and reviews have been published by
Michaelson (1969) and by Brent (1977). Michaelson gives a
discussion of why the energy from these sources is too small
regardless of dose to produce the type of excitation
necessary for ionization, consequently, there seems to be
agreement that any damage from these sources would be
related to hyperthermia which may be teratogenic under
certain conditions (see Hyperthermia). Radiation at
frequencies below 1000 megaHertz causes heat primarily in
deep tissues; while with increasing frequencies and
especially over 3000, proportionally more surface heating
occurs. Most microwave ovens and diathermy generate
approximately 2450 mega Hertz, and according to Brent
(1977), even at the maximum permissible level of 1 to 10 mW,
no hazard to the human embryo would be expected.

Hofmann and Dietzel (1966) reported that diathermy treatment
of rats on the 13th or 14th gestational day produced defects
of the tail and extremities. They used a 70 or 100 watt
intensity at 27 mega Hertz for 10 minutes. Pregnancy in the
rabbit was interrupted especially by treatment on the 10th
day. Umeda (1941) applied diathermy to rabbits for 20
minutes at various times during pregnancy and produced fetal
death and some histological changes in the viscera of
surviving fetuses. Mannor et al 1972) in the mouse used
levels of 164 to 1050 mW per square cm at 2.28 mega Hertz
for up to 60 minutes for varying periods of gestation. Four
hundred and ninety mW did not cause critical temperature
rises and higher intensity produced tissue defects identical
to those from overheating. No defects were produced and
postnatal fertility and chromosomal findings in the offspring were normal. Shoji et al(1975) treated mice for 5
hours during day 8 with 2.25 mega Hertz and power of 40 mW
per square cm. They found a low but significant increase in
severe brain and facial defects in one of two strains.

page 299

885

Fetal heart detectors used in human pregnancy monitoring produce 5 to 20 mW per square cm (Mannor et al, 1972). Tachibana (1977) exposed 2 strains of mice to up to 10 minutes of 200 mW per square cm at a frequency of 2 megahertz from the 7th to the 13th day of gestation. Although there was no increase in fetal loss or significant increase in malformations, a few exencephalies and umbilical hernias occurred in the treated group. Nawrot et al (1981) exposed mice on multiple days to 8 hour daily periods of 2.45-GH2 CW at 5-30mWCMSq. The higher energy levels raised body temperature. At the highest energy 3.2 percent of the fetuses were malformed; this was significantly (P 0.05) more than in the hyperthemic control group which had 1.7 percent defects. Decreased implantation was found when treatment was given on days 1-6. Lary et al (1982) exposed pregnant rats to 27.12 mega Hertz radiations at 300 volts per meter and found malformations of the central nervous system, skeleton and palate when treatment was on days 9, 11, 13, or 15. The defects were related to measured hyperthermia to 43.0 degrees C. Preimplantation exposures were followed by some increase in defects.

Rubin and Erdman (1959) reported four case histories of pregnant women inadvertently treated with microwave for chronic pelvic infection. The dose was 2450 mega Hertz with a 100-W machine. One miscarried after 10 days treatment; the others delivered normal infants. The women who miscarried became pregnant again, treatment was continued and she gave birth to a normal child.

Brent, R.L.: Radiations and other physical agents, In Handbook of Teratology, Vol. 1 edited by Wilson, J.G. and Fraser, F.C.; Plenum Press, 1977, pp. 153-223.

Hofmann, D. and Dietzel, F.: Aborte und Missbildungen nach Kurwellendurchflut-ung in der Schwangerschast. Geburts. Frauen Heilk. 26: 378-390, 1966.

Lary, J.M.; Conover, D.L.; Fole, E.D. and Hanser, P.L.: Teratogenic effects of 27.12 MHz radiofrequency radiation in rats. Teratology 26:299-309, 1981.

Mannor, S.M.; Serr, D.M.; Tamari, I.; Meshorer, A. and Frei, E.H.: The safety of ultrasound in fetal monitoring. Am. J. Obstet. Gynecol. 113:653-661, 1972.

Michaelson, S.M.: Biological effects of microwave exposure, in Biological Effects and Implications of Microwave Radiation. Symposium Proceedings, Richmond, Virginia, Sept. 17-19, edited by S.F. Cleary, U.S. Public Health Service, Richmond, Virginia, 1969, pp. 35-58.

Nawrot, P.S.; McRee, D.I.; Staples, R.E.: Effects of 2.4 GHz CW microwave radiation on embryofetal development in mice. Teratology 24: 303-314, 1981.

Rubin, A. and Erdman, W.J.: Microwave exposure of the human female pelvis during early pregnancy and prior to conception. Case rep. Am. J. Phys. Med. 38: 219:220, 1959.

Shoji, R.; Murakami, U. and Shimizu, T.: Influence of low-intensity ultrasonic irradiation on prenatal dvelopment of two in-bred mouse strains. Teratology 12:227-232, 1975.

Tachibana, M.: Effects of irradiation of high-energy continuous-wave ultrasounds on the fetuses of mice (dd-I and Ch3He strains). (Japanese) Acta Obst. Gynaec Jpn. 29:1097-1105, 1977.

Umeda, S.: Supplementary information on the biological effects of short waves. The effects on the course of pregnancy and development of fetuses. Sanka Fujinka Kiyo 24:265-346, 1941.

886 Miloxacin

Yamada et al (1980) studied this antibiotic in the rat before mating and during organogenesis in doses of up to 300 mg per kg daily. Fetal weight was reduced at doses above 37.5 mg per kg but no defects were found. At the highest dose some decrease in viability and fetal weight occurred when treatment was given on days 17-21.

Yamada T.; Tarumoto, Y.; Hosoda, K.; Koike, M.; Furasawa, S.; Sasajima, M.; Ohzeki, M.: Reproductive studies of miloxacin in rat fertility, teratogenicity and peri and postnatal studies. Oyo Yakuri 19 651-662, 815-831, 833-844, 1980.

887 Mimosine

Dewreede and Wayman (1970) fed rats diets containing this amino acid extracted from Leucaena leucocephala. With diets containing 0.7 percent the resorption rate was increased, and 3.5 percent of the fetuses were deformed. The deformities were associated with uterine perforations which caused constriction of the protruding fetal parts.

Dewreede, S. and Wayman, O.: Effect of mimosine on the rat fetus. Teratology 3: 21-28, 1970.

888 Minocycline

Jackson et al (1975) administered 8.7 -17.4 mg per kg orally to Rhesus monkeys during embryogenesis and the period of fetal skeletal formation. No adverse effects were observed.

Jackson, B.A.; Rodwell, D.E.; Kanegis, L.A.; Noble, J.F.: Effect of maternally administered minocycline on embryonic and fetal development in the Rhesus monkey. (abstract) Toxicol. Appl. Pharmacol. 33:156 (only) 1975.

889 Miracil-D

Karnofsky and Lacon (1962) briefly report that at the LD-50 of 2 to 4 mg per egg a slight feather inhibition was noted in the chick embryo.

889

Karnofsky, D.A. and Lacon, C.R.: Survey of cancer chemotherapy service center compounds for teratogenic effect in the chick embryo. Cancer Res. 22: 84-86, 1962.

890 Mirex-R

This polychlorinated insecticide was given in the diet at 5 PPM to mice by Ware and Good (1967). They found that this low dosage produced a significant reduction in litter size and the numbber of offspring produced. Congenital defects were not studied.

Khera et al (1976) studied this compound in rats at levels of 6 an 12.5 mg per kg which were toxic to the mother. Gavaging the mothers on days 6 through 15, they found decreased fetal survival with an increased incidence of cleft palate, subcutaneous edema along with several other types of defects. Grabowski (1982) gave 1 mg per kg on days 15 through 21 and found fetuses with respiratory distress, heartblock and cataracts.

Grabowski, C.T.: Functional testing for the effects of very low doses of the insecticide, Mirex (abstract). Teratology 25: 44A, 1982.

Khera, K.S.; Villeneuve, D.C.; Terry, G.; Panopio, L.; Nash, L. and Trivett, G.: Mirex: A teratogenicity, dominant lethal and tissue distribution study in rats. Fd. Cosmet. Toxicol. 14:25-29, 1976.

Ware, G.W. and Good, E.E.: Effects of insecticides on reproduction in the laboratory mouse. Toxicol. Appl. Pharmacol. 10: 54-61, 1967.

891 Miroprofen (2-(p-imidazo(1,2-a)pyridyl)phenyl proprionic acid)

Hamada and Imanishi (1981) in a series of papers studied this antiinflammatory agent in rats and rabbits. Doses of 25 mg per kg before mating had no adverse effect in the rat. During organogenesis both rabbits and rats received up to 100 mg per kg and no increase in major defects was found. These higher doses were particularly toxic in the rabbit where fetal death and lumbar ribs were more common. At 5 and 25 mg per kg given on day 17 through day 21 postnatally there was prolongation of gestation, parturition and excessive maternal vaginal bleeding. Neonates and suckling pups had a higher mortaliy rate. Studies done after weaning showed no changes in behavioral tests.

Hamada, Y.; Imanishi, M.: Fertility, teratogenicity and perinatal and postnatal studies of microprofen in rats. Iyakuhin Kenkyu 12:802- 841, 1981.

892 Mithramycin

Chaube and Murphy (1968) report that this antibiotic which inhibits nucleic acid and protein synthesis was not terato-

genic in the rat. Single doses of less than the fetal
LD-100 were given on the 5th through the 12th day.

Chaube, S. and Murphy, M.L.: The teratogenic effects of
the recent drugs active in cancer chemotherapy. In,
Woollam, D.H.M. (ed.): Advances in Teratology, Vol. 3.
New York: Logos and Academic Press, 1968. pp. 181-237.

893 Mitomycin C

This growth inhibitor isolated from streptomyces caespitosus
produces defects in the mouse when given 5 to 10 mg per kg
on single gestational days 7 through 13 (Tanimura, 1968).

Skeletal defects were most common with some defects of the
palate and brain. Chaube and Murphy (1968) found that in
the rat both the maternal and fetal LD-50 were 2 to 2.5 mg
per kg and no teratogenicity was found.

Chaube, S. and Murphy, M.L.: The teratogenic effects of
the recent drugs active in cancer chemotherapy. In,
Woollam, D.H.M. (ed.): Advances in Teratology, Vol. 3.
New York: Logos and Academic Press, 1968. pp. 181-237.

Tanimura, T.: Effects of mitomycin C administered at
various stages of pregnancy upon mouse fetuses. Okajimas
Folia Anat. Jap. 44: 337-355, 1968.

894 Molybdenum

Ridgway and Karnofsky (1952) found that the LD-50 for the
4-day chick embryo was 0.8 mg. No defects were found.
Schroeder and Mitchener (1971) fed mice a diet containing
0.45 PPM and found some runting in the offspring of the
third generation.

Ridgway, L.P. and Karnofsky, D.A.: The effects of metals
on the chick embryo: toxicity and production of abnormalities in development. Ann. N. Y. Acad. Sci. 55:
203-215, 1952.

Schroeder, H.A. and Mitchener, M.: Toxic effects of trace
elements on the reproduction of mice and rats. Arch.
Environ. Health 23: 102-106, 1971.

895 Monomethylaminobenzene (see Aminoazobenzene)

896 Monomethylformamide [N-Methylformamide]

Thiersch (1971) demonstrated that this compound was highly
toxic to rat fetuses even when it was administered by means
of tail painting. Tail painting on days 7 through 14
produced fetal death in 87 percent, and all of the survivors
were malformed. The malformations consisted of hydronephrosis, hydrocephalus, along with hydramnion. An oral
dose of 1.0 cc per kg produced similar results in the rat.
Oettel and Frohberg (1964) injected 0.1 ml per kg on the

11th and 12th day and produced a 50 percent mortality rate in the rat fetus. Tuchmann-Duplessis and Mercier-Parot (1965) demonstrated by skin application that the most sensitive period for teratogenicity was between the 10 and 12th day of gestation.

Oettel, H. and Frohberg, H.: Teratogene Wirkung einfacher Saureamide im Tierversuch. Naunyn-Schmiedebergs Arch. Pharmakol. Exp. Pathol. 247: 363-364, 1964.

Thiersch, J.B.: Investigations into the differential effect of compounds on rat litter and mother. In, Tuchmann-Duplessis, H. (ed.): Malformations Congenitales Des Mammiferes. Paris: Masson, 1971. pp. 95-113.

Tuchmann-Duplessis, H. and Mercier-Parot, L.: Production chez le rat, d'anomalies apres applications cutanees d'un solvent industriel: la mono-methyl-formamide. C. R. Acad. Sci. (Paris) 261: 241-243, 1965.

897 Monosodium Glutamate

Murakami and Inouye (1971) injected mice on the 17th or 18th day of gestation with 5 mg per kg. Nuclear pyknosis was found in the cells of the arcuate and ventromedial nuclei of the fetuses after 3 hours. Examination of treated fetuses after a 24-hr period did not show any abnormal lesion. Olney (1969) reported that immature mice injected with substantial doses of monosodium glutamate developed brain lesions.

Murakami, U. and Inouye, M.: Brain lesions in the mouse fetus caused by maternal administration of monosodium glutamate (preliminary report). Congenital Anomalies 11: 171-177, 1971.

Olney, J.W.: Brain lesions, obesity and other disturbances in mice treated with monosodium glutamate. Science 164: 719-721, 1969.

898 Moquizone   [1-Morpholino-acetyl-3-phenyl-2,3-dihydro-
       -4(1H)quinazolinone hydrochloride]

Setnikar and Magistretti (1970) gave mice, rabbits and rats up to 60 mg per kg daily by mouth during active organogenesis and found no increase in congenital defects.

Setnikar, I. and Magistretti, M.J.: Maternal and fetal toxicity of moquizone. Arzneim. Forsch. 20: 1559-1561, 1970.

899 Morphine

Friedler and Cochin (1972) pretreated rats with morphine, and then after a 5-day non-treatment interval pregnancy was initiated. Although there were no reported changes in the litters, the fetuses after a 3 to 4-week period exhibited significant but transient growth retardation. The effect was not eliminated by cross-foster feeding, excluding a long-term effect through maternal nutrition. In subsequent work with mice treated pregestationally postnatal behavioral effects were found in the offspring (Friedler, 1978). Friedler and Wheeling (1979) also treated males with opioids prior to mating and found behavioral effects in the offspring.

Iuliucci and Gautieri (1971) gave 200 to 400 mg of morphine per kg on gestational day 8 or 9 of the mouse and produced a few exencephalic and axial skeletal defects. The authors point out that the hypoxic effect alone of such large doses could account for the defects. Johannesson and Becker (1972) were unable to produce fetal changes in rat fetuses exposed to maternal doses of 20 mg per kg for periods before and during organogenesis. Harpel and Gautieri (1968) produced exencephaly and skeletal defects in mice by injecting 300 mg and 400 mg per kg subcutaneously on day 8. Treatment with smaller doses and food deprivation caused no fetal malformations.

Geber and Schramm (1975) injected 35 to 322 mg per kg subcutaneously into hamsters on day 8 of gestation and produced with the higher doses 20-30 percent congenital defects in the day 12 embryos. Cranioschisis was the predominant type of defect. Morphine antagonists nalorphine, naloxone and cyclazocine blocked the teratogenic activity when given concurrently. Eleven other narcotic analgesics including codeine, heroin and meperidine were studied and found to produce similar teratogenicity.

Friedler, G.: Pregestational administration of morphine sulfate to fetal mice: long term effects on development of subsequent progeny. J. Pharmacol. Exp. Therap. 205:33-39, 1978.

Friedler, G. and Cochin, J.: Growth retardation in off-spring of female rats treated with morphine prior to conception. Science 175: 654-655, 1972.

Friedler, G.; Wheeling, H.S.: Behavioral effects on offspring of males injected with opioids prior to mating. Pharmacol. Biochem. 11 (suppl): 23-28, 1979.

Geber, W.F. and Schramm, L.C.: Congenital malformations of the central nervous system produced by narcotic analgesics in the hamster. Am. J. Obstet. Gynecol. 123: 705-713, 1975.

Harpel, H.S. and Gautieri, R.F.: Morphine-induced fetal malformations: exencephaly and skeletal fusions. J. Pharm. Sci. 57:1590-1597, 1968.

Iuliucci, J.D. and Gautieri, R.F.: Morphine-induced fetal malformations II. Influence of histamine and diphenhydramine. J. Pharm. Sci. 60: 420-424, 1971.

Johannesson, T. and Becker, B.A.: The effects of maternally-administered morphine on rat foetal development and resultant tolerance to the analgesic effect of morphine. Acta Pharm. Toxicol. 31: 305-313, 1972.

900

900 Mumps Virus

A number of studies of the offspring of mothers having mumps during gestation have demonstrated no increase in congenital defects (Hill et al.; 1958; Siegel et al.; 1966; Korones et al.; 1970).

An intriguing hypothesis that intrauterine mumps virus might cause congenital endocardial firbroelastosis has been tested by St. Geme et al. (1971) who have produced persistent virus infection in the chick embryo with associated myocarditis. Direct inoculation of the virus into fetal monkey brains did not produce any adverse effects (Moreland et al, 1979). Shone et al. (1966) observed a very high incidence of positive mumps skin tests in patients with either fibroelastosis or congenital mitral stenosis but could not show a rise in mumps serum antibodies in 23 patients with fibroelastosis. Gersony et al. (1966) using a more rigorous criterion for skin test interpretation could not show an increased incidence in this condition. St. Geme et al (1974) have extended their testing to the monkey but could not detect the persistence of virus in the fetuses. Delayed hypersensitivity without neutralizing antibody was demonstrated in this monkey fetal model. They report that during gestation the risk of endocardial fibroelastosis is less than 2 percent of the exposed fetuses.

Gersony, W.M.; Katz, S.L. and Nadas, A.S.: Endocardial fibroelastosis and the mumps virus. Pediatrics 37: 430-434, 1966.

Hill, B.; Doll, R.; Galloway, T.M. and Hughes, J.P.W.: Virus diseases in pregnancy and congenital defects. Br. J. Prev. Soc. Med. 12: 1-7, 1958.

Korones, S.B.; Todaro, J.; Roane, J.A. and Sever, J.L.: Maternal virus infection after the first trimester of pregnancy and status of offspring to 4 years of age in a predominantly Negro population. J. Pediatr. 77: 245-251, 1970.

Moreland, A.F.; Gaskin, J.M.; Schimpff, R.D.; Woodard, J.C.; Olson, G.A.: Effects of influenza, mumps and Western equine viruses on fetal rhesus monkeys (Macaca mulatta). Teratology 20:53-64, 1979.

Shone, J.; Armas, S.M.; Manning, J.A. and Keith, J.D.: The mumps antigen skin test in endocardial fibroelastosis. Pediatrics 37: 423-429, 1966.

Siegel, M. and Fuerst, H.T.: Low birth weight and maternal virus diseases: A prospective study of rubella, measles, mumps, chickenpox, and hepatitis. J.A.M.A. 197: 680-684, 1966.

St. Geme, J.W.; Peralta, H.; Farias, E.; Davis, C.W.C. and Noren, G.R.: Experimental gestational mumps virus infection and endocardial fibroelastosis. Pediatrics 48: 821-826, 1971.

St. Geme, J.W.; Davis, C.W.C. and Noren, G.R.: An overview of primary endocardial fibroelastosis and chronic viral cardiomyopathy. Perspectives in Biology and Medicine. Summer: 495-505, 1974.

901 Mycoplasma Pneumonia

There is increasing interest in the role of this organism in spontaneous abortion. Bray and Hackett (1976) reported an infant whose mother had mycoplasma pneumonia at 2 months of gestation. The infant had unexplained hydrocephalus with evidence of intrauterine infection. In addition, pedunculated skin tags of the eyelids, alopecia and punctate skin defects of the scalp were present.

Bray, P.F. and Hackett, T.N.: Multiple birth defects in a newborn exposed to mycoplasma pneumoniae in utero. Am. J. Dis. Child. 130:312-314, 1976.

902 Myesthema gravis

Holmes et al (1980) reported the case of a newborn with congenital contractures. The mother had myesthema gravis during her entire pregnancy. Several similar cases are cited.

Holmes, L.B.; Driscoll, S.G.; Bradley, W.F.: Contractures in a newborn infant of a mother with myesthema gravis. J. Pediat. 96: 1067-1069, 1980.

903 Myleran (see Busulfan)

904 Nafcillin

Schardein (1976) cites Mizutani et al who studied this antibiotic in mice and rats and found no teratogenicity.

Mizutani, M.; Ihara, T.; Kanamori, H.; Takatani, O.; Kaziwara, K.: Influence of sodium nafcillin upon the development of fetuses of mice and rats. Takeda Kenkyusho Ho 29:283-296, 1970.

Schardein, J.L.: Drugs as Teratogens, CRC Press, Cleveland, 1976, p.157.

905 Naphthalene

Van der Hoeve (1913) administered a metabolite of naphthalene, 2-naphthol to pregnant rabbits and found cataracts and retinal damage in the offspring. He gavaged the dams with 1 gm per kg on days 20, 22 and 24 of gestation.

Van der Hoeve, J.: Wirkung von Naphthol auf die und auf fotale Augen. Graele Arch. Ophthal 85:305-315, 1913.

906

906   Naproxen (D-2(6-methoxy-2-naphthyl) proprionic acid)

Wilkinson et al (1979) reported persistent pulmonary hypertension in three prematures born to mothers receiving this prostoglandin synthetase inhibitor.

Wilkinson, A.R.; Aynsley-Green, A.; Mitchell, M.D.: Persistent pulmonary hypertension and abnormal prostoglandin E levels: in preterm infants after maternal treatment with naproxen. Arch. Dis. Childhood 54:942-945, 1979.

907   Naltrexone

Kennedy et al (1975) studied this drug in pregnant rats and rabbits using up to 200 mg per day orally during active organogenesis. No fetal changes or teratogenicity occurred.

Kennedy, G.L.; Smith, S.; Keplinger, M.L. and Calandra, J.C.: Reproductive and teratogenic studies with naltrexone in rats and rabbits. (abstract) Toxicol. Appl. Pharm. 33: 173-174, 1975.

908   Natural Gas (see Methane)

909   Nebularine [9-beta-D-ribofuranosyl-9H-purine]

This compound isolated from mushrooms inhibits tumor cell growth. It was administered to mice in doses of greater than 800 mg per kg (the maternal LD-50) and did not produce fetal defects (Chaube and Murphy, 1968).

Chaube, S. and Murphy, M.L.: The teratogenic effects of the recent drugs active in cancer chemotherapy. In, Woollam, D.H.M. (ed.): Advances in Teratology, Vol. 3. New York: Logos and Academic Press, 1968. pp. 181-237.

910   Nefopam HCL

The analgesic was given orally to pregnant mice and rabbits in maximum doses of 75 or 80 mg per kg per day of active organogenesis and no teratogenic activity was observed (Case et al, 1975).

Case, M.T.; Smith, J.K. and Nelson, R.A.: Reproductive, acute and subacute toxicity studies with nefopam in laboratory animals. Toxicol. Appl. Pharm. 33: 46-51, 1975.

911   Neguvon (Metrifonatum)

Kronevi and Backstrom (1977) have reported a possible connection between maternal treatment with this organophophorous compound and congenital tremor with hypoplasia of the cerebellum in the piglet.

Kronevi, T. and Backstrom, L.: Kongenital tremor
(Skaksjuka) hos gris. Sartryck ur Svensk Veterinartidning
21:837-841, 1977.

912 Neopyrithiamine

This analogue of thiamine was injected into chick eggs in
amounts of 0.25 to 2.0 mg by Naber et al. (1954). Doses
above 0.5 mg were lethal to the embryos if given at the
start or at 5 days of incubation. Injection on the 10th or
15th day produced ataxia, paralysis and polyneuritis in the
hatched chicks. Kosterlitz (1960) administered an unstated
amount to pregnant rats and found fetal weight reduction but
no malformations.

Kosterlitz, H.W.: In, Wolstenholme, G.W.E. and O'Connor,
C.M. (eds.): Ciba Foundation Symposium on Congenital Malformations. Boston: Little Brown, 1960. P. 275 only.

Naber, E.C.; Cravens, W.W.; Baumann, C.A. and Bird, H.R.:
The effect of thiamine analogues on embryonic development
and growth of the chick. J. Nutr. 54: 579-591, 1954.

913 Neosynephrine

Gatling (1962) dropped neosynephrine on the chorio-allantoic
membrane of the chick once on the 10th, 11th or 12th day of
incubation and produced hemorrhages of the head, skin and
extremities.

Gatling, R.R.: The effect of sympathomimetic agents on the
chick embryo. Am. J. Pathol. 40: 113-127, 1962.

914 Nerve Growth Factor

Purified salivary nerve growth factor was injected in
microgm amounts into 7 to 10 day chick embryo yolk sacs and
3 to 4 days later the embryos were shown to have
hypertrophic and hyperplastic sensory and sympathetic nerve
ganglia. The viscera and skin were flooded with nerve
fibers. The same results were found in rat and
embryo-fetuses after maternal injection. Explanted ganglia
of human fetuses also responded to the material with a dense
growth of nerve fibers.

Levi-Montalcini, R. and Cohen, S.: Effects of the extract
of the mouse submaxillary salivary glands on the sympathetic
system of mammals. Ann. N. Y. Acad. Sci. 85: 324-341,
1960.

915 Netilmicin

This aminoglycoside antibiotic was given by Nomura et al
(1982) and Furuhashi et al (1982) to rats and rabbits
intramuscularly in amounts of up to 100 mg per kg daily.
Fertility, teratogenicity and postnatal studies were done in
rats and the only significant finding was reduced fetal

915

weights when 50 or 100 mg per kg was given during
organogenesis. No changes were produced in the rabbit
except for reduced weight of the fetuses at 35 and 100 mg
per kg.

Nomura, A.; Furuhashi, T.; Komura, E.; Uehara, M.; Miyoshi,
K.; Nakayoshi, H.: Reproductive study on Netilmicin in
rats. Japanese J. Antibiotics 35:614-629, 630-642, 1982.

Furuhashi, T.; Nomura, A.; Nakayoshi, H.: Reproductive
study on Netilmicin in rabbits. Japanese J. Antibiotics
35:659-666, 1982.

916 Newcastle Disease Virus

Robertson et al. (1955) inoculated chicken eggs with live
virus at 1.5 to 3.5 days of incubation and found that the
neural tube, lens, auditory vesicles, visceral arches and
limb buds were effected. Cytoplasmic degeneration followed
by nuclear disintegration was seen in the ectodermal tissues
of these structures. Williamson et al (1965) have studied
the pathogenesis of this virus in the chick model.

Robertson, G.G.; Williamson, A.P. and Blattner, R.J.: A
study of abnormalities in early chick embryos inoculated
with Newcastle disease virus. J. Exp. Zool. 129: 5-43,
1955.

Williamson, A.P.; Blattner, R.J. and Robertson, G.G.: The
relationship of viral antigen to virus-induced defects in
chick embryos. Newcastle disease virus. Dev. Biol. 12:
498-519, 1965.

917 Niagra Blue

Beck and Lloyd (1966) have reviewed the chemistry and
experimental work done with this series of azo dyes. Niagra
blue 2B was not teratogenic in experiments on rats by
Beaudoin (1962) but Beck and Lloyd (1966) injecting 150 mg
per kg on the 8.5th day found 25 percent abnormalities.
Doses of 200 mg per kg caused 100 percent resorptions.
Wilson (1955) found that niagra blue 4B and 6B were slightly
teratogenic. The syndrome of malformation is similar to
that seen with trypan blue. Kernis and Marshall (1969) have
shown an effect of niagra 2B on ionic absorption by the yolk
sac.

Beaudoin, A.R.: Interference of niagra 2b with teratogenic
action of trypan blue. Proc. Soc. Exp. Biol. Med. 109:
709-711, 1962.

Beck, F. and Lloyd, J.B.: The teratogenic effects of azo
dyes. In, Woollam, D.H.M. (ed.): Advances in Teratology,
Vol. 1. New York: Logos and Academic Press, 1966. pp.
131-193.

Kernis, M.M. and Johnson, E.M.: Effects of trypan blue and
niagra blue 2B on the in vitro absorption of ions by the rat
visceral yolk sac. J. Embryol. Exp. Morphol. 22:

115-125, 1969.

Wilson, J.G.: Teratogenic activity of several azo dyes chemically related to trypan blue. Anat. Rec. 123: 313-326, 1955.

918 Nialamide [Isonicotinic Acid 2-[2-(benzylcarbamoyl)-ethyl-]-hydrazide]

Tuchmann-Duplessis and Mercier-Parot (1963) maintained female rats on 10 mg per kg per day for 6 to 10 months before gestation. During gestation the same dose of this monoamine oxidase inhibitor was maintained. After weaning the newborns were given 5 mg per kg per day. Although the newborns and young rats showed no external changes, their fertility was markedly reduced and the females had an abnormal tendency to mount each other while refusing to accept males. Reserpine did not produce this effect.

Tuchmann-Duplessis, H. and Mercier-Parot, L.: Modifications du comportement sexual chez des descendants de rats traites par un inhibiteur des monoamine-oxydases. C. R. Acad. Sci. (Paris) 256: 2235-2237, 1963.

919 Nicardipine

Sejima and Sado (1979) gave this vasodilator orally to rats in maximum doses of 100 mg per kg on days 7-17 of gestation and found no adverse fetal effects. Sato et al (1979) gave the same dose before mating to male and female rats and during the first 7 days of gestation and observed no fertility decrease. Treatment on days 17-21 did not adversely affect postnatal function and fertility of the offspring. Rabbits given 150 mg per kg during organogenesis had fetuses which were not different from controls.

Sato, T.; Nagaoka, T.; Fuchigami, K.; Ohsuga, F.; Hatano, M.: Reproductive studies of 2-(N-benzyl-N-methylamino) ethyl methyl 2,6-dimethyl-4-m-nitrophenyl)-1,4-dihydropyridine-3,5-dicarboxylate hydrochloride (YC-93) in rats and rabbits. Kiso to Rinsho 13:1160- 13:1160-1176, 1979.

Sejima, Y.; Sado, T.: Teratological study of 2-(n-benzyl-N-methylamino) ethyl methyl 2,6-dimethyl-4-m-nitrophenyl)-1,4-dihydropyridine-3,5-dicarboxylate hydrochloride (YC-93) in rats. Kiso to Rinsho 13: 1149-1159, 1979.

920 Nickel

Ridgway and Karnofsky (1952) found no defects in chick embryos using the hydrated chloride salt at the estimated LD-50 dose of 0.2 mg on the 4th day of incubation. In a three-generation study of rats fed 5 ppm in their water an increase in number of newborn runts was found by Schroeder and Mitchener (1971). Sunderman et al (1979) produced anophthalmia and microphthalmia in rat fetuses exposed to

0.08 to 0.3 mg of nickel carbonyl per liter of air for 15
minute periods on either day 7 or day 8 of gestation. Very
few extraocular anomalies occurred. Lu et al (1974) found
teratogenic results when they injected pregnant mice with
nickel chloride (1-6.9 mg per kg) on individual days from
the 7th through the 11th day of gestation. Nadeenko et al
(1979) gave nickel in drinking water to rats for 7 months
before pregnancy and during pregnancy and some increase of
preimplantation mortality was found. Some cases of
malformed fetuses were noted.

Lu, C.; Matsumoto, N. and Iijime, S.: Teratogenic effects
of nickel chloride on embryonic mice and its transfer to
embryonic mice. Teratology 19:137-142, 1979.

Nadeenko, V.G.; Lenchenko, B.T.; Arkhipenko, G.A. and
Saichenko, S.P.: Embryotoxic effect of nickel getting by
organism with drinking water. Gig. i Sanit. (USSR)
6:86-88, 1979.

Ridgway, L.P. and Karnofsky, D.A.: The effects of metals
on the chick embryo: toxicity and production of abnormalities in development. Ann. N. Y. Acad. Sci. 55:
203-215, 1952.

Schroeder, H.A. and Mitchener, M.: Toxic effects of trace
elements on the reproduction of mice and rats. Arch.
Environ. Health 23: 102-106, 1971.

Sunderman, F.W.; Allpass, P.R.; Mitchell, J.M.; Basett, R.C.
and Albert, D.M.: Eye malformations in rats: Induction by
prenatal exposure to nickel carbonyl. Science 203:550-553,
1979.

921 Nicotinamide Deficiency (also see 6-Aminonicotinamide)

Although 6-aminonicotinamide, a nicotinamide antagonist, has
been shown to be teratogenic, the effect on fetal development of maternal diets deficient in nicotinamide does not
appear to have been reported. Fratta et al. (1964) fed
rats a diet deficient in nicotinamide and its precursors,
nicotinic acid and tryptophan, from day 2 through day 13 of
gestation and found no viable fetuses. Chlorpromazine or
imipramine protected the fetuses exposed to this regime. No
defects were described.

Fratta, I.; Zak, S.B.; Greengard, P. and Sigg, E.B.: Fetal
death from nicotinamide-deficient diet and its prevention by
chlorpromazine and imipramine. Science 145: 1429-1430,
1964.

922 Nicotine (also see Cigarette Smoking)

Essenberg et al. (1940) reduced the size of rat offspring
by exposing the mothers to nicotine or smoke. Schoeneck
(1941) using rabbits found an increased stillbirth rate and
reduced fetal size. Nishimura and Nakai (1958) produced
skeletal defects and occasional cleft palates in the mouse
fetus when the mother was injected with 25 mg per kg of

nicotine on the 9th, 10th and 11th day. The fetal size was reduced but not statistically so. In the rat Mosier and Armstrong (1964) used 0.05 mg per ml of drinking water and found a reduced size in the newborn. Menges et al. (1970) reported an epidemic of limb deformities in the offspring of swine which fed on tobacco stalks containing 1058 PPM of nicotine and 115 PPM of maleic hydrazide.

Mosier and Jansons (1972) using tritiated-labelled nicotine in mice showed that the substance and its breakdown product cotinine equilibrated at a higher concentration in fetal than in maternal plasma during one period after administration. Sieber and Fabro (1971) observed a 4 fold increase in concentration of nicotine in the rabbit blastocyst.

Essenberg, J.M.; Schwind, J.V. and Patras, A.R.: The effects of nicotine and cigarette smoke on pregnant female albino rats and their offspring. J. Lab. Clin. Med. 25: 708-716, 1940.

Sieber, S.M. and Fabro, S.M.: Identification of drugs in the preimplantation blastocyst and in the plasma, uterine secretion and urine of the pregnant rabbit. J. Pharmacol. and Expt. Therap. 176:65-75, 1971.

Menges, R.W.; Selby, L.A.; Marienfeld, C.J.; Ave, W.A. and Greer, D.L.: A tobacco related epidemic of congenital limb deformities in swine. Environ. Res. 3: 285-302, 1970.

Mosier, H.D. and Armstrong, M.K.: Effects of maternal intake of nicotine on fetal newborn rats. Proc. Soc. Exp. Biol. Med. 116: 956-958, 1964.

Mosier, H.D. and Jansons, R.A.: Distribution and fate of nicotine in the rat fetus. Teratology 6: 303-312, 1972.

Nishimura, H. and Nakai, K.: Developmental anomalies in offspring of pregnant mice treated with nicotine. Science 127: 877-878, 1958.

Schoeneck, F.J.: Cigarette smoking in pregnancy. N. Y. State J. Med. 41: 1945-1948, 1941.

923 Nicotinic Acid

Hansborough (1947) replaced 2 ml of egg white of chick eggs with a solution containing 20 mg of nicotinic acid at 2, 3 or 4 days of incubation. The embryos were found to have a high incidence of neural tube closure defects, abnormal neural development and abnormalities of the cardiovascular system.

Takaori et al (1973) gave 3-(0-methoxyphenoxy)-2-hydroxypropyl nicotinate, a nicotinic acid derivative, orally to pregnant rats and rabbits in doses of 100 or 1,000 mg per kg during the days of active organogenesis. No gross or skeletal defects were found.

Hansborough, L.A.: Effect of increased nicotinic acid in the egg on the development of the chick embryo. Growth 11:

923

177-184, 1947.

Takaori, S.; Usui, H. and Kondo, M.: Studies of a new
nicotinic acid derivative, 3-(0-methoxyphenoxy)-2-hydro-
propyl nicotinate (H-1) teratogenicity in rats and rabbits.
(Japanese) Oyo Yakuri 7: 441-447, 1973.

924 Nicotinic Acid Deficiency [Niacin Deficiency] (see
Nicotinamide Deficiency)

925 Nidroxyzone. [5-Nitro-2-furaldehyde 2-(2-hydroxyethyl-
)-semicarbazone] [Furadroxyl]

Nelson and Steinberger (1953) reported that 1.5 gm per kg of
diet fed to pregnant rats caused termination of pregnancy in
about 70 percent. No comment was made about associated congenital defects. Nomura et al (1975) gave pregnant mice 300
microgm per gm of body weight on day 10 of gestation. An
increase in limb reduction defects was found.

Nelson, W.O. and Steinberger, E.: Failure of pregnancy in
rats treated with furadroxyl. (abstract) Anat. Rec. 115:
352-353, 1953.

Nomura, T.; Kimura, S.; Isa, Y.; Tanaka, H. and Sakamoto,
Y.: Teratogenic and carcinogenic effects of nitrofurazone
on the mouse embryo and new born. (abstract) Teratology 12:
206-207, 1975.

926 Nifurtimox [Lampit-R] [3-Methyl-4-(5-nitrofurfurylidene-
amino)-tetrahydro-4H-1,4-thiazin

NE-1,1-dioxide]

Lorke (1973) tested this drug used in chagas disease in mice
and rats and found no evidence of teratogenicity although at
the highest doses fetal weight was reduced. Doses up to 125
mg per kg were given orally during organogenesis. 600 PPM
in the diet of male rats impaired their fertility.

Lorke, D.: Embryotoxicity studies of fertility and general
reproductive performance. Arzneim-Forsch 22: 1603-1607,
1972.

927 Nilvdipine

Hamada et al (1981) gave this vasodilator orally to mice,
rats and rabbits during their respective organogenesis
periods. Maternal toxicity occurred at 250 mg per kg in the
rats and rabbits. Some increase in fetal deaths occurred in
the rat at 250 mg per kg. No evidence of teratogenic
activity was found in any species. Postnatal studies in the
rat were done and no differences from control were found.

Hamada, Y.; Imanishi, M.; Hashiguchi, M.: Reproductive
study of nilvdipine 1 and 2. Ikukuhin Kenkyu 12:1082-1109,
1981.

928 Niridazole

Fantel et al (1982) found that this antischistosomal agent added directly to an in vitro culture of rat embryos produced right-sided hypoplasia and eye defects at concentrations of 25 and 50 micrograms per ml of medium. Reports of animal studies could not be located.

Fantel, A.G.; Greenaway, J.C.; Walker, E.A.: Axial assymetry resulting from exposure of rat embryos to niridazole in vitro (abstract) Teratology 25:39A, 1982.

929 Nitrilotriacetic Acid [NTA]

This amino acid chelating agent has been recommended as a partial substitute for phosphates as a detergent-building agent. Nolen et al. (1971) have tested the material in rabbits and rats and found no evidence for teratogenicity. The pregnant rats received up to 0.5 percent of NTA in their diet, and the rabbits were intubated with up to 250 mg per kg per day. Negative findings have been observed in the mouse (Tjalve, 1972).

Nolen, G.A.; Klusman, L.W.; Black, D.L. and Buehler, E.U.: Reproduction and teratology of trisodium nitrilotriacetate in rats and rabbits. Food Cosmet. Toxicol. 99: 509-518, 1971.

Tjalve, H.: A study of the distribution and teratogenicity of nitrilotriacetic acid (NTA) in mice. Toxicol. Appl. Pharm. 23: 216-221, 1972.

930 Nitrite

Sleight et al (1972) produced severe toxicosis in pregnant sows with 21 to 35 mg of sodium nitrite per kg subcutaneously. The treatment performed on various single days during the first 100 days of gestation did not produce any fetal defects. Fetal methemoglobin remained at a very much lower level than that in the mother. Globus and Samuel (1978) administered 0.5 mg of sodium nitrite to mice during pregnancy and found no adverse effects. Fetal erythropoiesis was stimulated.

Globus, M. and Samuel, D.: Effect of maternally adminis-tered sodium nitrite on hepatic erythropoiesis in fetal CD-1 mice. Teratology 18: 367-378, 1978.

Sleight, S.D.; Sinha, D.P. and Uzoukwu, M.: Effect of sodium nitrite on reproductive performance of pregnant sows. J.A.V.M.A. 161: 819-823, 1972.

931 2-Nitro-1,4-diaminobenzene

Marks et al (1979) studied the effect of this hair dye in pregnant mice and found at 160 mg per kg daily subcutaneously from days 6 through 15, an increase in cleft palate, resorptions and intrauterine growth retardation.

931

The no effect level was 64 mg per kg per day. Some alizarin red staining spots were found in the heart ventricles of the fetuses.

Marks, T.A.; Gupta, B.N.; Ledoux, T.A.; Staples, R.E.: Teratogenic evaluation of N-nitro-p-phenylenediamine, 4-nitro-0- phenylenediamine and 2,5-toluenediamine sulfate in the mouse. Teratology 24:253-265, 1981.

932 4-Nitro-1,2-diaminobenzene

This hair dye was given subcutaneously to pregnant mice from days 6 through 15 at levels of 256 mg per kg per day and an increase in cleft palate and major blood vessel anomalies were found. Maternal and fetal weights were reduced. At 128 mg per kg no fetal effects occurred.

Marks, T.A.; Gupta, B.N.; Ledoux, T.A.; Staples, R.E.: Teratogenic evaluation of N-nitro-p-phenylenediamine, 4-nitro-0- phenylenediamine and 2,5-toluenediamine sulfate in the mouse. Teratology 24:253-265, 1981.

933 Nitrofen (2,4-Dichlorophenyl)

Francis and Metcalf (1982) administered 18 mg per kg transcutaneously to mice and rats from implantation through organogenesis and produced a high incidence of eye defects. No increase in fetal mortality was found. Kavlock and Gray (1982) gave rats 75 mg per kg orally per day on day 11 and found hydronephrosis and reduced renal function in the offspring.

Francis, B.M.; Metcalf, R.L.: Percutaneous teratogenicity of nitrofen. (abstract) Teratology 25:41A, 1982.

Kavlock, R.J.; Gray, L.E.: Postnatal evaluation of the mophological and functional effects of prenatal nitrofen exposure (abstract) Teratology 25:53A, 1982.

934 Nitrofurantoin

Heinonen et al (1977) list 83 pregnant women who took this medication in the first 4 lunar months and they found 5 malformations which was not a significant increase.

Heinonen, O.P.; Slone, D.; Shapiro, S.: Birth Defects and Drugs in Pregnancy. Publishing Sciences Group, Inc., 1977.

935 Nitrogen Mustard [2,2-Dichloro-N-methyldiethylamine N-oxide Hydrochloride] [Methyl-bis(beta-chloroethyl)amine hydrochloride]

This alkylating agent has been used as a teratogen in rats and mice (see Reviews by Chaube and Murphy, 1968 and kalter, 1968). Skeletal defects, cleft palate, exencephaly and encephalocele have been reported; Kalter has emphasized that many of the neural closure type of defects have occurred following treatment given relatively late in pregnancy, at times when the neural tube is apparently already normally closed. The dose given in the rat is 0.5 to 0.7 mg per kg on the 11th or 12th gestational day. The maternal rat LD-50 is 2.0 mg per kg. Jurand (1961) using electron microscopy has studied histologic changes which occur in the central nervous system. Muller (1966) could produce defects by direct intrauterine injection. Salzgeber (1969) has studied in detail the action of nitrogen mustard on the production of limb defects in the chick embryo. Sanyal et al (1982) exposed rat embryos in vitro to 1-5 micrograms per ml and retarded growth severely.

Chaube, S. and Murphy, M.L.: The teratogenic effects of the recent drugs active in cancer chemotherapy. In, Woollam, D.H.M. (ed.): Advances in Teratology, Vol. 3. New York: Logos and Academic Press, 1968. Pp. 181-237.

Jurand, A.: Further investigations on the cytotoxic and morphogenetic effects of some nitrogen mustard derivatives. J. Embryol. Exp. Morphol. 9: 492-506, 1961.

Kalter, H.: Teratology of the central nervous system. Chicago: University of Chicago Press, 1968. pp. 139-140.

Muller, M.: Does nitrogen mustard affect the foetus directly or secondarily by its effect on the mother? Experientia 22: 247 only, 1966.

Salzgeber, B.: Etude comparative des effets de l'yperite azotee sur les constituants, mesodermique et ectodermique, des bourgeons de membres de l'embryon de poulet. J. Embryol. Exp. Morphol. 22: 373-394, 1969.

Sanyal, M.K.; Kitchin, K.T.; Dixon, R.L.: Rat conceptus development in vitro. Comparative effects of alkalating agents. Toxicol. Appl. Pharmacol. 57:14-19, 1981.

936 Nitroglycerin

Oketani et al (1981) administered up to 4 mg daily on days 6-18 to rabbits and found no adverse fetal effects. Rats were given up to 20 mg per kg intraperitoneally before mating, during organogenesis or during late gestation. No adverse effects were reported.

Oketai, Y.; Mitsuzona, T.; Ichikawa, K.; Itono, Y.; Gojo, T.; Gofuku, M.; Konoha, N.: Teratological studies in rabbits and reproductive and teratological studies in rats. Oyo Yakuri 22:633-648, 737-763, 1981.

937 P-Nitrophenyl-beta-D-xyloside (see Beta-D-xylosides)

938 4-Nitroquinoline 1-oxide

Nomura (1977) injected pregnant mice subcutaneously on day 9, 10 or 11 with 15 micrograms per gm of body weight. At this maximum tolerated dose, no increased malformations or fetal deaths occurred. When one microgram was injected directly into the amniotic cavity on day 11 cleft palate, tail and leg defects were found.

Nomura, T.: Similarity of the mechanism of chemical carcinogen- initiated teratogenesis and carcinogenesis in mice. Cancer Research 37: 969-973, 1977.

939 Nitrosomethylaniline

Alexandrov (1968 and 1973) reported that this carcinogen given to rats intraperitoneally (140 mg per kg) produced an increase in congenital defects in the offspring. The most sensitive days were the 9th and the 13th and the malformations included microophthalmos hydrocephaly, exencephaly and reduction defects of the forelimbs. Nitrosoethylaniline was also teratogenic at 180 mg per kg given on the 9th day.

Alexandrov, V.A.: Effect of N-nitroso-N-methyl-aniline and N-nitroso-N-ethylaniline on the rat embryo. Vop. Onkol. 14: 37-38, 1968.

Alexandrov, V.A.: Embryotoxic and teratogenic effects of chemical carcinogens. in Tomatis, L. and Mohr, U. Eds Transplacental Carcinogenesis. International Agency For Research in Cancer, Lyons, 1973, Pp 112-126.

940 Nitrosoethylenethiourea

Khera and Iverson (1980) gave single oral doses of 120 to 240 mg per kg on day 13 of rat gestation. At the higher doses there was maternal lethality but at 120 and 160 mg per kg hydrocephalus and other defects were found.

Khera, K.S.; Iverson, F.: Hydrocephalus induced by N-nitrosoethylene- thiourea in the progeny of rats treated during gestation. Teratology 21:367-370, 1980.

941 Nitrosourea (see Ethylnitrosourea) (see methylnitrosourea)

942 Nitrous Oxide (see also anesthetics)

Fink et al. (1967) using 50 percent nitrous oxide exposure for 2, 4 or 6 days starting on gestational day 8 produced rib and vertebral defects in nearly all surviving rat fetuses. A low incidence of hydrocephalus, cardiac and renal defects was observed. In later work 24-hour exposure on day 9 to 70 percent nitrous oxide was shown to produce the greatest number of defects (Shepard and Fink, 1968). Gofmecler et al (1977) using an exposure of 0.34-0.8 mg per cubic meter during the entire gestation produced some developmental anomalies and increased number of non viable rat fetuses. Rector and Eastwood (1964) and Smith et al. (1965) have shown that nitrous oxide causes lethality in chick eggs. Mazze et al (1982) found no reproductive ill effects in male mice treated for long periods.

Cohen et al (1980) analyzed questionnaires from 30,650 dentists and 30,547 chairside assistants. The chairside assistants reported a rate of 19 abortions among heavy users while the non-users had a rate of 8. In the same group there were 7.7 percent defects compared to 3.6 percent in the controls. These defects were mainly of the nervous and musculoskeletal systems.

Lane et al (1980) exposed rats on day 9 to 70-75 percent nitrous oxide and found increased malformations. Xenon, another anesthetic, did not produce defects.

Cohen, E.N.; Brown, B.W.; Wu, M.L.; Whitcher, C.E.; Brodsky, J.B.; Gift, H.C.; Greenfield, W.; Jones, T.W.; Driscoll, E.J.: Occupational decrease in dentistry and chronic exposure to trace anesthetic gases. J. Am. Dent. Ass. 101:21-31, 1980

Fink, B.R.; Shepard, T.H. and Blandau, R.J.: Teratogenic activity of nitrous oxide. Nature 214: 146-148, 1967.

Gofmecler, V.A.; Brekhman, I.I.; Golotin, V.G.; Sheparev, A.A.; Krivelevich, E.B.; Kamynina, L.N.; Dobryakova, A.I. and Gonenko, V.A.: Embryotoxic effect of nitrous dioxide and atmosphere pollution. Gigiena i Sanitariya (USSR) 12:22-25, 1977.

Lane, G.A.; Nahrwold, M.L.; Taylor-Busch, M.; Cohen, P.J.: Anesthetics as teratogens: Nitrous oxide is fetotoxic, Xenon is not. Science 210:899-901, 1980.

Mazze, R.I.; Wilson, A.I.; Rice, S.A.; Braden, J.M.: Reproduction and fetal development in mice chemically exposed to nitrous oxide. Teratology 26:11-16, 1982.

Rector, G.H.M. and Eastwood, D.W.: The effects of an atmosphere of nitrous oxide and oxygen on the incubating chick. Anesthesiology 25: 109 only, 1964.

Shepard, T.H. and Fink, B.R.: Teratogenic activity of nitrous oxide in rats. In, Fink, B.R. (ed.): Toxicity of Anesthetics. Baltimore: Williams and Wilkins, 1968. pp. 308-323.

Smith, B.E.; Gaub, M.L. and Moya, F.: Teratogenic effects of anesthetic agents: nitrous oxide. Anesth. Analg. (Cleve) 44: 726-732, 1965.

943 Noise [See Emotional Stress]

944 Nonachlazine

Smolnikova and Strekalova reported that nonachlazine given orally to rats from day 1 through day 17 of pregnancy in a dose of 35 mg per kg (one-eighth LD-50) produced no adverse effect on embryogenesis.

Smolnikova, N.M. and Strekalova, S.N.: Results of studies on embryotoxic and teratogenic action of nonachlazine.

944

Formakol. i. Toksokol. (USSR) 42.3:302-303, 1979.

945 Nonachlazine

Smolnikova and Strekalova reported that nonachlazine given orally to rats from day 1 through day 17 of pregnancy in a dose of 35 mg per kg (one-eighth LD-50) produced no adverse effect on embryogenesis.

Smolnikova, N.M. and Strekalova, S.N.: Results of studies on embryotoxic and teratogenic action of nonachlazine. Farmakol. i Toksikol. (USSR) 42.3:302-303, 1979.

946 Nonoxynol-9 (Vaginal spermicides)

This non-ionic surfactant commonly used in vaginal spermicidal formulations was studied in the rat by intravaginal application of 4 and 40 mg per kg on days 6 through 15 of gestation (Abrutyn et al, 1982). No maternal or fetal changes were observed. In similar experiments up to 400 mg per kg produced no fetal effects (Shiota and Shepard, unpublished data). Buttar (1982) has shown that 44 percent of the intravaginal dose is absorbed.

Jick et al (1982) have observed a rate of 5.8 percent for early spontaneous abortion among vaginal spermicide users while among oral contraceptive users and those who used nothing the rate was 3.1 and 3.3 percent respectively. A higher proportion of recovered abortuses were abnormal in the spermicide user group. Other factors in reproduction of the spermicide user could easily account for these differences. Polednak et al (1982) compared the offspring of 302 women using spermicides to those of 715 women using no contraceptives. The exposed female newborns were lighter and a non-significant increase in hypospadias and limb reduction defects occurred in the user's group.

Abrutyn, D.; McKenzie, B.E.; Nadaskay, N.: Teratology study of intravaginally administered nonoxynol-9 containing contraceptive cream in rats. Fertility and Sterility 37:113-117, 1982.

Buttar, H.S.: Transvaginal absorption and disposition of nonoxynol-9 in gravid rats. Toxicol. Letters 13:211-216, 1982.

Jick, H.; Shiota, K.; Shepard, T.H.; Hunter, J.R.; Stergachis, A.; Madsen, S.; Porter, J.B.: Vaginal spermicides and miscarriage seen primarily in the emergency room. Teratogenesis, Mutagenesis and Carcinogenesis. 2:205-210, 1982.

Polednak, A.P.; Janerich, D.T.; Glebatis, D.M.: Birthweight and birth defects in relation to maternal spermicide use. Teratology 26:27-38, 1982.

947 Noradrenalin

Pitel and Lerman (1962) injected 25 microgm of noradrenalin
directly into rat fetuses at 16 or 17 days of gestation and
produced a 50 percent incidence of cataract. The mechanism
of action was postulated to be by spasm of the hyoid
arteries. Similar results were obtained using adrenalin.

Pitel, M. and Lerman, S.: Studies on the fetal rat lens.
Effects of intrauterine adrenalin and noradrenalin. Invest.
Ophthalmol. 1: 406-412, 1962.

948 Norchlorcyclizine (also see Meclizine)

This antihistamine belongs to the benzhydrylpiperazine
series of compounds. It is the teratogenically active
breakdown product of several other compounds, and the
experimental studies in rats are described more fully under
meclizine. Wilk (1969) applied this substance directly over
the amniotic sac of the rat and produced cleft palates.

Wilk, A.L.: Production of fetal rat malformations by
norchlorcyclizine and chlorcyclizine after intrauterine
application. Teratology 2: 55-66, 1969.

949 Norea
(1-[5-(3a,4,5,6,7,7a-hexahydro-4,7-methanoindanyl]-3,3-dimethyl
urea)

This organophosphate cholinesterase inhibitor was tested by
Robens (1969) in hamsters using 2000 mg per kg by mouth on
days 6 through 8 and no adverse effect on reproduction were
found.

Robens, J.F.: Teratologic studies of carbaryl, diazinon,
norea, disulfiram and thiram in small laboratory animals.
Toxicol. Appl. Pharm. 15:152-163, 1969.

950 Norepinephrine

Gatling (1962) dropped norepinephrine on the
chorio-allantoic membranes of the chick once on the 10th,
11th or 12th day of incubation and produced cephalic, skin
and extremity hemorrhages.

Gatling, R.R.: The effect of sympathomimetic agents on the
chick embryo. Am. J. Pathol. 40: 113-127, 1962.

951 Norethandrolone (see 17-Alpha-ethinyl-19-nor-testosterone)

952 Norethynodrel (see Oral Contraceptives)

953 Norfloxacin

Irikura et al (1981) gave this chemotherapeutic agent orally
to rats and rabbits during organogenesis. Maximum doses of
500 in rats and 100 mg per kg in rabbits failed to produce

953

any increase in defects. At 100 mg per kg in the rabbit there was embryolethality.

Irikura et al (1981) gave up to 500 mg per kg daily before mating and during the first 6 days of gestation, on days 6-15 and on days 15 through the 21st postnatal day in the mouse. No adverse effects were found on fertility, the fetuses or on the postnatal function of the offspring.

Irikura, T.; Imada, O.; Suzuki, H.; Abe, Y.: Teratological study of 1-ethyl-6-fluoro-1,4-dihydro-4-oxo-7-(1-piperazinly)-3-quinolinecarboxilic acid (AM-715). Kiso to Rinsho 15: 5251-5263, 1981.

Irikura, T.; Suzuki, H.; Sugimoto, T.: Reproductive studies of AM-715. Chemotherapy 29:886-894, 895-914, 915-931, 1981.

954 Normethandrone (see 17 Alpha-ethinyl-testosterone)

955 Occupation (see solvents, also)

The teratogenesis of occupational chemicals has been reviewed. (Hemminki et al, 1980; Hemminki, 1980; and Hunt, 1977). A preliminary report shows some increase in defects of the abdominal wall of infants born to mothers in the printing industry (Erickson, 1978)

Peters et al (1981) reported an increase in the rate of brain tumors among the offspring of mothers exposed to chemicals, fathers exposed to solvents and fathers employed in the aircraft industry. The 92 cases were carefully matched but not to children with congenital health problems.

Erickson, J.D.; Cochran, W.M.; Anderson, C.E.: Birth defects and printing. Lancet 1:385 (only) 1978.

Hemminki, K.: Occupational chemicals tested for teratogenicity. Int. Arch. Occupational Environ. Health 47:191-207, 1980.

Hemminki, K.; Mutanen, P.; Luoma, K.; Saloniemi, I.: Congenital malformations by parental occupation in Finland. Int. Arch. Occup. Environ. Health 46:93-98, 1980.

Hunt, V.R.: Work and the Health of Women, CRC Press, Boca Raton, Florida, 1979.

Peters, J.M.; Preston-Martin, S.; Yu, M.C.: Brain tumors in children and occupational exposure of parents. Science 213:235-237, 1981.

956 Ochratoxin A

This mycotoxin was studied in pregnant mice by Hayes et al (1974). Intraperitoneal injection with 5 mg per kg on one of gestation days 7 through 12 resulted in fetal growth retardation and malformations. Exencephaly and anomalies of the eyes, face, digits and tail were found most commonly. Hood et al (1976) found teratogenicity in hamsters using 5 to 20 mg per kg intraperitoneally on days 7, 8 or 9.

Hayes, A.W.; Hood, R.D. and Lee, H.L.: Teratogenic effects of ochratoxin A in mice. Teratology 9: 93-98, 1974.

Hood, R.D.; Naughton, M.J.; Hayes, A.W.: Perinatal effects of ochratoxin A in hamsters. Teratology 13:1-14, 1976.

957 Alph-olefin Sulfonate (also see Surfactants)

958 Oral Contraceptives [Contraceptives, Oral]

No increase in congenital defect rate has been shown in the offspring of 1250 women having used oral contraceptives (Robinson, 1971). Similar negative findings were reported in 5,530 pregnancies reported to the Royal College of General Practitioners (1976). Janerich et al (1974) found a higher incidence of oral contraceptive users among mothers of children with limb defects and all these children were males. Jaffe et al (1975) did not observe an increase in inadvertent oral contraception continuance in seven cases where limb reduction was found. Nora and Nora (1973) have suggested that congenital heart disease was more common in pregnancies during which birth control pills were continued. Heinonen et al (1976) studied 1042 women who received female hormones during early pregnancy and found a heart defect rate of 18 per 1000 which was compared to a control of 7.8 per 1000. After controlling the data for confounding factors, the difference was significant at the probability level of 0.05. Savolainen et al (1981) reported no significant differences in malformation rates among 800 users as compared to matched controls. Harlap et al studied prospectively 11,468 pregnancies in Israel and found 5 with heart disease when the expected rate was 2.6. Neither limb reduction nor esophageal atresia occurred in the studied group. Goujard and Rumeau-Rouquette (1971) reported on a prospective study of 830 women receiving mostly hormonal pregnancy tests. General malformation rates, limb and heart defects were not increased but a microcephaly rate of 3.4 per 1000 as compared to a control of 0.6 was found. Ferencz et al (1980) studied mothers of 110 children with heart disease and found no association with maternal hormone therapy. Reports which did not find significantly associated teratogenicity are available (Mulvihill et al, 1974; Yasuda and Miller, 1975; Rothman et al, 1979). A Well balanced discussion of this important unsolved problem has been published (Anonymous, 1974, Yerushalmy, 1972).

Janerich et al (1980) have listed 18 papers reporting the rate of malformation in the offspring of women exposed to oral contraceptives. Approximately one-half found no increase. Wilson and Brent (1981) reviewed the literature and concluded there was no proof that exogenous sex hormones produce non genital malformations. Schardein (1980) has reviewed the clinical data on birth defects and hormones during pregnancy and concludes there is little hazard.

958

Carr (1967) reported six abnormal karyotypes in eight
specimens from mothers previously taking oral
contraceptives; the overall incidence and especially that of
triploidy was significantly higher than that found in
abortuses of mothers not taking contraceptives. Boue (1970)
reporting on studies from 333 unselected spontaneous abortions found a 61.6 percent incidence of abnormal chromosomes
with no increase in abortuses from mothers who took oral
contraceptives. Boue observed a much higher incidence of
abnormal karyotypes in the younger specimens and pointed out
that the apparent increase in Carr's series may have been
related to the presence of older specimens in the control
group. Nelson et al. (1971) and Dhadial et al. (1970)
also failed to observe an increase in abnormal karyotypes
from abortuses of mothers taking contraceptives. Boue et al
(1975) have reported no increase in chromosome aberrations
among 520 spontaneous abortions following the use of birth
control pills. Janerich et al (1976) found no increase in
oral contraception use among 103 mothers giving birth to
children with Down's syndrome. Jagiello and Lin (1974)
studied the effect of a large number of oral contraceptives
on the oocyte of several species. In over 175 human ova
from oral-contraceptive-taking women about one-third divided
in vitro a result similar to the control group. Poland and
Ash (1973) found a significantly higher incidence of
'disorganized' abortuses from women who took oral
contraceptives as compared to women using other forms of
contraception.

Tuchmann-Duplessis and Mercier-Parot (1972) using 1 mg per
kg per day of both norethyndrel and mestranol in the rat
either before or during gestation observed no congenital
defects. Treatment during two generations did not cause any
functional or histologic abnormalities of the fetal genital
tracts.

Anonymous: Synthetic sex hormones and infants. Brit. Med.
J. 4: 485-486, 1974.

Boue, J.: Etude chromosomique des avortements spontanes
apres inhibition physiologique or therapeutique de
l'ovulation. In, Netter, A. (ed.): L'inhibition De
L'ovulation. Paris: Masson, 1970. pp. 349-356.

Boue, J.; Boue, A. and Lazar, P.: Retrospective and
prospective epidemiological studies of 1500 karyotyped
spontaneous human abortions. Teratology 12: 11-26, 1975.

Carr, D.H.: Chromosomes after oral contraceptives. Lancet
2: 830-831, 1967.

Dhadial, R.K.; Machin, A.M. and Tait, S.M.: Chromosomal a-
nomalies in spontaneously aborted human fetuses. Lancet 2:
20-21, 1970.

Ferencz, C.; Matanoski, G.M.; Wilson, P.D.; Rubin, J.D.;
O'Neill, C.A.; Gutberlet, R.: Maternal hormone therapy and
congenital heart disease. Teratology 21:225-239, 1980.

Goujard, J. and Rumeau-Rouquette, C.: First trimester
exposure to progestagenoestrogen and congenital abnormali-

ties. Lancet 1:482-483, 1977.

Harlap, S.; Prywes, R. and Davies, A.M.: Birth defects and oestrogens and progesterones in pregnancy. Lancet 1: 682-683, 1975.

Heinonen, O.P.; Slone, D.; Monson, R.R.; Hook, E.B. and Shapiro, S.: Cardiovascular birth defects in antenatal exposure to female sex hormones. New Eng. J. Med. 296:67- 70, 1976.

Jaffe, P.; Liberman, M.M.; McFadyen, I. and Valman, H.B.: Incidence of congenital limb-reduction deformities. Lancet 1: 526-527, 1975.

Jagiello, G. and Lin, J.S.: Oral contraceptive compounds and mammalian oocyte meiosis. Am. J. Obstet. Gynec. 120: 390-406, 1974.

Janerich, D.T.; Flink, E.M. and Keogh, M.D.: Down's syndrome and oral contraceptive usage. Brit. J. Obstet. Gynecol. 8:617-620, 1976.

Janerich, D.T.; Piper, J.M. and Glebatis, D.M.: Oral contraceptives and congenital limb reduction defects. N. Eng. J. Med. 291: 697-700, 1974.

Janerich, E.T.; Piper, E.M.; Glebatis, D.M.: Oral contraceptives and birth defects. Am. J. Epidem. 112:73-79, 1980.

Levy, E.P.; Cohen, A. and Fraser, F.C.: Hormone treatment during pregnancy and congenital heart disease. Lancet 1: 611 (only), 1973.

Mulvihill, J.J.; Mulvihill, C.G. and Neill, C.A.: Congenital heart defects and prenatal sex hormones. Lancet 1:1168, 1974.

Nelson, T.; Oakley, G.P. and Shepard, T.H.: A centralized laboratory for collection of human embryos and fetuses: Seven years experience: II. Classification and tabulation of conceptual wastage with observations on type of malformations, sex ratio and chromosome studies. In, Hook, E.B.; Janerich, D.T. and Porter, I.H. (eds.): Monitoring, Birth Defects and Environment, The Problem of Surveillance. New York: Academic Press, 1971. pp. 45-81.

Nora, J.J. and Nora, A.H.: Can the pill cause birth defects? New Eng. J. Med. 291: 731-732, 1974.

Poland, B.J. and Ash, K.A.: The influence of recent use of an oral contraceptive on early intrauterine development. Am. J. Obstet. Gynecol. 116: 1138-1142, 1973.

Robinson, S.C.: Pregnancy outcome following oral contraceptives. Am. J. Obstet. Gynecol. 109: 354-358, 1971.

Rothman, K.J.; Fyler, D.C.; Goldblatt, A. and Kreidberg, M.B.: Exogenous hormones and other drug exposures of

958

children with congenital heart disease. Am. J.
Epidemiology 109:433-439, 1979.

Royal Coll. of Gen. Pract.: The outcome of pregnancy in
former contraceptive users. Brit. J. Obstet. Gynecol.
83:608-616, 1976.

Savolainen, E.; Saksela, E.; Saxen, L.: Teratogenic hazards
of oral contraceptives analyzed in the National Register.
Am. J. Obst. & Gynecol. 140:521-524, 1981.

Schardein, J.L.: Congenital abnormalities and hormones
during pregnancy: A clinical review. Teratology 22:251-270,
1980.

Shapiro, S.; Slone, D.: Effects of Exogenous female
hormones on the fetus. Epidemiologic Reviews 1:110-123,
1979.

Tuchmann-Duplessis, H. and Mercier-Parot, L.: Action d'un
steroide anticonceptionnel sur la descendance. J. Gynecol.
Obstet. Biol. Repr. 1: 141-159, 1972.

Wilson, J.G.; Brent, R.L.: Are female sex hormones
teratogenic? Am. J. Obst. & Gynecol. 141:567-580, 1981.

Yasuda, M. and Miller, J.R.: Prenatal exposure to oral
contraceptives and transposition of the great vessels in
man. Teratoloy 12:239-244, 1975.

Yerushalmy, J.: Methodologic problems encountered in
investigating the possible teratogenic effects of drugs, in
Drugs and Fetal Development, edited by Klingberg, M.A.;
Abramovici, A. and Chemke, J.; Plenum Press, New York,
1972, pp. 427-440.

959 Oxacillin

Korzhova et al (1981) gave rats 40,000 units orally on the
4th through 13th day of gestation. Growth retardation,
mortality and hemorrhages of the brain and kidneys were
increased in the treated fetuses. No disturbances of
central nervous system function were found in the living
young.

Korzhova, V.V.; Lisitsyna, N.T.; Mikhailova, E.G.: Effect
of ampicillin and oxacillin on fetal and neonatal
development. Bull Exp. Biol. Med. (USSR) 91:169-171,
1981.

960 Oxolamine [5-(2-Diethyl-aminoethyl)-3-phenyl-1,2,4-oxadiazo-
le Citrate]

This antiinflammatory drug was tested in pregnant mice by
Nilsson (1967). No significant gross defects occurred with
2 mg daily injections although some increase in number of
ribs and abnormal centers in the sternum occurred in the
treatment and sham injected groups.

Nilsson, L.: Teratogenic studies on mice with an antiphlogistic substance, 5-(2-diethyl-aminoethyl-)-3-phenyl-1,2,4-oxadiazole citrate. Arzn. Forsch. 17: 781-782, 1967.

961 Delta-hydroxy-gamma-oxo-L-norvaline

This asparagine analogue was studied by Mizutani and Ihara (1973) in mice, rats, hamsters and rabbits. The minimal dose by mouth or intraperitoneally that produced defects in rats and rabbits was 500 mg per kg and 1000 mg per kg in mice and hamsters. In all species digital defects were produced. In addition, neural tube closure defects and cleft palate were produced in mice and rats, hydrocephalus in hamsters and cleft palate in rabbits.

Mizutani, M. and Ihara, T.: Teratogenicity of delta-hydro-xy-gamma-oxo-L-norvaline. 1. Studies in mice, rats, hamsters and rabbits. (abstract). Teratology 8: 99 (only), 1973.

962 Oxomemazine (see Phenothiazines)

963 Oxonate, Potassium

Gralla et al (1975) used this uricase inhibitor in the diet of pregnant mice and rats in amounts of 3 percent of the diet and found embryolethality. A low incidence of congenital defects was found when sodium urate injections were added to the treatment.

Gralla, E.J.; Crelin, E.S. and Osbald, G.W.: The embryotoxic effects of a uricase inhibitor and IV sodium urate in rats and mice (abstract). Teratology 11: 19a (only), 1975.

964 Oxophenarsine Hydrochloride [Mapharsen-R]

Mosher (1938) administered ten 1 mg doses in 9 hours to a pregnant guinea pig. Hemorrhages in the fetal scala vestibuli and vestibule were found.

Mosher, H.P.: Does animal experimentation show similar changes in the ear of the mother and fetus after the ingestation of quinine by the mother? Laryngoscope 48: 361-395, 1938.

965 Oxygen (see Hyperoxia) (see Hypoxia)

966 5-Oxymethyl Uracil

Kosmachevskaya and Tichodeeva (1968) injected 4 mg of this substance into chick eggs at 24 hours of incubation and found no lethal effect but 15 percent of the embryos had malformations which included microphthalmia, rumplessness, beak and skeletal defects and celosomia.

Kosmachevskaya, E.A. and Tichodeeva, I.I.: Relation between embryotoxic activity of some pyrimidine derivatives and their chemical structure. Chick embryo test. Pharmacol. Toxicol. (Russian) No. 5: 618-620, 1968.

967 Oxytetracycline [Terramycin-R]

This antibiotic is capable of crossing the placenta and causing staining of the deciduous teeth. It stains to a lesser degree than tetracycline (Baden, 1970).

Baden, E.: Environmental pathology of the teeth. In, Gorlin, R.J. and Goldman, H.M. (eds.): Oral Pathology, Vol. 1. St. Louis: C.V. Mosby, 1970. P. 190 only.

968 Oxythiamine

This analogue of thiamine was used by Naber et al. (1955) in the chick. With 0.25 to 2.0 mg injected at the start or after 5 days of incubation a high mortality was found. Hemorrhage, edema and abdominal hernias were found in the dying embryos.

Naber, E.C.; Cravens, W.W.; Baumann, C.A. and Bird, H.R.: The effect of thiamine analogues on embryonic development and growth of the chick. J. Nutr. 54: 579-591, 1954.

969 Ozone

Kavlock et al (1979) exposed rats to up to 1.97 ppm during parts or all of organogenesis and produced no defects in the offspring. Resorption rates were increased. Veninga (1967) reported blepharophimosis and jaw anomalies in mouse fetuses exposed in utero to 0.2 ppm for 7 hours five days a week.

Kavlock, R.; Daston, G. and Grabowski, C.T.: Studies on the developmental toxicity of ozone 1. Prenatal effects. Toxicol. Appl. Pharmacol. 48: 19-28, 1979.

Veninga T.S.: Toxicity of ozone in comparison with ionizing radiation. Strahlentherapie 134:469- 477, 1967.

970 Palladium

Ridgway and Karnofsky (1952) tested the chloride salt in chick eggs and found it non-teratogenic. The LD-50 was greater than 20 mg per egg on the 4th day of incubation.

Ridgway, L.P. and Karnofsky, D.A.: The effects of metals on the chick embryo: Toxicity and production of abnormalities in development. Ann. N. Y. Acad. Sci. 55: 203-215, 1952.

971 Palm Oil

Singh (1980) gave this food substance which contains carotene (32-48 mg per 100 ml) to rats in amounts of 1-3 ml daily on days 5 through 15 of pregnancy. Exencephaly was found at 1,2 and 3 mg levels. At 3 mg levels eye defects and cleft palate occurred.

Singh, J.D.: Palm oil induced congenital anomalies in rats. Cong. Anom. 139-142, 1980.

972 Palmotoxin

Bassir and Adekunle (1970) injected chick eggs with 0.2 to 0.6 microgm of the B(O) form and 2.0 to 6.3 microgm of the G(O) form and observed an increased death rate and twisting of the lower extremities, crossed beak and roughness of plumage.

Bassir, O. and Adekunle, A.: Teratogenic action of aflatoxin B(1), palmotoxin B(O) and palmotoxin G(O) on the chick embryo. J. Pathol. 102: 49-51, 1970.

973 Paludrine-R

Dyban et al. (1966) using 5 to 30 mg of paludrine between days 8 to 13 detected no toxic or teratogenic effect in the offspring of rats.

Dyban, A.P.; Udalova, L.D. and Akimova, I.M.: Correlation between teratogenic activity and chemical structure of drugs. Experiments with chloridine and paludrine. Dokl. Acad. Sci. of U.S.S.R. (Russian) 167: No. 1, 228-231, 1966.

974 Pantothenic Acid Deficiency

Kalter and Warkany (1959) reviewed and summarized the literature about this experimental model in rodents. Boisselot (1948) was the 1st to feed a pantothenic acid-deficient diet and observe defective rat offspring. Nearly all organ systems can be effected, and a deficiency lasting 36 hours during active embryogenesis may produce specific defects (Nelson et al.; 1957). A dietary level in the rat below 10 microgm per day produces complete litter resorption, while a level of 20 to 25 microgm produces a large number of defective offspring; the minimal amount required to prevent fetal defects in the rat is 50 microgm (Giroud et al.; 1954; Lefebvres, 1954). Three chemical antagonists have been used to augment the deficiency state (X-methylpantothenic, sodium omega methyl pantothenic and pantoyltaurine).

Boisselot, J.: Malformations congenitales provoquees chez le rat par une insuffisance en acide pantothenique du regime maternel. C. R. Soc. Biol. (Paris) 142: 928-929, 1948.

Giroud, A.; Levy, G. and Lefebvres, J.: Recherches sur le taux de l'acide pantothenique chez les meres et les foetus normaux et chez les meres carencees. Int. Z.

974

Vitaminforschung 25: 148–153, 1954.

Kalter, H. and Warkany, J.: Experimental production of congenital malformations in mammals by metabolic procedure. Physiol. Rev. 39: 69–115, 1959.

Lefebvres, J.: Influence d'une deficience pantothenique legere sur les resultats de la gestation chez la ratte. C. R. Acad. Sci. (Paris) 238: 2123–2125, 1954.

Nelson, M.M.; Wright, H.V.; Baird, C.D.C. and Evans, H.M.: Teratogenic effects of pantothenic acid deficiency in the rat. J. Nutr. 62: 395–406, 1957.

975 Pantoylaurine

This pantothenic acid antagonist has been used by Zunin and Borrone to produce defects in the offspring of treated rats.

They used 0.5 to 1.5 mg by injection daily during various periods of gestation. The syndrome of defects resembled that seen with pantothenic acid deficiency. Generalized edema, hemorrhage and neural tube closure defects were seen.

Zunin, C. and Borrone, C.: Embriopatie da carenza di acido pantotenico. Acta Vitaminol. Enzymol. (Milano) 8: 263–268, 1954.

976 Papaverine

Neural tube closure defects have been found in the chick after culture in medium containing 50 micrograms per ml of medium (Lee and Nagele, 1979).

Lee, H.; Nagele, R.G.: Neural tube closure defects caused by papaverine in explanted early chick embryos. Teratology 20:321– 332, 1979.

977 Paradimethylaminobenzene

Pizzarello and Ford (1968) injected chick eggs at 48 hours of incubation with 6 mg of this carcinogen and produced shortening of the legs and feather defects in the survivors.

Pizzarello, D.J. and Ford, R.V.: Effects of paradimethyl-aminoazobenzene and the antioxidant N,N-diphenyl-P-phenylene diamine in developing chicks. Experientia 24: 621–622, 1968.

978 Paramethadione (see Trimethadione)

979 Paraquat [1,1-Dimethyl-4,4-dipyridilium Dichloride]

This herbicide was given to hens in their drinking water at a concentration of 40 ppm and about 0.1 ppm was found in their eggs (Fletcher, 1967). A small but significant

979

increase in the number of abnormal eggs was found in the treated group. The type of defect was not described. Khera et al. (1970) reported a small increase in incidence of costal cartilage defects in the offspring of rats injected with 0.5 mg per kg per day.

Fletcher, K.: Production and viability of eggs from hens treated with paraquat. Nature 215: 1407-1408, 1967.

Khera, K.S.; Whitta, L.L. and Clegg, D.J.: Embryopathic effects of diquat and paraquat. In, Deichmann, W.B.; Radomski, J.L. and Penalver, R.A. (eds.): Pesticides Symposia, Interamerican Congress on Toxicology and Occupational Medicine. Miami: Halos and Ass. Inc.; 1970. pp. 257-261.

980 Parathion (Diethyl-0-4-nitrophenyl Phosphorothiote)

Fish (1966) gave rats 3.8 mg per kg on days 8, 9, 15 or 16 of gestation and found no abnormalities in the offspring. The perinatal death rate was increased and some subcutaneous hemorrhages were found. The weight gain post-delivery was slower in the treated group. Fetal cerebral cortical cholinesterase was decreased. Postnatal studies in the mouse exposed prenatally to 3 mg per kg were negative (Al-Hachim and Fink, 1968).

Al-Hatchim, G.M.; Fink, G.B.: Effect of DDT or parathion on condition avoidance response from DDT or parathion treated mothers. Psychopharmacologia 12:424-427, 1968.

Fish, S.A.: Organophosphorus cholinesterase inhibitor and fetal development. Am. J. Obstet. Gynecol. 96: 1148-1154, 1966.

981 Passiflora Incarnata Extract

Hirakawa et al (1981) fed up to 400 mg per kg to rats on days 7-17 and found no adverse fetal effects.

Girakawa, T.; Suzuki, T.; Sano, Y.; Kamata, T.; Nakamura, M.: Reproductive studies of Passiflora Incarnata extract. Teratological study. Kiso to Rinsho 15:3431-3451, 1981.

982 Patulin

This mycotoxin was given in doses of up to 2.0 mg per kg on days 6 through 17 to mice and although fetal weight reduction occurred, no teratogenicity was detected.

Reddy, C.S.; Chan, P.K. and Hayes, A.W.: Teratogenicity and dominant lethal studies of patulin in mice. Toxicology 11:219-223, 1978.

983 PCB (see Kanechlor)

page 331

984   Penbutolol Sulfate

This beta adrenergic blocker was administered orally to mice
at doses of 6 to 60 mg per day. Dosing before mating,
during organogenesis or on the last portion of gestaion had
no adverse effect on the fetuses. Behavioral studies were
also negative (Sagisaki et al, 1981).

Sagisaki, T.; Takagi, S.; Seshimo, M.; Hayashi, S.;
Miyamoto, M.: Reproductive studies of penbutolol sulfate
given orally to mice. Oyo Yakuri 22:289-305, 1981.

985   Penfluridol   (4-(4-chloro,alpha,alpha,alpha-trifluoro-m-
tolyl)-1-(4,4,bis(p-fluorophenyl)butyl)-4-piperidinol)

Asano et al (1979) gave orally 0.5 to 8 mg per kg to rats on
days 15 through 20 of gestation. At doses of 2 mg per kg
and above an increase in stillbirths and a decrease in body
weight and neonatal survival were found.

Asano, Y.; Ariyuki, F.; Higaki, K.: Peri and postnatal
studies of penfluridol (TLP-607) in rats. Oyo Yakuri
17:849-857, 1979.

986   D-Penicillamine

A single case report of a newborn with signs of
Ehlers-Danlos syndrome has been recorded following administration of large doses of penicillamine (2,000 mg per day)
to a mother with cystinuria (Mjolnerod et al.; 1971).
Solomon et al (1977) reported that a woman with rheumatoid
arthritis receiving 900 mg per day until the 16th week of
gestation gave birth to a 2,000 gm infant with lax skin,
inguinal hernias and flexion contractures of the knees and
hips. The infant died of an undiagnosed abdominal
obstruction.

Scheinberg and Sternlieb (1975) have summarized 29 pregnancies in women being treated for Wilson's disease with
approximately 1000 mg of penicillamine per day and they
reported no adverse fetal effects. The possibility has been
raised that in Wilson's disease the effective penicillamine
exposure is reduced due to its loss in the urine.

Merker et al (1975) have observed skeletal alterations in
rat fetuses whose mothers received 200 mg per animal
intraperitoneally on days 15 through 19. Rib fusions,
incomplete mineralization and swelling of collagen fibrils
was found. Kilbourn and Hess gavaged rats on days 9-14 of
gestation with 250 mg per kg and found tracheobronchomegaly
in 40 percent of the offspring. Yamada et al (1979) found
no increase in defects after giving 500 mg per kg orally to
rats.

Kilbourn, K.H.; Hess, R.A.: Neonatal deaths and pulmonary
dysplasia due to d-penicillamine in the rat. Teratology
26:1-9, 1982.

Merker, H.J.; Franke, L. and Gunther, T.: The effect of

D-penicillamine on skeletal development of rat foetuses. Naunyn Schmiedbergs Arch. Pharm. 287:359-376, 1975.

Mjolnerod, O.K.; Rassmussen, K.; Dommerud, S.A. and Gjeruldsen, S.T.: Congenital connective-tissue defect probably due to penicillamine treatment in pregnancy. Lancet 1: 673-675, 1971.

Scheinberg, I.H. and Sternlieb, I.: Pregnancy in penicillamine-treated patients with Wilson's disease. N. Engl. J. Med. 293:1300-1302, 1975.

Solomon, L.; Abrams, G.; Dinner, M. and Berman, L.: Neonatal abnormalities associated with D-penicillamine treatment during pregnancy. N. Engl. J. Med. 296: 54-55, 1977.

Yamada, T.; Otome, S.; Tanaka, Y.; Sasajima, M.; Ohzeki, M.: Reproductive studies of d-penicillamine in rats. Fertility study. Pharmacometrics 18:553-560, 1982.

987 Penicillin

Boucher and Delost (1964) failed to produce defects in the mouse fetus after giving the mother 50 or 500 units per gm on the 14th gestational day. They found that the treated fetuses grew more rapidly in early post-natal life. Brown et al. (1968) maintained pregnant rabbits on penicillin G or V (100 mg per kg per day) and found no abortions or evidence of teratogenic action.

Boucher, D. and Delost, P.: Developpement post-natal des descendents issus de meres traitees par la penicilline au cours de la gestion chez la souris. C. R. Soc. Biol. (Paris) 158: 528-532, 1964.

Brown, D.M.; Harper, K.H.; Palmer, A.K. and Tesh, S.A.: Effects of antibiotics upon pregnancy in the rabbit. (abstract) Toxicol. Appl. Pharmacol. 12: 295 only, 1968.

988 Pentachlorophenyl

Schwetz et al (1974) administered oraly 5, 15, 30 and 50 mg per kg to rats on days 6-15. No effect was seen at 5 mg but embryolethality and toxicity occurred at 15 mg and higher. Hinkle (1973) found resorptions and embryotoxicity at oral levels of 1.25 to 20 mg per kg in the hamster. Small amounts have been shown to cross the placenta (Larsen et al, 1975).

Hinkle, D.K: Fetotoxic effects of pentachlorophenol in the golden Syrian hamster. Toxicol. Appl. Pharmacol. 25:455, only, 1973.

Larsen, R.V.; Boin, G.S.; Kessler, W.V.; Shaw, S.M.; Von Sickle, D.C.: Placenta transfer and teratology of pentachlorophenyl in rats. Envir. Lett. 10:21-128, 1975.

Schwetz, B.A.; Keeler, P.A.; Gehring, P.J.: The effect of

988

purified and commercial grade pentachlorophenol on rat
embryonal and fetal development. Tox. Appl. Pharm.
28:151-161, 1974.

989 Pentachoronitrobenzene

Jordan et al (1975) administered this compound orally to
pregnant rats during the active period of organogenesis in
doses up to 125 mg per kg per day and found no fetal
toxicity or teratogenicity.

Jordan, R.L.; Sperling, F.; Klein, H.H. and Borzelleca,
J.F.: A study of the potential teratogenic effects of
pentachloronitrobenzene in rats. Toxicol. Appl.
Pharmacol. 33: 222-230, 1975.

990 Pentobarbital (see Barbituric Acid)

991 Pentoxifylline (1-(5-oxohexyl)theobromine)

Sugisaki et al (1981) administered this xanthine derivative
intravenously in daily doses of up to 25 mg per kg on days 6
through 18 in the rabbit. No adverse fetal effects were
found. Sugisaki et al (1981) gave this xanthine vasodilator
intravenously to mice before mating and during the first 7
days or on days 6-15 of gestation. Maximum doses of 50 mg
failed to produce changes in fertility or in the fetuses.

Sugsaki, T.; Hayashi, S.; Miyamoto, M.: Teratological study
of pentoxifylline in rabbits by the intravenous route. Oyo
Yakuri 22:451-458, 1981.

992 Perflavon

This drug used in humans for angina was given by Ito et al
(1972) to pregnant mice and rats in amounts up to 250 mg per
kg per day orally. At the highest dose the mice had delayed
partuition with dead fetuses. No teratogenicity was found.

Ito, R.; Kawamura, H.; Tokoro, Y.; Tosaka, K.; Nakagawa, S.;
Toida, S.; Matsuura, S.; Ozaki, M. and Hiyama, T.: 1,3-di-
methylxanthine-7-acetic acid-7(beta-dimethyl) (amino-ethoxy)
flavon (perflavon). (Japanese) J. Med. Soc.. Toho Japan
19: 116-125, 1972.

993 Perphenazine

This phenothiazine neuroleptic was administered by gavage to
pregnant rats during days 7 through 14 in doses of 20 to 150
mg per kg (Druga, 1976). Significant increases in cleft
palate, retrognathia and micromelia occurred at all dose
levels. Single doses of 90 mg per kg on days 9 through 12
also produced defects, compared to a chemical derivative,
methophenazine, the drug was more teratogenic in the rat.

Druga, A.: The effect of perphenazine treatment during the

organogenesis in rats. Acta Biol. Acad. Sci. Hung.
27:15-23, 1976.

994   Phaltan [N-(Trichloromethylthio)phthalimide]

Fabro et al. (1966) fed 80 mg per kg daily to rabbits on
days 7 through 12 and found no defects in the offspring.

Fabro, S.; Smith, R.L. and Williams, R.T.: Embryotoxic
activity of some pesticides and drugs related to
phthalimide. Food Cosmet. Toxicol. 3: 587-590, 1966. |ag
Phenacetin

Heinonen et al (1977) found no increase in the defect rate
among 5,546 exposed pregnancies.

Heinonen, O.P.; Slone, D.; Shapiro, S.: Birth Defects and
Drugs in Pregnancy. Publishing Sciences Group, Inc., 1977.

995   Phenazepam
(7-Brom-t(0-Chlorphenyl)-1,2-Dehydro-3H-1,4-benziazepin-
2-OH)

Smolnikova and Strekalova (1980) showed that this drug (100
mg per kg daily during the entire pregnancy) did not damage
fetal development but caused some behavioral abnormalities
in the offspring. Different doses were also tested in
pregnant mini-pigs, dogs and guinea pigs but no congenital
malformations were observed (Lyubimov et al, 1979).

Lyubimov, B.I.; Smolnikova, N.M.; Strekalova, S.N.; Boiko,
S.S.; Yavorsky, A.N.; Dushkin, V.A. and Poznakhirev, P.R.:
Study of the embryotropic action of phenazepam in mini pigs,
a new species of experimental animals. Byull. Eksp. Biol.
Med. (USSR) 88, 11:557-560, 1979.

Lyubimov, B.I.; Smolnikova, N.M.: Strekalova, S.N.;
Kurochkin, I.G.; Mitrofanov, V.S.; Porfirieva, R.P.; Markin,
V.A. and Sharow, P.A.: Preclinical trials of the new
tranquilizer phenazepam safety. Farmakol. Toksikol.
(USSR) 42,5:464-467, 1979.

Smolnikova, N.M. and Strekalova, S.N.: Development of the
progeny in antenatal exposure to phenazepam. Farmakol.
Tokisol. (USSR) 43,3:293- 302, 1980.

996   Phencyclidine (PCP)

Jordan et al (1978) injected 25 to 30 mg per kg into rats of
gestational days 6 through 15 and produced skeletal
dysplasias and cleft palates in the offspring. Marks et al
(1980) gavaged mice on days 6-15 with 60 to 120 mg per kg.
At the highest level some maternal mortality occurred and a
6 percent rate of defective offspring was found.

Jordan, R.L.; Young, T.R. and Harry, G.J.: Teratology of
phencyclidine in rats: Preliminary results. (abs)
Teratology 17:40A (only), 1978.

996

Marks, T.A.; Worthy, W.C.; Staples, R.E.: Teratogenic
potential of phencyclidine in the mouse. Teratology
21:241-246, 1981.

Tonge, S.R.: Neurochemical teratology: 5-hydroxyindole
concentations in discrete areas of the rat brain pre- and
neonatal administration of phencyclidine and imipramine.
Life Sci. 12:481-486, 1972.

997 Phenelzine [Beta-phenylethylhydrazine Hydrogen Sulfate]

This monoamine oxidase inhibitor decreases implantation in
mice when given during the 1st 6 days of gestation in
amounts of 25 mg per kg per day (Poulson and Robson, 1964).
Heinonen et al (1977) reported 3 defects among 21 women
taking monoamine oxidase inhibitors. Three of these women
took phenelzine in the first 4 lunar months.

Heinonen, O.P.; Slone, D.; Shapiro, S.: Birth Defects and
Drugs in Pregnancy. Publishing Sciences Group, Inc., 1977.

Poulson, E. and Robson, J.M.: Effect of phenelzine and
some related compounds on pregnancy and on sexual development. J. Endocrinol. 30: 205-215, 1964.

998 Phenglutarimide [Aturban-R] [2-(2-Diethylaminoethyl-
)-2-phenylglutarimide]

Tuchmann-Duplessis and Mercier-Parot (1964) administered 50
to 60 mg per kg to rats, mice and rabbits during
organogenesis and produced no defective fetuses.

Tuchmann-Duplessis, H. and Mercier-Parot, L.: Action sur
la gestation et le developpement foetal d'un derive
glutarimique, 1 aturbane. C. R. Acad. Sci. (Paris) 258:
2666-2669, 1964.

999 Phenmetrazine (Preludin-R)

Milkovich and Van den Berg (1977) did a prospective study of
406 children exposed in utero to phenmetrazine and found no
increase in serious defects. Heinonen et al (1977) reported
no increase in congenital defect rate among 58 women who
took the drug during the first 4 months.

Heinonen, O.P.; Slone, D.; Shapiro, S.: Birth Defects and
Drugs in Pregnancy. Publishing Sciences Group, Inc., 1977.

Milkovich, L. and Van den Berg, B.J.: Effects of antenatal
exposure to anorectic drugs. Am. J. Obstet. Gynecol.
129:637-642, 1977.

1000 Phenobarbital (also see Barbaturic Acid)

McColl et al. (1963) found double vertebral centra in the
offspring of mice fed 0.16 percent phenobarbital; this
skeletal finding could be due to a nutritional effect

causing delayed ossification rather than representing a true congenital defect. McColl et al. (1967) reported skeletal and aortic arch defects in the offspring of rabbits treated with 50 mg per kg from days 8 through 16.

Gupta and Yaffee (1981) administered 40 mg per kg subcutaneously to pregnat rats during the last several days of gestation. The female offspring had delay in onset of puberty, disorders of the estrus cycle and a 50 percent infertility rate.

Gupta, C.; Yaffee, S.J.: Reproductive dysfunction in female offspring after prenatal exposure to phenobarbital: critical period of action. Pediatric Res. 15:1488-1491, 1981.

McColl, J.D.; Globus, M. and Robinson, S.: Drug induced skeletal malformations in the rat. Experientia 19: 183-184, 1963.

McColl, J.D.; Robinson, S. and Globus, M.: Effect of some therapeutic agents on the rabbit fetus. Toxicol. Appl. Pharmacol. 10: 244-252, 1967.

1001 Phenol

Minor and Becker (1971) injected rats intraperitoneally on days 8-10 or 11-13 with up to 200 mg per kg. No adverse fetal effects were found.

Minor, J.L.; Becker, B.A.: A comparison of the teratogenic properties of sodium salicylate, sodium benzoate and phenol (abstract) Toxicol. Appl. Pharmacol. 19:373 (only) 1971.

1002 Phenothiazines (Acetylpromazine, Chlorpromazine, Pipamazine, Promethazine, Promazine, Prochlorpromazine, Methotrimeprazine, Trimeprazine, Oxomemazine)

This group of antipsychotic and antinauseant drugs consists of over two dozen structurally related chemicals. Rumeau-Rouquette et al (1977) studied prospectively 12,764 pregnancies and observed eleven malformed children from 304 women who took phenothiazines during the first 3 months. The rate in this group was 3.5 percent which was significantly higher than the 1.6 percent found in mothers not taking the drugs. The 3- carbon side chained phenothiazines (chlorpromazine, methotri- meprazine, trimeprazine and oxomemazine) were taken by 133 mothers and 8 malformed infants occurred in the offspring. Other forms with 2-carbon, piperazine or piperidine side chains were taken by fewer women but were not associated with significant increases in defects.

In another larger group of pregnancies in which phenothiazines were taken during the first four lunar months, 66 malformed infants were found among 1,309 exposed women (Heinonen et al, 1977). Of this large group, 877 took prochlorperizine. When the exposed group was matched carefully for parity, age and social class, no significant difference from the controls was found. It is of interest that this study found approximately a 5.0 percent defect

1002

rate in both control and treated groups while the study
reported above found 3.5 percent in the exposed and 1.6
percent in the control group. This study is also reported
by Slone et al (1976). Milkovich and Van den Berg (1976)
studied 543 pregnancies exposed to phenothiazines and 433
exposed to prochlorthiazine and found no significant
increases in serious congenital malformations in the offspring at birth, one year or at 5 years. Mellin (1975) in
another study did not identify an increased defect rate in
74 women who took prochlorperazine. The general subject is
reviewed by Nahas and Goujard (1979).

Animal studies and some additional clinical data on these
agents are reported under their individual headings
(chlopromazine, prochlorperazine, promazine, methophenazine
and trifluoperazine). The role of the piperazine ring in
teratogenicity in th rat has been studied by Druga et al
(1980).

Minor and Becker (1971) injected rats intraperitoneally on
days 8-10 or 11-13 with up to 200 mg per kg. No adverse
fetal effects were found.

Minor, J.L.; Becker, B.A.: A comparison of the teratogenic
properties of sodium salicylate, sodium benzoate and phenol.
(abstract) Toxicol. Appl. Pharmacol. 19:373 (only) 1971.

Druga, A.; Nyitra, M.; Szaszovszky, E.: Experimental
teratogenicity of structurally similar compounds with or
without piperazine-ring: a preliminary report. Pol. J.
Pharmacol. Pharm. 32:199-204, 1980.

Heinonen, O.P.; Slone, D. and Shapiro, S.: Birth Defects
and Drugs in Pregnancy. Publishing Sciences Group Inc.;
Littleton, Mass.; 1977.

Mellin, G.W.: Report of prochlorperazine utilization during
pregnancy from fetal life study data bank (abs). Teratology
11:28A, 1975.

Milkovich, L. and Van den Berg, B.J.: An evaluation of the
teratogenicity of certain antinauseant drugs. Am. J.
Obstet. Gynecol. 125:244-248, 1976.

Nahas, G. and Goujard, J.: Phenothiazines,
benzodiazepines, and the fetus, in Reviews in Perinatal
Medicine, edited by E.M. Scarpelli and E.V. Cosmi, Raven
Press, New York, 1979, pp.243-280.

Rumeau-Rouquette, C.; Goujard, J. and Huel, G.: Possible
teratogenic effect of phenothiazines in human beings.
Teratology 15:57-64, 1977.

Slone, D.; Siskind, V.; Heinonen, O.P.; Monson, R.R.;
Kaufman, D.W.; Shapiro, S.: Antenatal exposure to
phenothiazines in relation to congenital malformations,
perinatal mortality rate, birth weight, and intelligence
quotient scores. Am. J. Obstet. Gynecol. 128: 486-488,
1977.

1003 Phenoxyacetic Acid

Hood et al (1979) gavaged pregnant mice with 800-900 mg per kg on single days 8 through 15 or with 250-300 mg per kg on multiple days during organogenesis and observed no adverse fetal effects.

Hood, R.D.; Patterson, B.L.; Thacker, G.T.; Sloan, G.L.; Szczech, G.M.: Prenatal effect of 2,4,5-T,2,4,5-trichlorophenol and phenoxyacetic acid in mice. J. Envir. Sci. Health C13:189-204, 1979.

1004 Phenoxy-isobutyric Acid Ethyl Ester

Amels et al (1974) gave this anticholesterol compound to rats and mice at various periods during gestation. An oral dose for two days during early embryogenesis produced some fetuses with edema and hemorrhages in both species. The dose was 33 mg per kg, close to the presumptive human therapeutic dose.

Amels, D.; Fazekas-Todea, I. and Sandor, S.: The prenatal noxious effect of a blood cholesterin level lowering compound. Rev. Roum. Morphol. Embryol. 19: 37-43, 1974.

1005 Phenylalanine

The offspring of mothers with penylketonuria have shown a high frequency of mental retardation with microcephaly and intrauterine growth retardation (reviewed by Hsia, 1970, and Frankenburg et al.; 1968). Those mothers with hyperphenylalaninemia, but with serum phenylalanine levels below 15 mg per 100 ml during pregnancy, have produced 11 normal infants out of a total of 12 (Hsia, 1970). Lenke and Levy (1980) have reviewed 524 pregnancies in mothers with phenylketonuria. Among 34 women who were treated there was a tendency for higher IQ and normal head circumference with treatment begun earlier in gestation.

Other anomalies associated with these children have been congenital heart disease, dislocation of the hips and strabismus (Stevenson and Huntley, 1967). In a report of two families they found eight out of ten children had congenital heart disease which included coarctation of the aorta, patent ductus arteriosus and other types. Of 26 documented pregnancies, 16 (62 percent) terminated in abortion. Montenegro and Castro (1965) and Fisch et al. (1969) have reported similar types of defects in the offspring of phenylketonuric mothers. Gandier et al (1972) have summarized the literature and reported 3 new cases.

Kerr et al. (1968) fed phenylalanine to pregnant Rhesus monkeys and found mental retardation, but this was not associated with microcephaly or other congenital defects. They observed higher phenylalanine levels in the cord blood than in the maternal blood.

Fisch, R.O.; Doeden, D.; Lansky, L.L. and Anderson, J.A.: Maternal phenylketonuria. Detrimental effects on

1005

embryogenesis and fetal development. Am. J. Dis. Child.
118: 847-858, 1969.

Frankenburg, W.K.; Duncan, B.R.; Coffelt, R.W.; Koch, R.;
Coldwell, J.G. and Son, C.D.: Maternal phenylketonuria:
implications for growth and development. J. Pediatr. 73:
560-570, 1968.

Gandier, B.; Ponte, C.; Duquennoy, G.; Callens, M. and
Ballester, L.: Retard de croissance intra-uterin avec
microcephalie chez trois enfants nes de mere
hyperphenylalaninemique. Ann. Pediatr. (Paris) 19:
269-276, 1972.

Hsia, D.Y.: Phenylketonuria and its variants. In,
Steinberg, A.G. and Bearn, E.G. (eds.): Progress in
Medical Genetics, Vol. 7. New York: Grune and Stratton,
1970. pp. 53-68.

Kerr, G.R.; Chamove, A.S.; Harlow, H.F. and Waisman, H.A.:
'Fetal PKU' the effect of maternal hyperphenylalaninemia
during pregnancy in the Rhesus monkey (Macaca mulatta).
Pediatrics 42: 27-36, 1968.

Lenke, R.R.; Levy, H.L.: Maternal phenylketonuria and
hyperphenylalaninemia. New. Eng. J. Med. 303:1202-1208,
1980.

Montenegro, J.E. and Castro, G.L.: Fenilcetonuria materna:
anomalieas en la descendencia. Acta Med. Venezolana 12:
233-236, 1965.

Stevenson, R.E. and Huntley, C.C.: Congenital malformations in offspring of phenylketonuric mothers. Pediatrics
40: 33-45, 1967.

1006 2-Phenyl-5-benzothiazole Acetic Acid

This non-steroidal anti-inflammatory agent was given orally
to rabbits in doses of up to 200 mg per kg on days 8 through
16 of gestation (Ito et al, 1977). At the highest dose
level which was toxic to the mother, fetal death was
increased significantly. No increase in malformations was
found although two dead fetuses at the highest dose level
had exencephaly. There were 86 live normal fetuses in this
group. They cite their previous work stating that no
teratogenicity was found in mice but cleft palate occurred
in exposed rat embryos.

Ito, T.; Yamamoto, M. and Kamimura, K.: Teratogenicity of
a non-steroidal anti-inflammatory agent in rabbits. Acta
Medica et Biologica 24:173-178, 1977.

1007 Phenylbutazone

Schardein et al. (1969) found no teratogenic action in rats
and rabbits using 42 and 50 mg per kg respectively daily
during organogenesis.

Kato et al (1979) gave the drug orally to rabbits at maximum doses of 120 mg per kg per day on days 6 through 18 of gestation. An increase in fetal lethality occurred but defects were not increased.

Kato, M.; Matsuzawa, K.; Enjo, H.; Malsita, T. and Hashimoto, Y.: Reproductive studies of feprazone 2. Teratogenicity study in rats and rabbits. Iyakuhin Kenkyu 10:149-164, 1979.

Schardein, J.L.; Blatz, A.T.; Woosley, E.T. and Kaup, D.H.: Reproductive studies on sodium meclofenamate in comparison to aspirin and phenylbutazone. Toxicol. Appl. Pharmacol. 15: 46-55, 1969.

1008 1-Phenyl-3,3-dimethyl-triazene

Druckrey (1973) has reviewed work with the triazenes. In the rat 1-phenyl-3,3-dimethyl-triazene, produced postnatal brain tumors when given in single parenteral doses of up to 110 mg per kg during the last part of gestation or at birth. The 3-dimethyl-aryltriazenes were teratogenic after the 10th day when skeletal defects and cleft palates were produced. Pyridyl-dimethyltriazene given in a dose of 5 mg per kg on the 14th day produced microcephaly.

Druckrey, H.: Specific carcinogenic and teratogenic effects of indirect alkylating methyl and ethyl compounds and their dependency on stages of ontogenic developments. Xenobiotica 3: 271-303, 1973.

Druckrey, H.; Ivankovic, S.; Preussmann, R.; Zulch, K. and Mennel, H.D.: Selective induction of malignant tumors of the nervous system by resorptive carcinogens In, Kirsch, W.M.; Paoletti, E.G. and Paoletti, P. (eds): The Experimental Biology of Brain Tumors. Springfield: C.C. Thomas, 1972, pp. 111-112.

1009 2-Phenyl-1,3-dioxolan-4-yl-methyl)piperidinium Iodide

Takai and Nakada (1970) reported no teratogenicity or fetal changes in mice and rats treated orally during organogenesis. The maximal dose in the rat was 50 mg per kg and in the mouse 100 mg per kg per day.

Takai, A. and Nakada, H.: Teratological studies on N-methyl-N-(2-cyclohexyl-2-phenyl-1,3-dioxolan-4-yl-methyl-)piperi

idinium iodide (SH-100). (Japanese) Oyo Yakuri 4: 109-112, 1970.

1010 Phenylephrine

Heinonen et al (1977) found no increase in defect rate among 1,249 exposed pregnancies. There were 8 eye and ear malformations as compared to an expected number of 2.9; the difference was not significantly increased.

1010

Heinonen, O.P.; Slone, D.; Shapiro, S.: Birth Defects and
Drugs in Pregnancy. Publishing Sciences Group Inc., 1977.

1011 O-Phenylenediamine

Karnofsky and Lacon (1962) report 0.5 ml of this material
injected into the yolk sac of the 4-day old chick produced
facial coloboma, cleft palates and skeletal defects.

Karnofsky, D.A. and Lacon, C.R.: Survey of cancer
chemotherapy service center compounds for teratogenic effect
in the chick embryo. Cancer Res. 22: 84-85, 1962.

1012 Phenylglycidyl Ether

Terrill et al (1982) exposed rats to 2 to 11 ppm (6 hours
daily five days a week) in a two generation study and during
organogenesis. No adverse fetal or reproductive changes
were found.

Terrell, J.B.; Lee, K.P.; Culik, R.; Kennedy, G.L.:
Inhalation toxicity of phenylglycidyl ether: Reproductive,
mutagenic, teratogenic and cytogenic studies. Toxicol.
Appl. Pharm. 64:204-212, 1982.

1013 Phenylhydrazine

Tamaki et al (1974) studied postnatal function of rat
fetuses made icteric by administering the mother 10 mg per
kg intraperitoneally on the 17th, 18th and 19th days of
gestation. Conditioned avoidance learning was found to be
significantly retarded. Studies of the brains of these
animals did not show kernicterus (Yamamura et al, 1973).

Yamamura, H.; Semba, H.; Keino, H.; Ohta, K. and Murakami,
U.: Experimental studies on developmental disorder due to
Icterus gravis neonatorum: perinatal hemolytic jaundice and
its effect on postnatal development. (abstract) Teratology
8: 110 (only), 1973.

Tamaki, Y.; Ito, M.; Semba, R.; Yamamura, H. and Kiyono,
S.: Functional disturbances in adult rats suffered from
Icterus gravis neonatorum due to maternal application of
phenylhydrazine hydrochloride. Cong. Anom. 14: 95-103,
1974.

1014 Phenylmercuric Acetate (see Mercury)

1015 Phenyl-beta-Naphtilamine (Neozon-D)

This antioxidant was given intragastrically to SHK strain of
mice during all of gestation and postnatally (9 mg per
animal). Malignant tumors in the offspring were observed.
Salnikova et al (1979) did not detect any embryotoxic action
of this substance.

Salnikova, L.C.; Vorontsov, R.S.; Pavlenko, G.I.   and
Kotosova, L.D.: Mutagenic, embryotropic and blastomogenic
effect of neozon-D (Phenyl- beta-naphtilamine). Gigiena tr.
prof. zabol. (USSR) 9:57, 1979.

1016 Phenylpropanolamine

Heinonen et al (1977) studied the offspring of 726 women
exposed to this drug in the first 4 months and reported 71
defects which included malformations of the eye, ear and
hypospadias. The rate was 1.40 times higher than the
control and this was a statistically significant increase
(p>0.01).

Heinonen, O.P.; Slone, D.; Shapiro, S.: Birth Defects and
Drugs in Pregnancy. Publishiing Sciences Group, Inc., 1977.

1017 L-Phenylsemicarbazide (see Semithiocarbazide)

1018 Phleomycin

In explanted chick embryos Lee et al (1972) found that
concentrations above 0.05 microgram per ml inhibited mitosis
and neural tube closure.

Lee, H-Y.; Cortes, J.L.   and Levin, M.A.: Teratogenic
effects of phleomycin in early chick embryos. Teratology 6:
201-206, 1972.

1019 Phosalone

Khera   et   al   (1979)   administered   this   cholinesterase-
inhibiting insecticide to rats by gavage in amounts of up to
50 mg per kg from day 6-15 and found no teratogenicity.

Khera, K.S.; Whalen, C.; Angers, G.   and Trivett, G.:
Assessment of the teratogenic potential of piperonyl
butoxide, biphenyl, and phosalone in the rat. Toxicol.
Appl. Pharmacol. 47:353-358, 1979.

1020 Phosphonacetyl-L-aspartic Acid

This antitumor agent was studied by Seiber et al (1980) in
mice at doses of 0.75 to 6.25 mg per kg given
intraperitoneally on days 7-11 of gestation or on single
days. The 4-day regime at 1.5 mg per kg was associated with
53 percent fetal lethality. Increased malformation rates
were found after treatment on days 7 and 8. Skeletal, heart
and renal defects were most common.

Sieber, S.M.; Botkin, C.; Soong, P.; Lee, E.C.; Whang-Peng,
J.: Embryotoxicity in mice of phosphonacetyl-L-aspartic
acid (PALA), a new antitumor agent 1. Embryolethal,
teratogenic and cytogenetic effects. Teratology 22:311-319,
1980.

1021 Phosphoramide Mustard (see Cyclophosphamide)

1022 Photodieldrin

This photo-degradation product of dieldrin was given by intubation to pregnant rats and mice on days 7 through 16 in doses up to 0.6 mg per kg and neither fetal effects nor teratogenic action were found (Chernoff et al, 1975).

Chernoff, N.; Kavlock, R.J.; Katherein, J.R.; Dunn, J.M. and Haseman, J.K.: Prenatal effects of dieldrin and photodieldrin in mice and rats. Toxicol. Appl. Pharm. 31: 302-308, 1975.

1023 Photomirex

This photodegradation product of mirex was fed in the diet to rats in amounts of 5-40 ppm. At 40 and 20 ppm the survival indices of pups were decreased (Chu et al, 1981).

Chu, I.; Villeneuve, D.C.; Secours, V.F.; Valli, V.E.; Becking, G.C.: Effects of photomirex and mirex on reproduction in the rat. Toxicol. Appl. Pharm. 60:549-556, 1981.

1024 Phthalamudine   [3-(4-Chloro-3-sulphamoyl)-3-hydro-xyphthalimidine]

Fabro et al. (1966) found no teratogenic action of this compound when it was fed to rabbits in amounts of 150 mg per kg per day during days 7 through 12 of gestation.

Fabro, S.; Smith, R.L. and Williams, R.T.: Embryotoxic activity of some pesticides and drugs related to phthalimide. Food Cosmet. Toxicol. 3: 587-590, 1966.

1025 Phthalate Esters (Di(2-ethylhexyl)phthalate, Di-n-buyl phthalate)

Singh et al. (1972) using the rat studied eight phthalate esters. Injections were made intraperitoneally on gestational days 5, 10 and 15. Doses were generally from about 0.2 ml to 1.0 ml per kg. Few or no defects occurred in the groups receiving the following esters: dimethyl, di-ethyl, bibutyl, diisobutyl, butyl carbobutoxy methyl and di-2-ethylhexyl. The dimethoxyethal and dioctyl forms were associated with congenital defects which included absence of the tail, anophthalmia, twisted hind legs and hematomas. Bower et al. (1970) have studied the effect of various phthalic esters on the development of the chick embryo. Dibutoxyethyl (0.05 to 0.1) injected into the yolk at 2.5 to 3 days of incubation was associated with crania bifida and anophthalmia.

Shiota et al (1980) gave mice diets containing 0.05 - 1.0 percent di-2-ethylhexyl (DEHP) or di-n-butyl phthalate (DBP) throughout gestation. In the group treated with 0.4 and 1.0

percent DEHP all the implanted oval died. At 0.2 percent
there was an increase in defects which was of borderline
significance (4 out of 77 implants). With 1.0 percent DBP
two of the 181 implants had exencephaly. They estimated
that the maximum no effect level was 70 mg per kg per day
far higher than current estimated human intake.

Bower, R.K.; Haberman, S. and Minton, P.D.: Teratogenic
effects in the chick embryo caused by esters of phthalic
acid. J. Pharmacol. Exp. Ther. 171: 314-324, 1970.

Shiota, K.; Chou, M.J.; Nishimura, H.: Embryotoxic effects
of di-2-ethylhexyl phthalate (DEHP) and di-n-butyl phthalate
(DBP) in mice. Env. Res. 22:245-255, 1980.

Singh, A.R.; Lawrence, W.H. and Autian, J.: Teratogenicity
of phthalic esters in rats. J. Pharm. Sci. 61: 51-55,
1972.

1026 Phthalazinol
     (7-ethoxycarbonyl-4-hydroxymethyl-6,8-dimethyl-1-1
     (2H)-phthalazinone)

This analgesic was given orally by Matsuzaki et al (1982) to
rats and rabbits in maximum doses of up to 800 and 400 mg
respectively. No effects on fertility or postnatal function
were found in the rat. During organogenesis doses of 800 mg
per kg were associated with increased malformations which
included hematomas, edema and skeletal abnormalities. Heart
defects were also found. The rabbit fetuses after exposure
during organogenesis to 200 mg per kg had an increase in
heart and skeletal defects.

Matsuzaki, M.; Akutsu, S.; Karwana, K.; Kato, M.; Shimamura,
T.; Nagami, K.: Reproductive studies of phthalazinol in
rats and rabbits. Kiso to Rinsho 16:6357-6364, 6365-6380,
6381-6388, 6389-6396, 1982.

1027 Phthalic acid

Verrett et al. (1969) reported a 4 percent incidence of
congenital defects in chicks receiving 3 to 20 mg of this
material via the yolk sac or air cell before incubation.
Tetrahydrophthalimide, phthalimide and phthalamide were
similarly teratogenic. Defects of the head and eyes and
phocomelia or amelia were noted. The compound, which is
related to thalidomide, was not teratogenic in rabbits when
used in amounts of 150 mg per kg on days 7 through 12 of
pregnancy (Smith et al.; 1965).

Smith, R.L.; Fabro, S.; Schumacher, H.J. and Williams,
R.T.: Studies on the relationship between chemical
structure and embryotoxic activity of thalidomide and
related compounds. In, Robson, J.M.; Sullivan, F.M. and
Smith, R.L. (eds.): Embryopathic Activity of Drugs.
Boston: Little Brown, 1965. pp. 194-209.

Verrett, M.J.; Mutchler, M.K.; Scott, W.F.; Reynaldo, E.F.
and McLaughlin, J.: Teratogenic effects of captan and

related compounds in the developing chicken embryo. Ann.
N. Y. Acad. Sci. 160: 334-343, 1969.

1028 Phthalimide

This chemical structurally related to thalidomide was tested
in rabbits and found not to be teratogenic. Smith et al.
(1965) gave 150 mg per kg on days 7 through 12 of pregnancy.

Smith, R.L.; Fabro, S.; Schumacher, H.J. and Williams,
R.T.: Studies on the relationship between chemical
structure and embryotoxic activity of thalidomide and
related compounds. In, Robson, J.M.; Sullivan, F.M. and
Smith, R.L. (eds.): Embryopathic Activity of Drugs.
Boston: Little Brown, 1965. pp. 194-209.

1029 4-Phthalimidobutyric Acid

Kohler et al (1973) found fetal skeletal defects when this
chemical was given to mice in doses of 800 mg per kg
intraperitoneally on day 9 of gestation.

Kohler, F.; Ockenfels, H. and Meise, W.: Teratogene
Aktivitat von N-Phthalylglycin und 4-Phthalimidobuttersaure.
Pharmazie 28: 680-681, 1973.

1030 Phthalimidoethanesulphon-N-isopropylamide

This taurine derivative proposed as an anticonvulsant was
tested in mice orally from the 6th through the 12th day of
gestatiousingng doses of up to 1040 mg per kg. No adverse
fetal effects were found (Lankinen et al, 1982).

Lankinen, S.; Linden, I.-B.; Gothoni, G.: Teratological
studies on a new anticonvulsive taurine derivative in mice.
(abstract) Teratology 26:19A, 1982.

1031 Phthalophose

Kagan et al (1978) observed teratogenic and embryotoxic
action of this pesticide in rats treated during all the
gestation (0.3-15 mg per kg). These doses were non-toxic
for the maternal organism. Abbasov et al (1980) obtained
similar results.

Abbasov, T.G.; Karavaeva, G.H. and Makhno, P.M.:
Embryotoxic effect of phthalophose. Veterinariya. (USSR)
1:62-63, 1980.

Kagan, Yu. S.; Voronina, V.M. and Akkerman, G.A.: Effect
of phthalophose on the embryogenesis and its metabolism in
the body of albino rats and their embryos. Gig i Sanit.
(USSR) 9:28-31, 1978.

1032 N-Phthalylglycine

Kohler et al (1973) found fetal skeletal defects when this chemical was given to mice in doses of 200 mg per kg intraperitoneally on day 9 of gestation.

Kohler, F.; Ockenfels, H. and Meise, W.: Teratogene Aktivitat von n-Phthalylglycin und 4-Phthalimidobuttersaure. Pharmazie 28: 680-681, 1973.

1033 Phthorotanum

Anisimova (1981) treated by inhalation (1024 plus or minus 10.4 mg per cubic meter) pregnant rats during the entire gestation and observed gonadotoxic effects. Embryotoxic and teratogenic effects were not found.

Anisimova, I.G.: Gonadotoxic and embryotoxic effect of phthorotanum. Gig. i Sanit. (USSR) 4:21-24, 1981.

1034 Physostigmine [Eserine]

Landauer (1954) injected this material into the yolk sac Aktivitat von n-Phthalylglycin und 4-Phthalimidobuttersaure. syndactylism and clubbed down.

Bueker and Platner (1956) injecting 0.05 to 15.0 mg into the yolk sac during the 1st 12 days of incubation produced severe vertebral defects and micromelia in chicks. Ancel (1946) used 0.05 mg at 26 hours to produce brachymelia and spina bifida in the chick.

Ancel, P.: Reserche experimentale sur le spina bifida. Arch. Anat. Microscop. 36: 45-68, 1946.

Bueker, E.D. and Platner, W.S.: Effect of cholinergic drugs on development of chick embryo. Proc. Soc. Exp. Biol. Med. 91: 539-543, 1956.

Landauer, W.: On the chemical production of developmental abnormalities and of phenocopies in chicken embryos. Cell Comp. Physiol. 43: 261-305, 1954.

1035 Picloram (4-Amino-3,5,6-trichloropicolinic Acid (Picloram-R)

Thompson et al (1972) found no teratogenic action of this compound in rats fed up to 100 mg per kg on gestational days 6 through 15. No neonatal adverse affects were noted.

Thompson, D.J.; Emerson, J.L.; Strebing, R.H.; Gerbig, C.G.; Robinson, V.B.: Teratology and postnatal studies on 4-amino-3,5,6- trichloropicolinic acid (Picloram) in the rat. Food Cosmet. Toxicol. 10:797-803, 1972.

1036 Picosulfate, Sodium

This laxative was given by gastric intubation to rats and rabbits during organogenesis. At 100 mg per kg no increase in malformations occurred, but in the rabbit, early

resorptions were increased (Nishimura, 1977). At 10,000 mg
per kg in the rat and 1,000 mg per kg in the rabbit, there
was no increase in malformations. In both species, maternal
treatment postnatally was associated with increased death in
the offspring.

Nishimura, M.; Kast, A. and Tsunenari, Y.: Reproduction
studies of sodium picosulfate (DA-1773, Laxoberon) on rats
and rabbits. (Japanese) Iyakuhin Kenkyu 8:366-396, 1977.

1037 Pilocarpine

Landauer (1953) used this parasympathomimetic drug to
produce defects in chick embryos. He injected 3 to 12 mg
into the yolk at 24 to 96 hours of incubation. Rumplessness
occurred in some of the early injected embryos; injection at
a later period was associated with tarsometatarsus, beak and
other skeletal defects. Nicotinamide given concurrently
protected against the teratogenic effects.

Landauer, W.: on teratogenic effects of pilocarpine in
chick development. J. Exp. Zool. 122: 469-483, 1953.

1038 Pimeprofen   (2-pyridylmethyl   2-(P-(2-methylpropyl)phenyl)
       proprionate)

Fuchigami et al (1982) gave rats up to 75 mg per kg
subcutaneously on days 7-17 of gestation and observed no
adverse fetal effects. Postnatal studies with doses to 150
mg per kg produced no significant changes. Using rabbits
and a subcutaneous dose of up to 40 mg per kg during
organogenesis they observed no adverse fetal effects.

Fuchigami, K.; Hatano, M.; Shimamura, K.; Iwaki, M.; Aoyama,
T.; Tsuji, M.; Noda, K.: Reproductive studies on
2-pyridylmethyl 2- (p-(2-methylpropyl)phenyl) proprionate
(pimeprofen). Oyo Yakuri 23:883-893, 24:1-47, 1982.

1039 Pimozide

Fukuhara et al (1980) gave this diphenylbutyl piperidine
drug to rats orally in amounts of up to 3.2 mg per kg daily
from 3 weeks of age through pregnancy and found no ill
effects on fertility or the offspring.

Fukuhara, Y.; Fujii, T.; Kado, Y.; Watanabe, N.:
Reproductive studies of pimozide administered from young age
in rats. Kiso to Rinsho 14:2163-2170, 1980.

1040 Pine Needles

Chow et al. (1972) have summarized the work in cattle and
mice on the effect of pine needle ingestion on pregnancy.
In cows abortions or weak non-viable calves followed pine
needle consumption. Mice fed after the 4th, 10th or 15th
day of pregnancy had reduction in litter-size as well as
fetal weight. No congenital defects were reported. An

aqueous fraction of the pine needles was the most active.

Subsequent work by this group has indicated that the active agent was heat labile product of fungi associated with the pine needles (Chow et al, 1974).

Chow, F.C.; Hamar, D.W. and Udall, R.H.: Myotoxic effect on fetal development: Pine needle abortion in mice. J. Reprod. Fert. 40: 203-204, 1974.

Chow, F.C.; Hanson, K.J.; Hamar, D.W. and Udall, R.H.: Reproductive failure of mice caused by pine needle ingestion. J. Reprod. Fertil. 30: 169-172, 1972.

1041 Pipamazine (see Phenothiazines)

1042 Pipemidic Acid

Nishimura et al (1976) gave this antibacterial agent to pregnant rats by gavage in doses of up to 3,200 mg per kg on days 8 through 14 of gestation. At the highest dose, a slight decrease in fetal weight and delay in ossification occurred. Dilation of the ureters and renal pelves were significantly more common in the fetuses exposed to 800 and 3,200 mg per kg. Postnatally 8 of 132 pups in the 3,200 mg per kg group showed dilation of the renal pelves.

Nishimura, K.; Nanto, T.; Mukumoto, K.; Yasuba, J.; Sasaki, H.; Terada, Y.; Fukagawa, S.; Shigematsu, K. and Tatsumi, H.: Reproduction studies of pipemidic acid in rats 2. Teratogenicity study (Japanese) Iyakuhin Kenkyu 7:321-329, 1976.

1043 2-(1-Piperidino)-ethyl Benzilate Ethylbromide (PB-106)

This anticholinergic and ganglion-blocking agent was tested in pregnant rats and mice by Ohata and Nomura (1970). Treatment was given during active organogenesis using the oral, intraperitoneal or subcutaneous route. Oral doses of up to 1000 mg per kg were used. No teratogenicity or fetal effects were observed.

Ohata, K. and Nomura, A.: Influence of 2-(1-piperidino)-ethyl benzilate ethylbromide (PB-106) on pregnant mice and rats, and on their fetuses. (Japanese) Oyo Yakuri 4: 59-68, 1970.

1044 Piperonyl Butoxide

Khera et al (1979) administered this compound to rats by gavage at doses up to 500 mg per kg on days 6-15 of gestation and found no evidence of teratogenicity. KenNedy et al (1977) also had negative findings at dose of 1000 mg per kg.

Kennedy, G.L.; Smith, S.H.; Kinoshita, F.K. and Keplinger, M.L.: Teratogenic evaluation of piperonyl butoxide in the rat. Food Cos. Toxicol. 15:337-339, 1977.

Khera, K.S.; Whalen, C.; Angers, G. and Trivett, G.:
Assessment of the teratogenic potential of piperonyl
butoxide, biphenyl, and phosalone in the rat. Toxicol.
Appl. Pharmacol. 47:353-358, 1979.

1045 Pipobroman [1,4-Bis(3-bromopropionyl)piperazine]

Nagai (1972) injected this anti-neoplastic agent into
pregnant mice. At doses of 30 mg per kg given on days 11
through 14 of gestation brachygnathia and small noses
occurred.

Nagai, H.: Effects of transplacentally injected alkalating
agents upon development of embryos. Bull. Tokyo Dent.
Coll. 13: 103-119, 1972.

1046 Piquizium

Tsuruzaki et al (1981) gave this anticholinergic to rats
daily in amounts of up to 250 mg per kg before mating and
during the first 7 days and found no decrease in
reproduction. Up to 500 mg per kg was given during
organogenesis and no adverse fetal effects were observed.
Postnatal function was unaffected.

Tsuruzaki, T.; Inui, H.; Kato, H.; Yamamoto, M.: Effects of
3-(di-2-thienyl-methylene)-5-methyl-trans-quinolizidinium
bromide on reproduction. Kiso to Rinsho 15:6183-6193,
6194-6244, 6251-6233, 1981.

1047 Pirbuterol Hydrochloride

Sakai et al (1980) gave rats up to 300 mg per kg orally
before mating and for 7 days of gestation, on days 7-17 or
on days 17-21. The only ill effect was growth retardation
when 300 mg per kg was given during organogenesis.
Postnatal effects were not seen. The rabbits received up to
300 mg per kg orally on days 6-18. At the highest dose
abortion occurred in 4 of 13 litters. Body weight of the
fetuses was reduced at 30, 100, and 300 mg per kg.

Sakai, T.; Owaki, Y.; Noguchi, Y.: Reproduction studies of
pirbuterol hydrochloride. Yakuri to Chiro 8:731-743, 1980.

1048 Pirenzepine (Gastrozepin-R)

Iida et al (1980) gave this anti-ulcer medication to rats
and rabbits preconceptually, during organogenesis and
perinatally and found no adverse effects on reproduction.

Iida, H.; Matsuo, A.; Kast, A.; Tsunenari, Y.: Reproductive
studies with pirenzepine (LS519Cl(2)) in rats and rabbits.
Ihakuhin Kenkyu 11:424-436, 1980.

1049 Piroxicam

Sakai et al (1980) studied this non-steroidal antiinflammatory in rabbits and rats using maximum oral doses of up to 10 and 70 mg per kg respectively. At 2.5 mg per day on days 7-17 there was decreased fetal growth. At 10 mg per kg 11 of 39 dams died. No fetal malformation increase was found. After perinatal studies, growth retardation was found at 10 mg per kg. Studies of rabbits during organogenesis were negative except most of the dams died at 70 mg per kg.

Sakai, T.; Ofsuki, I.; Noguchi, F.: Reproduction studies on piroxicam. Yakuri to Chiryo 8:4655-4671, 1980.

1050 Piretenide (4-phenoxy-3-(1-pyrrolidynyl-5-sufamoylbenzoic Acid)

Kitantani et al (1980) gave this diuretic drug to mice and rabbits by both oral and intravenous routes. With oral doses of up to 500 mg per kg in the rat, no adverse effects were found except that the pregnancy rate was reduced when treatment was on the first 7 days of gestation. The intravenous daily dose (60 mg per kg) did not alter postnatal growth or produce increased defects in the rat. Doses of 1.25 mg or 1.0 mg per kg were given intravenously or by mouth respectively during organogenesis and rabbit fetuses were similar to controls.

Kitantani, T.; Sugisaki, T.; Takagi, S.; Hayashi, S.; Miyamoto, M.: Reproductive studies of piretanide. Kiso to Rinsho 14:4330-4347, 4348- 4363, 4364-4366, 4367-4373, 1980.

1051 Pitressin (see Vasopressin)

1052 Pituitary Growth Hormone (see Somatotropin)

1053 Podophyllinic Acid Ethylhydrazide (see 1-Methyl-formylhydrazine)

1054 Podophyllotoxin

This chemical derived from the American May-apple is an antitumor agent. Chaube and Murphy (1968) report that single injections of 0.3 to 1.0 mg per kg into pregnant rats once from the 9th to the 12th day produced no fetal changes. Litter resorption occurs if the drug is used earlier than the 9th day in the rat (Thiersch, 1963) or mouse (Wiesner and Yudkin, 1955).

Thiersch (1963) reported no congenital defects in the rat fetuses.

Chaube, S. and Murphy, M.L.: The teratogenic effects of the recent drugs active in cancer chemotherapy. In, Woollam, D.H.M. (ed.): Advances in Teratology, Vol. 3.

New York: Logos and Academic Press, 1968. pp. 181-237.

Thiersch, J.B.: Effect of podophyllin (P) and podophyllotoxin (PT) on the rat litter in utero. Proc. Soc. Exp. Biol. Med. 113: 124-127, 1963.

Wiesner, B.P. and Yudkin, J.: Control of fertility by antimitotic agents. Nature (Lond.) 176: 249-250, 1955.

1055 Poliomyelitis Vaccine (see SV-40 virus)

1056 Polybrominated Biphenyls (Firemaster BP-60)

Corbett et al (1978) fed mice and rats up to 1,000 parts per million during gestation and produced no significant increase in defects in the offspring.

Fisher (1980) administered the compound to rats 24 hours before explanting their embryos. He found chemical growth retardation and malformations in these embryos when their were grown in vitro.

Corbett, T.H.; Simmons, J.L. and Endres, J.: Teratogenicity and tissue distribution studies of polybromated biphenyls (Firemaster BP-6) in rodents (abs) Teratology 17:37A (only), 1978.

Fisher, D.L.: Effects of polybrominated biphenyls on the accumulation of DNA, RNA, and protein in cultured rat embryos following administration. Envir. Res. 23:334-340, 1980.

1057 Polychlorcamphen

This chlororganic pesticide was administered per os to pregnant rats for 2 weeks at doses of 12 mg per kg daily (Badaeva, 1979). It was demonstrated that the substance in question decreased cholinesterase activity of fetal neural structures and hampered differentiation of cardiac neural elements. Martson and Shepelskaya (1980) gave this compound to rats from 6 through 15 days (40 mg per kg) or from day 1 through 20 (4 mg per kg) and to hamsters in the same doses from days 7 through 11 or on days 1 through 15. The compound showed slightly teratogenic and gonadotoxic activities.

Badaeva, L.N.: The effect of some pesticides on cholinesterase activity in the cardiac neural elements of pregnant animals and fetuses. Arkh. Anat. Gistol. Embryol. (USSR) 67,4:68-71, 1979.

Martson, L.V. and Shepelskaya, N.R.: Study of the generative function in animals exposed to polychlorocamphene. Gig. i Sanit. (USSR) 5:14-16, 1980.

1058 Polychlorobiphenyls (see Chlorobiphenyls and Kanechlor)

1059 Polyriboinosinic: Polyribocytidylic Acid [Poly l-poly-c]

This synthetic double stranded RNA was injected into rabbits in amounts of 1 or 2 mg per kg on days 8 and 9 or 11 and 12 (Adamson and Fabro, 1969). A very high resorption rate occurred but the number of defects in the survivors was not greater than in the control fetuses.

Adamson, R.H. and Fabro, S.: Embryotoxic effect of poly l-poly-C. Nature 223: 718 only, 1969.

1060 Polyvinyl Chloride (see vinyl chloride)

1061 Potassium

Crocker and Vernier (1970) showed in organ culture of fetal mouse kidney that lowered concentrations of potassium produced abnormal branching of tubules and occasional cystic dilatations of the ureteral buds.

Wilson et al. (1968) have shown that potassium deficiency does not account for the limb defects associated with acetazolimide administration.

Crocker, J.F.S. and Vernier, R.L.: Fetal kidney in organ culture: abnormalities of development induced by decreased amounts of potassium. Science 169: 485-487, 1970.

Wilson, J.G.; Maren, T.H.; Takano, K. and Ellison, A.C.: Teratogenic action of carbonic anhydrase inhibitors in the rat. Teratology 1: 51-60, 1968.

1062 Potato Blight

Renwick in 1972 published a hypothesis that anencephaly and spina bifida were associated with maternal exposure to an unknown substance in blighted potatoes. A geographical and temporal correlation between the severity of the late-blight of potatoes and the incidence of neural tube closure defects was made. An explanation for the higher incidence of these defects in the lower socioeconomic groups could have been explained by this hypothesis. This work has stimulated a large number of studies which have not been supportive (see Below). Renwick (1974) has modified his approach to the hypothesis suggesting long term storage in the body of some component from potatoes. Other types of moldy foods perhaps containing cytochalasins might be involved (Shepard, 1973). Tea drinking (Fedrick, 1974) and corned beef consumption (Knox, 1974) have also been shown to be more commonly found in the diets of mothers producing anencephalics. A comprehensive review of potato ingestion and anencephaly can be found in Lemire et al (1977).

The following paragraph lists the negative evidence against Renwick's hypothesis. Macmahan et al (1973) in Maine, Elwood (1973) in Eastern Canada, Field and Kerr (1973) in Australia, Smith et al, (1973) and Kinlen and Hewitt (1973) in Scotland have not been able to associate blighted potato

epidemics with neural tube closure defects. Clarke et al
(1973) and Roberts et al (1973) have studied the dietary
intake and storage methods of potatoes used by mothers
giving birth to children with neural tube closure defects
and neither could support the hypothesis that blighted
potatoes was a causative factor. Emanuel (1972) has pointed
out that in Taiwan where potato eating is more common in the
economically richer groups a higher rate of neural defects
persists in the poorer population.

Although Poswillo et al (1972) reported midline skull
defects in marmosets after maternal feeding of blighted
potato, these workers were unable to duplicate their
experiment (Poswillo et al, 1973). Allen et al (1977) fed
phytophthora blighted potatoes to pregnant rhesus monkeys
and marmosets and produced no neural tube defects. Two of
32 rhesus fetuses had hydrocephalus. The feeding of
blighted potato to rats has produced no congenital defects
(Ruddick et al, 1974; Swinyard and Chaube, 1973). Keeler et
al (1975) found no teratoenicity from blighted or aged
potatoes fed to pregnant rabbits, hamsters, rats and mice.
A few neural defects are reported in the pig and rabbit by
Sharma et al (1978).

Allen, J.R.; Marlar, R.J.; Chesney, C.F.; Helgeson, J.P.;
Kelman, A.; Weckel, K.G.; Traisman, E. and White, J.W.:
Teratogenicity studies on late blighted potatoes in
non-human primates (Macaca mulatta and Saguinus labiatus).
Teratology 15:17-24, 1977.

Clarke, C.A.; McKendrick, D.M. and Sheppard, P.M.: Spina
bifida and potatoes. Brit. Med. J. 3: 251-254, 1973.

Elwood, J.M.: Anencephaly and potato blight in Eastern
Canada. Lancet 1: 769 (only), 1973.

Emanuel, I.: Non-tuberous neural tube defects. Lancet 2:
879 only, 1972.

Fedrick, J.: Anencephalus and maternal tea drinking:
evidence for a possible association. Proc. Roy. Soc.
Med. 67: 356-359, 1974.

Field, B. and Kerr, C.: Potato blight and neural-tube
defects. Lancet 2: 507-508, 1973.

Keeler, R.F.; Douglas, D.R. and Stallknecht, G.F.: The
testing of blighted, aged, and control Russett Burbank
potato tuber preparations for ability to produce spina
bifida and anencephaly in rats, rabbits, hamsters and mice.
Am. Potato J. 52:125-132, 1975.

Kinlen, L. and Hewitt, A.: Potato blight and anencephalus
in Scotland. Brit. J. Prev. Soc. Med. 27: 208-213,
1973.

Knox, E.G.: Anencephalus and dietary intakes. Proc. Roy.
Soc. Med. 67: 355-356, 1974.

Lemire, R.J.; Beckwith, J.B. and Warkany, J.: Anencephaly,
chapter 2, Incidences, Etiology and Epidemiology. Raven

Press, New York, 1977, pp. 12-47.

MacMahon, B.; Yen, S. and Rothman, K.J.: Potato blight and neural-tube defects. Lancet 1: 598-599, 1973.

Poswillo, D.E.; Sopher, D. and Mitchell, S.: Experimental induction of foetal malformation with blighted potato: A preliminary report. Nature 239: 462-464, 1972.

Poswillo, D.E.; Sopher, D.; Mitchell, S.J.; Coxon, D.T.; Curtis, R.F. and Price, K.R.: Further investigations into the teratogenic potential of imperfect potatoes. Nature 244: 367-368, 1973.

Renwick, J.H.: Hypothesis. Anencephaly and spina bifida are usually preventable by avoidance of a specific but unidentified substance present in certain potato tubers. Br. J. Prev. Soc. Med. 26: 67-88, 1972.

Renwick, J.H.; Possamai, A.M. and Munday, M.R.: Potatoes and spina bifida. Proc. Roy. Soc. Med. 67: 360-364, 1974.

Roberts, C. J.; Revington, C.J. and Lloyd, S.: Potato cultivation and storage in South Wales and its relation to neural tube malformation prevalence. Brit. J. Prev. Soc. Med. 27: 214-216, 1973.

Ruddick, J.A.; Warwig, J. and Scott, P.M.: Nonteratogenicity in rats of blighted potatoes and compounds contained in them. Teratology 9: 165-168, 1974.

Sharma, R.P.; Willhite, C.C.; Wu, M.T. and Salunkhe, D.K.: Teratogenic potential of blighted potato concentrate in rabbits, hamsters and miniature swine. Teratology 18: 55-62, 1978.

Shepard, T.H.: Anencephaly and potatoes. Lancet 1: 79 (only), 1973.

Smith, C.; Watt, M.; Boyd, A.E.W. and Holmes, J.C.: Anencephaly, spina bifida and potato blight in the Edinburgh area. Lancet 1: 269 (only), 1973.

Swinyard, C.A. and Chaube, S.: Are potatoes teratogenic for experimental animals? Teratology 8: 349-358, 1973.

1063 Prazosin Hydrochloride

Noguchi and Ohwaki (1979) gave this hypotensive drug orally up to 300 mg per kg to pregnant rats on days 9-14 and observed no adverse effects in the fetuses. In rabbits on days 8-16 at 200 mg per kg some fetal weight reduction and kinky tails was found. No teratogenic effects were found at this dose which was toxic to the dams. Late gestational treatment in the rat was associated with slight reduction in fetal weight and survival.

Noguchi, Y.; Ohwaki Y.: Reproductive and teratologic studies with prazosin hydrochloride in rats and rabbits.

Oyo Yakuri 17:57-62, 1979.

1064 Preclampsia (see Hypertension)

1065 Prednisolone (also see Cortisone)

Pinsky and DiGeorge (1964) gave 0.5 mg daily to A-JAX mice during mid-pregnancy and produced a 77 percent incidence of cleft palate in the offspring. In clinically equivalent doses these authors felt that hydrocortisone had less ability to produce cleft palate than predinisolone. Balika and Kartasheva (1979) gave 30 mg daily to rats on days 10-15 of gestation. Clinicaly equivalent doses caused a stimulation of erythropoiesis, but retardation of myelopoiesis in the offspring. The disturbance observed was considered to be a result of drug transplacental passage.

Hasegawa et al (1974) studied beta-methasone,17,21-dipropionate, a long-acting derivative of prednisolone in pregnant rats and mice. Doses up to 2.5 mg per kg were given subcutaneously during midpregnancy. Adrenal hypertrophy and hemorrhage along with decreased viability occurred in the rat fetus. Also cleft palates and umbilical hernias were increased in the rat fetus. In the mouse fetus at the 2.5 mg dose level, 96 percent of the fetuses had cleft palates compared to a 11 percent incidence in those treated with 20.0 mg prednisolone.

Koga et al (1980A&B) studied the 17 valerate 21-acetate form of prednisolone in the pregnant rat and rabbit. Using up to 10 mg per kg subcutaneously on days 7 through 17 in the rat they found growth retardation and omphaloceles in the fetuses. In the rabbit using 0.1 and 0.25 mg per kg subcutaneously on days 6 through 18 they found increased resorptions and cleft palates in the fetuses. Fertility studies in the rat using 1.0 mg per kg were done and no adverse effects were found (Koga et al, 1980C).

Balika, Yu.D. and Kartasheva, V.E.: Transplacental action of prednisolone on fetuses blood-forming system. Akush. Ginekol. (USSR) 9:29-30, 1979.

Koga, T.; Ota, T.; Aoki, Y.; Nishigaki, K.; Suganuma, Y.: Reproductive studies of prednisolone 17-valerate 21-acetate teratologic studies in the rats. Oyo Yakuri 20:67-86, 1980A.

Koga, T.; Ota, T.; Aoki, Y.; Suganuma, Y.: Reproductive studies of prednisolone 17-valerate 21-acetate teratologic studies in rabbits. Oyo Yakuri 20:87-98, 1980B.

Koga, T.; Ota, T.; Nishigaki, K.; Aoki, Y.; Suganuma, Y.: Fertility study in rats of prednisolone 17-valerate 21 acetate. Yakuri to Chiryo 8:2169-2181, 1980C.

Hasegawa, Y.; Yoshida, T.; Kozen, T.; Ohara, T.; Okamoto, A.; Sakaguchi, I. and Kozen, T.: Teratology studies on betamethasone 17,21-diproprionate, prednisolone and beta-methasone 21-disodium phosphate in mice and rats.

(Japanese) Oyo Yakuri 8: 705-720, 1974.

Pinsky, L. and DiGeorge, A.M.: Cleft palate in the mouse: a teratogenic index of glucocorticoid potency. Science 147: 402-403, 1965.

1066 Prednisone (see Also cortisone)

Renisch et al (1978) gave mice 100 or 400 micrograms subcutaneously from day 13 until day 18 and observed significant weight reduction in the offspring. They also reported reduced weight in the newborns of 119 women treated with 10 mg daily for infertility problems. The newborn infants weighed approximately 300 gm less than the controls. Unfortunately, in neither the mouse nor the human study was the important effect of maternal weight gain reported or discussed.

Renisch, J.M.; Simon, J.N.; Karow, W.G. and Gandelman, R.: Prenatal exposure to prednisone in humans and animals retards intrauterine growth. Science 202: 436-438, 1978.

1067 Pregnancy Test Tablets

Gal (1972) has summarized the evidence that oral hormone pregnancy test tablets (Primodos-R or Amenorone Forte-R) are associated with neural tube malformations. From a group of 100 mothers giving birth to defective children 19 had been given the hormone pregnancy test. In a matched control of 100 only four women had been tested. Maternal age and the number of infections in the test group were also increased significantly but were shown not to account for the increased malformation rate. Smithells (1965) found only three congenital defects (cardiac) among 189 infants whose mothers were pregnancy tested with tablets. Oakley et al (1973) have reported a survey which gave no definite evidence for teratogenicity of this treatment. Dubowitz (1962) has reported a single case of a virulized female with a cloaca following pregnancy testing sometime after about the 35th gestational day. Neither Smithells (1965) nor Kullander and Kallen (1976) found hypospadius in the male offspring of 253 exposed mothers.

Dubowitz, V.: Virulisation and malformation of a female infant. Lancet 2: 405-406, 1962.

Gal, I.: Hormonal imbalance in human reproduction. In, Woollam, D.H.M. (ed.): Advances in Teratology, Vol. 5. New York: Academic Press, 1972. pp. 161-173.

Kullander, S. and Kallen, B.: A prospective study of drugs and pregnancy. Acta Obstet. Gynecol. Scand. 55:221-224, 1976.

Oakley, G.P.; Flynt, J.W. and Falek, A.: Hormone pregnancy tests and congenital anomalies. Lancet 2: 256-257, 1973.

Smithells, R.W.: The problem of teratogenicity. Practitioner 194: 104-110, 1965.

1068 Primethamine   (see   2,4-Diamino-5-chlorophenyl-6-ethyl-
     pyrimidine)

1069 Primidone (Mysoline-R)

     This anticonvulsant has a major metabolite which is a
     barbiturate. Myhre and Williams (1981) have reported two
     children exposed solely to the drug during gestation. Both
     had low nasal bridges and ocular hypertelorism. One had
     pulmonic stenosis and the other developmental delay. Rudd
     and Freedom (1979) have reported another case. More
     clinical data is needed to assess the associated risk.

     Myhre, S.A.; Williams, R.: Teratogenic effects associated
     with maternal primidone therapy. J. Pediat. 99:160-162,
     1981.

     Rudd, N.L.; Freedom, R.M.: A possible primidone
     embryopathy. J. Ped. 94:835-837, 1979.

1070 Procarbazine   (N-Isopropyl-alpha-(2-methyl-
     hydrazino)-p-toluamide)

     Tuchmann-Duplessis and Mercier-Parot (1967) administered
     this hydrazine orally to rats on the 8th to 14th days of
     gestation in a dose of 5 to 10 mg per kg. Treatment before
     the 12th day produced almost exclusively eye defects whereas
     after the 12th day they found defects of the limbs. Chaube
     and Murphy (1968) did teratologic studies in the rat and
     found that five 1-methyl-2-benzyl hydrazines derivatives
     were similarly teratogenic. Ivankovic (1972) produced
     neurogenic tumors in the offspring of rats given 125 mg per
     kg intravenously on day 22 of gestation. Thompson et al
     (1982) found a dose-related reduction in fetal brain weight
     when 1-10 mg per kg was given gravid rats on days 12-15. No
     obvious behavioral changes occurred.

     In the human Mennuti et al (1975) report a woman treated
     with 100 mg daily of this drug from the 28th through the
     35th gestational days was found to have a fetus with small
     pelvic kidneys. She also received as treatment of her
     Hodgkin's disease

     a single intravenous dose of nitrogen mustard and
     vincristine on the 28th day. Wells et al (1968) report a
     normal infant from a woman treated in early pregnancy.

     Chaube, S. and Murphy, M.L.: The teratogenic effects of
     the recent drugs active in cancer chemotherapy. In,
     Woollam, D.H.M. (ed.): Advances in Teratology, Vol. 3.
     New York: Academic Press, 1968. pp. 181-237.

     Ivankovic, S.: Erzengung von Malignomen bei Ratten nach
     Transplazentarer Einwirkung von N-isopropyl-alpha-2-(methyl-
     -hydrazino)-P-tolvamid HCl. Arzneim-Forsch 22: 905-907,
     1972.

     Mennuti, M.T.; Shepard, T.H. and Mellman, W.J.: Fetal
     renal malformation following treatment of Hodgkin's disease

during pregnancy. Obst. and Gynecol. 46: 194-196, 1975.

Thompson, D.J.; Dyke, I.L.; Lower, C.L.; Johnson, J.M.; Solomon, J.L.; Burek, J.D.: Spectrum of teratogenic effects of procarbazine HCl in the rat. Teratology 25:79A, 1982.

Tuchmann-Duplessis, H. and Mercier-Parot, L.: Production chez le rat de malformations oculaires et squelettiques par administration d'une methyl-hydrazine. C. R. Soc. Biol. (Paris) 161: 2127-2131, 1967.

Wells, J.H.; Marshall, J.R.; Carbone, P.P.: Procarbazine therapy for Hodgkin's disease in early pregnancy. JAMA 205: 935-937, 1968.

1071 Procaterol (5-(1-Hydroxy-2-isopropylaminobutyl)-8- Hydro-xycarbostyril Hydrochloride Hemihydrate)

This beta adrenergic stimulant was administered orally to rats on days 7 through 17 in doses as high as 250 mg per kg daily (Minami et al, 1979). Retarded ossification occurred in the treated fetuses. At 250 mg per kg there was an increase in number of enlarged renal pelves in the fetuses. This occurred in 52 percent of the treated and 28.7 percent of the controls. In the rabbit, doses of up to 500 mg per kg on days 6 through 18 were given orally (Tamagawa et al, 1979). The fetal weight was reduced and fetal deaths increased at the 150 mg per kg level. No increase in defects was found.

Minami, J.; Hatori, M. and Tanaka, N.: Reproduction studies of procaterol 2. Teratogenicity study in rats. (Japanese). Iyakuhin Kenkyu 10:102-111, 1979.

Tamagawa, M.; Kita, K.; Okabe, M. and Tanaka, N.: Reproduction studies of procaterol 3. Teratogenicity study in rabbits. Iyakuhin Kenyku 10:80-101, 1979.

1072 Prochlorperazine [Prochlorpemazine, Compazine-R, see Phenothiazines)

Roux (1959) administered this tranquilizer to pregnant mice and rats and found an increased incidence of cleft palate. A few anencephalic defects and one double monster were observed. The rats received 2.5 to 10 mg per day parenterally or 10 to 20 mg per day orally.

In a group of 4,295 pregnant women, Mellin (1975) identified 74 who took Compazine-R during their pregnancy. No increase in malformation rate or pattern of malformations was found. Among the 543 offspring of mothers taking this medication in the first 84 days of gestation, Milkovich and Van den Berg (1976) found no increase in malformations. Heinonen et al (1977) found 877 mothers who took the drug during the first lunar months and no increased defect rate was found. Vorhees et al (1979) gave 20 mg per kg orally to rats from day 7 to 20 and found a significant postnatal weight decrease and increase in fetal mortality. Only minor behavioral changes occurred.

1072

Vorhees, C.V.; Brunner, R.L. and Butcher, R.E.: Psychotropic drugs as behavioral teratogens. Science 205:1220-1225, 1979.

Heinonen, O.P.; Slone, D.; and Shapiro, S.: Birth Defects and Drugs During Pregnancy. Publishing Sciences Group Inc. Littleton, Mass.; 1977.

Mellin, G.W.: Report of prochlorperazine utilization during pregnancy from fetal life study data bank. (abstract) Teratology 11: 28a, 1975.

Miilkovich, L. and Van den Berg, B.J.: An evaluation of the teratogenicity of certain antinauseant drugs. Am. J. Obst. Gynecol. 125:244-248, 1976.

Roux, C.: Action teratogene de la prochlorpemazine. Arch. Fr. Pediatr. 16: 968-971, 1959.

1073 Progesterone

Neither progesterone nor 17-hydroxyprogesterone have been shown to masculinize the external genitalia of female fetuses from experimental animals. Johnstone and Franklin (1964) injected 0.25 mg from day 16 to day 19 in mice with negative results. In the rat Revesz et al. (1960) using up to 200 mg reported no virilization of the female fetuses. Suchowsky and Junkmann (1961) found no virilizing effects in the rat fetus exposed to progesterone or 17-hydroxyprogesterone.

Although there are many reports in the human of masculinization by the synthetic progestins (see 17-alpha--ethinyl-testosterone), the use of progesterone itself has been infrequently reported. Hayles and Nolan (1958) reported two masculinized female infants whose mothers received progesterone (10 mg by injection on 3 days and in the 2nd case up to 60 mg by mouth).

Aarskog (1979) has reported evidence that progesterone at doses of 5 to 250 mg per day may be associated occasionally with hypospadias. Among 130 patients with hypospadias, there were 11 whose mothers were exposed during pregnancy to progestins (medroxyprogesterone, hydroxyprogesterone, nor-ethisterone). In the control group of mothers giving birth to infants with facial clefts there were only 2 of 111 with similar exposures. He summarizes two similar studies of infants with hypospadias, both of which found a slight increased number of exposed mothers (Sweet et al, 1974 and Kupperman, 1961). Mau (1981) studied 33 males with hypospadias and found that eight were exposed to progestins during early pregnancy. This was not a significant increase over the 11 percent of control mothers exposed to progestins. The degree of hypospadias was not related to the period in pregnancy during which the medication was taken.

Yerushalmy (1972) in an analysis of hormones used for bleeding concluded that the bleeding was associcated with an increase in malformation rate but the hormone treatment without bleeding caused no increase.

Aarskog, D.: Maternal progestins as a possible cause of hypospadias. N. Eng. J. Med. 300:75-78, 1979.

Hayles, A.B. and Nolan, R.B.: Masculinization of the female fetus, possibly related to administration of progesterone during pregnancy. Proceedings of Staff Meeting, Mayo Clinic 32: 200-203, 1957.

Johnstone, E.E. and Franklin, R.R.: Assay of progestins for fetal virilizing properties in the mouse. Obstet. Gynecol. 23: 359-362, 1964.

Kupperman, H.S.: Progesterone and related steroids in the management of abortion. Brook Lodge Symposium, edited by A.K. Barnes, Brook Lodge Press, Augusta, 1961, pp. 105-107.

Mau, G.: Progestins during pregnancy and hyposadias. Teratology 24:285-287, 1981.

Revesz, C.; Chappel, C.I. and Gaudry, R.: Masculinization of female fetuses in the rat by progestational compounds. Endocrinology 66: 140-144, 1960.

Suchowsky, G.K. and Junkmann, K.: Study of the virilizing effect of progestogens on the female rat fetus. Endocrinology 68: 341-349, 1961.

Sweet, R.A.; Schrott, H.G.; Kurland, R. and Culp, A.S.: Study of the incidence of hypospadias in Rochester, Minnesota, 1940-1970, and a case-control comparison of possible etiologic factors. Mayo Clin. Proc. 49:52-58, 1974.

Yerushalmy, J.: Methodologic problems encountered in investigating the possible teratogenic effects of drugs, in Drugs and Fetal Development, edited by Klingberg, M.A. Abramovici, A. and Chemke, J.; Plenum Press, New York, 1972, pp. 427-440.

1074 Proglumide [D-L-4-Benzamido-N-N-dipropylglutaramic Acid]

This compound used in peptic ulcer therapy was given orally to pregnant rats and mice during major organogenesis. At the highest doses (rats 3,350 mg per kg, mouse 225 mg per kg) no gross defects or postnatal changes were found, but an increase in extra ribs and abnormal vertebrae was observed. (Ishizaki et al, 1971).

Ishizaki, O.; Saito, G. and Kagiwada, K.: The pharmacological study on proglumide 4. Effects of proglumide (KXM) on pre- and post-natal developments of the offsprings. Oyo Yakuri 5: 225-237, 1971.

1075 Proguanil (see Cycloguanil)

1076 Prolinomethyltetracycline

Fujita et al (1972a and 1972b) injected this compound in amounts up to 300 mg per kg intraperitoneally into mice and rats during major organogenesis. Pyrrolidion-methyl tetracycline was also tested in the mouse and both drugs produced some maternal toxicity and death at doses of 150 mg or more per kg as well as an increase in the incidence of polydactyly in the mice. Polydactyly of the hindlimbs was also found in tetracycline-treated mice (150 mg per kg). Post-natal studies were done in both species without major findings.

Fujita, M.; Moriguchi, M. and Koeda, T.: Teratological studies on prolinomethyltetracycline (PM-TC) in mice. Iyakuhin Kenkyu 3: 75-81, 1972a.

Fujita, M.; Moriguchi, M. and Koeda, T.: Teratological studies on prolinomethyltetracycline (PM-TC) in rats. Iyakuhin Kenkyu 3: 69-74, 1972b.

1077 Promazine (see Phenothiazines)

Murphree et al. (1961) observed an increased post-natal mortality in rats when the mother was given 5 mg per kg during 18 days of gestation.

Murphree, O.D.; Monroe, B.L. and Seager, L.D.: Survival of offspring of rats administered phenothiazines during pregnancy. J. Neuropsychiatry 3: 295-297, 1962.

1078 Propanediol-1,3

Gebhardt (1968) tested a number of glycols in the developing chick and found that propanediol-1,3 caused micromelia if given by injection into the air or yolk sac on the 4th day. He used 0.05 ml of the compound. It also produced micromelia if injected at the beginning of incubation. Similar amounts of propylene glycol (propanediol-1,2) butanediols, glycerol and diethyl and ethyl glycol were not teratogenic. Glycerol, propylene glycol and propanediol-1,3 were all moderately lethal when injected into the air cell on the 4th day.

Gebhardt, D.O.E.: The teratogenic action of propylene glycol (propanediol-1,2) and propanediol-1,3 in the chick embryo. Teratology 1: 153-162, 1968.

1079 Propanolol (and Phenylpropanolamine)

Although this drug has been shown to cross the placenta and produce respiratory depression, hypoglycemia and bradycardia in the neonate (Gladstone et al, 1975), there have been no reports of the production of congenital defects. Propanolol has been shown to be pharmacologically active during the early somite stages of the explanted rat embryo (Robkin et al, 1974).

A derivative of propanolol, phenylpropanolamine, was used in 726 pregnancies during the first 4 lunar months and 71 offspring were malformed (Heinonen et al, 1978). The general increase was significant statistically and included defects of the CNS, hypospadias and eye and ear defects. This drug is added to many proprietary preparations used to test upper respiratory diseases.

There is evidence that propanolol is associated with decreased fetal growth in the rat (Redmond, 1981) and suggestive evidence in humans (Redmond, 1982).

Injection of 10 mg per kg intravenously on day 13 of the mouse produced no fetal defects (Fujii and Nishimura, 1974).

Gladstone, G.R.; Hardof, A. and Gersony, W.M.: Propanolol administration during pregnancy: Effects on the fetus. J. Pediat. 86: 962-964, 1975.

Fujii, T.; Nishimura, H.: Reduction in frequency of fetopathic effects of caffeine in mice by pretreatment with propranolol. Teratology 10:149-151, 1974.

Heinonen, O.P.; Slone, D.; Shapiro, S.: Birth Defects and Drugs in Pregnancy. Publishing Sciences Group, Inc., 1977.

Redmond, G.P.: Propanolol inhibits brain and somatic growth in the rat. Pediat. Res. 15:645 (only) 1981.

Redmond, G.P.: Propanolol and fetal growth retardation. Seminars in Perinatalogy. 6:142-147, 1982.

Robkin, M.A.; Shepard, T.H. and Baum, D.: Autonomic drug effects on the heart rate of early rat embryos. Teratology 9: 35-44, 1974.

1080 Propoxyphene Napsylate (Darvon-R)

Emmerson et al. (1971) studied the effect of the analgesic compound in the pregnant rat and rabbit and found no terato-genic action. The rats receiving 200 and 400 mg per kg per day had some reduced fertility, fetal deaths and stunting of fetuses, but these doses produced about a 20 percent maternal death rate. The rabbits were given up to 80 mg per kg per day. Mineshita et al (1970) administered the drug by gavage to pregnant mice and rats during active organogenesis and no teratogenic or postnatal effects were found. The mice received up to 600 mg per kg and the rats 100 mg per kg per day. Vorhees et al (1979) reported behavioral changes in rats whose mothers received 75 mg per kg daily during most of gestation. Barrow and Souder (1971) have reported a single case of a newborn with arthrogryposis and Pierre Robin syndrome following maternal ingestion of the drug. Heinonen et al (1977) report that in over 600 exposed women there was no increase in malformation rate.

Barrow, M.V. and Souder, D.E.: Propoxyphene and congenital malformations. J.A.M.A. 217: 1551-1552, 1971.

Emmerson, J.L.; Owen, N.V.; Koenig, G.R.; Markham, J.K. and

1080

Anderson, R.C.: Reproduction and teratology studies on propoxyphene napsylate. Toxicol. Appl. Pharmacol. 19: 471-479, 1971.

Heinonen, O.P.; Slone, D.; Shapiro, S.: Birth Defects and Drugs in Pregnancy. Publishing Sciences Group, Inc., 1977.

Mineshita, T.; Hasegawa, Y.; Yoshida, T.; Kozen, T.; Maeda, T.; Sakaguchi, I. and Yamamoto, A.: Teratological effects of dextropropoxyphene napsylate on foetuses and suckling young of mice and rats. (Japanese) Oyo Yakuri 4: 1031-1038, 1970.

Vorhees, C.V.; Brunner, R.L. and Butcher, R.E.: Psychotropic drugs as behavioral teratogens. Science 205:1220-1225, 1979.

1081 Propylene Glycol (see Propanediol-1,3)

1082 Propylthiouracil

Klevit (1969) has reviewed the goitrogenic action of this drug on the human fetus. Freiesleben and Kjerulf-Jensen (1947) reviewed some clinical cases of goiter and reported that feeding 2000 mg Per kg of diet to maternal rats produced fetuses which were then fed to untreated rats and produced thyroid hypertrophy.

Freiesleben, E. and Kjerulf-Jensen, K.: The effect of thiouracil derivatives on fetuses and infants. J. Clin. Endocrinol. 7: 47-51, 1947.

Klevit, H.D.: Iatrogenic thyroid disease. In, Gardner, L.I. (ed.): Endocrine and Genetic Diseases of Childhood. Philadelphia: W.B. Saunders, 1969. pp. 243-252.

1083 Prostoglandin A-1

Jackson and Persaud (1976) treated rats on day 9 through 12 or 12 through 15 with 200 microgms subcutaneously and found no growth retardation or increase in resorptions or malform- ations. Using intrauterine injections on day 17, a significant increase in resorptions was found.

Jackson, C.W. and Persaud, T.V.N.: Pregnancy and progeny in rats treated with prostoglandin A-1. Acta Anat. 95:40-49, 1976.

1084 Prostoglandin E-1 (16,16-Dimethyl-trans-delta-2)

Ichikawa et al (1982) administered this compound intravaginally to the rat on days 0-7 and found decreased implantations but when pregnancy was established there was no adverse fetal effect. The dose was 1.0 mg per kg. Second pregnancies were not abnormal. They also gave up to 0.5 mg per kg intraperitoneally on days 17-21 and for 20 days postnatally to dams. Labor was complicated and fetal viability was reduced.

Ichikawa, Y.; Ozeki, K.; Yamamoto, Y.; Suzuki, Y.; Toh, A.: Studies of the administration of 16, 16-dimethyl-trans-Delta-2-prostoglandin E-1 in the pregnant rat. Gendai Iryo 14:593-618, 809-829, 1982.

1085 Prostoglandin E-2 methylhesperidin

Fujita et al (1973) gave this compound orally to mice and rats during active organogenesis in the maximum dose of 240 mg per kg daily and found an increase in resorptions but no malformation increase. Mercier-Parot and Tuchmann-Duplessis (1977) confirmed these findings in the rat but at intraperitoneal doses of 12.5 or more per kg on days 6 to 10, malformations occurred. The defects included anophthalmia, anencephaly, cleft lip and shortening of the mandible.

Daidohji et al (1981) gave oral doses of up to 2000 mg per kg to rats and mice during organogenesis and found no significant fetal effects. Postnatal function and reproduction in the rat offspring were normal. Administration on days 17 through weaning in the rat was associated with a decreased survival rate.

Daidohji, S.; Ishizaki, O.; Horiguchi, T.; Kimura, K.; Shibuya, K.; Ohmori, Y.: Reproductive studies of prostoglandin E-2-methylhesperidin complex (KPE). Yakuri to Chiryo 9:1369-1394, 1395-1411, 1981.

Fujita, T.; Suzuki, Y.; Yokohama, H.; Yonezawa, H.; Ozeki, Y.; Ichikawa, Y.; Yamamoto, Y. and Matsuoka, Y.: Toxicity and teratogenicity of prostaglandin E-2. (Japanese) Oyo Yakuri 8: 787-796, 1973.

Mercier-Parot, L. and Tuchmann-Duplessis, H.: Action of prostoglandin E-2 on pregnancy and embryonic development of the rat. Toxicology Letters 1:3-7, 1977.

1086 Prostoglandin F-2-alpha

Matsuoka et al (1971) gave this compound to pregnant mice intraperitoneally and intravenously to rats during active organogenesis. In the mice no significant changes were found in the fetuses. The maximum daily dose in mice was 0.25 mg per kg and in rats 2.0 mg per kg. At the highest dose in the rat, an increase in short tails was found.

Chang and Hunt (1972) studied the effect of this prostaglandin on the uterus, fallopian tube and embryo of the rabbit. 5 mg per kg soon after ovulation caused the disappearance of eggs and administration during the next 5 days disturbed development of the corpus leuteum and embryo. Abortion was produced with 2 to 5 mg per kg given subcutaneously on day 21. The effective dose was close to the lethal dose in the rabbit.

Chang, M.C. and Hunt, D.M.: Effect of prostaglandin F-2-

alpha on the early pregnancy of rabbits. Nature 236: 120-121, 1972.

Matsuoka, Y.; Fujita, T.; Nozato, T.; Yokohama, H.; Onishi, Y. and Ohta, K.: Toxicity and teratogenicity of prostaglandin F-2 alpha. (Japanese) Iyakuhin Kenkyu 2: 403-413,

1087 Prozyme

Tsutsumi et al (1978) fed this protease to pregnant rats and mice on days 7 through 13 in amounts up to 2,500 mg per kg per day. No adverse fetal effects were found.

Tsutsumi, S.; Yamamoto, R.; Tamura, A.; Sakuma, N. and Fuikiage, S.: Investigations on the possible teratogenicity of prozyme in mice and rats (Japanese) Clinical Report 12: 767-774, 1978.

1088 D-Prunasin (see Laetrile)

1089 Pteroylglutamic Acid Deficiency (see Folic Acid deficiency)

1090 Pyrantel Pamoate [Trans-1,4,5,6-tetrahydro-1-methyl--2-[-2(2-thienyl)vinyl] pyrimidine Pamic Acid Salt]

Owaki et al (1971) fed this anthelminthic to pregnant rats on days 9 through 14 of gestation in the highest dose of 3,000 mg per kg. No teratogenic or postnatal effects were seen. The same authors (1971) found no changes in fetuses from treated rabbits (1,000 mg per kg).

Owaki, Y.; Sakai, T. and Momiyama, H.: Teratological studies on pyrantel pamoate in rats. Oyo Yakuri 5: 41-50, 1971.

Owaki, Y.; Sakai, T. and Momiyama, H.: Teratological studies on pyrantel pamoate in rabbits. Oyo Yakuri 5: 33-39, 1971.

1091 Pyrazole (and derivatives)

Pyrazole (6 mg per kg), 4-methylpyrazole (6 mg per kg) or decyclopyrazole (6 mg per kg) were injected intraperitoneally on days 8, 10, 12 and 14 of the mouse gestation (Giknis and Damjanov, 1982). Malformations did not increase but each of the two derivatives increased embryo lethality when combined with ethanol.

Giknis, M.L.A.; Damjanov, I.: The effects of pyrazole and its derivatives on the transplacental embryotoxicity of ethanol (abstract) Teratology 25:43A-44A, 1982.

1092 Pyrethrum Extract

Lutz-Ostertag and Lutz (1970) applied an extract containing pyrethrum and piperonyl butoxide to the chorio-allantoic membrane and produced damaged testes with absence of gonadocytes in the surviving chicken embryo. Khera et al gavaged rats on days 6-15 with 50, 100 and 150 mg per kg and found increased resorptions at the 100 and 150 mg levels No significant increase in defect rate was found.

Khera, K.S.; Whalen, C.; Angers, G.: Teratogenicity study on pyrethrum and rotenone (natural origin) in pregnant rats. J. Toxicol. & Envir. Health 10:111-119, 1982.

Lutz-Ostertag, Y. and Lutz, H.: Action teratogene et sterilisante des pyrethrines synergisees sur l'embryon de poulet. C. R. Soc. Biol. 164: 777-779, 1970.

1093 Pyridine, Substituted (also see 6-Aminonicotinamide)

Landauer and Salam (1974) injected pyridine (20 mg per egg) into the developing chick egg at 96 hours and found muscular hypoplasia of the legs. Landauer and Salam (1973) have summarized their studies on chick teratogenicity of 12 substituted pyridines. 3-hydroxypridine and 3-hydroxy-6-methyl pyridine are highly teratogenic, producing micromelia and beak defects at doses of 2.5 mg injected at 96 hours of incubation. 2-hydroxypyridine caused the same type of malformations but at a lower frequency and higher dose. 4-hydroxypyridine was non-teratogenic.

2-amino-3hydroxypyridine was highly teratogenic and produced acromelia. 2,3-dihydroxypyridine was teratogenic at 1.0 mg levels and produced microphthalmia and rumplessness. 2,6-dihydroxypyridine was non-teratogenic.

The teratogenic effects were felt due to interference with pyridine nucleotide utilization with substitutions at the 3-position playing a dominant role.

Landauer, W. and Salam, N.: The experimental production in chicken embryos of muscular hypoplasia and associated defects of beak and cervical vertebrae. Acta Embryol. Experimentalis 1: 51-66, 1974.

Landauer, W. and Salam, N.: Quantitative and qualitative distinctions in developmental interference produced by various substituted pyridines. Molecular shape and teratogenicity as studied on chicken embryos. Acta Embryol. Experimentalis, 179-197, 1973.

1094 Pyridine-2-thiol-1-oxide [Omadine-R]

The zinc salt of this compound was applied to pregnant pigs daily from day 8 through 32 of gestation and no teratogenic effects were found. The concentration of the ointment was as high as 400 mg per kg (Wedig et al, 1975).

Wedig, J.H.; Kennedy, G.L.; Jenkins, D.H.; Henderson, R. and Keplinger, M.L.: Teratologic evaluation of zinc omadine when applied dermally on Yorkshire pigs. (abstract)

1094

Toxicol. Appl. Pharmacol. 33: 123 (only), 1975.

1095 Pyridoxine Deficiency [Vitamin B6 Deficiency]

Davis et al. (1970) produced defects in the offspring of rats maintained during pregnancy on a pyridoxine deficient diet and with 4-deoxypyridoxine added to the drinking water (0.1 mg per ml). Reduction defects of the digits, cleft palate, omphalocele and exencephaly were found. The treated fetuses had significant reductions in the weight of their spleen and thymus but not their kidney. The effects of the experimental regime were prevented by adding 1.0 mg pyridoxine to each ml of drinking water.

Davis (1974) has produced a post-natal immune deficiency by prenatal deficiency in the rat. The deficiency was terminated on day 21 of gestation. Runting syndrome occurred in some of the offspring. The non-runted offspring at 6 weeks of age were immunized with mycobacterium tuberculosis and when skin-tested had significantly less response than the controls.

Davis, S.D.: Immunodeficiency and runting syndrome in rats from congenital pyridoxine deficiency. Nature 251: 548-550, 1974.

Davis, S.D.; Nelson, T. and Shepard, T.H.: Teratogenicity of vitamin B(6) deficiency: omphalocele, skeletal and neural defects, and spleenic hypoplasia. Science 169: 1329-1330, 1970.

1096 1-Pyridyl-3,3-diethyltriazine (see 1-Phenyl-3,3

1097 Pyrimethamine (see 2,4-Diamino-5-p-chorophenyl-6- ethyl-pyrimidine) Dimethyl Triazine)

1098 Pyrithione

The zinc salt of this antidandruff agent was applied to the skin of pregnant rabbits from days 7 through 18 and no embryotoxicity or teratogenicity was observed (Nolen et al, 1975).

Nolen, G.A.; Patrick, L.F. and Dierckman, T.A.: A percutaneous teratology study of zinc pyrithione in rabbits. Toxicol. Appl. Pharmacol. 31: 430-433, 1975.

1099 Q Fever Agent (see Coxiella Burnetti)

1100 Quinacillin [3-Carboxy-2-quinoxalinylpenicillin]

Bough et al. (1971) injected pregnant rats and rabbits with 250 and 100 mg per kg respectively and found no fetal changes. The rats were injected from day 1 through day 20 and the rabbits from day 1 through day 16 of gestation. They demonstrated that the antibiotic reached the fetal serum and amniotic fluid.

Bough, R.G.; Everest, R.P.; Hale, L.J.; Lessel, B.; Mason, C.G. and Spooner, D.F.: Chemotherapeutic and toxicological properties of quinacillin. Chemotherapy 16: 183-195, 1971.

1101 Quinacrine

Rothschild and Levy (1950) injected 120 mg per kg of quinacrine subcutaneously into rats on the 13th through the 19th gestational days. Fetal death was increased but no defective fetuses were found. The level of quinacrine in the fetal liver was only 9 microgm as compared to the maternal liver level of 549 microgm.

Rothschild, B. and Levy, G.: Action de la quinacrine sur la gestation chez la rate. C. R. Soc. Biol. 144: 1350-1352, 1950.

1102 2-Quinoline Thioacetamide

In doses as high as 400 mg per kg on day 8 to 14, no teratogenic activity was found in rats. However, when the drug was given in doses of 200 mg per kg after organogenesis, a single dose produced a high incidence of digital abnormalities. This phenomenon was associated with protracted fetal vascular spasm (Sugitani et al, 1976).

Sugitani, T.; Ihara, T. and Mizutani, M.: Teratologic study of 2-quinoline thioaetamide in the rat (abs). Teratology 14: 254-255, 1976.

1103 Quinine

Mosher (1938) using guinea pigs gave quinine at different times during pregnancy. The average total dose was 1.8 gm. Hemorrhages, practically always localized to the scala tympani of the fetal inner ear, were found. Covell (1936) reported histologic changes in the cochlea of fetal guinea pigs after maternal treatment with 200 mg per kg.

Robinson et al. (1963) reported quinine ingestion during early pregnancy in two out of 200 mothers giving birth to congenitally deaf children. Tanimura (1972) has reviewed the human literature and reported that from 21 attempted abortions 10 central nervous system defects (6 hydrocephalics), 8 limb, 6 face, 5 digestive and 3 urogenital malformations resulted. The same author summarizes results in experimental animals and reports the absence of defects or abortions in pigtail monkeys receiving up to 200 mg per kg for 3 days.

Covell, W.P.: A cytologic study of the effects of drugs on the cochlea. Arch. Otolaryngol. 23: 633-641, 1936.

Mosher, H.P.: Does animal experimentation show similar

1103

changes in the ear of mother and fetus after the ingestion
of quinine by the mother? Laryngoscope 48: 361-395, 1938.

Robinson, G.C.; Brommitt, J.R. and Miller, J.R.: Hearing
loss in infants and preschool children. II. Etiological
Considerations. Pediatrics 32: 115-124, 1963.

Tanimura, T.: Effects on macaque embryos of drugs reported
or suspected to be teratogenic to humans. In Diczfalusy, E.
and Standley, C.C. (eds) The Use of Non-human Primates in
Research on Human Reproduction: Stockholm: WHO Research and
Training Centre on Human Reproduction, 1972, pp. 293-308.

1104 Rabbit Serum Protein

Adachi (1979) injected rabbit serum intraperitoneally into
mice in 1 and 2 ml amounts on days 10, 12 or 14. Treatment
on day 12 was followed by increases in cleft palate and
skeletal defects. The average number of live fetuses was
also reduced in the treatment groups.

Adachi, K.: Congenital malformations induced by
heterologous protein. Cong. Anom. 19:57-64, 1979.

1105 Radar

Sigler et al (1965) studied the radiation exposures of
parents of children with Down's syndrome. In the study
group 8.7 percent of the fathers had been intimately exposed
to radar. This was significantly greater than exposures in
a matched healthy control group (3.3 percent).

Sigler, A.T.; Lilienfeld, A.M.; Cohen, B.H. and Westlake,
J.E.: Radiation exposures in parents of children with
mongolism (Down's syndrome). Johns Hopkins Hosp. Bull.
117:374-399, 1965.

1106 Radiation [X-irradiation]

A large body of information is available on the adverse
effects of irradiation on the human and animal embryo and
fetus. Several reviews are available; Hicks and D'Amato
(1966), Yamazaki (1966), Kalter (1968) and Brent (1972:
1977) give general summaries, Jacobsen (1970) reviews data
related to low dose irradiation and Sikov and Mahlum (1969)
have edited a large symposium on radiation biology of the
fetal mammal. The main concentration has been on gene
mutation and development of the central nervous system.

Among commonly used animal models the mouse has been studied
extensively by Russell (1950). She reported that
preimplantation irradiation tended to be lethal or to have
no effect. Exposure on days 6.5 through 13.5 produced
little or no prenatal death but a high incidence of growth
retardation and abnormalities which in general were related
to dose and time of administration. Eye defects
(microophthalmia and coloboma) were most common after
treatment on days 7.5 through 9.5, while renal changes were

associated with treatment at day 9.5 and skeletal changes
appeared after exposure during days 9.5 to 12.5. After
treatment on day 14.5 abnormalities were uncommon, but
cataracts, hydrocephalus and skin defects did develop in
later life. Dr. Lillian Russell used radiation doses of
100 to 400 r.

Hicks and D'amato (1966) have concentrated their studies in
rats and mice on the central nervous system effects
occurring when treatment is given in the late embryonic and
fetal periods.

Wilson et al. (1953) have reported the effect of timed
radiation on type of defect including those of the
cardiovascular system. The effect of radiation on the
skeletal system of mouse fetuses has been detailed by
Degenhardt and Franz (1969) and Murakami and Kameyama
(1964). Rugh et al. (1964a and 1964b) have carried out
studies of the association of x-rays with cataract formation
and skeletal retardation. The cataracts developing in mice
were most common after exposure immediately after
fertilization and were interpreted as over-all damage rather
than direct effects on the organ primordia. Kalter (1968)
reviews the work that has been done in the rabbit and
hamster.

The effects of radiation on the human conceptus has centered
on (1) damage to the fetal central nervous system, (2) early
embryonic death with sex ratio changes and (3) long-term
effects on carcinogenesis. The effects of accidental
x-radiation on the developing fetus are well documented.
Driscoll et al. (1963) report on histologic changes
occurring in human fetuses following dosages of about 500 r.
Plummer (1952) observed that microcephaly was a common
complication of intrauterine radiation after the atomic bomb
explosion at Hiroshima, and that the degree of microcephaly
was directly related to the distance the mother was from the
epicenter. Blot and Miller (1973) found mental retardation
after 50 r doses in Hiroshima but 200 r doses in Nagasaki
and suggested the lower dose effect may have been due to a
higher neutron exposure in Hiroshima. Miller (1956) and
Neel and Schull (1956) did not find further health problems
in survivors or significant increases in defects in the offspring of parents exposed to the Japanese atomic bomb
explosions. Miller (1956) did find a subsequent leukemia
incidence of 1 in 1000 in children who were under 10 years
of age and were within 1500 meters of the epicenter of the
atomic bomb explosion. Macht and Lawrence (1955) surveyed
the offspring of radiologists and could detect no increase
in congenital defects. Wagner and Hayman (1982) summarized
the relative safety of pregnancy in female radiologists. An
association between Down's syndrome and maternal x-ray
exposure has been suggested by three retrospective studies
(Uchida and Curtis, 1961; Sigler et al.; 1965; Alberman et
al.; 1972a), but Carter et al. (1961) could not show a
connection. Uchida (1977) has recently summarized 11
studies of which 9 showed an increase in radiation exposure
of the mothers giving birth to Down's infants. Although
Neel and Schull did not report significant sex ratio changes
in the offspring of irradiated parents, Scholte and Sobels
(1964) offered some evidence for a change in sex ratio after

1106

parents were given radiation therapy. Brent (1980) has
reviewed the subject of radiation teratogenesis.

Boue et al (1975) reported an increase in chromosomally
abnormal abortuses from fathers who were occupationally
exposed to xray.

Long term effect of maternal radiation on the incidence of
malignancies in the offspring has been reported by MacMahon
(1962). The extensive data of the Oxford Survey of
Childhood Cancers (Bithell and Stewart, 1975) indicated a
relative risk estimate of 1.47 for mothers with prenatal
radiation exposure. Translated into numbers of childhood
cancers per 10,000, the increase would be from 10 to 15
cases. The risk was dependent on the number of films taken
and could be described as a linear relationship. Exposure
in the earlier months of pregnancy appeared to carry a much
higher risk. Other factors leading to maternal radiation
are hard to separate from the radiation effect. A special
committee of the United Nations (1972) has carefully
assessed the reports dealing with this subject. Diamond et
al (1973) studied 20,000 children exposed to radiation
during gestation and found a tripling of the leukemia death
rate in the treated white group but none was observed in an
equal-sized group of black children similarly exposed.

An increase in spontaneous abortion has been associated with
gonadal radiation (Alberman et al, 1972b). They reported
that matched controls received 180 mR while all forms of
spontaneously aborting women received 245 mR. Among the
group with abnormal karyotype the average exposure was 331.
Mothers of triploid embryos averaged 735 mR and these
authors point out that most of the increased risk is
expressed by non-viable conceptuses.

Schull et al (1981) have compared gonadal doses from atomic
bomb exposed parents with life expectancy, chromosomal
aneuploidy, and electrophoretic mutants of their offspring.
Their pregnancy outcomes were also studied. Although all
four indicators were found to be changed as expected there
was no statistical significance. The average genetic
doubling dose for the four indicators was 156 rems.

The teratogenic action of different isotopes such as
tritium, strontium, and I(131) are listed under their
separate headings. Okamoto et al. (1968) studied the
effect of fast neutron irradiation on the 7th through the
11th days in the rat fetus and found a dose-related increase
in congenital malformations. Cardiovascular anomalies were
the most frequent and an increased mortality of female
fetuses was observed. Hammer-Jakobsen (1961) gives
estimates for the mother's gonadal dose during pelvimetry of
822 mR.

Alberman, E.; Polani, P.E.; Fraser-Roberts, J.A.; Spicer,
C.C.; Elliott, M. and Armstrong, E.: Parental exposure to
x-irradiation and Down's syndrome. Ann. Hum. Genet.; Lond
36: 195-208, 1972a.

Alberman, E.; Polani, P.E.; Fraser-Roberts, J.A.; Spicer,
C.C.; Elliott, M.; Armstrong, E. and Dhadial, R.K.:

1106

Parental x-irradiation and chromosome constitution in their spontaneously aborted foetuses. Ann. Hum. Genet.; Lond 36: 185-194, 1972b.

Bithell, J.F. and Stewart, A.M.: Prenatal irradiation and childhood malignancy: A review of the British data from the Oxford survey. Br. J. Cancer 31: 271-287, 1975.

Blot, W.J. and Miller, R.W.: Mental retardation following in utero exposure to the atomic bombs of Hiroshima and Nagasaki. Radiology 106: 617-619, 1973.

Boue, J.; Boue, A. and Lazar, P.: Retrospective and prospective epidemiological studies of 1500 karyotyped spontaneous abortions. Teratology 12: 11-26, 1975.

Brent, R.L.: Irradiation in pregnancy. In, Lovinsky, J.J. (ed.): Gynecology and Obstetrics, Vol. 2, Chapter 32. Hagerstown, Maryland: Harper and Row, 1971. pp. 1-30.

Brent, R.L.: Radiation and other physical agents, in Handbook of Teratology, edited by F.C. Fraser and J.G. Wilson, Plenum Press, New York, 1977, pp. 153-201.

Brent, R.L.: Radiation teratogenesis. Teratology 21:281-298, 1980.

Carter, C.O.; Evans, K.A. and Stewart, A.M.: Maternal radiation and Down's syndrome (mongolism). Lancet 2: 1042 only, 1961.

Degenhardt, K.H. and Franz, J.: Models in comparative teratogenesis. Arch. Biol. (Liege) 80: 257-298, 1969.

Diamond, E.L.; Schmerler, H. and Lilienfeld, A.M.: The relationship of intra-uterine radiation to subsequent mortality and development of leukemia in children: A prospective study. Am. J. Epidemiol. 97: 283-313, 1973.

Driscoll, S.G.; Hicks, S.P.; Copenhaver, E.H. and Easterday, C.L.: Acute radiation injury to two human fetuses. Arch. Pathol. 76: 113-119, 1963.

Hammer-Jakobsen, E.: Gonad-doses in diagnostic radiology. J. Belge de Radiologie 44:253-276, 1961.

Hicks, S.P. and D'Amato, C.J.: Effects of ionizing radiations on mammalian development. In, Woollam, D.H.M. (ed.): Advances in Teratology, Vol. 1. New York: Academic Press, 1966. pp. 195-250.

Jacobsen, L.: Radiation induced foetal damage. A quantitative analysis of seasonal influence and possible threshold effect following low dose x-irradiation. In, Woollam, D.H.M. (ed.): Advances in Teratology, Vol. 4. New York: Academic Press, 1970. pp. 95-124.

Kalter, H.: Teratology of the central nervous system. Chicago: University of Chicago Press, 1968. pp. 90-138.

Macht, S.H. and Lawrence, P.S.: National survey of congenital malformations resulting from exposure to roentgen radiation. Am. J. Roentgenol. Radium Ther. Nucl. Med. 73: 442-466, 1955.

Macmahon, B.: Prenatal x-ray exposure and childhood cancer. J. Natl. Cancer Inst. 28: 1173-1191, 1962.

Miller, R.W.: Delayed effects occurring within the first decade after exposure of young individuals to the Hiroshima atomic bomb. Pediatrics 18: 1-18, 1956.

Murakami, U. and Kameyama, Y.: Vertebral malformation in the mouse foetus caused by x-radiation of the mother during pregnancy. J. Embryol. Exp. Morphol. 12: 841-850, 1964.

Neel, J.V. and Schull, W.J.: The effect of exposure to the atomic bombs on pregnancy termination in Hiroshima and

Nagasaki. National Academy of Science, N. R. Council Publication 461, Washington, 1956.

Okamoto, N.; Ikeda, T.; Satow, Y.; Sawasaki, M. and Inoue, A.: Effects of fast neutron irradiation on the developing rat embryo. Hiroshima J. Med. Sci. 17: 169-190, 1968.

Plummer, G.: Anomalies occurring in children exposed in utero to the atomic bomb in Hiroshima. Pediatrics 10: 687-693, 1952.

Rugh, R.; Duhamel, L.; Chandler, A. and Varma, A.: Cataract development after embryonic and fetal x-irradiation. Radiat. Res. 22: 519-534, 1964a.

Rugh, R.; Duhamel, L.; Osborne, A.W. and Varma, A.: Persistent stunting following x-irradiation of the fetus. Am. J. Anat. 115: 185-198, 1964b.

Russell, L.B.: Xray induced developmental abnormalities in the mouse and their use in the analysis of embryological patterns. J. Exp. Zool. 114: 545-602, 1950.

Scholte, P.J.L. and Sobels, F.H.: Sex ratio shifts among progeny from patients having received therapeutic x-radiation. Am. J. Human Genetics 16: 26-37, 1964.

Schull, W.J.; Otake, M.; Neal, J.V.: Genetic effect of the atomic bombs: A reappraisal. Science 213:1220-1227, 1981.

Sigler, A.T.; Lilienfeld, A.M.; Cohen, B.H. and Westlake, J.E.: Radiation exposure in parents of children with mongolism (Down's syndrome). Bulletin of Johns Hopkins Hospital 117: 374-399, 1965.

Sikov, M.R. and Mahlum, D.D.: (eds.) Radiation Biology of The Fetal and Juvenile Mammal. Proceedings of the 9th Annual Hanford Biology Symposium at Richland, Washington, May 5-8, 1969. U. S. Atom Energy Commission, Oakridge, Tenn.; Division of Technical Information, 1969.

Strobino, B.R.; Kline, J.; Stein, A.: Chemical and physical exposures of parents: Effects on human reproduction and offspring. Early Human Dev. 1:371-399, 1978.

Uchida, I.: Maternal radiation and trisomy 21 in Population Cytogenetics, Studies in Humans, edited by E.B. Hook and I.H. Porter, Academic Press, New York, 1977, pp. 285-299.

Uchida, I. and Curtis, E.J.: A possible association between maternal radiation and mongolism. Lancet 2: 848-850, 1961.

U.N. Committee: Ionizing radiation: levels and effects. Volume II. Effects. United Nations, New York. 1972, pp 427-428.

Wagner, L.K.; Hayman, L.A.: Pregnancy and women radiologists. Radiology 145:559-562, 1982.

Wilson, J.G.; Brent, R.L. and Jordan, H.C.: Differentiation as a determinant of the reaction of rat embryos to x-irradiation. Proc. Soc. Exp. Biol. Med. 82: 67-70, 1953.

Yamazaki, J.N.: A review of the literature on the radiation dosage required to cause manifest central nervous system disturbances from in utero and postnatal exposure. Pediatrics 37: 877-903, 1966.

1107 Radioiodine (see Iodine(131))

1108 Rat Virus (H-1 Strain)

Ferm and Kilham injected guinea pigs intravenously with the H-1 strain of rat virus on days 6, 7 or 8 of pregnancy. The virus was cultured from the fetuses the tissues of which had widespread intranuclear inclusions. Exencephaly, microcephaly and spina bifida were found in the embryos examined. Some enlarged livers and hearts were also reported.

Ferm, V.H. and Kilham, L.: Histopathologic basis of the teratogenic effects of H-1 virus on hamster embryos. J. Embryol. Exp. Morphol. 13: 151-158, 1965.

1109 Rauwolfia Alkaloids (see Deserpidine) (see Reserpine)

1110 Remantadine
(alpha-Methyl-1-Adamanthylmethylaminohydrochloride)

Alexandrov et al (1982) gave intragastrically to pregnant rats (500 mg per kg) and mice (300 mg per kg) on the 8, 9th or 13th day respectively and found no fetal damage. However, when the drug was given to rats on the 8th day of gestation embryonic mortality increased.

Alexandrov, V.A.; Pozharsky, K.M.; Likhachev, A.Ya.; Anisimov, V.N.: Okulov, V.B. and Ivanov, M.N.: The result of testing remantadine for carcinogenicity, teratogenicity and embryotoxicity. In: "Remantadine and other viruses inhibitors". (Riga, USSR) pp. 154-165, 1982.

1111

1111 Reovirus

Kilham and Margolis (1974) have reported the transplacental passage of reovirus type 3. In the hamster, inoculation during the first 5 days of gestation caused fetal death. On day 9 through 11 the fetuses became infected but survived and developed normally. The pathogenesis and fetal recovery after this virus infection in the rat has been described by these authors (1973).

Kilham, L. and Margolis, G.: Congenital infections due to reovirus type 3 in hamsters. Teratology 9: 51-64, 1974.

Margolis, G. and Kilham, L.: Pathogenesis of intrauterine infections in rats due to reovirus type 3. Pathologic and Fluorescent Antibody Studies. Lab Inv. 28: 605-613, 1973.

1112 Reserpine

Sobel (1960) reported pregnancy outcome from 15 women treated with reserpine. One stillborn and one pair of twins with congenital lung cysts resulted. Budnick et al. (1955) found nasal congestion with cyanosis, costal retraction and lethargy in newborns whose mothers were treated close to the time of partuition.

Kehl et al. (1956) reported that 0.75 to 4.5 mg administered during 6 to 10 day periods early in pregnancy prevented implantation in the rabbit. They found no effect on the fetus with treatment later in pregnancy. Tuchmann-Duplessis et al. (1957) studied the rat and found increased abortions. Goldman and Yakovac (1965) giving 1.5 mg per kg on the 9th or 10th day produced anophthalmia and other defects in slightly over 20 percent of the surviving rat fetuses. Kalter (1968) has reviewed the teratologic work on rauvolfia alkaloids.

Budnick, I.J.; Leiken, S. and Hoeck, L.E.: Effect in the newborn infant of reserpine administered ante partum. A.M.A. J. Dis. Child. 90: 286-289, 1955.

Goldman, A.S. and Yakovac, W.C.: Teratogenic action in rats of reserpine alone and in combination with salicylate and immobilization. Proc. Soc. Exp. Biol. Med. 118: 857-862, 1965.

Kalter, H.: Teratology of the central nervous system. Chicago: University of Chicago Press, 1968. pp. 147-148.

Kehl, R.; Audibert, A.; Gage, C. and Amarger, J.: Action de la reserpine a differentes periodes de la gestation chez la lapine. C. R. Soc. Biol. (Paris) 150: 2196-2199, 1956.

Sobel, D.E.: Fetal damage due to ECT, insulin coma, chlorpromazine or reserpine. A.M.A. Gen. Psychiatry 2: 606-611, 1960.

Tuchmann-Duplessis, H.; Gershon, R. and Mercier-Parot, L.: Troubles de la gestation chez la ratte, provoques par la reserpine et essais d'hormontherapie compensatrice. J. Physiol. 49: 1007-1019, 1957.

1113 Retinoic acid

This form of vitamin A is biologically more active than retinol or retinylesters but fails to protect a vitamin A deficient animal from blindness. Kochhar (1967) using pregnant rats and mice could produce the same defects as with excess retinyl acetate. A maternal oral dose of 50 mg per kg on day 9 or 10 produced over 40 percent malformations in the fetal mice. Shenefelt (1972) has used the material as a teratogen in the hamster. Wilson (1971) reported a Rhesus monkey with malformed face and ears and hydrocephalus following administration of 40 mg per kg on days 23, 24 and 25 of gestation. Fantel et al (1977) report oral-facial, limb and urogenital anomalies in a series of pigtail monkeys treated with 10 mg per kg per day from day 20 through 44.

Fantel, A.G.; Shepard, T.H.; Newell-Morris, L.L. and Moffett, B.C.: Teratogenic effects of retinoic acid in pigtail monkeys (Macaca nemestrina). Teratology 15: 65-72, 1977.

Kochhar, D.M.: Teratogenic activity of retinoic acid. Acta Pathol. Microbiol. Scand. 70: 398-404, 1967.

Shenefelt, R.E.: Morphogenesis of malformations in hamsters caused by retinoic acid: Relation to dose and stage of treatment. Teratology 5: 103-118, 1972.

Wilson, J.G.: Use of primates in teratological research and testing. In, Tuchmann-Duplessis, H. (ed.): Malformations Congenitales Des Mammiferes. Paris: Masson, 1971. pp. 277-280.

1114 Rheumatic Disease of Mother

Of 22 children with congenital heart block, 14 were born to mothers with rheumatic disease, primarily systemic lupus arythematosis (McCue et al, 1977).

McCue, C.M.; Mantakas, M.E.; Tingelstad, J.B. and Ruddy, S.: Congenital heart block in newborns of mothers with connective tissue disease. Circulation 56: 82-90, 1977.

1115 Rheumatoid Synovium Agent

Warren et al. (1970) injected pregnant mice with a raw slurry of synovial fluid from patients with rheumatoid arthritis and produced a redness and swelling in the joints of over one-half the offspring. The condition which resembled rheumatoid arthritis was transmitted to four generations without further injections.

Warren, S.L.; Marmor, L.; Liebes, D.M. and Hollins, R.L.: Congenital deformities of mice transmitted by a human rheumatoid synovium agent. In, Urist, M. (ed.): Clinical

1115

Orthopedics and Related Research, No. 70. Philadelphia:
J.B. Lippincott, 1970. pp. 216-219.

1116 Rhodium

Ridgway and Karnofsky (1952) exposed chick embryos at eight
days of incubation to Rh chloride (4.3 microatoms) and
caused stunting, mild micromelia and inhibition of feather
growth.

Ridgway, L.P. and Karnofsky, D.A.: The effects of metals
on the chick embryo: toxicity and production of abnormalities in development. Ann. N. Y. Acad. Sci. 55:
203-215, 1952.

1117 Ribavirin   (1-Beta-D-ribofuranosyl-1,2,4   triazole-3-
carboximide)

Kilham and Ferm (1977) gave single intraperitoneal doses of
1.25 to 6.15 mg per kg to hamsters on day 8 and found a high
incidence of defects which included the limbs, ribs, eyes,
and central nervous system. Anophthalmia and exencephaly
were found. In mice Kochhar et al (1980) produced
craniofacial bone defects when doses were 25 mg per kg daily
intraperitoneally for 3 days during organogenesis.

Kilham, L. and Ferm, V.H.: Congenital anomalies induced in
hamster embryos with ribavirin. Science 195:413-414, 1977.

Kochhar, D.M.; Penner, J.D.; Knudson, T.B.: Embryotoxc,
teratogenic and metabolic effects of ribavirin in mice.
Toxicol. Appl. Pharm. 52:99-112, 1980.

1118 Riboflavin Deficiency (also see Galactoflavin)

Experiments by Warkany and Nelson (1940) established for the
1st time that a syndrome of skeletal malformations could be
induced in mammals by withholding a single dietary factor.
A high number of offspring from deficient rats have short
mandibles, cleft palate, syndactylism and reduction defects
of the extremities. Hydronephrosis occurs also but defects
of the central nervous system and eye are uncommon. The
standard method for producing this experimental model is at
the beginning of pregnancy to place the rat on a riboflavin
deficient diet containing galactoflavin (60 mg per kg of
diet) a riboflavin analog. The mechanism of teratogenesis
is associated with a lack of the high energy generating
source, the terminal electron transport system (Aksu et al.;
1968). Warkany and Kalter (1959) have reviewed the general
subject. Kalter and Warkany (1957) have produced congenital
hydrocephalus in the mouse fetus made riboflavin deficient.
Romanoff and Bauernfeind (1942) produced micromelia and
mandibular hypoplasia and increased mortality in chicks from
hens maintained for three weeks on a riboflavin deficient
diet.

There is no compelling evidence that riboflavin deficiency
is a cause of congenital defects in the human fetus.

Aksu, O.; Mackler, B.; Shepard, T.H. and Lemire, R.J.:
Studies of the development of congenital anomalies in
embryos of riboflavin-deficient, galactoflavin fed rats.
II. Role of the terminal electron transport systems.
Teratology 1: 93-102, 1968.

Kalter, H. and Warkany, J.: Congenital malformations in
inbred strains of mice induced by riboflavin-deficient
galactoflavin-containing diets. J. Exp. Zool. 136:
531-566, 1957.

Romanoff, A.L. and Bauerfeind, J.C.: Influence of
riboflavin-deficiency in eggs on embryonic development
(Gallus domesticus). Anat. Rec. 82: 11-24, 1942.

Warkany, J. and Kalter, H.: Experimental production of
congenital malformations in mammals by metabolic procedure.
Physiol. Rev. 39: 69-115, 1959.

Warkany, J. and Nelson, R.C.: Appearance of skeletal abnormalities in the offspring of rats reared on a deficient
diet. Science 92: 383-384, 1940.

1119 Rifamycin [Methyl-4-piperazinyl-1 iminomethyl-3 rifamycine
S.V.]

Tuchmann-Duplessis and Mercier-Parot (1969) gave this
antibiotic by mouth to mice, rats and rabbits during the
active period of organogenesis. In the mice and rats doses
above 150 mg per kg produced spina bifida in both and cleft
palates in the mouse fetuses. Similar treatment of pregnant
rabbits had no effect on the fetuses. Anufrieva et al (1980
A and B) exposed by inhalation (in doses 6.1 and 0.81 mg per
cubic kilometer) Wistar rats during the entire gestation and
this drug produced no congenital malformations. Some
functional disturbances of the offspring's organs were
found. The authors thought that the drug did not affect the
structure or function of the placenta.

Warkany (1979) has reviewed this subject and 82 exposed
pregnancies where no increase in malformation rate occurred.
Steen and Stainton-Ellis (1977) reported nine malformations
among 202 exposed newborns. The malformations included
anencephaly (1), hydrocephalus (2), genitournary anomalies
(2), dislocated hip (1) and skeletal reduction anomalies
(3). The presence of three skeletal reduction defects in
such a small group is unusual. The method for selecting the
treated women was not given in the report and without this
knowledge about the total exposed population, evaluation is
difficult. In a personal communication from Dr. Steen the
writer was informed that the total number of treated
pregnancies was not known.

Greenaway et al (1981) produced open neural tubes in rat
embryos grown in vitro at concentrations of 12.5 to 50
micrograms per ml of medium. Bioactivation by a liver
monooxygenation was necessary to produce the defects but not
the reduction in growth measures.

Anufrieva, R.G.; Zeltser, I.Z.; Balabanova, E.L.;

Lapchinskaya, A.V.; Baru, R.V. and Svinogeeva, T.P.: Experimental study of rifampicin effect on albino rat embryogenesis. Antibiotiki (USSR) 25,4:280-284, 1980A.

Anufrieva, R.G.; Zeltser, I.Z. and Svinogeeva, T.P.: Placenta permeability by rifampicin. Antibiotiki (USSR) 25,3:199-201, 1980B.

Greenaway, J.C.; Fantel, A.G.; Shepard, T.H.: In vitro metabolic activation of rifampicin teratogenicity (abstract) Teratology 23: 37A, 1981.

Steen, J.S.M.; Stainton-Ellis, D.M.: Rifampicin in pregnancy. Lancet 2:604-605, 1977.

Tuchmann-Duplessis, H. and Mercier-Parot, L.: Influence d'un antibiotique, la rifampicine, sur le developpement prenatal des ronguers. C. R. Acad. Sci. (d) (Paris) 269: 2147-2149, 1969.

Warkany, J.: Antituberculous drugs. Teratology 20:133-138, 1979.

1120 Ronnel (Fenchlorphos)

This insecticide was administered by gavage in doses of 400, 600 and 800 Mg per kg to rats on days 6 through 15 (Khera et al, 1982). Extra ribs were increased in the 600 and 800 mg groups but fetal weight was not decreased.

Khera, K.S.; Whalen, C.; Angers, G.: Teratogenicity study on pyrethrum and rotenone (natural origin) and ronnel in pregnat rats. J. Toxicol. Envir. Health 10:111-119, 1982.

1121 Rotenone

This pesticide is known to be a specific and irreversible inhibitor of the electron transport chain between flavoprotein and cytochromes. Rao and Chauhan (1971) exposed early chick embryo explants for 15 minutes to 1 microgm per ml and observed after explantation various degrees of growth inhibition and neural tube defect. Khera et al (1982) gavaged rats on days 6 through 15 with 2.5, 5 or 10 mg per kg. Maternal and fetal weights were reduced at 5 and 10 mg. Minor skeletal defects were found in the 5 mg group and resorptions were 46 percent in the 10 mg group.

Khera, K.S.; Whalen, C.; Angers, G.: Teratogenicity study of pyrethrum and rotenone (natural origin) and ronnel in pregnant rats. J. Toxicol. and Envir. Health. 10-111-119, 1982.

Rao, K.V. and Chauhan, S.P.S.: Teratogenic effects of rotenone on the early development of chick embryos in vitro. Teratology 4: 191-198, 1971.

1122 Rubella Vaccines

The inadvertent vaccination of pregnant women with the rubella vaccines has not produced any part of the rubella syndrome in the offspring. Ebbin et al (1973) studied the pregnancy outcome of 60 women immunized in the first trimester and found no adverse fetal effects. Transplacental passage of the Cendehill virus has been shown (Ebbin et al, 1972; Bolognese et al, 1973) and the virus has been isolated from the fetus even 94 days after vaccination. Modlin et al (1975) have reviewed the effects of the vaccines.

Plotkin (1979) reported negative virus cultures from 12 products of conception after vaccination with RA27-3.

Bolognese, R.J.; Corson, S.L.; Fuccillo, D.A.; Sever, J.L. and Traube, R.: Evaluation of possible transplacental infection with rubella vaccination during pregnancy. Am. J. Obstet. Gynecol. 117: 939-941, 1973.

Ebbin, A.J.; Wilson, M.G.; Chandor, S.B. and Wehrle, P.F.: Inadvertent rubella vaccination in pregnancy. Am. J. Obstet. Gynecol. 117: 505-512, 1973.

Ebbin, A.J.; Wilson, M.G.; Wehrle, P.F.; Chin, J.; Emmons, R.W. and Lennette, E.H.: Rubella vaccine and pregnancy (letter) Lancet 2: 481 (only), 1972.

Modlin, J.F.; Brandling-Bennett, D.; Witte, J.J.; Campbell, C. C. and Meyers, J.D.: A review of five years experience with rubella vaccine in the United States. Pediatrics 55: 20-29, 1975.

Plotkin, S.A.: Rubella vaccination. Lancet 1:382, 1979.

1123 Rubella Virus

The original rubella syndrome described by Gregg (1941) consisted of the triad of congenital heart disease, deafness and cataracts. Since the identification of the virus (Alford et al.; 1964) the syndrome has been expanded to include intrauterine growth retardation, encephalitis, thrombocytopenia, radiographic changes of the long bones and persistence of the virus in the infant for a number of months after birth (Banatvala et al.; 1965; Cooper and Krugman, 1967; Korones et al.; 1965; Plotkin et al.; 1965; Rudolph et al.; 1965). Menser et al. (1967) reported a 25 year follow-up of 50 congenital rubella patients in Australia and found deafness (96 percent), cataracts (52 percent), small stature (50 percent) and congenital cardiovascular defects (22 percent). Ninety percent of these patients were of normal intelligence. One congeni-tally infected mother gave birth to a child with proven con-genital rubella. Neurological abnormalities have been described by Desmond et al. (1967). Studies of the inner ear pathology (Ward et al.; 1968) and function (Keir, 1965) have been reported. The pathologic findings are discussed by Tondury and Smith (1966) and by Naeye and Blanc (1965). Menser and Reye (1974) have reviewed the pathology and

1123

discussed the several rare forms of late onset of the
disease which may represent an immunopathological mechanism.
Diabetes mellitus may be found more commonly in the adult
survivors.

The incidence of rubella syndrome is higher in women exposed
during the 1st 90 days of gestation, and after this period
clinical manifestations are less common (Micheals and
Mellin, 1960). Sever et al. (1965) reported from data
collected prospectively from the collaborative study of
cerebral palsy that 10 percent of women with clinical
rubella in the 1st trimester had offspring with rubella
syndrome diagnosed within the 1st month. Because of
relative late registration of these mothers in the study
program it is reasonable to expect a higher incidence for
the total 1st-trimester-exposure women. Of mothers with
first trimester exposure but no clinical illness, 0.6
percent had a child with the congenital rubella syndrome.
Increased attack rates among Japanese women are best
explained by preexisting antibodies in the population.
(Ueda et al, 1978).

The production of virologic model syndromes in monkeys
(Parkman et al.; 1965; Delahunt and Rieser, 1967), rabbits
(Kono et al.; 1969) and rats (Cotlier et al.; 1966) have
been reported.

Ueda et al (1979) have reported the correlation between type
of defect and the time in gestation of the maternal rubella.
Among 55 patients, all 13 with cataract were exposed within
the first 60 days after the last normal menstrual period.
The occurrence of intrauterine growth retardation in the
same group of patients occurred only when the infection was
within the first 100 days of gestation; it was not related
to the type of defects that were present (Ueda et al, 1981).

Alford, C.A.; Neva, F.A. and Weller, T.H.: Virologic and
serologic studies on human products of conception after
maternal rubella. N. Engl. J. Med. 271: 1275-1281,
1964.

Banatvala, J.E.; Horstmann, D.M.; Payne, M.B. and Gluck,
L.: Rubella syndrome and thrombocytopenic purpura in
newborn infants. N. Engl. J. Med. 273: 474-478, 1965.

Cooper, L.Z. and Krugmann, S.: Clinical manifestations of
postnatal and congenital rubella. Arch. Ophthalmol. 77:
434-439, 1967.

Cotlier, E.; Fox, J.; Bohigian, G.; Beaty, C. and Dupree,
A.: Pathogenic effects of rubella virus on embryos and
newborn rats. Nature 217: 38-40, 1968.

Delahunt, C.S. and Rieser, N.: Rubella-induced
embryopathies in monkeys. Am. J. Obstet. Gynecol. 99:
580-588, 1967.

Desmond, M.M.; Wilson, G.S.; Melnick, J.L.; Singer, D.B.;
Zion, T.E.; Rudolph, A.J.; Pineda, R.G.; Ziai, M. and
Blattner, R.J.: Congenital rubella encephalitis. Course
and early sequalae. J. Pediatr. 71: 311-331, 1967.

1123

Gregg, N.M.: Congenital cataract following German measles in the mother. Trans. Ophthalmol. Soc. Aust. 3: 35-46, 1941.

Keir, E.H.: Results of rubella in pregnancy: II. Hearing defects. Med. J. of Aust. 2: 691-698, 1965.

Kono, R.; Hayakawa, Y.; Hibi, M. and Ishii, K.: Experimental vertical transmission of rubella virus in rabbits. Lancet 1: 343-347, 1969.

Korones, S.B.; Ainger, L.E.; Monif, G.R.G.; Roane, J.A.; Sever, J.L. and Fuste, F.: Congenital rubella syndrome: New clinical aspects with recovery of virus from infants. J. Pediatr. 67: 166-181, 1965.

Menser, M.A. and Reye, R.D.K.: The pathology of congenital rubella: A review written by request. Pathology 6: 215-222, 1974.

Menser, M.A.; Dods, L. and Harley, J.D.: A twenty-five-year follow-up of congenital rubella. Lancet 2: 1347-1350, 1967.

Micheals, R.H. and Mellin, G.W.: Prospective experience with maternal rubella and associated congenital malformations. Pediatrics 26: 200-209, 1960.

Naeye, R.L. and Blanc, W.: Pathogenesis of congenital rubella. J.A.M.A. 194: 1277-1283, 1965.

Parkman, P.D.; Phillips, P.E. and Meyer, H.M.: Experimental rubella virus infection in pregnant monkeys. Am. J. Dis. Child. 110: 390-394, 1965.

Plotkin, S.A.; Oski, F.; Hartnett, E.M.; Hervada, A.R.; Friedman, S. and Gowing, J.: Some recently recognized manifestations of the rubella syndrome. J. Pediatr. 67: 182-191, 1965.

Rowe, R.D.: Maternal rubella and pulmonary artery stenosis. Report of eleven cases. Pediatrics 32: 180-185, 1963.

Rudolph, A.J.; Yow, M.D.; Phillips, C.A.; Desmond, M.M.; Blattner, R.J. and Melnick, J.L.: Transplacental rubella infection in newly born infants. J.A.M.A. 191: 139-845, 1965.

Sever, J.L.; Nelson, K.B. and Gilkeson, M.R.: Rubella epidemic, 1964: effect on 6,000 pregnancies. Am. J. Dis. Child. 110: 395-407, 1965.

Tondury, G. and Smith, D.W.: Fetal rubella pathology. J. Pediatr. 68: 867-879, 1966.

Ueda, K.; Hisanga, S.; Nishida, Y.; Shepard, T.H.: Low-birth weight and congenital rubella syndrome: Effect of gestational age at time of maternal gestation. Clinical Pediatrics (in press)

Ueda, K.; Nishida, Y.; Oshima, K.; Yoshikama, H. and

Nonaka, S.: An explanation for high incidence of congenital rubella in Ryukyu. Am. J. Epid. 107:344-351, 1978.

Ueda, K.; Nishida, Y.; Oshima, K. and Shepard, T.H.: Congenital rubella syndrome: Correlation of gestational age at time of maternal rubella with type of defect. J. Pediatr. 94:763-765, 1979.

Ward, P.H.; Honrubia, V. and Moore, B.S.: Inner ear pathology in deafness due to maternal rubella. Arch. Otolaryngol. 87: 40-46, 1968.

1124 Rubeola

In a prospective study of the offspring of 60 mothers with rubeola during pregnancy Siegel and Fuerst (1966) found no increase in the incidence of congenital defects.

Siegel, M. and Fuerst, H.T.: Low birth weight and maternal disease. A prospective study of rubella, measles, mumps, chicken pox and hepatitis. J.A.M.A. 197: 680-684, 1966.

1125 Rubidomycine

Roux and Taillemite (1969) injected 1 to 3 mg per kg of this antibiotic into rats starting on the 7th day of gestation. With the higher dose which was given for 3 days by intraperitoneal route they found that 45 percent of the fetuses were defective. Ocular anomalies were the most common but defects of the heart, kidney and brain were present also. Using 1 mg daily from the 7th through the 14th day they obtained a malformation rate of 16 percent. Julou et al. (1967) did not produce congenital defects in the chick, mouse and rabbit. Although their dose in the rabbit was 0.25 mg per kg the mice received subcutaneous doses of 1.25 mg per kg during pregnancy.

Julou, L.; Ducrot, R.; Fournel, J.; Ganter, P.; Maral, R.; Populaire, P.; Koenig, F.; Myon, J.; Pascal, S. and Pasquet, J.: Un nouvel antibiotique doue d' activite antitumorale: la rubidomycine (13.057 R.P.). Arzneim. Forsch. 17: 948-954, 1967.

Roux, C. and Taillemite, J.L.: Action teratogene de la rubidomycine chez le rat. C. R. Soc. Biol. 163: 1299-1302, 1969.

1126 Rubratoxin B

Hood et al (1973) studied this mold metabolite in pregnant mice. Treatment consisted of single intraperitoneal injections on one of days 6 through 12 of gestation. At doses of 0.6 mg per kg malformations were produced and generally above this dose embryo lethality was found. The malformations found were exencephaly, open eye and umbilical hernia. Evans and Harbison (1977) found that the structural requirement for toxicity was an alpha-beta unsaturated lactone ring.

Evans, M.A. and Harbinson, R.D.: Prenatal toxicity of rubratoxin B and its hydrogenated analog. Toxicol. Appl. Pharm. 39:13-22, 1977.

Hood, R.D.; Innes, J.E. and Hayes, A.W.: Effects of rubratoxin B on prenatal development in mice. Bull. Environ. Contamination and Toxicology 10: 200-207, 1973.

1127 Rufocromomycin

Maraud et al. (1963) added 1 or 3 microgm to the vascular area of the chick embryo on the 3rd day of incubation and produced defects of the eye and skeleton. Thyroxine reduced the teratogenicity of this antimitotic antibiotic.

Maraud, R.; Coulaud, H. and Stoll, R.: Sur l'action tera-togene, chez l'embryon de poulet de la rufocromomycine associee ou non a la thyroxine. C. R. Soc. Biol. (Paris) 157: 1566-1569, 1963.

1128 Saccharin

Lorke (1969) tested pregnant mice with saccharin and found no evidence of teratogenicity. The mice received up to 25 mg per kg daily from the 6th through the 15th day. Cyclamate up to 250 mg per kg was also given without producing fetal changes. Fritz and Hess (1968) reported no teratogenic effects in the rat fetus when the mother received 25 mg per kg from day 6 through 15 of gestation. Kroes et al (1977) also found no teratogenicity in long term studies in mice. In the male offspring of rats maintained on a diet of 7.5 percent saccharin an increase in bladder neoplasms was found (Taylor et al, 1980). No increase was found with a diet containing 5 percent saccharin.

Lederer (1977) studied embryofetotoxicity of possible intermediates or contaminants of commercially prepared saccharin. Administered orally to rats at 0.1 percent of the diet, 0-toluenesulfonamide was devoid of toxicity, 0-sulfobenzoic acid increased the number of fetal resorptions sightly, but 0-sulfamoylbenzoic acid, and especially NH-4 0-sulfobenzoic acid markedly increased resorptions.

The general subject of saccharin toxicity is reviewed in detail by Cranmer (1980).

Kline et al (1978) found no increase in spontaneous abor-tions among women taking saccharin.

Cranmer, M.F.: Saccharin, a report. American Drug Institute Inc. and Pathotox Publishers Inc., 1980.

Fritz, H. and Hess, R.: Prenatal development in the rat following administration of cyclamate, saccharin and sucrose. Experientia 24: 1140-1141, 1968.

Kline, J.; Stein, Z.A.; Susser, M. and Warburton, D.: Spontaneous abortion and the use of sugar substitutes. Am.

1128

J. Obstet. Gynecol. 130: 708-711, 1978.

Kroes, R.; Peters, P.W.J.; Berkvens, J.M.; Verschuuren, T.D. and Van Esch, G.J.: Long term toxicity and reproduction study (including a teratogenicity study) with cyclamate, saccharin and cyclohexylamine. Toxicology 8:285-300, 1977.

Lederer, J.: Problem of saccharin. Med. Nutr. 13:23-32, 1977.

Lorke, D.: Untersuchungen von Cyclamat und Saccharin auf embryotoxische und teratogene wirkung an der Maus. Arzneim. Forsch. 19: 920-922, 1969.

Taylor, J.M.; Weinberger, M.A.; Friedman, L.: Chronic toxicity and carcinogenicity to the urinary bladder of sodium saccharin in the utero-exposed rat. Toxicol. & Appl. Pharm. 54:57-75, 1980.

1129 Salicylamide

This analgesic drug was fed as 2 percent of the diet to rats from the 5th to 11th or 12th to eighteenth days and a high proportion of the fetuses had skeletal defects of the ribs, spine and extremities (Knight and Roe, 1978).

Knight, E. and Roe, D.A.: Effect of salicylamide and protein restriction on the skeletal development of the rat. Teratology 18:17-22, 1978.

1130 Salicylate (Methyl, Sodium and Acetyl Forms)

Warkany and Takacs (1959) using methyl or sodium salicylate in the rat produced craniorachischisis, exencephaly, hydrocephaly, facial clefts, eye defects, gastroschisis and irregularities of the vertebrae and ribs. The methyl salicylate in doses of 0.1 to 0.5 ml was injected on the 9th, 10th and 11th gestational day. The sodium salicylate was injected on the same days in doses of 60 to 180 mg. These dose levels caused some maternal deaths. Since this work appeared numerous workers have confirmed and extended it (for summary see Kalter, 1968). Goldman and Yakovac (1963) showed that treatment on the 10th day with 300 mg per kg was non-teratogenic but 400 and 500 mg per kg caused defects in the rat fetus. Larsson and Eriksson (1966) gave mice 10 mg of sodium salicylate on various days of of gestation and found skeletal defects and hemorrhages of the extremities with a few cases of exencephaly. Trasler (1965) gave acetylsalicylic acid (with a trace of tween 80) to mice on the 9th and 10th or 10th and 11th day of pregnancy and produced cleft lip, exencephaly, microcephaly and spina bifida.

Lepointe and Harvey used salicylamide (d-hydroxybenzamide) in the hamster and produced 'cranial blisters' in the offspring. Wilson (1971) gave monkeys 250 mg per kg twice daily for three days at various times between the 18th to 26th day of gestation and produced two abortions, two small normal fetuses, one normal and two fetuses with malformations (one multiple and both with heart defects). At doses of 100 or 150 mg per kg per day on days 22 through 32 in the monkey, Wilson et al (1977) observed two fetuses of 41 with defects (cystic kidney and cranioschisis). They compared the pharmacodynamics in the rat and monkey and found higher concentrations and larger duration of concentrations in the rat. Gulienetti et al. (1962) found increased amniotic fluid volume in treated rats. Goldman and Yakovac (1964, 1965) have published a series of studies attempting to determine the mechanism of teratogenic action. Adrenalectomy did not change the abnormality rate but sodium carbonate and chloride and central nervous system depressants protected the fetuses. Larsson (1971) has reviewed his work on the action of salicylate on the fetus.

Chebotar (1967) reported that both immobilization and ammonium chloride intensified while sodium bicarbonate reduced the teratogenic effects of sodium salicylate in the rat. Both ammonium chloride and immobilization caused the maternal salicylate level to increase. Beall and Klein (1977) found that aspirin teratogenicity was increased in rats which were also food restricted. Salicylate added directly to culture at 600 microgram per ml of medium produced dilation of the rhombencephalon and mesoncephalon of the rat embryos (McGarrity et al, 1978 and Greenaway et al, 1982). Saglo (1982) reported that female Wistar rats after receiving one intragastric dose of 700 mg per kg salicylate delivered fetuses with numerical and structural chromosome aberrations. The same effect was observed after treatment of male rats with the same dose of this substance. Vasilenko et al (1979) established that administration of this substance (one-tenth LD-50) to male rats during 1.5 months seriously damaged spermatogenesis and repeated inhalations (25 mg per cubic meter) during 4 months produced pathological changes in spermatogenic epithelium of offspring.

In humans Turner and Collins (1975) studied 144 mothers taking salicylates regularly. The stillbirth rate was increased and the birth weight was reduced as compared to matched controls. No increase in congenital defects was noted. They confirmed the findings of Lewis and Schulman (1973) that therapeutic doses of salicylate are often associated with the post-maturity syndrome. Nelson and Forfar (1971) reported 8 anomalies in 458 pregnancies where salicylates were taken in the first 28 days of gestation. Although this was higher than the 3 malformations in 911 controls, the exposed group included achondroplasia and Down's syndrome, two defects of probable preconceptual origin. Richards (1969) studied 833 pregnancies with anomalies in the offspring and matched these against pregnancies with normal offspring. For the women ingesting salicylates during the first trimester, the rate was 22 and the control 14, a difference which was significant at the 0.1 percent level. The author did not find an increase in the number of salicylate exposed malformation pregnancies during the second and third pregnancies. Crombie et al (1977) queried 10,000 and found no excess of aspirin users among those who had malformed infants. Slone et al (1976) found no increase in malformation rates among nearly 14,000 offspring of heavy or occasional aspirin users. Corby (1978) has reviewed the

1130

effect of aspirin on the mother and fetus.

Rumack et al (1981) studied intracranial hemorrhage in 108 infants born at 34 weeks gestation or earlier. The incidence of hemorrhage was 71 percent (12 of 17) among the offspring of mothers who took aspirin within a week of delivery. This was significantly more common than in the control group (31 of 71 infants). Ten of twenty infants exposed to acetaminophen had bleeding and this rate did not differ from the control.

Beall, J.R. and Klein, M.F.: Enhancement of aspirin-induced teratogenicity by food restriction in rats. Toxicol. Appl. Pharmacol. 39: 489-495, 1977.

Chebotar, N.A.: Peculiarities of action of sodium salicylate at various stages of embryogenesis in rats and the influence of certain shifts in the female organism on its teratogenic activity. Pharmacol. Toxicol. (Russian) No. 2: 221-225, 1967.

Corby, D.G.: Aspirin in pregnancy: Maternal and fetal effects. Pediatrics 62:930-945, 1978.

Crombie, D.L.; Pinsent, K. and Slater, B.C.: Teratogenic drugs R.C.G.P. survey. Brit. Med. J. 4: 178-179, 1970.

Goldman, A.S. and Yakovac, W.C.: The enhancement of salicylate teratogenicity by maternal immobilization in the rat. J. Pharmacol. Exp. Ther. 142: 351-357, 1963.

Goldman, A.S. and Yakovac, W.C.: Prevention of salicylate teratogenicity in immobilized rats by certain central nervous system depressants. Proc. Soc. Exp. Biol. Med. 115: 693-696, 1964.

Goldman, A.S. and Yakovac, W.C.: Teratogenic action in rats of reserpine alone and in combination with salicylate and immobilization. Proc. Soc. Exp. Biol. Med. 118: 857-862, 1965.

Greenaway, J.C.; Shepard, T.H.; Fantel, A.G.; Juchau, M.R.: Sodium salicylate teratogenicity in vitro. Teratology 26:167-171, 1982.

Gulienetti, R.; Kalter, H. and Davis, N.C.: Amniotic fluid volume and experimentally-induced congenital malformations. Biol. Neonate 4: 300-309, 1962.

Kalter, H.: Teratology of the central nervous system. Chicago: University of Chicago Press, 1968. pp. 153-154.

Lapointe, R. and Harvey, E.B.: Salicylamide-induced anomalies in hamster embryos. J. Exp. Zool. 156: 197-200, 1964.

Larsson, K.S.: Action of salicylate on prenatal development. In, Tuchmann-Duplessis, H. (ed.): Malformations Congenitales Des Mammiferes. Paris: Masson, 1971. pp. 171-186.

Larsson, K.S. and Eriksson, M.: Salicylate-induced fetal death and malformations in two mouse strains. Acta Paediatr. 55: 569-576, 1966.

Lewis, R.B. and Schulman, J.D.: Influence of acetylsalicylic acid, an inhibitor of prostoglandin synthesis, on the duration of human gestation and labour. Lancet 2: 1159, 1973.

McGarrity, C.; Samani, N.J.; Beck, F.: The in vivo and in vitro action of sodium salicylate on rat embryos. J. Anat. 127:646 (only), 1978.

Nelson, M.M. and Forfar, J.O: Associations between drugs administered during pregnancy and congenital anomalies of the fetus. Brit. Med. J. 1:523-527, 1971.

Richards, I.D.G.: Congenital malformations and environmental influences in pregnancy. Brit. J. Prev. Med. 23:218-225, 1969.

Rumack, C.M.; Guggenheim, M.A.; Rumack, B.H.; Peterson, R.G.; Johnson, M.L.; Braithwaite, W.R.: Neonatal intracranial hemorrhage and maternal use of aspirin. Obstetrics and Gynecology 58(5):52-S-56-S, 1981.

Saglo, V.J.: Effect of sodium salicylate on the chromosome apparatus of rat somatic and embryonal cells. Farmakol. Toksikol. (USSR) 5:88-89, 1982.

Slone, D.; Heinonen, O.P.; Kaufman, D.; Siskind, V.; Monson, R.R. and Shapiro, S.: Aspirin and congenital malformations. Lancet 1:1373-1375, 1976.

Trasler, D.G.: Aspirin-induced cleft lip and other malformation in mice. Lancet 1: 606-607, 1965.

Turner, G. and Collins, E.: Fetal effects of regular salicylate ingestion during pregnancy. Lancet 2: 338-339, 1975.

Vasilenko, N.M.; Manzhelay, E.S. and Gnezdilova, A.J.: Gonadotoxic action of acetylsalicylic acid. Farmakol. Toksikol. (USSR) 4:421-423, 1979.

Warkany, J. and Takacs, E.: Experimental production of congenital malformations in rats by salicylate poisoning. Am. J. Pathol. 35: 315-331, 1959.

Wilson, J.G.: Use of Rhesus monkeys in teratological studies. Fed. Proc. 30: 104-109, 1971.

Wilson, J.G.; Ritter, E.J.; Fradkin, R.: Comparative distribution and embryotoxicity of acetylsalicylic acid in pregnant rats and Rhesus monkeys. Toxicol. Appl. Pharmacol. 41:67-68, 1977.

1131 Sarkomycin

Takaya (1965) injected rats with 5 to 11 mg per kg daily on

1131

the 6th through 10th day and produced 10 percent malformations in the offspring. The malformations included hydronephros and microophthalmia.

Takaya, M.: Teratogenic effects of antibiotics (Japanese). J. Osaka City Medical Center 14: 107-115, 1965.

1132 Sauna Bathing

Saxen et al (1982) studied the sauna habits of 100 women giving birth to children with neural defects and 202 giving birth to children with orofacial defects. Their habits did not differ from the control Finnish women. The authors point out that nearly every woman in Finland visited the sauna bath, and yet, the central nervous system defect rate in Finland is among the lowest.

Harvey et al (1981) concluded from their studies that remaining in a hot tub at 39 degrees for at least 15 minutes and 41.1 degrees for least 10 minutes was unlikely to damage a human pregnancy. None of the volunteers were able to remain in the sauna for a long enought time to significantly increase body temperature.

Harvey, M.A.S.; McRorie, M.M.; Smith, D.W.: Suggested limits to the use of hot tub and sauna in pregnant women. Canad. M. A. J. 125: 50-53, 1981.

Saxen, L.; Holmberg, P.C.; Nurminen, M.; Koosma, E.: Sauna and congenital defects 25:309-313, 1982.

1133 Schizophyllan

This antitumor glycan was given by Ishizaki et al (1982) subcutaneously to rats and rabbits during organogenesis. The highest dose in the rat was 50 mg per kg and in the rabbit 25 mg per day. No significant changes were produced in the fetuses of either species.

Ishizaki, O.; Daidohji, S.; Ohmori, Y.; Saito, G.: Reproductive studies of schizophyllan (SPG). Oyo Yakuri 23:935-951, 1982.

1134 Scopoletin (see Solanine)

1135 Selenium

Franke et al. (1936) applied 0.5 mg per kg (of egg) to the air cell of the chick and produced eye or beak defects in about 50 percent of the survivors. Ridgway and Karnofsky (1952) produced head and beak defects and cysts of the rump in chick embryos treated with 0.01 to 0.08 mg of selenious acid during the 1st 8 days of incubation. Schroeder et al. (1971) fed 3 ppm in the drinking water to mice and observed a significant increase in the number of runts produced, and by the third generation the treatment group became reduced in number.

Franke, K.W.; Moxon, A.L.; Poley, W.E. and Tully, W.C.: Monstrosities produced by the injection of selenium salts into hens eggs. Anat. Rec. 65: 15-22, 1936.

Ridgway, L.P. and Karnofsky, D.A.: The effects of metals on the chick embryo: toxicity and production of abnormalities in development. Ann. N. Y. Acad. Sci. 55: 203-215, 1952.

Schroeder, H.A. and Mitchener, M.: Toxic effects of trace elements on the reproduction of mice and rats. Arch. Environ. Health 23: 102-106, 1971.

1136 Semicarbazide HCl

Neuman et al. (1956) injected 2.0 mg of this chemical on the 6th day into the yolk and observed bent tarsometatarsal and tibiotarsal bones and malformed beaks in the 14-day-chick embryos. P-hydrazinbenzoic acid and thiosemicarbazide produced similar defects, but 1-phenylsemicarbazide produced shortening of the leg bones with moderate edema and whitish areas in the liver. No defects were found with benzoic hydrazide. Stoll et al. (1970) were able to show that vitamin B-6 administration reduced the number of defects in the semicarbazide-treated chick and that desoxypyridoxamine enhanced this teratogen.

Neuman, R.E.; Maxwell, M. and McCoy, T.A.: Production of beak and skeletal malformations of chick embryo by semicarbazide. Proc. Soc. Exp. Biol. Med. 92: 578-581, 1956.

Stoll, R.; Bodit, F. and Maraud, R.: Sur l'action teratogene de la semi-carbizide. Role de la vitamine B-6 et des amines biogenes. C. R. Soc. Biol. 164: 1011-1013, 1970.

1137 Sendai Virus [Parinfluenza 1 virus]

Coid and Wardman (1971) have reported fetal wastage in rats infected with Sendai virus. No malformations were detected. Tuffrey et al (1972) demonstrated the virus by immunofluorescence in fertilized mouse ova.

Coid, R. and Wardman, G.: The effect of para-influenza type 1 (Sendai) virus infection on early pregnancy in the rat. J. Reprod. Fert. 24: 39-43, 1971.

Tuffrey, M.; Zisman, B. and Barnes, R.D.: Sendai (parainfluenza 1) infection of mouse eggs. Br. J. Exp. Path. 53: 638-640, 1972.

1138 Sennaglucosides

Mizutani et al (1980) studied the reproductive effects of this vegetable laxative on rats. They gave up to 90 mg per kg daily either before mating and during the first 7 days of gestation or on days 7-17. There were no reproductive problems or adverse fetal effects found.

1138

Mizutani, M.; Izutsu, M.; Hoshimoto, Y.; Nagao, T.; Matsuda, H.: Effects of sennaglucosides on reproductive function and fetal development and differentiation in rats. Kiso to Rinsho 14:380-396, 1980.

1139 Septra-R (see Trimethoprim)

1140 Serotonin [5-Hydroxytryptamine]

Poulson et al. (1963) injected 2 ml of the creatine sulfate form into mice on the 8th, 9th or 10th day of gestation and produced defects of the eye, limbs and tail. Some skull and central nervous system abnormalities were found also. From earlier work (Poulson et al.; 1960) they propose that the mechanism of action of this substance is through placental hemorrhagic changes. Marley et al. (1967) performed detailed equilibrium studies in the rat on day 9 and 10 and showed that 5-hydroxytryptamine greatly slowed the transfer of radioactive sodium to the embryo.

Reddy et al. (1963) injected rats with 0.5 to 5.0 mg daily during pregnancy and at the 1.5 mg level found abnormalities in 4 of 17 live fetuses. The congenital defects consisted of anophthalmia, hydrocephalus, exencephaly and omphalocele. Vacuolization of the myocardial cells was found also. They report that a woman with a carcinoid tumor gave birth to three infants who died of neonatal respiratory distress and a 4th infant with undetermined multiple defects. Thompson and Gautieri (1969) injected mice subcutaneously with 5 or 10 mg per kg on days 7 through 12 and produced defects including hydrocephalus, exencephalus, hydronephrosis, renal agenesis and gastroschisis.

Marley, P.B.; Robson, J.M. and Sullivan, F.M.: Embryotoxic and teratogenic action of 5-hydroxytryptamine: mechanism of action in the rat. Br. J. Pharmacol. Chemother. 31: 494-505, 1967.

Poulson, E.; Botros, M. and Robson, J.M.: Effect of 5-hydroxytryptamine and iproniazid on pregnancy. Science 131: 1102-1103, 1960.

Poulson, E.; Robson, J.M. and Sullivan, F.M.: Teratogenic effect of 5-hydroxytryptamine in mice. Science 141: 717-718, 1963.

Reddy, D.V.; Adams, F.H. and Baird, C.D.C.: Teratogenic effects of serotonin. J. Pediatr. 63: 394-397, 1963.

Thompson, R.S. and Gautieri, R.F.: Comparison and analysis of the teratogenic effects of serotonin, angiotensin-2 and bradykinin in mice. J. Pharm. Sci. 58: 406-412, 1969.

1141 Shortwave (see Microwave Radiations)

1142 Silver

Ridgway and Karnofsky (1952) using AgNO(3) determined that the LD-50 was 0.10 mg in chick eggs. No defects were reported.

Ridgway, L.P. and Karnofsky, D.A.: The effects of metals on the chick embryo: toxicity and production of abnormalities in development. Ann. N. Y. Acad. Sci. 55: 203-215, 1952.

1143 Silymarin

This antihepatotoxic substance from the plant silybum marianum was tested in rats and rabbits by Hahn et al. (1968) and no evidence for teratogenicity was found. The pregnant rats received 1 gm per kg and the rabbits 100 mg per kg during the active period of organogenesis.

Hahn, G.; Lehmann, H.D.; Kurten, M.; Uebel, H. and Vogel, G.: Zur Pharmacologie und Toxikologie von Silymarin des Antihepatotoxischen Wirkprinzipes aus Silybum Marianum (1.) Gaertn. Arzneim. Forsch. 18: 698-704, 1968.

1144 Sisomycin

Esaki et al (1978) administered this antibiotic to pregnant mice on days 6 through 15 in doses up to 120 mg per kg and found no adverse fetal changes. Tanioka et al (1978) gave up to 30 mg per kg to monkeys on days 23 through 36 and found no teratogenic changes.

Esaki, K.; Ohshio, K. and Yoshikawa, K.: Effects of subcutaneous administration of sisomycin on reproduction in the mouse. Experiments on drug administration during the development period in fetuses. (Japanese) CIEA Preclin Rpt 4: 157-164, 1978.

Tanioka, Y.; Koizumi, H. and Inaba, K.: Teratogenicity test by intramuscular administration of sisomycin in Rhesus monkeys. CIEA Preclin Rpt 4:57-71, 1978.

1145 Small Pox Vaccination

Vaccination against small pox during pregnancy has not been associated with increased defects in the human. Saxen et al. (1968) found no effect of a mass population vaccination on fetal wastage and congenital defects in the Finnish population. Over 300,000 persons were vaccinated during a 5-month period.

Green et al. (1966) have reviewed experience with fetal vaccinia infection which may occur after vaccination of the mother during pregnancy.

Thalhammar (1957) reported that cataracts could be produced experimentally in the fetal mouse by maternal injection of the virus; however, no lesions could be found by Theiler (1966).

1145

Green, D.M.; Reid, S.M. and Rhaney, K.: Generalized vaccinia in the human fetus. Lancet 1: 1296-1298, 1966.

Saxen, L.; Cantell, K. and Hakama, M.: Relation between small pox vaccination and outcome of pregnancy. Am. J. Public Health 58: 1910-1921, 1968.

Thalhammer, O.: Die Vakzine-virusembryopathie der weissen Maus. Wien. Z. Inn. Med. 38: 4-72, 1957.

Theiler, K.: Gibt es eine Vakzine-virusembryopathie? Pathol. Microbiol. 29: 825-836, 1966.

1146 Smoking (see Cigarette Smoking)

1147 Snake Oil

Hashimoto et al (1979) gave this oil extracted from the digestive tract of the cobra to mice orally from day 6 through 15 in amounts of 4,500 mg per kg and found no adverse fetal effects.

Hashimoto, T.; Takeuchi, K.; Nagase, M. and Akatuka, K.: Pharmacological studies of snake oil. Teratology test in mice. (Japanese) Clinical Report 13:808-814, 1979.

1148 Sodium Chloride

Nishimura and Miyamoto (1969) injected 1900 or 2500 mg per kg into mice on the 10th or 11th day of pregnancy and produced up to 18 percent skeletal defects. Clubfoot was the most frequently found defect. The type of defect was different than found with fasting.

Nishimura, H. and Miyamoto, S.: Teratogenic effects of sodium chloride in mice. Acta Anat. (Basel) 74:121-124, 1969.

1149 Soforalcone
(2-carboxymethoxy-4,4-bis(3-methyl-2-butenyloxy)- chalcone)

Yamada et al (1980) administered up to 1000 mg per kg daily orally before mating, during the first week or during all of gestation and found no adverse effects on the fetuses or offspring. Maternal weight gain was reduced at the highest dose.

Yamada, T.; Tanaka, Y.; Suzuki, H.; Nogariya, T.; Nakone, S.; Sasajima, M.; Ohzeki, M.: Reproductive studies of 2-(carboxymethoxy- -4,4-bis(3-methyl-2-butenyloxy)chalcone. Fertlity perinatal and postnatal study in rats. Oyo Yakuri 19:515-553, 1980.

1150 Solanine

Solanine, a toxic alkaloid isolated from both deadly

nightshade and from shoots of stored potatoes, has been tested for teratogenicity in chick embryos by Nishie et al. (1971). Ten to 25 mg was administered on the 4th day of incubation to the chick and no increase in congenital mal- formations was found.

The embryonic LD-50 was 19 mg. Kline et al. (1961) fed rats a diet containing 10 percent potato sprouts from the time pregnancy was indicated by increased weight gain. No defects were detected but the pups died before weaning. Ruddick et al (1974) found no congenital defects in rats after they administered up to 25 mg per kg on days 8 through 11. Ruddick et al (1974) also fed rats scopoletin and alpha-chaconine with negative teratogenic findings.

Kline, B.E.; Elbe, H.U.; Dahle, N.A. and Kupchan, S.M.: Toxic effects of potato sprouts and of solanine fed to pregnant rats. Proc. Soc. Exp. Biol. Med. 107: 807-809, 1961.

Nishie, K.; Gumbmann, M.R. and Keyl, A.C.: Pharmacology of solanine. Toxicol. Appl. Pharmacol. 19: 81-92, 1971.

Ruddick, J.A.; Harwig, J. and Scott, P.M.: Nonteratogen- icity in rats of blighted potatoes and compounds contained in them. Teratology 9: 165-168, 1974.

1151 Solvents, Organic (see Toluene, Xylene, Trichlorethylene, Methyl ethyl Ketone, 2-Ethoxyethanol and Methyl Chloride)

Holmberg (1979) found solvent exposure in 14 mothers of 132 offspring with neural tube closure defects or hydrocephaly. Since only two of the matched controls had exposure he reported that there was a signifcant increase in exposure. The type of solvent was variable and included denatured alcohol, acetone, styrene, toluene, xylene, ethylene oxide, benzene and methylethylketone. Syrovadko and Malsheva (1977) studied 311 female enamelers who were exposed to 2-ethoxyethanol, chlorobenzene, tricresol and solvent naphtha. Congenital anomalies including heart defects and tallipes were significantly increased (10.0 vs 3.9 percent). The control workers were from a regional hospital, silica plant and elsewhere.

Holmberg, P.C.: Central-nervous-system defects in children born to mothers exposed to orgaic solvents during pregnancy. Lancet 2:177-179, 1979.

Syrovadko, D.N.; Malsheva, Z.U.: Work conditions and their effect on certain specific functions among women who are engaged in the production of enamel-insulated wire (Russian) Gig Tr. Prof. Zabol. 4:25-28, 1977.

1152 Somatotrophin

Hultquist and Engfeldt (1949) using two preparations from the anterior pituitary were able to produce enlarged rat fetuses. The preparations used, Phyol-R (80 to 120 units) or antuitrin G (120 to 180 units), were contaminated with other endocrine substances, and the effect of litter size and duration of gestation complicated the analysis of fetal growth. Clendinnen and Eayrs (1961) injected 3.2 mg of purified somatotropin into rats from the 7th to the 19th day of gestation and observed a significant increase in birth weight over the control animals. The duration of the gestation periods in the control and treated was not stated. The treated group of fetuses showed enhancement of corttically-mediated behavior, and this was supported by histologic studies showing hypertrophy of neurones. Zamenof et al. (1971) have extended this work and shown that growth hormone reverses the adverse effect of starvation on brain development.

Croskerry and Smith (1975) have presented convincing evidence that human somatotrophin prolongs pregnancy in the rat and they believe that this postmaturity along with an increase in maternal weight may explain the increases in brain growth and learning observed by others after growth hormone therapy during pregnancy.

Clendinnen, B.G. and Eayrs, J.T.: The anatomical and physiological effects of prenatally administered somatotrophin on cerebral development in rats. J. Endocrinol. 22: 183-193, 1961.

Croskerry, P.G. and Smith, G.K.: Prolongation of gestation by growth hormone: A confounding factor in the assessment of its prenatal action. Science 189: 648-650, 1975.

Hultquist, G.T. and Engfeldt, B.: Giant growth of rat fetuses produced experimentally by means of administration of hormones to the mother during pregnancy. Acta Endocrinol. 3: 365-376, 1949.

Zamenof, S.; Mathens, E.V. and Gravel, L.: Prenatal cerebral development: Effect of restricted diet, reversal by growth hormone. Science 174: 954-955, 1971.

1153 Spermine

Butros (1972) has studied the effect of this polyamine on chick embryos. Injecting 2.6 to 10 mg per egg at 0 to 7 days of incubation he observed a general arrest of development at 2.5 days. A striking finding was an over production of immature erythrocytes which at times packed the brain vesicles.

Butros, J.: Action of spermine on early chick development. I. Morphogenesis and histogenesis. Teratology 6: 181-190, 1972.

1154 Spironolactone (see Aldactone-R)

1155 Spray Adhesives

in 1973 DR. J.r. Seely reported publically that 10 persons exposed to spray adhesives had significant increases in the number of chromosomal breaks and gaps in peripheral lymphocytes and two of these persons were infants with multiple anomalies. Reanalysis of the slides by an ad hoc committee failed to reach definitive conclusions (Anonymous, 1973). Separate studies of humans exposed to spray adhesives (see Murphy et al for review, 1975) and epidemiologic studies failed to find that spray adhesives were associated with chromosomal damage or birth defects.

No defects were found in fetal hamsters exposed from day 5 through 10 of gestation to inhalation of foil art adhesive (Murphy et al, 1975).

Anonymous: Adhesive spray studies are inconclusive so far. Prod. Safety Lett. 2: 2 (only), 1973.

Murphy, J.C.; Collins, T.F.X.; Black, T.N. and Osterberg, R.E.: Evaluation of teratogenic potential of a spray adhesive in hamsters. Teratology 11: 243-246, 1975.

Oakley, G.P.; Nissim, J.E.; Hanson, J.W.; Boyce, J.M. and Roberts, M.: Epidemiologic investigations of possible teratogenicity of spray adhesives (abstract). Teratology 9: 31a-32a, 1974.

1156 Staphlococcal Phage Lysate

Hirayama et al (1980) gave this product subcutaneously to pregnant rats before gestation, during the first 7 days, during days 6 through 16 and during days 17 through 7 postnatal days. The maximum dose was 2.0 ml (400 microunits) per kg per day. No ill effects were found on fertility, the fetuses or postnatal development. Rabbits were given up to 0.5 ml daily during gestation with no ill effects being found in the fetuses.

Hirayama, H.; Wada, S.; Kimura, T.; Enokuya, Y.; Ohkuma, H.; Hikita, J.: Reproductive evaluation of staphlococcal phage lysate (SPL). Oyo Yakuri 20:487-499, 575-594, 595-608, 1980.

1157 Starvation (see Fasting)

1158 Stelazine-R (see Trifluoperizine)

1159 Stilbestrol-R (see Diethylstilbesterol)

1160 Streptomycin

Two case reports have questioned the association of streptomycin medication with congenital nerve deafness. Leroux (1950) reported a deaf infant following treatment of the mother with 30 gm of streptomycin during the 8th month, and Kern (1962) reported deafness of an infant whose mother was given 20 gm of dihydrostreptomycin during the 1st 4 months of pregnancy. Robinson and Cambon (1964) reported

1160

two congenitally deaf children whose mothers were treated
with 1 gm per day during the last 4 months in one case and
during the 6th to 14th week in the other. Varpela et al.
(1969) found normal hearing in 50 children who had been
exposed in utero to dihydrostreptomycin or streptomycin.
Conway and Birt (1965) examined 13 children exposed to the
drugs in utero and found no disability but the caloric test
in six and audiograms in four were abnormal.

Suzuki and Takeuchi (1961) were unable to detect deafness in
mice or rats exposed to 200 to 600 mg per kg during pregnancy. Boucher and Delost (1964) gave 25 or 250 mg per kg to
mice on the 14th gestational day and detected growth failure
for a month after birth. Warkany (1979) has recently
reviewed the teratogenicity of this and other
antituberculous drugs.

Boucher, D. and Delost, P.: Developpement post-natal des
descendants issus de meres traitees par la streptomycine au
cours de la gestation chez la souris. C. R. Soc. Biol.
(paris) 158: 2065-2069, 1964.

Conway, N. and Birt, B.D.: Streptomycin in pregnancy:
effect on the fetal ear. Br. Med. J. 2: 260-263, 1965.

Kern, G.: Zur Frage der Intrauterinen Streptomycin
Schadigung. Schweiz. Med. Wochenschr. 92: 77-79, 1962.

Leroux, M.L.: Existe-t-il une surdite congenitale acquise
due a la streptomycine? Ann. Otolaryngol. 67: 194-196,
1950.

Robinson, G.C. and Cambon, K.G.: Hearing loss in infants
of tuberculous mothers treated with streptomycin during
pregnancy. N. Engl. J. Med. 271: 949-951, 1964.

Suzuki, Y. and Takeuchi, S.: Etude experimentale sur
l'influence de la streptomycine sur l'appareil auditif du
foetus apres administration de doses variees a la mere
enceinte. Keio J. Med. 10: 31-41, 1961.

Varpela, E.; Hietalahti, J. and Aro, M.J.T.: Streptomycin
and dihydrostreptomycin medication during pregnancy and
their effect on the child's inner ear. Scand. J. Resp.
Dis. 50: 101-109, 1969.

Warkany, J.: Antitubeerculous drugs. Teratology
20:133-138, 1979.

1161 Streptonigrin

Warkany and Takacs (1965) injected rats intraperitoneally
with 0.25 mg per kg on the 9th, 10th or 11th day of
gestation. Following treatment on the 10th day 96 percent
of the fetuses were abnormal. A wide variety of defects
occurred; omphalocele, exencephaly, hydrocephaly and defects
of the eye and skeleton predominated. The axial skeleton
was commonly involved and the authors describe in detail one
fetus with iniencephalus. Chaube et al. (1969) confirmed
the findings and found that methyl ester streptonigrin and

isopropylidine azastreptonigrin were equally teratogenic.

Chaube, S.; Kuffer, F.R. and Murphy, M.L.: Comparative teratogenic effects of streptonigrin (NSC-45383) and its derivatives in the rat. Cancer Chemother. Rep. 53: 23-31, 1969.

Warkany, J. and Takacs, E.: Congenital malformations in rats from streptonigrin. Arch. Pathol. 79: 65-79, 1965.

1162 Streptozotocin (see Diabetes)

1163 Stress, Psychological (see Emotional Stress)

1164 Strontium [Sr-90]

Nilsson and Henricson (1969) injected pregnant mice on the 11th or 16th gestational day with 20 microcuries of Sr(90). A general reduction of fetal oocytes was found. Finkel and Biskis (1969) concluded from dog experiments that the fetal dog was not more sensitive than the adult to either the lethal or the oncogenic effect of radiostrontium. Underdeveloped jaws, disproportionate growth of the long bones and many fractures were found in fetuses after administration of 1 millicurie per kg to the mother 6 days before delivery. Hiraoka (1961) injected 5 to 10 microcuries intraperitoneally into pregnant mice at various times during pregnancy and found an increase in skeletal defects.

Sternglass (1969) has compared excess fetal death rate with the Sr(90) content of fetal bone and was of the opinion that a strong correlation existed between the two measurements. This assertion by Sternglass has been clearly refuted by Lindop and Rotblat (1969) who pointed out that he had manipulated the data to fit his conclusions and many better explanations than radiation effects could account for the diminished decline in infant mortality.

Finkel, M.P. and Biskis, B.O.: Pathological consequences of radiostrontium administered to fetal and infant dogs. In, Sikov, M.R. and Mahlum, D.D. (eds.): Radiation Biology of the Fetal and Juvenile Animal. Oak Ridge, Tennessee: United States Atomic Energy Commission, 1969. pp. 543-566.

Hiraoka, S.: The transplacental effects of the radio-strontium-90 upon the mouse embryos. Acta Anatomica Nipponica 36: 161-171, 1961.

Lindop, P.J. and Rotblat, J.: Strontium-90 and infant mortality. Nature 244: 1257-1260, 1969.

Nilsson, A. and Henricson, B.: Effect of Sr(90) on the ovaries of fetal mice. In, Sikov, M.R. and Mahlum, D.D. (eds.): Radiation Biology of The Fetal and Juvenile Animal. Oak Ridge, Tennessee: United States Atomic Energy Commission, 1969. Pp. 313-324.

1164

Sternglass, E.J.: Evidence for low-level radiation effects on the human embryo and fetus. In, Sikov, M.R. and Mahlum, D.D. (eds.): Radiation Biology of the Fetal and Juvenile Animal. Oak Ridge, Tennessee: United States Atomic Energy Commission, 1969. pp. 693-718.

1165 Styrene

Murray et al (1978) studied the effect of inhalation and gavage in the pregnant rat and rabbit during organogenesis. At doses of 600 ppm for 7 hours daily, no fetal changes were produced in either species. Rats were given up to 150 mg per kg without fetal effects.

Murray, F.J.; John, J.A.; Balmer, M.F. and Schwetz, B.A.: Teratologic evaluation of styrene given to rats and rabbits by inhalation and by gavage. Toxicology 11:335-343, 1978.

1166 Sucrose

Seta (1931) produced skeletal changes in the guinea pig fetus by feeding the mother 5 to 10 gm per kg during the later half of pregnancy. Hirata (1936) added 5 to 7 gm per kg of body weight to the diet of pregnant rabbits. Although the results in the first litters were almost absent treatment was continued and the fetuses from the second and third litters were reported to have cataract, microphthalmia and hydrocephalus. Furukawa (1939) confirmed this work.

Furukawa, S.: Experimental production of malformation. Nisshin Igaku (Japanese) 28: 1119-1160, 1939.

Hiruta, M.: Experimental study on congenital hydrocephaly. Part I. Relationship between production of congenital hydrocephaly and maternal diet. Nisshin Igaku (Japanese) 25: 1980-2004, 1936.

Seta, S.: Effect of maternal nutrition during pregnancy on the skeletal development of the fetus. Nisshin Igaku (Japanese) 21: 486-504, 1931.

1167 Sulfaguanol   [N-[(4,5-Dimethyl-
-2-oxazolyl)amidino]-sulfanilamide

Kuhne et al (1973) fed this antibiotic to pregnant rats and rabbits during organogenesis in amounts up to 250 mg per kg and found no fetal changes.

Kuhne, J.; Leuschner, F. and Neumann, W.: Untersuchungen zur Toxikologie von Sulfaguanol. Arzneim-Forsch 23: 178-184, 1973.

1168 Sulfamethazine (see Sulphonamides)

1169 Sulfamethoxazole (see also Trimethoprim)

Sulfamethoxazole crosses the human placenta and reaches a peak at 10 hours. After a few gestational weeks, the concentration of sulfamethoxazole is lower in amniotic fluid and in the foetus than in maternal serum (Reid et al, 1975). Williams et al (1969) treated 120 pregnant women and found no increase in defects in their offspring; only 10 of the women were treated before the 16th week. Heinonen et al (1977) reported no increase in malformation rates in the offspring from 46 pregnancies when treatment was given in the first 4 lunar months.

Heinonen, O.P.; Slone, D.; Shapiro, S.: Birth Defects and Drugs in Pregnancy. Publishing Sciences Group, Inc.. 1977.

Reid, D.W.J.; Caille, G.; Kaufmann, N.R.: Maternal and transplacental kinetics of trimethoprim and sulfamethoxazole, separately and in combination. Can. Med. Assoc. J. 112:67S-72S, 1975.

Williams, J.D.; Brumfitt, W.; Condie, A.P.; Reeves, D.S.: The treatment of bacteriuria in pregnant women with sulphamethoxazole and trimethoprim. A microbiological, clinical and toxicological study. Postgrad. Med. J. Suppl. 45, 71-76, 1969.

1170 2-Sulfamonyl-4,4-diaminodiphenylsulfone

Asano et al (1975) gave pregnant rats up to 4,000 mg per kg orally from day 9 through 14 of gestation and found no significant increase in fetal defects. Post-natal studies were negative.

Asano, Y.; Susami, M.; Ariyuki, F. and Higaki, K.: The effects of administration of 2-sulfamonyl-4,4-diamino-diphenylsulfone (SDDS) on rat fetuses. (Japanese) Oyo Yakuri 9: 695-707, 1975.

1171 0-Sulfamoylbenzoic Acid (see Saccharin)

1172 Sulfanilylurea

Bariliak (1968) using 1000 mg per kg on the 10th day produced death in 44 percent of rat fetuses but no congenital defects.

Bariliak, I.R.: Comparison of antithyroidal and teratogenic activity of some hypoglycemic sulphonamides. Problems of Endocrinology (Russian) 14: No. 6, 89-94, 1968.

1173 0-Sulfobenzoic Acid (see Saccharin)

1174 Sulfuric Acid Aerosol

John et al (1979) exposed mice and rabbits to up to 20 mg per square meter of air for 7 hours daily during major organogenesis and found no teratogenic effects.

1174

John, J.A.; Murray, F.J.; Murray, J.S.; Schwetz, B.A. and
Staples, R.E.: Evaluation of environmental contaminants,
tetrachloroacetone, hexachlorocyclopentadiene and sulfuric
acid aerosol for teratogenic potential in mice and rabbits
(abs) Teratology 19:32A-32B, 1979.

1175 Sulgin-R

This oral hypoglycemic was tested by Bariliak (1968) in rats
using 3.0 gm per kg on the 10th day of gestation. Although
a 10 percent fetal mortality occurred no congenital defects
were noted.

Bariliak, I.R.: Comparison of antithyroidal and teratogenic
activity of some hypoglycemic sulphonamides. Problems of
Endocrinology (Russian) 14: No. 6, 89-94, 1968.

1176 Sulphamoprine (also see Sulphonamides)

Paget and Thorpe (1964) found that dietary levels of 0.025
percent produced dental anomalies in the offspring of rats
and mice but had no effect on rabbits.

This long-acting sulfonamide drug was given orally to rats
on the 11th, 13th, 14th and 16th days of gestation, and
postnatally the offspring developed short snouts with
positional defects of the incisors (Goultschin and Ulmansky,
1971). The dosage was 75 mg per kg daily.

Goultschin, J. and Ulmansky, M.: Skull and dental changes
produced by sulfonamide in rats. Oral Surg. 31: 290-294,
1971.

Paget, G.E. and Thorpe, E.: A teratogenic effect of a
sulphonamide in experimental animals. Brit. J. Pharmacol.
23: 305-312, 1964.

1177 Sulphanilamide (also see Sulphonamides)

Bariliak (1968) gave 3000 mg per kg of body weight to rats
on the 10th day of gestation and found no lethal or teratogenic properties.

Bariliak, I.R.: Comparison of antithyroidal and teratogenic
activity of some hypoglycemic sulphanylamides. Problems of
Endocrinology (Russian) 14: No. 6, 89-94, 1968.

1178 N-Sulphanilylacetamide (see Sulphonamides)

1179 Sulphisoxozole (Gantrisin-R, Sulfafurazole)

When mice and rats were administered 1000 mgkg bw
sulfafurazole orally on days 7-12 and 9-14 of pregnancy,
respectively, a significant increase in cleft palate and
skeletal defects was found in offspring of both species; in
addition mandibular defects were present in the rat fetuses

(Kato and Kitagawa, 1973).

Sulfafurazole has been shown to transfer into the amniotic fluid during early fetal life (Blum et al, 1975). Mellin (1964) found no increase in the defect rate when mothers were treated in the first trimester. Heinonen et al (1977), who examined records of 796 offspring of mothers treated in the first 4 lunar months of pregnancy, also found no increase in malformation rate.

Blum, M.; Elian, I.; Ben-Tovim, R.: Transfer of antibiotics across the placenta in early pregnancy (Heb.). Harefuah 88:510-512, 1975.

Heinonen, O.P.; Slone, D.; Shapiro, S.: Birth Defects and Drugs in Pregnancy. Publishing Sciences Group, Inc., 1977.

Kato, T.; Kitagawa, S.: Production of congenital skeletal anomalies in the fetuses of pregnant rats and mice treated with various sulfonamides. Congenital Anomalies 13:17-23, 1973.

Mellin, G.W.: Drugs in the first trimester of pregnancy and the fetal life of Homo sapiens. Am. J. Obst. Gynecol. 90:1169-1180, 1964.

1180 Sulphapyridine (see Sulphonamides)

1181 Sulphonamides

Landauer and Wakasugi (1968) have summarized their extensive work with sulphonamides as teratogens in the chick embryo. Using acetazolamide, dichlorphenamide and methazolamide with doses of 0.5 to 2.0 mg given at 96 hours incubation they produced short upper beaks and syndactylism. P-sulphamoylbenzoic acid was non-teratogenic. For a more detailed description of the very specific teratogenic lesions found in mammals after administration of the strong carbonic anhydrase inhibiting sulfonamides reference should be made to the entry under acetazolamide.

Various sulphanilamides with bacteriostatic properties were shown by Ancel (1945) to be teratogenic in the chick. He showed that sulphanilamide, sulphapyridine and N-sulphanilylacetamide produced a syndrome of micromelia, syndachtylism and parrot beak. Doses of 1 mg per egg at 96 hours of incubation were used by Landauer and Clark (1962) to produce the syndrome. Landauer concluded that these agents interfered with purine synthesis or with functions of NAD-linked dehydrogenases, resulting in local deficiency of folic acid.

Paget and Thorpe (1964) reported that sulfadimethoxy pyrimidine treatment led to skeletal and dental defects in rats.

Bertazzoli et al. (1965) reported that sulfamethazine in doses of 50 mg per kg daily from the 11th through the 20th gestational day was associated with maloccluded incisors in

1181

the weaned rat offspring. Kalter and Warkany (1959) list a number of references to studies where large doses of sulfonamides given to pregnant animals caused only fetal resorption. Using 8 separate sulfonamides Kato and Kitagawa (1973a, 1973b) administered orally 500-1,000 mg per kg per day to mice on the 7th to the 12th day and to rats on the 9th through the 14th days of gestation. In both species cleft palate was produced by sulfamonomethoxine, sulfamethoxine, sulfamethomidine, sulfamethoxypyridazine, sulfisoxazole and sulfadiazine. Sulfanilamide and sulfisomidine did not produce defects. Using sulfamethopyrazine Suzuki et al (1973) produced an increase in cleft palates in rat and mouse fetuses by giving mice 1,000 or 2,000 mg per kg per day of organogenesis and had similar results in the rat at 700 mg per kg. At 685 and 865 mg of sulfamethazine per kg on days 6-15 Wolkowski-Tyl et al (1982) found cleft palate, hydroureter and hydronephrosis in rat fetuses.

There is no conclusive evidence that these compounds are teratogenic in man (Smithells, 1966). Slone et al have reported no increase in defects among 1,400 pregnancies exposed during the first 4 months. At 4 years, no IQ differences were found.

Ancel, P.: L'achondroplasie. Sa realisation experimentale - sa pathogene. Ann. Endocrinol. 6: 1-24, 1945.

Bertazzoli, C.; Chieli, T. and Grandi, M.: Absence of tooth malformation in the offspring of rats treated with a long-acting sulphonamide. Experientia 21: 151-152, 1965.

Kalter, H. and Warkany, J.: Experimental production of congenital malformations in mammals by metabolic procedure. Physiol. Rev. 39: 69-115, 1959.

Kato, T. and Kitagawa, S.: Production of congenital anomalies in fetuses of rats and mice with various sulfonamides. Cong. Anom. 13: 7-15, 1973.

Kato, T. and Kitagawa, S.: Production of congenital skeletal anomalies in fetuses of pregnant rats and mice treated with various sulfonamides. Cong. Anom. 13: 17-23, 1973.

Landauer, W. and Clark, E.M.: On the teratogenic nature of sulfanilamide and 3-acetylpyridine in chick development. J. Exp. Zool. 156: 313-322, 1964.

Landauer, W. and Wakasugi, N.: Teratological studies with sulfonamides. J. Embryol. Exp. Morphol. 20: 261-284, 1968.

Paget, G.E. and Thorpe, E.: A teratogenic effect of sulphonamide in experimental animals. Br. J. Pharmacol. 23: 305-312, 1964.

Slone, D.; Shapiro, S.; Monson, R.R.; Kaufman, D.W.; Siskind, V. and Heinonen, O.P.: Antenatal exposure to the sulfonimides in relation to congenital malformation, birth weight and intelligence quotient. J. Inf. Dis. (in press).

Smithells, R.W.: Drugs and human malformations. In, Woollam, D.H.M. (ed.): Advances in Teratology, Vol. 1. New York: Academic Press, 1966. pp. 251-278.

Suzuki, Y.; Wakita, Y.; Kondo, S.; Okada, F.; Suzuki, I.; Asano, F.; Matsuo, M. and Chiba, T.: Effects of sulfamethopyrazine administered to pregnant animals upon the development of their fetuses and neonates. Oyo Yakuri 7: 1005-1019, 1973.

Wolkowski-Tyl, R.; Jones-Price, C.; Kimmel, C.A.; Ledoux, T.; Reel, J.R.; Langhoff,-Paschke, L.:Teratologic evaluation of sulfamethazine in CD rats (abstract) Teratology 25:81A-82A, 1982.

1182 Sulfonamide CS-61 (3,6-Dimethoxy-4-sulfanilamidopyridazine)

Kato and Kitagawa (1974) studied this compound in pregnant rats and mice. At doses of 750 and 1000 mg per kg in the rat on days 9 through 14, a significant increase in absence of the kidney occurred in the fetuses. At the same dose range in the mouse, there was an increase in cleft palate.

Kato, T. and Kitagawa, S.: Effects of a new antibacterial sulfonamide (CS-61) on mouse and rat fetuses. Toxicol. Appl. Pharmacol. 27:20-27, 1974.

1183 Supidimide (CG-3033, EM-87)

This structural analog of thalidomide was tested in pregnant baboons (Hendrickx and Helm, 1980) and monkeys (Scott et al, 1980) at up to 40 and 15 mg per kg respectively. Treatment was during organogenesis; no defects were produced.

Hendrickx, A.G.; Helm, F.CH.: Nonteratogenicity of a structural analog of thalidomide in pregnant baboons (Papio cynocephalus). Teratology 22:179-182, 1980.

Scott, W.J.; Wilson, J.G.; Helm, F.CH.: A metabolite of a structural analog of thalidomide lacks teratogenic effect in pregnant rhesus monkeys. Teratology 22:183-185, 1980.

1184 Surfactants

Palmer et al (1975a and 1975b) studied the effect of linear alkylbenzene sulfonate, alcohol sulfate, sodium dodecylethoxysulfate and alpha-olefin sulfonate on pregnancy in the rat, mouse and rabbit. At maternal toxic doses total litter resorptions increased and a few minor skeletal defects were found. The toxic doses in mg per kg in the rat were: linear alkylbenzene sulfonate, 600; alcohol sulfate, 600; and alpha-olefin sulfonate, greater than 600.

Palmer, A.K.; Readshaw, M.A. and Neuff, A.M.: Assessment of the teratogenic potential of surfactants part 1-LAS, AS, CLD. Toxicology 3: 91-106, 1975a.

1184

Palmer, A.K.; Readshaw, M.A. and Neuff, A.M.: Assessment
of the teratogenic potential of surfactants part 2 AOS.
Toxicology 3: 107-113, 1975b.

1185 Surgery (see Trauma)

1186 Suxibbuzone

This antiinflammatory compound was studied in pregnant mice,
rats and rabbits by Yoshida et al (1980). In the rat at
oral doses of 284 mg per kg no adverse effects on fertiliy
were found. Decreased fetal weight was found with doses of
142 mg per kg or above. At 284 mg per kg resorptions were
increased. No external defects were found. In the mouse a
dose of 800 mg per kg was associated with decreased body
weight and delayed ossification in the fetuses.
Phenylbutazone was also studied in both rats and mice. In
the rabbit Yoshida et al (1980) found an increase in
resorptions at 36 mg per kg orally and at 142 mg decreased
implantation was found.

Yoshida, R.; Asanoma, K.; Kurokawa, M.; Morita,
K.:Reproductive studies of suxibuzone
(4-butyl-4)beta-carboxypropionyl-oxymethyl-1,2-diphenyl-3,
5-pyrazolidinedione. Oyo Yakuri 20:281-288, 289-298,
377-386, 387-392, 1980.

1187 SV-40 Virus

Farwell et al (1979) reported an increase in central nervous
system tumors among the offspring of mothers given
poliomyelitis vaccine contaminated with SV-40 virus between
1955 and 1961. Of 15 children with meduloblastoma 10 had
been exposed to the contaminated vaccine and this was a
statistically significant increase over matched controls.
Suggestive association was made for gliomas. Heinonen et al
(1973 and 1977) list 8 CNS tumors in the offspring of polio
vaccinated mothers and this was 17.9 times the hospital
standardized relative risk.

Farwell, J.W.; Dohrmann, G.J.; Marrett, L.D.; Meigs, J.W.:
Effect of SV-40 virus-contaminated polio vaccine on the
incidence and type of CNS neoplasm in children. A
population-based study. Trans. Am. Neurological Ass.
104:1-4, 1980.

Heinonen, O.P.; Slone, D.; Shapiro, S.: Birth Defects and
Drugs in Pregnancy. Publishing Sciences Group, Inc., 1977.

Heinonen, O.P.; Shapiro, S.; Monson, R.R.; Hartz, S.C.;
Rosenberg L.; Slone, D.: Immunization during pregnancy
against poliomyelitis and influenza in relation to childhood
malignancy. Int. J. Epid. 2:229- 235, 1973.

1188 Swaddling

Swaddling of young infants has been shown to be related to

congenital dislocation of the hips. A higher incidence of the defect occurring in infants born during the colder months was noted by Record and Edwards (1958) who postulated that during the colder months the infant was exposed to more swaddling which held the hips in adduction predisposing toward dislocation. The use of craddle boards by Inddians has the same effect (Salter, 1968).

Record, R.G. and Edwards, J.H.: Environmental influences related to the aetiology of congenital dislocation of the hip. Br. J. Prev. Soc. Med. 12: 8-12, 1958.

Salter, R.B.: Etiology, pathogenesis and possible prevention of congenital dislocation of the hip. Can. Med. Assoc. J. 98: 933-945, 1968.

1189 Swine Fever Virus

Harding et al. (1966) produced some circumstantial evidence that swine fever led to cerebellar hypoplasia and spinal hypomyelinogenesis in newborn piglets. An association between the congenital defect and the presence of immunity to the agent was made in 32 of 33 herds studied.

Harding, J.D.J.; Done, J.T. and Darbyshire, J.H.: Congenital tremors in piglets and their relation to swine fever.

Vet. Rec. 79: 388-390, 1966.

1190 Syphilis

The causative organism, Treponema pallidum, can be transmitted transplacentally and produces characteristic pathologic findings in the human fetus (Ingall and Norris, 1976; Grossman, 1977). Although Harter and Benirschke (1976) have demonstrated the organisms in abortus material of less than 12 weeks, the pathologic picture does not appear before the 4th to 5th month of gestation, and may evolve primarily as a result of maturation of the fetuses' immune system. The infection spreads hematogenously from the placenta which is charateristically large and pale. The visceral and skin lesions resemble those seen in the postnatally acquired disease.

Grossman, J.: Congenital syphilis. Teratoloy 16:217-224, 1977.

Halter, C.A. and Benirschke, K.: Fetal syphilis in the first trimester. Am. J. Obstet. Gynecol. 124:705-711, 1976.

Ingall, D. and Norris, L.: Syphilis Chapter 9 in, Infectious Diseases of the Fetus and Newborn Infant, edited by J.S. Remington and J.O. Klein, Saunders Co.; Philadelphia, 1976, pp. 414-463.

1191 T-1220

This new penicillin analog was given intravenously in amounts of up to 2,000 mg per kg daily to mice on days 6 through 15 and no teratologic or postnatal growth changes occurred. (Takai et al, 1977A). The same authors (1977B) found no teratogenicity in the rat given 1,000 mg per kg daily on days 7 through 17 of gestation.

Takai, A.; Yoneda, T.; Nakada, H.; Nakamura, S. and Inaba, J.: Toxicity tests of T-1220 6. Reproduction study in mice. (Japanese) Chemotherapy 25:915-927, 1977.

Takai, A.; Yoneda, T.; Nakada, H.; Nakamura, S. and Inaba, J.: Toxicity tests of T-1220 7. Teratology tests in rats. (Japanese) Chemotherapy 25:928-933, 1977.

1192 T-2 Toxin

This mold metabolite of Fusarium tricinctum given in amounts of 0.5 mg per k intraperitoneally to mice on days 8 or 10 produced tail and limb abnormalities (Hood et al, 1978).

Hood, R.D.; Kuczuk, M.H. and Szczech, G.M.: Effects in mice of simultaneous prenatal exposure to ochratoxic A and T-2 toxin. Teratology 17; 25-30, 1978.

1193 2,4-5T (see Trichlorophenoxyacetic Acid)

1194 TA1-284 (6-Chloro-5-cyclohexyl-1-indancarboxylic Acid)

Kusanagi et al (1977) gavaged pregnant mice with 10, 30 and 90 mg per kg per day from day 7 through day 15. At 90 mg per kg, skeletal defects involving fused ribs and irregular vertebral bodies occurred. Other defects were not increased over the controls.

Kusanagi, T.; Ihara, T. and Mizutani, M.: Teratogenic effects of non-steroidal anti-inflammatory agents in mice. (Japanese) Cong. Anom. 17:177-185, 1977.

1195 Tamoxifen

This antineoplastic agent was given orally to rabbits in doses of 0.25 to 4.0 mg per kg daily. A high fetal loss was found at 4 mg per kg. Some fetal death increase was found at 0.5 and 2.0 mg per kg but no defect increase occurred with treatment on days 6-18.

Esaki, K.; Sakai, Y.: Influence of oral administration of tamoxifen in the rabbit fetus. Preclin. Rep. Cent. Inst. Exp. Animal 6:217-238, 1980.

1196 Taurine

Takahashi et al (1972) gave 4 gm per kg orally for 7 days starting on the 7th day in the pregnant mouse and found no alterations in the treated fetuses.

Yamada et al (1981) administered this compound orally to rats on days 7-17 in amounts of up to 3000 mg per kg and reported no adverse fetal effects.

Takahashi, H.; Kaneda, S.; Fukuda, K.; Fujihira, E. and Nakazawa, M.: Studies on the teratology and three generation reproduction of taurine in mice. Oyo Yakuri 6: 535-540, 1972.

Yamada, T.; Nogariya, T.; Nakane, S.; Sasajima, M.: Reproductive studies of taurin. Kiso to Rinsho 15: 4229-4240, 1981.

1197 Tecoram

Van Steenis and Van Logten (1971) inoculated chick eggs with 0.01 to 10 mg of the dithiocarbamate of tecoram on day 7 of incubation. With doses over 1.0 mg paralysis, shortening of extremities and muscular atrophy was found at the 19th day.

Van Steenis, G. and Van Logten, M.J.: Neurotoxic effect of dithiocarbamate tecoram on the chick embryo. Toxicol. Appl. Pharmacol. 19: 675-686, 1971.

1198 Tegafur-Uracil (UFT)

Tegafur(1-(2-tetrahydrofuryl)5-fluorouracil) was mixed in a 1:4 molar ratio with uracil to produce an antineoplastic agent. Asanoma et al (1980) gave it orally to rabbits on days 6-18 of geestation in amounts of up to 12.96 mg per kg daily and found no significant fetal differences. At 81 mg orally in the rat during days 7-17 some fetal weight decrease, increase in resorptions and delay in fetal ossification was found. Postnatal function was not affected. Pre-mating dosing of the males and females did not alter fertility.

Asanoma, K.; Matsubara, T.; Morita, K.: Effect of UFT on reproduction. Oyo Yakuri 20:1001-1007, 22:85-107, 109-129, 1980, 1981.

1199 Tegratol-R (see Carbamazepine)

1200 Tellurium

Garro and Pentschew (1964) fed pregnant rats diets containing 500 to 2,500 parts per million and observed a dose related increase in postnatal hydrocephalus. Agnew and Curray (1972a) found the most vulnerable time for induction of hydrocephalus was day 9 and 10 in the rat and reported on the distribution of tellurium-127M in the pregnant rat (1972b). Duckett (1971) fed a diet with 3000 ppm throughout the rat gestation period. Although communicating hydrocephalus was present at birth, it became converted to an obstructive type within a few days. Of 237 newborn rats 179 developed hydrocephalus within 3 days. Duckett presents evidence that the element was present in fetal brain tissue.

Agnew, W.F. and Curry, E.: Period of teratogenic vulnerability of rat embryo to induction of hydrocephalus by tellurium. Experientia 2: 14441445, 1972a.

Agnew, W.F.: Transplacental uptake of tellurium-127M studied in whole-body radioautography. Teratology 6: 331-338, 1972b.

Duckett, S.: The morphology of tellurium-induced hydrocephalus. Exp. Neurol. 31: 1-16, 1971.

Garro, F. and Pentschew, A.: Neonatal hydrocephalus in the offspring of rats fed during pregnancy non-toxic amounts of tellurium. Arch. Psychiat. Neurol. 206: 272-280, 1964.

1201 Telodrin

Ware and Good (1967) fed this polychlorinated insecticide in the diet to mice. A dietary level of 1 ppm had no effect on fertility or litter size.

Ware, G.W. and Good, E.E.: Effects of insecticides on reproduction in the laboratory mouse. Toxicol. Appl. Pharmacol. 10: 54-61, 1967.

1202 Tenuazonic Acid

This metabolite of alternaria tenus inhibits tumor growth but has little growth retarding effect in the chick embryo (Gitterman et al, 1964).

Gitterman, C.O.; Dulaney, E.L.; Kaczka, E.A.; Campbell, G.W.; Hendlin, D. and Woodruff, H.B.: The human tumor-egg host system. 3. Tumor-inhibitory properties of tenuazonic acid. Cancer Res. 24: 440-443, 1964.

1203 Testosterone

Masculinization of the external genitalia of female infants has been observed following maternal administration of testosterone, even in amounts small enough to have no effect in the mother (Van Wyk and Grumbach, 1968). Methyltestosterone and testosterone proprionate have been associated with clitoromegaly with or without fusion of the labia minora. Moncrieff (1958) reported dosage levels of methyltestosterone as low as 6 mg daily. Hoffman et al. (1955) reported a masculinized fetus following administration to the mother of testosterone enanthate from the 4th to the 9th month. Grumbach and Ducharme (1960) have summarized the human reports. Drawing from the more numerous examples of masculinization by the use of progestins, Grumbach et al. (1959) have observed that labioscrotal fusion is more commonly found when treatment is given the mother before the 80th to 90th day of gestation. Clitoromegaly may result from treatment at any period.

An extensive literature on experimental production of masculinization led to the above-described human observations. Greene et al. (1939) carried out detailed studies in the rat; the mouse was used by Raynaud (1947); Bruner and Witschi (1946) utilized the hamster; and Jost's work (1953) in the rabbit is well known. Wells and Van Wagenen (1954) produced pseudohermaphroditism in the female monkey. Grumbach et al. (1960) and Jost (1953) have reviewed the subject. To briefly summarize, the urogenital sinus and its derivatives and the external genitalia can be masculinized. Except in the hamster the wolffian ducts do not regress and form seminal vescicles, epididymides and to a variable extent vasa deferentia. The mullerian ducts are not appreciably affected, and inversion of ovarian development does not occur.

Bruner, J.A. and Witschi, E.: Testosterone-induced modifications of sexual development in female hamsters. Am. J. Anat. 79: 293-320, 1946.

Greene, R.R.; Burrill, M.W. and Ivy, A.C.: Experimental intersexuality. The effect of antenatal androgens on sexual development of female rats. Am. J. Anat. 65: 415-469, 1939.

Grumbach, M.M. and Ducharme, J.R.: The effects of androgens on fetal sexual development. Fertil. Steril. 11: 157-180, 1960.

Grumbach, M.M.; Ducharme, J.R. and Moloshok, R.E.: On the fetal masculinizing action of certain oral progestins. J. Clin. Endocrinol. Metab. 19: 1369-1380, 1959.

Hoffman, F.; Overzier, C. and Uhde, G.: Zur Frage der Hormonalen erzeugung Fotaler Zwittenbildungen beim Menschen. Geburtshilfe Frauenheilkd. 15: 1061-1070, 1955.

Jost, A.: Problems of fetal endocrinology: The gonadal and hypophyseal hormones. Recent Progr. Horm. Res. 8: 379-418, 1953.

Moncrieff, A.: Non-adrenal female pseudohermaphroditism associated with hormone administration in pregnancy. Lancet 2: 267-268, 1958.

Raynaud, A.: Observations sur le developpement normal des ebauches de la glande mammaire des foetus males et femelles de souris. Ann. Endocrinol. 8: 349-359, 1947.

Van Wyk, J. and Grumbach, M.M.: Disorders of sex differentiation. In, Williams, R.H. (ed.): Textbook of Endocrinology. Philadelphia: W.B. Saunders, 1968. pp. 537-612.

Wells, L.J. and Van Wagenen, G.: Androgen-induced female pseudohermaphroditism in the monkey (Macaca mulatta) anatomy of the reproductive organs. Carnegie Institute Contributions Embryol. 35: 93-106, 1954.

1204 Tetrachloroacetone

John et al (1979) gave oral doses to mice and rabbits during

1204

active organogenesis and observed major malformations in mice at 15 and 50 mg per kg per day. A low incidence of malformations was found in rabbits at 1 to 10 mg per kg per day.

John, J.A.; Murray, F.J.; Murray, J.S.; Schwetz, B.A. and Staples, R.E.: Evaluation of environmental contaminants, tetrachloroacetone, hexachlorocyclopentadiene and sulfuric acid aerosol for teratogenic potential in mice and rabbits (abs) Teratology 19:32A-33A, 1979.

1205 3,3,4,4-Tetrachlorobiphenyl (see Kanechlor and Chlorobiphenyls)

Wardell et al (1982) gave rats orally up to 10 mg per kg on days 6-18 of gestation. At 3 and 10 mg per kg levels there was an increase in bloody amniotic fluid and blood in the fetal intestinal tract. Fetal mortality increase and growth retardation were found at the 3 and 10 mg levels.

Wardell, R.E.; Seegmiller, R.E.; Bradshaw, W.S.: Induction of prenatal toxicity in the rat by diethylstilbestrol, zeranol, 3,4,3,4-Tetrachlorobiphenyl, cadmium and lead. Teratology 26: 229- 236, 1982.

1206 2,3,7,8-Tetrachlorodibenzo-P-dioxin [TCDD]

Sparschu et al. (1971) found that very small amounts of this material were embryotoxic to the rat embryo. They produced death, resorptions and fetal gastrointestinal hemorrhage with doses of 0.125 to 8.0 microgm per kg given orally on days 6 through 15 of gestation. Courtney and Moore (1971) using TCDD subcutaneously in amounts of 3 microgms per kg daily from day 6 through day 15 of mouse gestation produced cleft palate and renal malformations in the offspring. Cleft palates did not appear in the rat but renal defects were found with a dose of 0.5 microgm per kg daily. Neubert et al (1973) have reviewed the embryotoxic effects of this compound and Golberg (1971) has summarized the general area of herbicide toxicity.

Courtney, K.D. and Moore, J.A.: Teratology studies with 2,4,5-trichlorophenoxyacetic acid and 2,3,7,8-tetra-chorodibenzo-P-dioxin. Toxicol. Appl. Pharmacol. 20: 396-403, 1971.

Golberg, L.: Trace chemical contaminants in food: potential for harm. Food Cosmet. Toxicol. 9: 65-80, 1971.

Neubert, D.; Zens, P.; Rothenwallner, A. and Merker, H.J.: A survey of the embryotoxic effects of TCDD in mammalian species. Environmental Health Perspectives 5: 67-79, 1973.

Sparschu, G.L.; Dunn, F.L. and Rowe, V.K.: Study of the teratogenicity of 2,3,7,8-tetrachlorodibenzo-P-dioxin in the rat. Food Cosmet. Toxicol. 9: 405-412, 1971.

1207 Tetrachloroethylene (Perchloroethylene)

Schwetz et al (1975) exposed pregnant mice and rats to concentrations of 300 ppm. Both species were exposed for 7 hours daily periods on days 6 through 15 of gestation. No fetal toxicity or teratogenicity was found. Nelson et al (1980) performed behavioral tests on the offspring of rats exposed to 100 ppm for 7 hours daily on days 14-20 of gestation and found no changes from the control pups. At exposure levels of 900 ppm the maternal animals gained less weight and the offspring performed less well on neuromotor tests and had lower levels of brain acetylcholine and dopamine. Pair fed controls were not used.

Nelson, B.K.; Taylor, B.J.; Setzer, J.V.; Hornung, R.W.: Behavioral teratology of perchloroethylene in rats J. Envir. Path. Toxicol. 3:233-250, 1980.

Schwetz, B.A.; Leong, B.K.J.; Gehring, P.J.: The effect of maternally inhaled trichloroethylene, perchloroethylene, methyl chloroform and methylene chloride on embryonal and fetal development in mice and rats. Toxicol. Appl. Pharmacol. 32:84-96, 1975.

1208 Delta-9-Tetrahydrocannibinal (see Cannibis and Marihuana)

1209 Tetracycline

Baden (1970) has reviewed the literature on tetracycline staining of deciduous teeth. Brownish staining of the teeth may result following administration after the 4th month of pregnancy. Generally only the deciduous teeth are involved although with administration close to term the crowns of the permanent teeth may be stained. Although Fillippi (1967) reported cleft palate and shortened extremities in rat fetuses whose mothers received 5 mg daily from the 5th to 20th day, two other studies did not confirm the findings. Bevelander and Cohlan (1962) produced stunting but no defects in the rat fetus by injecting 40 to 80 mg per kg on the 10th through the 15th gestational day. Hurley and Tuchmann-Duplessis (1963) could not produce defects in the rat fetus. McColl et al. (1965) found only an increase in hydroureters in rat fetuses exposed to 500 mg daily.

Baden, E.: Environmental pathology of the teeth. In, Gorlin, R.J. and Goldman, H.M. (eds.): Thomas Oral Pathology. St. Louis: C.V. Mosby Co.; 1970, 6th Ed. pp. 189-191.

Bevelander, G. and Cohlan, S.Q.: The effect on the rat fetus of transplacentally acquired tetracycline. Biol. Neonate 4: 365-370, 1962.

Fillippi, B.: Antibiotics and congenital malformations: evaluation of the teratogenicity of antibiotics. In, Woollam, D.H.M. (ed.): Advances in Teratology, Vol. 2. New York: Academic Press, 1967. pp. 237-256.

Hurley, L.S. and Tuchmann-Duplessis, H.: Influence de la tetracycline sur le developpement pre- et post-natal du rat. C. R. Acad. Sci. (Paris) 257: 302-304, 1963.

McColl, J.D.; Globus, M. and Robinson, S.: Effect of some therapeutic agents on the developing rat fetus. Toxicol. Appl. Pharmacol. 7: 409-417, 1965.

1210 N-(2-Tetrahydrofuryl) 5-Flourouracil

Morita et al (1971) gave this anticancer agent intravenously to pregnant mice and rats once daily during active organogenesis. The highest dose in the rat was 150 mg per kg and 90 mg per kg in the mouse. Some fetal growth retardation and increased resorptions were found in both species but no teratogenic action was found.

Morita, K.; Watanabe, S.; Mizuno, T.; Takikawa, K. and Harima, K : Teratogenic study of N-(2-tetrahydrofuryl)-5-fluorouracil. Oyo Yakura 5: 555-568, 1971.

1211 Delta-9-Tetrahydrocannabinol (see Marihuana)

1212 Tetrahydrophthalimide

Verrett et al. (1969) injected this material into chick eggs and produced congenital defects in 4.8 percent of the survivors. Doses of 3 to 20 mg per kg (of egg) were used. The type of defect included micromelia of the legs, skull defects and ectopia of the viscera. The mortality rate was 38 percent at the 20 mg level. DMSO or absolute ethanol were used as vehicles.

Verrett, M.J.; Mutchler, M.K.; Scott, W.F.; Reynaldo, E.F. and McLaughlin, J.: Teratogenic effects of captan and related compounds in the developing chicken embryo. Ann. N. Y. Acad. Sci. 160: 334-343, 1969.

1213 Tetrahydro-2-pyrimidinethiol (see Ethylenethiourea)

1214 1,1,3,3-Tetramethyl-2-thiourea (see Ethylenethiourea)

1215 Tetramethylthiuramdisulfide

Vasilos et al (1978) showed this compound in subtoxic maternal doses induced subcutaneous hematomes and a decrease in fetal weight. It also caused embryonic resorptions.

Vasilos, A.F.; Anisimova, L.A.; Todorova, E.A. and Dmitrienko, V.D.: The reproductive function of rats in acute and chronic intoxication with tetramethylthiuramdisulfide. Gig. i Sanitariya (USSR) 6:37-40, 1978.

1216 Thalidomide   [Alpha-phthalimidoglutarimide]   [Distaval-R] [Kevadon-R] [Contergan-R]

This sedative became the most notorious teratogen known to

man. Although these events are becoming part of medical history, several teratologic principles were forcefully illustrated by observations made of the outbreak. The 1st point was that there existed extreme variability in species susceptibility to thalidomide and the 2nd was that there was a very sharp relationship between the time of exposure and the presence and type of congenital defect. Further comments will be made here about the epidemiology of the problem and about the relationship between configuration of the compound and its teratogenic action.

Lenz (1962) and McBride (1961) were the 1st to report that thalidomide was the source of an almost world-wide epidemic of phocomelia. A number of general reviews of the subject have appeared (Lenz, 1962; Taussig, 1962; Mellin and Katzenstein, 1962; Cahen, 1966).

Species variability: The mouse and rat embryo are relatively insensitive to thalidomide while the rabbit, monkey and man are sensitive. Cahen has listed 14 separate publications dealing with the mouse; nearly all reported negative findings or else a few defects which did not resemble the thalidomide syndrome. A similar outcome was found from studies in the rat which included many strains. The New Zealand rabbit has been shown to be teratologically the most sensitive small animal and doses of 250 mg per kg on days 8 to 10 are suitable to produce limb defects. The early pathology in rabbit limb buds indicated a defect of cartilage condensation; no increased cell necrosis was found (Vickers, 1967). Axelrod (1970 has summarized the experimental work done in monkeys in which a single dose of 8 to 10 mg per kg on the 25th to 30th day produces the thalidomide syndrome. Salzgeber and Salaun (1965) have produced defects in the extremity of the chick. Cahen (1966) has tabulated the results with treatment of many species tested.

The type of defect observed in children has been well correlated with the time of treatment. German workers (Lenz and Knapp, 1962; Knapp et al.; 1962) were able to trace the date of prescription in 86 cases and of this group the approximate date of conception was known in 32 mothers. None of these mothers giving birth to limb defective children were known to have taken the drug only before the 27th day or only after the 40th day. Accordingly the critical period appeared to be no longer than 14 days. Furthermore administration of the drug from the 27th to the 30th days was associated most often with only the arms affected while treatment during the 30th to 33rd days caused leg deformity with less involvement of the arms. These findings correlate with the appearance of the lower limb buds in the human embryo at about the 30th day. The previously quoted time of 27 to 28 days for appearance of the lower limbs has been increased by 2 or 3 days to the 30th day (Iffy et al.; 1968; Schumacher, 1975; Jonsson, 1972). Defects of the external ears are the earliest occurring of the thalidomide anomalies. (approximately day 21 to day 27). Other anomalies associated with phocomelia are facial hemangioma, atresia of the esophagus or duodenum, tetrology of Fallot and renal agenesis. Cleft palate is a rare complication and the central nervous system is not adversely affected. It is estimated that defective children resulted in about 20 percent of mothers ingesting the drug during the sensitive period. A single dose of this sedative has been documented to produce human defects.

Although much careful work has been done in an attempt to understand the mechanism of action, the reason for the chemical and species specificity remains an intriguing pharmacologic riddle (Jonsson, 1972; Schumacher, 1975). The work of Smith et al. (1965), Keberle et al. (1965) and Wuest et al. (1968) give the numerous studies of compounds chemically related to thalidomide. The embryotoxic properties of the compound do not appear to be due to the simple chemical subunits such as phthalimide, phthalic acid, 3-aminoglutarimide and glutamine. Dyban and Akimova (1966) were able to produce eye and palate defects in the rat with thalidomide when the mothers were deficient of riboflavin and folic acid. Staples and Holtkamp (1963) reported that riboflavin therapy ameliorated the limb defects produced in the rabbit. McBride (1974) has found neuronal degeneration and reduction in cell number in the dorsal root ganglia of newborn rabbits with thalidomide defects. McBride (1977) has summarized the evidence that the mechanism of action in the embryo is via changes in the peripheral nerves of the limbs. Evidence that an arene oxide metaboolite may be associated with thalidomide toxicity in a cell culture system has been presented (Gordon et al, 1981). Fabro (1981) has reviewed the mechanisms of action that have been proposed.

The comparable teratogenic doses on a mg per kg dose are approximately 1 mg for man and monkey and 50 mg for the rabbit.

The compound with the carbonyl group in the phthalimide ring changed to a methylene has been shown to retain teratogenicity (Schumacher et al.; 1972). Stockinger and Koch (1969) from studies of a new hypnotic suggested that the aromatic phthalidimide variety of thalimide was responsible for teratogenicity. Jonsson et al (1972) have studied some derivatives of isoindolinone, benzisothiazoline and 4(3H) quinazolinone and did not find thalidomide teratogenicity.

The epidemiologic aspects of the outbreak are covered by Taussig (1962). Lenz (1966) has shown the very close correlation between thalidomide sales and incidence rates of phocomelia. Over 5,000 cases were known in West Germany while only 17 were found in the United States where the drug was not permitted on the market. Speirs (1962) gave an interesting report of how an initial survey of the drug ingestion of mothers of phocomelic children gave no hint of a common agent; when thalidomide was later implicated eight of these ten mothers were shown to have ingested it.

Axelrod, L.R.: Drugs and nonhuman primate teratogenesis.

In, Woollam, D.H.M. (ed.): Advances in Teratology, Vol. 4. New York: Academic Press, 1970. pp. 217-230.

Cahen, R.L.: Experimental and clinical chemoteratogenesis. Adv. Pharmacol. 4: 263-349, 1966.

Dekker, A. and Mehrizi, A.: The use of thalidomide as a teratogenic agent in rabbits. Bulletin Johns Hopkins Hospital 115: 223-230, 1964.

Dyban, A.P. and Akimova, I.M.: Significance of vitamin B complex and genetic factors in reaction to thalidomide in rat embryos. Arch. Anat. (Russian) 51: No. 8, 3-17, 1966.

Fabro, S.: Biochemical basis of thalidomide teratogenicity. Chapter 5 in The BiochemicAl Basis of Chemical Teratogenesis edited by Mont R. Juchau, Elsevier-North Holland, New York, 1981, pp. 157-178.

Gordon, G.B.; Spielberg, S.P.; Blake, D.A.; Balasubramanian, V.: Thalidomide teratogenesis: Evidence for a toxic arene oxide metabolite. Proc. Natl. Acad. Sci. 78: 2545-2548, 1981.

Iffy, L.; Shepard, T.H.; Jakobovits, A.; Lemire, R.J. and Kerner, P.: The rate of growth in young human embryos of streeters horizons XIII to XXIII. Acta Anatomica 66: 178-186, 1967.

Jonsson, N.A.; Mikiver, L. and Selberg, U.: Chemical structure and teratogenic properties II synthesis and teratogenic activity on rabbits of some derivatives of phthalimide, isoindoline-1-one, 1,2-benzisothiazoline-3-onel,1-dioxide and 4(3H)quinazolinone. Acta Pharm. Suec. 9: 431-446, 1972.

Jonsson, N.A.: Chemical structure and teratogenic properties. 3. A review of available data on structure-activity relationships and mechanism of action of thalidomide analogues. Acta Pharm. Suecica 9: 521-542, 1972.

Keberle, H.; Faigle, J.W.; Fritz, H.; Knusel, F.; Loustalot, P. and Schmid, K.: Theories on the mechanism of action of thalidomide. In, Robson, J.M.; Sullivan, F.M. and Smith, R.L. (eds.): Embryopathic Activity of Drugs. Boston: Little Brown and Co.; 1965. pp. 210-233.

Knapp, K.; Lenz, W. and Nowack, E.: Multiple congenital abnormalities. Lancet 2: 725 only, 1962.

Lenz, W.: Malformations caused by drugs in pregnancy. Am. J. Dis. Child. 112: 99-106, 1966.

Lenz, W. and Knapp, K.: Thalidomide embryopathy. Arch. Environ. Health 5: 100-105, 1962.

McBride, W.G.: Thalidomide and congenital abnormalities.

Lancet 2: 1358 only, 1961.

McBride, W.G.: Fetal nerve cell degeneration produced by thalidomide in rabbits. Teratology 10: 283-292, 1974.

Mellin, G.W. and Katzenstein, M.: The saga of thalidomide. Neuropathy to embryopathy, with case reports of congenital anomalies. N. Engl. J. Med. 267: 1184-1193, 1238-1244, 1962.

Salzgeber, B. and Salaun, J.: Action de la thalidomide sur l'embryon de poulet. J. Embryol. Exp. Morphol. 13: 159-170, 1965.

Schumacher, H.J.; Terapane, J.; Jordan, R.L. and Wilson, J.G.: The teratogenic activity of a thalidomide analogue, EM(12) in rabbits, rats, and monkeys. Teratology 5: 233-240, 1972.

Schumacher, H.J.: Chemical structure and teratogenic properties in Shepard, T.H.; Miller, J.R. and Marois, M. (eds.): Methods For Detection of Environmental Agents That Produce Congenital Defects. Amsterdam: North Holland-American Elsevier, 1975, pp. 65-77.

Smith, R.L.; Fabro, S.; Schumacher, H.J. and Williams, R.T.: Studies on the relationships between chemical structure and embryotoxic activity of thalidomide and related compounds. In, Robson, J.M.; Sullivan, F.M. and Smith, R.L. (eds.): Embryopathic Activity of Drugs. Boston: Little Brown and Co.; 1965. pp. 194-209.

Speirs, A.L.: Thalidomide and congenital abnormalities. Lancet 1: 303-305, 1962.

Staples, R.E. and Holtkamp, D.E.: Effects of parental thalidomide treatment on gestation and facial development. Experimental and Molecular Path. Suppl. 2 pp. 81-106, 1963.

Stockinger, L. and Koch, H.: Teratologische Untersuchung einer Neuen, dem Thalidomid Strukturell Nahestehenden Sedativ-hypnotisch Wirksamen Verbindung (K-2004). Arzneim. Forsch. 19: 167-169, 1969.

Taussig, H.B.: A study of the German outbreak of phocomelia. The Thalidomide Syndrome. J.A.M.A. 180: 1106-1114, 1962.

Vickers, T.H.: Concerning the morphogenesis of thalidomide dysmelia in rabbits. Brit. J. Exptl. Pathol. 48:579-592, 1967.

Wuest, H.M.; Fox, R.R. and Crary, D.D.: Relationship between teratogenicity and structure in the thalidomide field. Experientia 24: 993-994, 1968.

1217 Thallium

Karnofsky et al. (1950) reported that chicks receiving 0.5 to 2.0 mg of thallium sulfate via the yolk sac on the 4th day of incubation developed an achondroplastic-like condition. Gibson and Becker (1970) administered the sulfate form intraperitoneally in amounts up to 10 mg per kg to pregnant rats during critical times of development. Some fetal weight reduction and a slight increase in hydro-nephrosis was reported.

Gibson, J.E. and Becker, B.A.: Placental transfer, embryo
toxicity and teratogenicity of thallium sulfate in normal
and potassium-deficient rats. Toxicol. Appl. Pharmacol.
16: 120-132, 1970.

Karnofsky, D.A.; Ridgway, L.P. and Patterson, P.A.:
Production of achondroplasia in the chick embryo with
thallium. Proc. Soc. Exp. Biol. . Med. 73: 255-259,
1950.

1218 Thebaine

Geber and Schramm found a 2 to 4 percent incidence of
cranioschisis in hamster fetuses exposed to 140 and 193 mg
per kg on day 8 of gestation. Maternal mortalities at these
two dose levels were 10 and 75 percent.

Geber, W.F. and Schramm, L.C.: Congenital malformations of
the central nervous system produced by narcotic analgesics
in the hamster. Am. J. Obstet. Gynecol. 123:705-713,
1975.

1219 Theophylline

Ishikawa et al (1978) applied 1.0 ml of 0.02 M theophylline
directly to the chorioallantoic membrane of stage 24 to 27
chick embryos and produced 63 percent aortic aneurysms, many
with ventricular septal defects and some with truncus
arteriosus. Robkin et al (1974) at doses of 50 microgram
per ml of medium could show cardiac acceleration in day 11
explanted rat embryos.

Heinonen et al (1976) found no increase in defects among 76
women exposed to the drug.

Heinonen, O.P.; Slone, D. and Shapiro, S.: Birth Defects
and Drugs in Pregnancy. Publishing Sciences Group. Inc.
Littleton, Mass.; 1977.

Ishikawa, S.; Gilbert, E.F.; Bruyere, H.J. and Cheung,
M.O.: Aortic aneurysm associated with cardiac defects in
theophylline stimulated chick embryos. Teratology 18;23-30,
1978.

Robkin, M. A.; Shepard, T.H. and Baum, D.: Autonomic drug
effects on the heart rate of early rat embryos. Teratology
9:35-49, 1974.

1220 Thiabendazole

Ogata et al (1981) gavaged mice on days 7-15 with amounts of
700- 2400 mg per kg. Fusion of vertebrae, cleft palate and
skeletal anomalies were increased as was the maternal
mortality.

Ogata, A.; Ando, H.; Kubo, Y.; Takahashi, H.; Hiraga, K.:
Teratogenicity of thiabendazole (TB2) in mice (abstract)
Teratology 24: 24A-25A, 1981.

1221

1221 Thiadiazole (see 2-Ethylamino-1-3,4, thiadiazole)

1222 Thiamine Deficiency

Nelson and Evans (1955) in an extensive analysis of the effect of thiamine deficiency on the pregnant rat could detect no increase in congenital defects in the offspring. Dietary intake which was reduced in the thiamine deficient animals was partly responsible for the increased death rate and small size of the fetuses. Pfaltz and Severinghaus (1956) reported that some rat fetuses from deficient mothers had hemorrhages, edema of the head and torso and sometimes exencephaly. Full details were not given.

Two chemically related antagonists, oxythiamine and neopyrithiamine, may be teratogenic and are discussed under their own separate headings.

Pfaltz, H. and Severinghaus, E.L.: Effects of vitamin deficiencies on fertility, course of pregnancy, and embryonic development in rats. Am. J. Obstet. Gynecol. 72: 265-276, 1956.

Nelson, M.M. and Evans, H.M.: Relation of thiamine to reproduction in the rat. J. Nutr. 55: 151-163, 1955.

1223 Thiamine Tetrahydrofurfuryl Disulfide [TTFD]

Mizutani et al (1972) fed this compound to pregnant monkeys and rabbits in maximum doses of 300 and 500 mg per kg respectively during organogenesis and found no increase in fetal malformations.

Mizutani, M.; Ihara, T. and Kaziwara, K.: Effects of orally administered thiamine tetrahydrofurfuryl disulfide on foetal development of rabbits and monkeys. Jap. J. Pharmacol. 22: 115-124, 1972.

1224 Thiamphenicol

Suzuki et al (1973) studied this antibiotic drug in pregnant rats and mice by giving it by gavage during organogenesis. Complete resorptions resulted in the rats receiving more than 50 mg per kg per day and in mice with more than 1,000 mg per kg. Fetal mortality and growth retardation were found at the highest doses but no teratogenic action was found. Bass et al (1978) studied respiration and replication in mitochondria from exposed embryos. Postnatal studies did not reveal differences between the treated and control groups. Nau et al (1981) demonstrated transplacental passage in the early human pregnancy.

Bass, R.; Detlef, O.; Krowke, R.; Spielman, H.: Embryonic development and mitochondrial function 3. Inhibition of resorptions and ATP generation in rat embryos by thiamphenicol. Teratology 18:93-102, 1978.

Nau, H.; Welsch, F.; Ulbrich, B.; Bass, R.; Lange, J.:

page 420

Thiamphenicol during the first trimester of human pregnancy: placental transfer in vivo, placental uptake in vitro and inhibition of mitochondrial function. Toxicol. Appl. Pharmacol. 60:131-141, 1981.

Suzuki, Y.; Kondo, S.; Okada, F.; Suzuki, I.; Asano, F.; Matsuo, M. and Chiba, T.: Effects of thiamphenicol administered to the pregnant animals upon the development of their fetuses and neonates. (Japanese) Oyo Yakuri 7: 41-51, 1973.

1225 Thiamphenicol Glycinate HCl

Suzuki et al (1973) gave this drug intraperitoneally to pregnant rats and mice in maximum oral doses of 100 mg and 700 mg per kg per day respectively. Fetal mortality was found increased in rats at the 100 mg level and in mice at the 700 mg level. Fetal growth inhibition also occurred at the higher doses, but no teratogenic activity occured. Both species were treated during active organogenesis.

Suzuki, Y.; Okada, F.; Kondo, S.; Suzuki, I.; Asano, F.; Matuo, M. and Chiba, T.: Effects of thiamphenicol glycinate hydrochloride administered to the pregnant animals upon the development of their fetuses and neonates. (Japanese) Oyo Yakuri 7: 859-870, 1973.

1226 Thiazolidine Carboxylic Acid

Bertrand and Piton (1972) gave 25 to 250 mg per kg by mouth to pregnant mice, rats and rabbits and found no fetal effects. The rats and mice were treated between the 3rd and 15th day and the rabbits between the second and twenty-seventh gestational day.

Bertrand, M. and Piton, Y.: Recherche du risque d'effet teratogene de l'acide thiazolidine carboxylique. Gazzetta Medica Italiana 131: 268-271, 1972.

1227 Beta-2-Thienylalanine

This structural analogue of phenylalanine inhibits differentiation of ectomesenchyme derived from cranial neural crest. It was added to organ culture medium of fusing palatal shelves in the concentration of 2 mm (Barrd and Verrusio, 1973) and the fusion was prevented.

Barrd, G. and Verrusio, A.C.: Inhibition of palatal fusion in vitro by beta-2-thienylalanine. Teratology 7: 37-48, 1973.

1228 Thymoxamine Hydrochloride

Shoji et al (1982) studied this adrenergic blocker in rats and rabbits using 120 mg per kg per day orally. No effects on fertility, fetal development or postnatal function were reported. Rabbit fetuses did not have demonstrable adverse

1228

effects.

Shoji, S.; Kida, M.; Wada, S.; Kurimoto, T.; Shikuma, N.;
Okuma, Y.; Harada, H.; Machida, N.,;Hirayama, Y.:
Reproductive studies of thymoxamine hydrochloride. Yakura
to Chiryo 10:589-602, 603-615, 617-627, 629-640, 1982.

1229 Thioguanine

Thiersch (1957) injected intraperitoneally pregnant rats
with 10 mg per kg. Complete resorption was found with
treatment on the 7th and 8th day while unspecified types of
malformation or runting were found after treatment on the
4th and 5th or 11th and 12th days.

Thiersch, J.B.: Effect of 2-6 diaminopurine (2-6 DP): 6
chlorpurine (CLP) and thioguanine (THG) on rat litter in
utero. Proc. Soc. Exp. Biol. Med. 94: 40-43, 1957.

1230 Thiopental Sodium (also see Barbituric Acid)

Tanimura et al. (1967) found no defects in the offspring of
female mice receiving 100 mg per kg by injection on day 11
of pregnancy. Some reduction in fetal weight was found with
doses of 50 mg or more per kg. Persaud (1965) injected 50
and 100 mg into pregnant rats on the 4th day of gestation
and found no defective offspring.

Persaud, T.V.N.: Tiererperimentelle Untersuchungen zur
Frage der teratogenen Wirkung von Barbituraten. Acta Biol.
Med. Ger. 14: 89-90, 1965.

Tanimura, T.; Owaki, Y. and Nishimura, H.: Effect of administration of thiopental sodium to pregnant mice upon the
development of their offspring. Okajimas Folia Anat. Jap.
43: 219-226, 1967.

1231 Thiophanate [1,2-Bis(3-ethoxycarbonyl-thioureido)-benzene]

Makita et al (1970) gave up to 1000 mg per kg orally to
pregnant mice during organogenesis and observed no increase
in malformations although some growth retardation was
recorded. A three generation test with 3,000 PPM in the
diet was negative.

Mikita, T.; Hashimoto, Y. and Noguchi, T.: Toxicological
evaluation of thiophanate. 2 Studies on the teratology and
three generation reproduction of thiophanate in mice. Oyo
Yakuri 4: 23-30, 1970.

1232 Thiophanate-methyl   Dimethyl   [4,4-0-Phenylene
     bis(3-thioallophanate)]

This systemic fungicide was given intraperitoneally to mice
on days 1 through 15 of gestation in doses up to 1000 mg per
kg. No teratogenic effect was found although fetal death
occurred at the highest dose (Makita et al, 1973).

Makita, T.; Hashimoto, Y. and Noguchi, T.: Mutagenic, cytogenetic and teratogenic studies on thiophanate-methyl. Toxicol. Appl. Pharm. 24: 206-215, 1973.

1233 Thiophenicol

Silva and Andrade (1970) gave rats intraperitoneal doses of 100 mg per kg on the 1st, 3rd, 5th and 7th days of gestation and found an increase in resorption rate over controls. Although some increase in congenital defects occurred, the number was not significantly greater than in the controls.

Silva, N.O.G. and Andrade, A.T.L.: The effects of thiophenicol upon the rat conceptus. Fertil. Steril. 21: 431-433, 1970.

1234 Thioridazine (Mellaril-R) (see Phenothiazines)

1235 Thiosemicarbazide (also see Semicarbazide)

Neuman et al. (1956) and Bodit et al. (1966) have produced beak abnormalities and skeletal defects of the legs in chick embryos. Bodit et al. (1966) used 0.5 to 1.0 mg applied to the vascular area on the 3rd day of incubation.

Bodit, F.; Stoll, R. and Maraud, R.: Action de l'hydro-xyuree, de la semicarbazide sur le developpement de l'embryon de poulet. C. R. Soc. Biol. (Paris) 160: 960-963, 1966.

Neuman, R.E.; Maxwell, M. and McCoy, T.A.: Production of beak and skeletal malformations of chick embryo by semicarbazide. Proc. Soc. Exp. Biol. Med. 92: 578-581, 1956.

1236 Thio-TEPA [Triethylene Thiophosphoramide]

Murphy et al. (1958) using the rat determined that the dose per kg which killed 50 percent of the fetuses on the 12th gestational day was 5.0 mg per kg. The maternal LD-50 was 1.75 times greater. Growth retardation, syndactyly and skeletal defects were frequent and encephaloceles were occasionally produced. They were unable to demonstrate teratogenicity by treating the 4-day chick embryo with 0.01 mg. Thiersch (1957) also reported that two daily injections of 5 mg per kg caused many resorptions if given on two consecutive days during the rat pregnancy. Many of the survivors were malformed. Tanimura (1968) has published an extensive study of the effect of this compound on the mouse embryo.

Murphy, M.L.; Delmoro, A. and Lacon, C.R.: The comparative effects of five polyfunctional alkalating agents on the rat fetus with additional notes on the chick embryo. Ann. N. Y. Acad. Sci. 68: 762-782, 1958.

Tanimura, T.: Relationship of dosage and time of adminis-

1236

tration to teratogenic effects of thio-TEPA in mice. Sonderabdruck Okajimas Folia Anatomica Japonica 44: 203-253, 1968.

Thiersch, J.B.: Effect of 2,4,6, triamin-S-triazine (TR), 2,4,6 tris (ethyleneimino)-S-triazine (TEM) and N,N, N-tri-ethylenephosphoramide (TEPA) on rat litter in utero. Proc. Soc. Exp. Biol. Med. 94: 36-43, 1957.

1237 Thiothixene [Navane-R]

Owaki (1969) gave up to 90 mg per kg per day to pregnant mice from days 7 through 12 and observed no teratogenic or postnatal effects. Similar findings were reported from rabbits (Owaki et al, 1969).

Owaki, Y.; Momiyama, H. and Yokoi, Y.: Teratological studies on thiothixene in mice. (Japanese) Oyo Yakuri 3: 315-320, 1969.

Owaki, Y.; Momiyama, H. and Yokoi, Y.: Teratological studies on thiothixene (navane) in rabbits. (Japanese) Oyo Yakuri 3: 321-324, 1969.

1238 Thiram [Tetramethyl-thiuram Disulfide]

Roll (1971) reported production of cleft palate, curved long bones and micrognathia in two strains of mice. Treatment with doses over 250 mg per kg on the 12th and 13th days of gestation produced the highest incidence of defects. Robens (1969) reported defects in the offspring of hamsters treated on the 7th or 8th day with 10 mg per kg. Fused ribs were found most frequently.

Robens, J.F.: Teratologic studies of carbaryl, diazinon, norea, disulfiram and thiram in small laboratory animals. Toxicol. Appl. Pharmacol. 15: 152-163, 1969.

Roll, R.: Teratologische Untersuchungen mit Thiram (TMTD) an zwei Mausestammen. Arch. Toxikol. 27: 173-186, 1971.

1239 Thorazine (see Chlorpromazine)

1240 Thyroid Antibodies

Maternal autoimmunization to thyroid has been implicated (Blizzard et al.; 1960) etiologically in athyrotic cretinism but the incidence of thyroid antibodies in the serum of the mothers of cretins was low (25 percent) (Chandler et al.; 1962). The possibility exists that the antibodies resulted from an unidentified agent which affected both mother and fetus, destroying the fetal thyroid and damaging the maternal gland sufficiently to produce a maternal antibody to thyroid.

Blizzard, R.M.; Chandler, R.W.; Landing, B.H.; Pettit, M.D. and West, C.D.: Maternal autoimmunization to thyroid as probable cause of athyrotic cretinism. N. Engl. J. Med. 263: 327-336, 1960.

Chandler, R.W.; Blizzard, R.M.; Hung, W. and Kyle, M.: Incidence of thyrocytotoxic factor and other antithyroid antibodies in the mothers of cretins. N. Engl. J. Med. 267: 376-380, 1962.

1241 Thyroidectomy (also see Hypothyroidism)

Langman and Van Faassen (1955) partially thyroidectomized rats before pregnancy and found in subsequently produced fetuses about a 50 percent abnormality rate in the lenses. Besides retinal folding various degrees of lenticular degeneration were present. Partial thyroidectomy early in pregnancy was not associated with defects.

The postnatal effects following maternal thyroidectomy were reported by Bakke et al, 1975. Persistently enlarged thyroids and elevated thyroid stimulating hormone levels were found in the male offspring.

Bakke, J.L.; Lawrence, N.L.; Robinson, S. and Bennett, J.: Endocrine studies of the untreated progeny of thyroidectomized rats. Pediat. Res. 9: 742-748, 1975.

Langman, J. and Van Faassen, F.: Congenital defects in the rat embryo after partial thyroidectomy of the mother animal: A preliminary report of eye defects. Am. J. Ophthalmol. 40: 65-76, 1955.

1242 Thyrotropin-Releasing-Hormone [TRH]

Asano et al (1974) injected this synthetic neuroendocrine substance intraperitoneally into pregnant rats and mice on days 7 through 16 and 6 through 15 respectively. Doses of 0.2 to 30 mg per kg were used. No teratogenicity or postnatal changes were found except for growth retardation in the rat offspring. A reduction in the weight of the fetal mouse thyroids was found.

Asano, Y.; Ariyuki, F. and Higaki, K.: Effects of adminis- tration of synthetic thyrotropin-releasing-hormone on mouse and rat fetuses. Oyo Yakuri 8: 807-816, 1974.

1243 Thyroxine

Giroud and Rothschild (1951) tube-fed 0.25 to 0.30 mg of thyroxine daily to rats and found cataracts in 38 percent of the offspring. Other types of defects were not seen. Stoll et al. (1966) using 3 to 24 microgm of L-thyroxine per egg on the 2nd, 3rd or 5th day of incubation produced a monstrosity characterized by eversion of the body wall and sac from which the legs, wings and head protrude. Triodothyronine (0.1 microgm) produced a similar type of defect.

1243

A decrease in cleft palate in the mouse associated with thyroxine administration was reported by Woollam and Miller (1960) and a possible explanation that the thyroxine causes an increasd fetal loss rate in the affected but not the normal litter mates was offered by Juriloff and Fraser (1977).

Giroud, A. and Rothschild, B.: Repercussions de la thyroxine sur l'oeil du foetus. C. R. Soc. Biol. (Paris) 145: 525-526, 1951.

Juriloff, D.M. and Fraser, F.C.: Differential mortality of the cleft lip embryos in response to maternal treatment with thyroxine (abs) Teratology 15:18-19A, 1977.

Stoll, R.; Coulaud, H.; Faucounau, N. and Maraud, R.: Sur l'action teratogene des hormones thyroidiennes chez l'embryon de poulet. Les Mechanisms Morphogenetiques De La Strophosomie. Arch. Anat. Microsc. Morphol. Exp. 55: 59-76, 1966.

Woollam, D.H.M. and Millen, J.W.: Influence of thyroxine on the incidence of hairlip in the "Strong A" line of mice. Br. Med. J. 1:1253-1254, 1960.

1244 Tiaprofenic Acid

Esaki and Oshio (1980) in a series of papers studied the effects of this antiinflammatory drug on breeding, prenatal and perinatal development in the mouse. Dosing up to 80 mg per kg orally produced some delay in fetal development but no other adverse effects were noted.

Esaki, K.; Oshio, K.: Effects of oral administration of tiaprofenic acid (RU-15060) on reproduction in the mouse. Preclin. Rep. Cent. Inst. Exp. Anim. 6:195-216, 1980.

1245 Ticlopidine Hydrochloride (5-(0-chlorobenzyl-4,5,6,7-tetrahydrothieno[3,2,c]pyridine hydrochloride

Watanabe et al (1980) gave up to 320 mg per kg orally to rats before and during pregnancy. Sedation and other side effects were noted in the adults but no adverse effects on reproduction were found. Some delay in oss;fication of;the fetus wa; observed.; ;

Watanbe, T.; Takagi, S.; Mochida, K.; Ohura, K.; Matsuhashi, K.; Morita, H.; Akimoto, T.: Reproductive studies of triclopidine hydrochloride Fertility studies in rats. Ikakuhin Kenkyu 11:255-264, 1980.

1246 Timebutino Maleate

Asano et al (1982) studied this digestive tract antimotility agent in rats and rabbits at oral doses of up to 1000 mg per kg. No fertility decrease or change in postnatal function was found in rats and in neither species was there any change in the fetuses.

Asano, Y.; Fujisawa, K.; Ono, T.; Ariyuki, F.; Higaki, K.: Reproductive studies of trimebutine maleate in rats and rabbits. Kiso to Rinsho 16:633-650, 1982.

1247 Timiperone
(4-(4-(2,3-dihydro-2-thioxo-1H-benzimidazol-1-yl)-1-piperidinyl)-1-(4-fluoro-phenyl)-1-butanone)

Nakashima et al (1981) found neither teratogenic effect nor changes in postnatal function in rat fetuses exposed to up to 10 mg per kg daily during organogenesis. Maternal and fetal weight reduction occurred. Similar treatment of rabbits revealed no significant differences from controls.

Nakashima, K.; Yamashita, N.; Morita, H.: Reproductive studies of timiperone. Ikakuhin Kenkyu 12:861-880, 1981.

1248 Tioconazole

Noguchi et al gave this antifungal agent which is an imidazole derivative subcutaneously to rats. When 30 and 100 mg per kg were given before mating and during the first 7 days of gestation a reduction in implantation and live fetuses was found. The same doses were associated after treatment on days 17-21 with decreased fetal survival and reduced lactation. No malformations were increased after treatment on days 7-17.

Noguchi, Y.; Tochibana, M.; Nabatake, H.; Iijima, M.; Horimoto, M.; Yamakawa, S.; Ishikawa, J.; Otsaki, I.: Preclinical safety evaluation of tioconazole. Yakuri to Chiryo 10:3849-3861, 1982.

1249 Tinidazole   [Ethyl[2-(2-methyl-5-nitro-1-imidazolyl)ethyl-]sulfone]

Owaki et al (1974) gave this compound orally to pregnant mice and rats in maximum doses of 2,000 mg per kg per day of organogenesis and found no teratogenic effects.

Owaki, Y.; Momiyama, H.; Sakai, T. and Nabata, H.: Effects of tinidazole on the fetuses and their postnatal development in mice and rats. (Japanese) Oyo Yakuri 8: 421-427, 1974.

1250 Tobacco (see Cigarette Smoking) (see Nicotine)

1251 Tobacco Stalks

Crowe and Swerczek (1974) fed aqueous tobacco leaf filtrates or tobacco stalks to sows and found congenital arthrogryposis in the offspring. The material was administered from the 4th through the 53rd day of gestation. The causative agent was not determined. Keeler and Crowe (1981) have isolated anabasine from these stalks and fed N. glauca,, a plant containing the chemical as its sole alkaloid, to cows and pigs and produced congenital defects.

1251

Crowe, M.W.; Swerczek, T.W.: Congenital arthrogryposis in offspring of sows fed tobacco (Nicotiana tabacum). Am. J. Vet. Res. 35:1071- 1073, 1974.

Keeler, R.F.; Crowe, M.W.: Congenital deformities in livestock induced by maternal Nicotiana ingestion. (abstract) Teratology 23:44A, 1981.

1252 Tobramycin

This aminoglycoside was given subcutaneously to rats and rabbits in doses of 100 mg and 20 or 40 mg per kg respectively. No effect on fetal development occurred (Welles et al, 1973).

Welles, J.S.; Emmerson, J.L.; Gibson, W.R.; Nickander, R.; Owen, N.V. and Anderson, R.C.: Preclinical toxicology studies of tobramycin. Toxicol. Appl. Pharm. 25: 398-409, 1973.

1253 Tofisopam

This benzodiazepin tranquilizer was tested by Hayashi et al (1981) in rats. They used oral doses of up to 100 mg per kg daily before conception and on days 71-7 and 17-21 of gestation. No adverse effects on reproduction was found.

Hayashi, Y.; Inoue, K.; Kasuys, S.; Tomita, K.; Ito, C.; Ohnishi, H.: Toxicological studies of tofisopam: Reproductive studies of tofisopam in rats. Iyakuhin Kenkyu 12:565-580, 1981.

1254 Tokishakuyaku-san

Aburada et al (1982) fed up to 800 mg per kg daily to rats during days 7-17 and found no adverse fetal or maternal effects. This material is an old Chinese medicine.

Aburada, M.; Akiyama, Y.; Ichio, Y.; Nakamura, A.; Ichikawa, N.: Teratological study of Tokishakuyaku-san in rats. Oyo Yakuri 23:981-997, 1982.

1255 Tolbutamide

Tuchmann-Duplessis and Mercier-Parot (1959) and Demeyer (1961) have produced congenital defects of the eye in the offspring of treated rats. Demeyer (1961) used 300 mg per day on the 8th and 9th days. Smithberg and Runner (1963) injected mice intraperitoneally 1 mg per gm of weight on the 9th gestational day and found exencephaly, rib and vertebral defects in many of the offspring. Lazarus and Volk (1963) injected 125 mg per kg twice daily into rabbits from the 7th through the 14th gestational day and found no evidence of teratogenicity. These authors review the available negative evidence for teratogenicity in man. Sterne (1963) reviewed 34 pregnancies treated with oral hypoglycemics and reported 28 normal births and six stillbirths but no congenital defects.

Demeyer, R.: Etude experimentale de la glycoregulation gravidique et de l action teratogene des perturbations du metabolisme glucidique. Paris: Masson Et Cie, 1961. pp. 175-183.

Lazarus, S.S. and Volk, B.W.: Absence of teratogenic effect of tolbutamide in rabbits. J. Clin. Endocrinol. 23: 597-599, 1963.

Smithberg, M. and Runner, M.N.: Teratogenic effects of hypoglycemic treatments in inbred strains of mice. Am. J. Anat. 113: 479-489, 1963.

Sterne, J.: Antidiabetic drugs and teratogenicity. Lancet 1:1165, only, 1963.

Tuchmann-Duplessis, H. and Mercier-Parot, L.: Influence de divers sulfamides hypoglcemiants sur le developpement de l'embryon. Etude experimentale chez le rat. Acad. Nat. De Medecine (Paris) 143: 238-241, 1959.

1256 Tolciclate

This topical antifungal agent was given subcutaneously to rats and rabbits in maximal doses of 100 mg per kg daily by Harakawa et al (1981). No ill effects were found on fetuses of either species. Fertility and postnatal studies also showed no ill effects.

Harakawa, T.; Suzuki, T.; Hayashizaki, A.; Nishimura, N.; Sano, Y.; Nishikawa, M.; Kato, M.; Sato, Y.; Iwasaki, K.; Kihara, T.: Reproductive studies of tolciclate. Kiso to Rinsho 15:2413-2425, 1981.

1257 Tolmetin, Sodium (see 1-Methyl-5-p- toluoylpyrrole-2-acetate Dihydrate, Sodium)

1258 Toluene

Hudak and Ungvary (1978) exposed rats to 1500 mg per square meter of air from day 1 through 8 or 1000 mg per square meter for 8 hours daily from day 1 through day 21 and found no teratogenic effect. Some fetal growth retardation occurred at the higher dose which also killed some of the mothers. Mice were exposed during days 6-13 to 1500 mg per square meter of air with similar results. Nawrot and Staples (1979) gavage fed mice 1.0 mg per kg on days 6 through 15 and found increased cleft palate in the offspring. Syrovadko (1977) reported a higher incidence of fetal asphyxia and low birth weight in the offspring of women working with "organosilicon" varnishes which increase the exposure to toluene and other agents.

Hudak, A. and Ungvary, G.: Embryotoxic effects of benzene and its methyl derivatives: toluene, xylene. Toxicology 11:55-63, 1978.

1258

Nawrot, P.S. and Staples, R.E.: Embryo-fetal toxicity and
teratogenicity of benzene and toluene in the mouse (abs)
Teratoloy 19:41A, 1979.

Syrovadko, O.N.: Working conditions and health status of
women handling organosilicon varnishes containing toluene.
g.g. Tr. Prof. Zabol. 12:15-19, 1977.

1259 2,5-Toluene diamine sulfate (see hair dyes)

1260 0-Toluene Sulfonamide (see Saccharin)

1261 Toxoplasmosis Gondii

Congenital toxoplasma gondii infection may be acquired
through asymptomatic maternal infection. The incidence
varies in the newborn population from 0.25 to 8 per 1000.
The maternal infection is acquired by ingestion of raw meat
or by oral contamination with infected cat fecies. A large
proportion of infected infants remain asymptomatic and
develop normally. Those with the syndrome may have
hepatosplenomegaly, icterus, maculopapular rash,
chorioretinitis and cerebral calcifications.

Hydrocephalus or microcephalus may develop and lead to
functional defects. The subject is reviewed by Feldman
(1968) and Warkany (1971).

The role of toxoplasmosis in the etiology of repeated
spontaneous abortion is controversial. Langer (1963) claims
that a high proportion of habitual or repeated abortions,
prematures and stillbirths in Germany are due to
toxoplasmosis. Other studies have shown a much lower
incidence. Kimball et al. (1971) in a prospective study of
5,000 New York women found that toxoplasma antibodies were
not associated with habitual abortion and could not culture
toxoplasma from 260 spontaneous abortions.

A significant increase from 31 to 38 percent positive dye
tests was observed in the group of women who reported
previous spontaneous abortions as compared to those without
abortions.

Feldman, H.A.: Toxoplasmosis. Medical Progress 279:
1371-1431, 1432-1437, 1968.

Kimball, A.C.; Kean, B.H. and Fuchs, F.: The role of
toxoplasmosis in abortion. Am. J. Obstet. Gynecol. III:
219-226, 1971.

Langer, H.: Repeated congenital infection with toxoplasma
gondii. Obstet. Gynecol. 21: 318-329, 1963.

Warkany, J.: Congenital Malformations Notes and Comments.
Chicago: Year Book Medical Publishers, 1971. pp. 78-81.

1262 Tranexamic Acid [Trans-4-(aminomethyl)cyclohexane-carboxylic

Acid]

This antifibrinolytic agent was given orally to mice and rats during organogenesis in doses as high as 1500 mg per kg per day. No fetal effects or teratogenicity occurred (Morita et al, 1971).

Morita, H.; Tachizawa, H. and Okimoto, T.: Evaluation of the safety of tranexamic acid (3) Teratogenic effects in mice and rats. Oyo Yakuri 5: 415-420, 1971.

1263 Trapymin

Ito et al (1976) gave pregnant rabbits up to 120 mg per kg orally on days 6 through 18. Maternal weight was reduced at the highest dose but no fetal changes occurred.

Ito, C.; Shibutani, Y.; Nakano, K. and Ohnishi, H.: Toxicological studies of trapymin 5. Teratological studies of trapymin in rabbits. (Japanese) Iyakuhin Kenkyu 7; 195-199, 1976.

1264 Trauma (also see Laporotomy)

There are only a small number of convincing case reports where trauma contributed to production of a human anomaly (Hinden, 1965).

Brent and Franklin (1960) reported the effect of uterine vascular clamping in the rat. With clamping for 1.5 to 3 hours on the 9th day they produced 16.7 percent malformations which included eye, kidney and vascular systems as well as anencephaly and omphalocele.

Brent, R.L. and Franklin, J.B.: Uterine vascular clamping: New procedure for the study of congenital malformations. Science 132: 89-91, 1960.

Hinden, E.: External injury causing foetal deformity. Arch. Dis. Child. 40: 80-81, 1965.

1265 Triacetyl-6-azauridine (see 6-Azauridine)

1266 Triamcinolone [Aristocort-R]

Walker (1965) was able to produce cleft palates in mice by administering daily as little as 1 microgm on days 11 through 14. The difference in cleft-palate producing doses between cortisone and triamcinolone was 200 times whereas their therapeutic effect in man differs by only about 6 times.

Walker, B.E.: Cleft palate produced in mice by human-equivalent dosage with triamcinolone. Science 149: 862-863, 1965.

1267 Triazine (see 1-Phenyl-3,3 dimethyl Triazine)

1268 Triazolam

Matsuo et al (1979) gave this tranquilizer by gastric gavage to rats and rabbits in maximum total daily doses of 300 and 50 mg per kg respectively. Given during organogenesis, there was no teratogenic effect in either species. In the rabbit, doses of 3 and 50 mg per kg daily caused a decrease in implantations viable fetuses and fetal weight.

Matsuo, A.; Kast, A. and Tsunenari, Y.: Reproduction studies of triazolam in rats and rabbits. (Japanese) Iyakuhin Kenkyu 10: 52-67, 1979.

1269 Tribromoethanol

This anesthestic has been tested in explanted rat embryos and at anesthetic dosage, a reduction in embryonic growth as measured by protein increase was found. (Kaufman and Steele, 1976).

Kaufman, M.H. and Steele, C.E.: Deleterious effect of an anesthetic on cultured mammalian embryos. Nature 260:782-783, 1976.

1270 Tricaprylin

Ohta et al (1970) gave 10 ml per kg to mice and observed no fetal effects. Studies with the pregnant rabbit were also negative for teratogenicity.

Ohta, K.; Matsuoka, Y.; Ichikawa, Y. and Yamamoto, K.: Toxicity, teratogenicity and pharmacology of tricaprylin. (Japanese) Oyo Yakuri 4: 871-882, 1970.

1271 1,1,1-Trichloroethane

Schwetz et al (1975) exposed pregnant mice and rats to this vapor in concentrations of 875 ppm. Both species were exposed for 7 hour daily periods on days 6 through 15 of gestation. No fetal toxicity or teratogenicity was found. Lane et al (1982) exposed mice to 1,000 mg per kg in drinking water and found no adverse effects on reproduction. York et al (1982) using 2100 ppm exposure (6 hours per day) during the rat gestation found some reduction in fetal weight and delay in osseous development. Their postnatal studies revealed no differences from controls.

Lane, R.W.; Riddle, B.L.; Borzelleca, J.F.: Effects of 1,1,1- trichloroethane in drinking water on reproduction and development in mice. Toxicol. Appl. Pharm. 63:409-421, 1982.

Schwetz, B.A.; Leong, B.K.J. and Gehring, P.J.: The effect of maternally inhaled trichorethylene, perchloroethylene, methyl chloroform and methylene chloride on embryonal and

fetal development in mice and rats. Toxicol. Appl. Pharm.
32: 84-96, 1975.

York, R.G.; Sowry, B.M.; Hastings, L.; Manson, J.M.:
Evaluation of teratogenicity and neurotoxicity with maternal
inhalation exposure to methyl chloroform. J. Toxicol.
Envir. Health 9:251-266, 1982.

1272 Trichloroethylene

Schwetz et al (1975) exposed pregnant mice and rats to 300
ppm. Both species were exposed to 7 hour daily periods on
days 6 through 15 of gestation No fetal toxicity or
teratogenicity was found. Dorfmueller et al (1979) exposed
female rats 6 hours daily for two weeks before pregnancy and
for the first 20 days of gestation to 1800 ppm and found
anomalies of skeletal and soft tissues which were considered
to be indicative of developmental delay. Behavioral
evaluation of the offsprng showed no effects from the
treatment. Sperm examination from mice exposed to 0.3
percent for 4 hours daily for 5 days revealed increased
abnormalities after 28 days (Land et al 1981).

Dorfmueller, M.A.; Henne, S.P.; York, R.G.; Bornschein,
R.L.; Manson, J.M.: Evaluation of teratogenicity and
behavioral toxicity with inhalation exposure of maternal
rats to trichloroethylene. Toxicology 14:153-166, 1979.

Land, P.C.; Owen, E.L.; Linde, H.W.: Morphological changes
in mouse spermatozoa after exposure to inhalational
anesthetics during early spermatogenesis. Anesthesiology
54:53-66, 1981.

Schwetz, B.A.; Leong, B.K.J. and Gehring, P.J.: The effect
of maternally inhaled trichorethylene, perchloroethylene,
methyl chloroform and methylene chloride on embryonal and
fetal development in mice and rats. Toxicol. Appl. Pharm.
32: 84-96, 1975.

1273 2,4,5-Trichlorophenoxyacetic Acid (2,4,5-T)

Emmerson et al. (1971) gave rats 1 to 24 mg by mouth on
days 6 through 15 and rabbits 10 to 40 mg on days 6 through
18. No effects on litter size, fetal weight or incidence of
congenital defects were found. Previous findings by
Courtney et al. (1970, 1971) about teratogenicity of
2,4,5-T may be explained by dioxin contaminants in the
material. Roll (1971) reported cleft palate production in
mice with a preparation contaminated with less than 0.1 ppm
of the dioxane. In a study by Chebotar et al (1978) female
rats received by gavage 2,4,5-trichlorphenoxyacetic acid in
the dose of 400 mg per kg, commercial sample of butyl ester
of 2,4,t-T in the dose of 50, 100, 200 mg per kg and
purified ester of 2,4,5-T in the dose of 800 mg per kg daily
on the 9,10,11,12,13 and 14th day of gestation. Embryotoxic
effect of 2,4,5-T was highest in the group of animals
treated on the 9th day of gestation, that of butyl ester of
2,4,5-T - on the 10th day. Immobilization of pregnant rats
(2 hours daily) significantly increased teratogenic action

of 2,4,5-T and butyl ester of 2,4,5-T.

Nelson et al (1979) have reviewed and contributed new data on the effect of 2,4,5-T on the human. By analysis of 1,201 cases of cleft palate over 32 years in the rice growing area of Arkansas, they could establish no relationship between 2,4,5-T use per county and incidence of clefts.

The rate of several congenital defects in Hungary did not change with the introduction and heavy use of 2,4,5T (Thomas, 1980). Field and Kerr (1979) noted that the neural tube defect rate in Australia was parallel to the amount of herbicides used. Smith et al (1981) in New Zealand and Townsend et al (1982) found no increase in defects or abortions among wives of exposed workers.

Chebotar, N.A.; Grebenic, L.A. and Kirilenko, A.I.: Effect of stress (immobilization) on embryotoxic and teratogenic action of 2,4,5-T-trichlorphenoxyacetic acid and its derivatives. Arkh. Anat. Gistol. Embryol. (USSR) 75,8:30-35, 1978.

Courtney, K.D.; Gaylor, D.W.; Hogan, M.D.; Falk, H.L.; Bates, R.R. and Mitchell, I.: Teratogenic evaluation of 2,4,5-T. Science 168: 864-866, 1970.

Courtney, K.D. and Moore, J.A.: Teratology studies with 2,4,5-trichlorophenoxyacetic acid and 2,3,7,8-tetrachloro-dibenzo-p-dioxin. Toxicol. Appl. Pharmacol. 20: 396-403, 1971.

Emmerson, J.L.; Thompson D.J.; Strebing, R.J.; Gerbig, C.G. and Robinson, V.B.: Teratogenic studies on 2,4,5-trichloro-phenoxyacetic acid in the rat and rabbit. Food Cosmet. Toxicol. 9: 395-404, 1971.

Field, B.; Kerr, C.: Herbicide use and incidence of neural tube defects. Lancet 1:1341-1342, 1979.

Nelson, C.J.; Holson, J.F.; Green, H.G. and Gaylor, D.W.: Retrospective study of the relationship between agricultural use of 2,4,5-T and cleft palate occurrence in Arkansas. Teratology 19:377-384, 1979.

Roll, R.: Untersuchungen u er die teratogene Wirkung von 2,4,5-T bei Mausen. Food. Cosmet. Toxicol. 9: 671-676, 1971.

Smith, A.H.; Matheson, D.P.; Fisher, D.O.; Chapman, C.J.: Preliminary report of reproductive outcomes among pesticide applications using 2,4,5-T. N.Z. Med. J. 93:177-179, 1981.

Thomas, H.F.: 2,4,5T use and congenital malformation rates in Hungary. Lancet 2:214-215, 1980.

Townsend, J.C.; Bodner, K.M.; Van Peenen, P.F.D.; Olson, R.D.; Cook, R.R.: Survey of reproductive events of wives of employees exposed to chlorinated dioxins. Am. J. Epid. 115:695-713, 1982.

1274 2,4,5-Trichlorophenol

Hood et al (1979) administered this compound by gavage to pregnant mice in single doses of 800-900 mg per kg or mutliple doses of 250- 300 mg per kg and found no significant fetal effects.

Hood, R.D.; Patterson, B.L.; Thacker, G.T.; Sloan, G.C.; Szeczech, G.M.: Prenatal effects of 2,4,5T, 2,4,5-trichlorophenol and phenoxyacetic acid in mice. J. Environ. Sci. Health C13:189-204, 1979.

1275 Triethanomelamine [TEM]

Thiersch (1957) reported that this compound was embryolethal in the rat. Chaube and Murphy (1968) injected 0.3 to 0.6 mg per kg on the 11th or 12th gestational day of the rat and produced defects of the central nervous system, palate and skeleton. Jurand (1959) has studied the embryopathogenesis of this drug in the mouse embryo and reports growth retardation, enlargement of the myocele, somite degeneration and other diverse defects. Kageyama and Nishimura (1961) have described the multiple defects found in the term mouse fetus. Sanyal et al (1982) exposed rat embryos in vitro to 1-5 micrograms per ml and retarded growth was found.

Chaube, S. and Murphy, M.L.: The teratogenic effects of the recent drugs active in cancer chemotherapy. In, Woollam, D.H.M. (ed.): Advances in Teratology, Vol. 3. New York: Academic Press, 1968. pp. 181-237.

Jurand, A.: Action of triethanomelamine (TEM) on early and late stages of mouse embryos. J. Embryol. Exp. Morphol. 7: 526-539, 1959.

Kageyama, M. and Nishimura, H.: Developmental anomalies in mouse embryos induced by triethylene melamine (T.E.M.). Acta Med. Univ. Kyoto 37: 318-327, 1961.

Sanyal, M.K.; Kitchin, K.T.; Dixon, R.L.: Rat conceptus development in vitro. Comparative effects of alkalating agents. Toxicol. Appl. Pharm. 57:14-19, 1981.

Thiersch, J.B.: Effect of 2,4,6, triamino-'s'-triazine (TR), 2,4,6, tris (ethereimino)-'s'-triazine (TEM) and N,N,N-triethylenephosphoramide (TEPA) on the rat litter in utero. Proc. Soc. Exp. Biol. Med. 94: 36-40, 1957.

1276 Trifluoperazine (also see Phenothiazines)

In a review of the literature on the teratogenicity of trifluoperizine, Moriarity (1963) reported the use of this drug in over 700 early pregnancies and could not find any increase in congenital malformations. Heinonen et al (1977) report the outcome of 42 pregnancies treated in the first four months with trifluoperizine. There was no significant increase in congenital defects.

Wheatley, 1974, reported 59 exposures with a 1.7% abnormality rate which was not increased over the normal. Schrire (1963) reported that there were no skeletal defects in 478 women who were treated with the drug during pregnancy. Hall (1963) reported one child with a reduction defect in the arm; the mother was treated with Stelazine for 2-3 days around the 25th day of gestation.

In the literature dealing with animal experimentation Vichi et al (1968) using doses of .05 to .8 milligrams per mouse during several four day periods in mid-pregnancy were able to produce an increase in cleft palate at the higher dose. Other defects were not mentioned. This dose, if converted to a per kilogram dose based upon an assumption that the mouse is about 20 grams, would be equivalent to 40 milligrams of the drug per kilogram per day. At this very high dose the mouse may be very sleepy and therefore have partial starvation. Starvation in the mouse is particularly prone to producing cleft palate.

Hall, G.: A case of phocomelia of the upper limbs. Med. J. Austr. 1:449-450, 1963.

Heinonen, O.P.; Slone, D.; Shapiro, S.: Birth Defects and Drugs in Pregnancy. Publishing Sciences Group, Inc., 1977.

Moriarity, A.J.: Trufluoperizine and congenital malformations. Can. Med. Assoc. J., 88:97, 1963.

Schrire, I.: Trifluoperizine and foetal anomalies. Lancet 1:174, 1963.

Vichi, F.; Pierleoni, P.; Orlando, S.; Tollaro, I.: Palatoschisi indolte da trifluoperidolo nel topo. Sperimentale 118:245-250, 1968.

Wheatley, D.: Drugs and the embryo. Br. Med. J. 1:630, 1964.

1277 5-Trifluoromethyl-2-deoxyuridine

Kury and Crosby (1967) injected the yolk sac of developing chick eggs once during the first 4 days of incubation with 0.1 to 3.0 microgm of this compound. Cleft palate, amelia and other skeletal defects as well as renal hypoplasias were produced.

Kury, G. and Crosby, R.J.: The teratogenic effect of 5-trifluoromethyl-2-deoxyuridine in chicken embryos. Toxicol. Appl. Pharmacol. 11: 72-80, 1967.

1278 1-[3,5-Bis-trifluoromethyl)phenyl]-4-methyl Thiosemicarbazide (Ciba 2696G0)

Rao et al (1973) gave 2.5 to 10 mg per day by gavage to rats from day 6 through day 15. A dose dependent increased incidence of exencephaly skeletal defects and resorptions was found.

Rao, R.R.; Bhat, N.G.; Nair, T.B. and Shukla, R.G.:
Toxicological and teratological studies with
1-[3,5-bis-trifluoromethyl)phenyl]-4-methylthiosemicarbazide
(Ciba 2696G0). Arzneim-Forsch 23: 797-800, 1973.

1279 Trifluperidol [Psicoperidol-R]

Vichi et al. (1968) produced cleft palates in the offspring
of mice treated with 0.1 to 0.8 mg per day from the 10th
through the 13th day of gestation.

Vichi, F.; Pierleoni, P.; Orlando, S. and Tollaro, I.:
Palatoschisi indotte la trifluperidolo nel topo.
Spermimentale 118: 245-250, 1968.

1280 Trifluralin-R (alpha,alpha,alpha-trifluoro-2,6-dinitro-
N,N-di N propyl-p-toluidine)

This herbicide was given by Beck (1981) to mice on days 6-15
of gestation. The dose was 1.0 gm per kg. On day 60
postnatally Alizarin red studies of the skeleton revealed an
increase in 14th ribs and other minor skeletal defects.

Beck, S.L.: Assessment of adult skeletons to detect
prenatal exposure to 2,4,5-T and trifluralin in mice.
Teratology 23:33-55, 1981.

1281 Trimethadione [3,5,5-Trimethyl-2,4-oxazolidinedione]

German et al (1970) reviewed 11 women treated during pregnancy with either trimethadione or paramethadione and found
an increased incidence of congenital defects in the 11
exposed children. These defects included cleft palate (4)
cardiac anomalies (3) and other types of conditions. Two
were normal. Zackai et al (1975) have described a specific
phenotype in children born in three families where the
mother took trimethadione. The syndrome included developmental delay, v-shaped eyebrows, low-set ears with
anteriorly folded helix, high-arched palate and irregular
teeth. Feldman et al (1977) have added four cases and
summarized the clinical picture from 53 pregnancies.
Feldman et al (1977) have added four cases and summarized
the clinical picture from 53 pregnancies.

Brown et al (1979) administered 543 to 858 mg per kg to mice
on days 8 through 10 or 11 through 13 and produced a high
incidence of visceral and skeletal malformations. Aortic
arch and vertebal defects were the most common.
Intraperitoneal routes gave the same results as oral dosing.
Fetal weight reduction occurred at dose levels of 35 mg per
kg.

Brown, N.A.; Shull, G.; Fabro, S.: Assessment of the
teratogenic potential of trimethadione in the CD-1 mouse.
Toxicol. Appl. Pharmacol. 51:59-71, 1979.

Feldman, G.L.; Weaver, D.D. and Lovrien, E.W.: The fetal
trimethadione syndrome. A. J. Dis. Child.

1281

131:1389-1392, 1977.

German, J.; Kowal, A. and Ehlers, K.H.: Trimethadione and human teratogenesis. Teratology 3: 349-362, 1970.

Zackai, E.H.; Melman, W.J.; Neiderer, B. and Hanson, J.W.: The fetal trimethadione syndrome. J. Pediat. 87: 280-284, 1975.

1282 Trimethobenzamide (Tigan-Rx)

This antinauseant qiven during the first 84 days in 193 pregnancies was associated with 2.6 percent serious congenital defects in the offspring studied at one year and in 5.8 percent at 5 years. The 5.8 percent incidence was borderline significant (p less than 0.05) as compared to non-treated control rates (3.2 percent). No pattern of malformation was identified.

Milkovich, L. and Van den Berg, B.J.: An evaluation of the teratogenicity of certain antinauseant drugs. Am. J. Obst. Gynecol. 125:244-248, 1976.

1283 Trimethoprim

Helm et al (1976) reported studies in the rat and rabbit using the drug in a 1 to 5 dose ratio with sulfamethoxazole. The rats received up to 600 mg per kg of the combination on days 8 through 15 and cleft palate, micrognathia and limb shortening were found in the fetuses. Doses of 180 mg per kg had no effect. In the rabbit treated on day 8 through 14 given 600 mg per kg, there were no malformations, but the fetal loss was increased. Sulfamethoxazole alone in corresponding doses was not embryotoxic.

Williams et al (1969) treated 120 pregnant women with combined sulfamethoxazole and trimethoprim and found no increase in defects in the offspring. Only 10 of the women were treated before 16 weeks of pregnancy. It has been pointed out that trimethoprim has an antifolic acid activity.

Helm, F.; Kretzschmar, R.; Leuschner, F. and Neumann, W.: Untersuchungen uber den Einfluss der Kombination Sulfamoxol-Trimethoprim (CN 3123) and Fertilitat und Embryonalentwicklung an Ratten und Kaninchen. Arzneim Forsch. 26:643-651, 1976.

Williams, J.D.; Condie, A.P.; Brumfitt, W. and Reeves, D.S.: The treatment of bacteriuria in pregnant women with sulphamethoxazole and trimethoprim. Postgrad. Med. J. Suppl. 45: 71-76, 1969.

1284 L-1-(3,4,5-Trimethoxybenzl)-6,7-dihvdroxy-1,2,3,4-tetra-hydroisoquinoline HCl

Kowa et al (1968) tested this drug in pregnant mice and rats using the oral and subcutaneous route during organogenesis at levels up to 500 mg per kg for rats and 1,000 mg per kg per day for mice. Some fetal growth retardation was found but no congenital defects were detected.

Kowa, Y.; Ariyuki, F.; Takashima, I. and Suma, M.: A teratological study of 1-1-(3,4,5-tetramethylbenzl)-6,7-dihydroxy-1,2,3,4-tetrahvdroisoquinoline HCl (AQL-208). (Japanese) Oyo Yakuri 2: 383-396, 1968.

1285 6,6,9-Trimethyl-9-azabicylo(3,3,1)non-3 beta-yl-alpha,alpha--di(2-thienyl) Glycolate HCl Monohydrate

Yamaguchi et al (1974) studied this compound in rat and mouse pregnancy and except for fetal weight reduction no fetal alterations were found. Dosage orally was up to 100 mg per kg in mice and 200 mg per kg in rats, and it was given during major organogenesis.

Yamaguchi, K.; Ishihara, H.; Ariyuki, F.; Noguchi, Y. and Kowa, Y.: Teratological study of 6,6,9-trimethyl--9-azabicyclo(3,3,1) non-3-beta-yl-alpha,alpha-di(2-thienyl) glycolate hydrochloride monohydrate (pg 501). Oyo Yakuri 8: 1213-1218, 1974.

1286 Trimetozine   (N-(3,4,5-Trimethoxybenzoyl)tetrahydro-1,4-oxazine)

Saito et al (1976) administered by mouth maximum doses of 1000 and 600 mg per kg daily to mice and rats respectively. The medication was given during organogenesis. At the highest doses, maternal and fetal weight were reduced. Resorptions were increased in the rat at 600 mg per kg. Some increase in 14th ribs was present in mouse fetuses exposed to 500 mg per kg. Internal malformations were not studied.

Saito, K.; Hikito, S.; Komori, A.; Matsubara, T.; Okuda, T.; Terashima, A.; Matsubara, T.; Okuda, T.; Terashima, A.; Saito, H.; Yamamoto, H. and Moritoki, H.: Studies on the toxicity of N-(3,4,5-trimethoxybenzoyl)tetrahydro-1, 4-oxazine (trimetozine) 3. Teratogenicity test in mice and rats. Yakuri to Chiryo 4:2526-274, 1976.

1287 Tri-0-cresyl Phosphate

Mele and Jensh (1977) produced no fetal changes in rat fetuses exposed via maternal intubation to 750 mg per kg on the 18th and 19th days of gestation.

Mele, J.M. and Jensh, R.P.: Teratogenic effects of orally administered tri-0-cresyl phosphate on Wistar albino rats (abs) Teratology 15:32A (only) 1977.

1288 Triparanol [MER-29]

Roux and Dupuis (1961) treated five rats with 1 gm per kg from the 7th through the 10th day of gestation. Three

litters were completely resorbed. Of the other two litters
all fetuses had facial defects and rachischisis of the
central nervous system was common. Later studies detailed
various forms of holoprosencephaly and genitourinary defects
(Roux, 1964).

Roux, C.: Action teratogene du triparanol chez l' animal.
Arch. Franc. Pediat. 21:451-464, 1964.

Roux, C. and Dupuis, R.: Action teratogene du triparanol.
C. R. Soc. Biol. (Paris) 155: 2255-2257, 1961.

1289 Tritium

During pregnancy rats were maintained at constant body
activities of tritiated water ranging through 1 to 100
microcuries per ml of body water (Cahill and Yuile, 1970).
Although gross defects were not seen the offspring exposed
to 10 microcuries or more were stunted and had microcephaly
and marked reduction in the size of the testes or ovaries.
Snow (1973) found that tritiated thymidine added to culture
medium containing mouse ova was associated with a reduction
in blastocyst cell number when concentrations over 0.01
microcuries were used.

Cahill, D.F. and Yuile, C.L.: Tritium: some effects of
continuous exposure in utero on mammalian development.
Radiat. Res. 44: 727-737, 1970.

Snow, M.H.L.: Abnormal development of preimplantation mouse
embryos grown in vitro with [H-3] thymidine. J. Embryol.
Exp. Morph. 29: 601-615, 1973.

1290 Triton-W.R. 1339 [P-Isooctylpolyoxyethylphenol polymer]

Roussel and Tuchmann-Duplessis (1968) injected mice on the
6th through 8th gestational day with 200 mg per kg and
produced 21 percent defective offspring. Neural tube
closure defects, microphthalmous and omphaloceles were
present. Concurrent administration of progesterone caused a
doubling in the defect rate.

Roussel and Tuchmann-Duplessis (1970) have suggested that
the teratogenic action of the compound is through
modification of lysosomal function in the yolk sac.

Roussel, C. and Tuchmann-Duplessis, H.: Dissociation des
actions embryotoxique et teratogene du triton w.r. 1339
Chez La Souris. C. R. Acad. Sci. (Paris) (d) 266:
2171-2174, 1968.

Roussel, C. and Tuchmann-Duplessis, H.: A propos des
actions embryotoxique et teratogene du 'triton wr-1339' chez
la souris: ufluence de la vitamine A. C. R. Acad. Sci.
(Paris) (d) 271: 215-218, 1970.

1291 Trypan Blue

This azo dye and its chemical related compounds have been the subject of a good deal of teratogenic investigation since Gilman et al. (1948) first noted that trypan blue had teratogenic activity in mammals and that it was produced without entry of the dye into the embryo proper. Beck and Lloyd (1966) have presented in detail the early work with trypan blue including the chemistry and relative teratogenicity of the other azo dyes and the types of defects obtained. Gilman et al. (1948) reported hydrocephalus, spina bifida, tail defects, eye defects and a few anomalies of other systems. Cleft lip and palate and skeletal defects were uncommon. Wilson (1959) later found 22 percent of the fetuses had cardiovascular defects. Fox and Goss (1958) extended the work and noted that transposition was common. Kreschover et al. (1957) described defects in dentition. Goldstein (1957) has described the urogenital defects. The mechanism producing hydrocephalus has been extensively studied (Warkany et al.; 1958; Wilson 1959; Gunberg, 1956; Vickers, 1961).

A dose of 50 mg per kg appears to be the optimum teratogenic dose. A characteristic observation with trypan blue is that with treatment after the 9th day of gestation defects are rare. This fact has supported other evidence that the mechanism of action was dependent on disruption of yolk sac nutrition.

The mouse (Hamburgh, 1954), hamster (Ferm, 1958), chick (Beaudoin and Wilson, 1958) and guinea pig (Hoar and Salem, 1961) are all susceptible to the teratogenic activity of trypan blue. In the monkey Wilson (1971) has caused abortions with doses of 50 mg per kg with single or two daily doses between the 20th to 25th day.

An interesting series of studies have produced evidence indicating a possible action of trypan blue on a nutritive function of the visceral yolk sac. The failure of trypan blue to act directly upon the embryo is generally held with the exception of Davis (1968) who has demonstrated some localization in the hindgut possibly due to incorporation through the yolk stalk. Experiments with ring-labelled radioactive trypan blue did not give evidence of any embryonic incorporation of the C(14) (Wilson et al.; 1963). The absence of teratogenic action after the initiation of chorio-allantoic placentation also indicated that yolk sac function was important in pathogenesis. The dye can be visualized in the cells of the visceral yolk sac.

Turbow (1965) has studied the production of defects in embryos isolated from the mother in an in vitro system.

Lloyd and Beck (1969) have summarized their work on the role of lysosomes of the visceral yolk sac in trypan blue teratogenesis. They have shown that both horseradish peroxidase and the protein-trypan blue complex are concentrated in lysosomes. Through disruption of the enzymatic digestive process in the yolk sac lysosome, trypan blue may interfere with normal embryonic nutritive processes. It seems likely that work on trypan blue will lead to more knowledge about the normal physiologic role of the yolk sac in the mammal.

Beaudoin, A.R. and Wilson, J.G.: Teratogenic effects of trypan blue on the developing chick. Proc. Soc. Exp. Biol. Med. 97: 85-92, 1958.

Beck, F. and Lloyd, J.B.: The teratogenic effects of azo dyes. In, Woollam, D.H.M. (ed.): Advances in Teratology, Vol. 1. New York: Academic Press, 1966. pp 131-193.

Davis, H.W. and Gunberg, D.L.: Trypan blue in the rat embryo. Teratology 1: 125-134, 1968.

Ferm, V.H.: Teratogenic effects of trypan blue on hamster embryos. J. Embryol. Exp. Morphol. 6: 284-287, 1958.

Fox, M.H. and Goss, C.M.: Experimentally produced malformations of the heart and great vessels in rat fetuses. Transposition complexes and aortic arch abnormalities. Am. J. Anat. 102: 65-92, 1958.

Gillman, J.; Gilbert, C.; Gillman, T. and Spence, I.: A preliminary report on hydrocephalus, spina bifida and other congenital anomalies in the rat produced by trypan blue. S. Afr. J. Med. Sci. 13: 47-90, 1948.

Goldstein, D.J.: Trypan blue induced anomalies in the genito-urinary system of rats. S. Afr. J. Med. Sci. 22: 13-22, 1957.

Gunberg, D.L.: Spina bifida and the Arnold-Chiari malformation in the progeny of trypan blue injected rats. Anat. Rec. 126: 343-367, 1956.

Hamburgh, M.: The embryology of trypan blue induced abnormalities in mice. Anat. Rec. 119: 409-427, 1954.

Hoar, R.M. and Salem, A.J.: Time of teratogenic action of trypan blue in guinea pigs. Anat. Rec. 141: 173-181, 1961.

Kreschover, S.J.; Knighton, H.T. and Hancock, J.A.: Influence of systemically administered trypan blue on prenatal development of rats and mice. J. Dent. Res. 36: 677-683, 1957.

Lloyd, J.B. and Beck, F.: Teratogenesis. In, Dingle, J.T. and Fell, H.B. (eds.): Lysosomes in Biology and Pathology. Amsterdam: North-Holland Publishing Comp.; 1969. pp. 333-449.

Turbow, M.M.: Teratogenic effect of trypan blue on rat embryos cultivated in vitro. Nature 206: 637 only, 1965.

Warkany, J.; Wilson, J.G. and Geiger, J.F.: Myeloschisis and myelomeningocele produced experimentally in the rat. J. Comp. Neurol. 109: 35-64, 1958.

Wilson, J.G.: Experimental studies on the mechanism of teratogenic action of trypan blue. J. Chron. Dis. 10: 111-130, 1959.

Wilson, J.G.: Use of Rhesus monkeys in teratological

studies. Fed. Proc. 30: 104-109, 1971.

Wilson, J.G.; Shepard, T.H. and Gennaro, J.F.: Studies on the site of action of C(14)-labeled trypan blue. (abstract) Anat. Rec. 145: 300 only, 1963.

Vickers, T.H.: Concerning the mechanism of hydrocephalus in the progeny of trypan blue treated rats. Arch. Entw. Mech. Org. 153: 255-261, 1961.

1292 Tryptophane

Naidu (1974) administered 2.0 mg of this amino acid to 72 hour chick embryos and produced limb deformities, rumplessness and visceral defects.

Naidu, R.C.M.: Teratogenic effects of tryptophane on the developing chick embryo. Experientia 30: 1462-1463, 1974.

1293 D-Tubocurarine (Curare)

Chandramohan Naaidu (1974) injected the yolk sac of developing chicks with 2.0 mg of tryptophane at 72 hours of gestation and produced defects in 70 percent of the survivors. Limb deformities, rumplessness and visceral

Chandramohan Naidu, R.: Teratogenic effects of tryptophane on the development of chick embryo. Experientia 30: 1462-1463, 1974. defects were found.

Jacobs (1971) administered 0.6 to 5 mg per kg intramuscularly to rats on day 15.3 of gestation. Although muscle flaccidity occurred in the fetuses their palates closed normally. Shoro (1972) produced club foot in 8 percent of rat fetuses injected in the intrascapular region between the 17th and 19th day of gestation.

Drachman and Coulombre (1962) produced clubfoot and arthrogryposis in chick embryos infused for 24 to 48 hour periods with 30 microgm per hour during the last quarter of incubation. This elegant experiment emphasizes the important role that prenatal movement plays in development of joints. Baker (1960) has reviewed the general lack of evidence for transplacental passage of this drug during partuition.

Jago (1970) reports arthrogryposis in an infant whose mother was treated for tetanus with D-tubocurarine for 19 days starting on about the 55th day of gestation.

Baker, J.B.E.: The effects of drugs on the foetus. Pharmacol. Rev. 12: 37-90, 1960.

Drachman, D.B. and Coulombre, A.J.: Experimental club foot and arthrogryposis multiplex congenita. Lancet 2: 523-526, 1962.

Jacobs, R.M.: Failure of muscle relaxants to produce cleft palate in mice. Teratology 4: 25-30, 1971.

1293

Jago, R.H.: Arthrogryposis following treatment of maternal tetanus with muscle relaxants. Arch. Dis. Child. 45: 227-279, 1970.

Shoro, A.A.: Club-foot and intrauterine growth retardation produced by tubocurarine in the rat fetus (abstract) j. Anat. 111: 506-508, 1972.

1294 U-600

Ito et al (1981) studied this anti-ulcer agent which was extracted from bovine spleen. Rats and rabbits were given up to 400 mg per kg per day subcutaneously during organogenesis and no adverse effects were found in the fetuses. Treatment of the rat in late gestation was done and no behavioral changes were found.

Ito, R.; Kajiwara, S.; Mori, S.; Ondo, T.; Miyamoto, K.; Sugimoto, T.: Fertiliy study on a new antiulcer agent U-600 in rats. Yakubutsu Ryoho (Medical Treatment) 14:43-56, 1981.

1295 Ubiquinone-9

Nakazawa et al (1969) gave this compound to rats and mice on days 9 through 14 and 7 through 12 respectively. Oral doses to 4,000 mg per kg daily in mice and 2,000 mg per kg per day in rats were used. Intravenous dosages were also used. No teratogenic action was observed.

Nakazawa, M.; Ohzeki, M.; Takahashi, N. and Tsuchida, T.: Toxicity tests of ubiquinone-9. 2 Teratogenicity (Japanese) Oyo Yakuri 3: 155-159, 1969.

1296 Ultrasound (also see Microwave Radiations)

McClain et al. (1972) exposed pregnant rats to ultrasound for either 0.5 or 2.0 hours daily from the 8th through the 10th day or from the 11th through the 13th day. They found no significant increase in resorptions or fetal congenital defects.

McClain, R.M.; Hoar, R.M. and Saltzman, M.B.: Teratogenic study of rats exposed to ultrasound. Am. J. Obstet. Gynecol. 114: 39-42, 1972.

1297 Uracil

Kosmachevskaya and Tichodeeva (1968) injected 0.25 to 4.0 mg of this chemical into chick eggs at 24 hours of incubation and found 24 percent of the surviving embryos deformed. Microphthalmia, rumplessness and axial skeletal defects were observed.

Kosmachevskaya, E.A.: Peculiarities of action of some pyrimidine derivatives on different stages of chicken embryogenesis. Bull. Expt. Biol. (Russian) No. 3:

109-113, 1968.

1298 Uracil Mustard (also see Nitrogen Mustard)

Chaube and Murphy (1968) reported that 0.3 to 0.6 mg per kg injected into rats on the 11th or 12th gestational day produced congenital defects in the offspring. Exencephaly or encephalocele and skeletal defects were observed.

Chaube, S. and Murphy, M.L.: The teratogenic effects of the recent drugs active in cancer chemotherapy. In, Woollam, D.H.M. (ed.): Advances in Teratology, Vol. 3. New York: Academic Press, 1968. pp. 181-237.

1299 Urethane [Ethylurethan] [Ethyl Carbamate]

Sinclair (1950) produced neural tube closure defects in the mouse fetus by injecting 15 mg on the 7th day of gestation. Nishimura and Kuginuki (1958) gave 1.5 gm per kg daily to mice from the 9th through 12th day of gestation and found skeletal and palate defects. Hall (1953) has demonstrated eye developmental defects in rats treated with this substance. Takaori et al. (1966) gave 1 gm per kg to rats on days 6 through 11 and produced a high incidence of skeletal defects. Gross defects were uncommon.

Hall, E.K.: Developmental anomalies in the eye of the rat after various experimental procedures. Anat. Rec. 116: 383-393, 1953.

Nishimura, H. and Kuginuki, M.: Congenital malformations induced by ethyl-urethane in mouse embryos. Okajimas Folia Anat. Jap. 31: 1-10, 1958.

Sinclair, J.G.: A specific transplacental effect of urethane in mice. Tex. Rep. Biol. Med. 8: 623-632, 1950.

Takaori, S.; Tanabe, K. and Shimamoto, K.: Developmental abnormalities of skeletal system induced by ethylurethan in the rat. Jap. J. Pharmacol. 16: 63-73, 1966.

1300 Urokinase

Akutsu et al (1974) used human purified urokinase in doses of 100,000 iu per kg in mice and rats during active organogenesis. Intraperitoneal doses did not produce any teratogenic action nor were differences produced in the off-spring during a 3 week post-natal period.

Akutsu, T.; Ito, C.; Sakai, K.; Arigaya, Y.; Ohnishi, H. and Ogawa, N.: Studies on teratogenicity of urokinase in mice and rats. Oyo Yakuri 8: 981-989, 1974.

1301 Urosulfan

Bariliak (1968) showed that urosulfan in doses of 1000 mg

1301

per kg of body weight on the 10th day of pregnancy caused
death in 44 percent of implanted fetuses but did not
manifest teratogenicity.

Bariliak, I.R.: Comparison of antithyroidal and teratogenic
activity of some hypoglycemic sulphanylamides. Problems of
Endocrinology (Russian) 14: No. 6, 89-94, 1968.

1302 D-Usnic Acid

Wiesner and Yudkin (1955) gave 1.5 mg to mice immediately
after copulation and prevented pregnancy. The litter size
was reduced in mice who were maintained on the compound for
long periods before pregnancy started.

Wiesner, B.P. and Yudkin, J.: Control of fertility by
antimitotic agents. Nature 176: 249-250, 1955.

1303 Uterine Clamping (see Trauma)

1304 Vaccinia Virus

Heath et al. (1956) injected chick eggs with this virus at
48 hours of incubation and found microcephaly and axial abnormalities in the embryos.

Heath, H.D.; Shear, H.H.; Imagawa, D.T.; Jones, M.H. and
Adams, J.M.: Teratogenic effects of herpes simplex,
vaccinia, influenza-A (NWS) and distemper virus infections
on early chick embryos. Proc. Soc. Exp. Biol. Med. 92:
675-682, 1956.

1305 Vaginal Spermicides (see Nonoxynol-9)

1306 Valexon

This insecticide caused gonadotoxic effects in male rats
(0.7 mg per kg daily during 10 weeks) but did not induce
damage of female gonads. Treatment of pregnant rats (90 mg
per kg daily) caused some congenital malformations in
offspring (abnormalities in heart ganglia and reduced
activity of cholinesterase).

Shepelskay, N.R.: The gonadotoxic effect of valexon in
experiments. Gig. i Sanit. (USSR) 7:77, 1980.

1307 Valium-R (see Diazepam)

1308 Valproic Acid

Suchestone et al (1979) administered this anticonvulsant to
mice orally on day 7 through 12 of gestation at doses of 225
to 560 mg per kg daily. Defects occurred at all dose levels
and consisted of neural closure defects and occasional limb

defects. In a monograph published by the manufacturer (1978) the teratogenic dose in mice, rats and rabbits was given as 150, 65 and 315 mg per kg. Cleft palate, skeletal as well as renal and other defects were found. Nau et al (1981) have reported on the pharmacodynamics of the drug. They also reported that among 12 exposed human pregnancies there were two offspring with microcephaly and four with head circumferences less than the 10th percentile. Dalens et al (1980) reported an infant with facial dysmorphology and congenital heart disease. The mother received 1000 mg daily during most of pregnancy. Clay et al (1981) reported an infant with microcephaly, facial dysmorphogenesis and ventricular septal defect. The mother and child had neurofibromatosis and the mother received 750 mg daily during pregnancy.

Robert and Guibaud (1982) found that among 72 women giving birth to offspring with caudal neural tube defects, 9 were taking valproic acid. The doses were usually over 1 gm daily. This would give an odds ratio of approximately 20 for the defect to occur among valproic acid using mothers. International studies are in progress (Bjerkedal et al, 1982).

Abbott Laboratory: Depakene, valproic acid Drug Monograph, 1978.

Bjerkedal, T.; Czeizel, A.; Goujard, J.; Kallen, B.; Mastroiacova, P.; Nevin, N.; Oakley, G.; Robert, E.: Valproic acid and spina bifida. Lancet 2:1096, 1982.

Clay, S.A.; McVie, R.; Chen, H.: Possible teratogenic effect of valproic acid. J. Peds. 99:828 only, 1981.

Dalens, B.; Raynaud, E-J.; Gaulme, J.: Teratogenicity of valproic acid. J. Ped. 97:332-333, 1980.

Nau, H.; Rating, D.; Koch, S.; Hauser, I.; Helge, H.: Valproic acid and its metabolites: Placental transfer, neonatal pharmacokinetics, transfer via mothers milk and clinical status in neonates of epileptic mothers. Pharmacol. and Experimenta Therapeutics 219:768-777, 1981.

Robert, E.; Guiband, P.: Maternal valproic acid and congenital neural tube defects. Lancet 2:937 (only), 1982.

Sucheston, M.E.; Hayes, T.G.; Paulson, R.B. and King, J.E.: Fetal malformations in valporate sodium treated CD-1 mice (abs) Teratology 19:49A, only, 1979.

1309 Vanadium

Roschin and Kazimov (1980) gave ortovanadate Na (0.85 mg per kg) intraperitoneally and subcutaneously to male rats and an alteration of spermatogenesis was found. Treating the pregnant rats with this substance caused increased preimplantation embryonic mortality.

Roschin, A.V. and Kazimov, M.A.: Effect of vanadium on the generative function of tested animals. Gig tr. i prof.

zabol. (USSR) 5:49-51, 1980.

1310 Varicella

Siegel and Fuerst (1966) made a prospective study of the offspring of 135 mothers with varicella during pregnancy and found no increase in congenital defect rate. The incidence of low birth weight was not increased. Savage et al (1973) report an infant exposed in utero to varicella at the 9th week with reduction defect of the extremity, Horner's syndrome, and meningo-encephalitis with defective swallowing. The presence of a depigmented depressed skin lesion on the deformed limb resembled those described in two other cited cases.

A case report by McKendry and Bailey (1973) describes a newborn whose mother had varicella at 11 weeks of pregnancy. The infant had focal skin and muscle defects, delayed growth and seizures. The clinical picture may include disorganization of the eye (Frey et al, 1976). A brief review of this congenital syndrome is given by Bai and John (1979).

The incidence of congenital defects following first trimester varicella is still unknown (Srabstein, et al, 1974) but an estimate of the fetal attack rate of 20 percent has been made. When there is maternal varicella within 4 days of delivery Herpes zoster immune serum should be given to protect the newborn from disseminated disease.

Bai, P.V.A. and John, J.: Congenital skin ulcers following varicella in late pregnancy. J. Pediatr. 94: 65-66, 1979.

Frey, H.M.; Bialkin, G. and Gershon, A.A.: Congenital varicella: Case report of a seralogically proved long-term survivor. Pediat. 59:110-112, 1977.

McKendry, J.B.J. and Bailey, J.D.: Congenital varicella associated with multiple defects. Can. Med. Assoc. J. 108: 66-67, 1973.

Siegel, M. and Fuerst, H.T.: Low birth weight and maternal virus diseases. A prospective study of rubella, measles, mumps, chicken pox and hepatitis. J.A.M.A. 197: 680-684, 1966.

Savage, M.D.; Moosa, A. and Gordon, R.R.: Maternal varicella infection as a cause of malformations. Lancet 1: 352-354, 1973.

Srabstein, J.C.; Morris, N.; Larke, R.B.B.; Derek, J.D.; Castelmo, B.B. and Sum, E.: Is there a congenital varicella syndrome J. Pediat. 84: 239-243, 1974.

1311 Vasopressin [Pitressin]

Jost (1951) injected rabbit fetuses intraperitoneally after 17 days of gestation with 5 to 500 milli units of Parke-Davis pitressin. With the lowest dose edema was produced and doses above 10 milli units were associated with hemorrhagic necrosis and amputations of the distal extremities. Davies and Robson (1970) injected the amniotic cavity of the mouse fetus on the 15th or 16th day and obtained lesions similar to those seen in the mouse. By direct observation they concluded that intensive arterial vasospasm occurred.

Davies, J. and Robson, J.M.: The effects of vasopressin, adrenaline and noradrenaline on the mouse fetus. Br. J. Pharmacol. 38: 446 only, 1970.

Jost, A.: Sur le role de la vasopressine et de la corticostimuline (A.C.T.H.) dans la production experimentale de lesions des extremities foetales (hemorragies, necroses, amputations congenitales). C. R. Soc. Biol. (Paris) 145: 1805-1809, 1951.

1312 Venezuelan Equine Encephalitis

London et al (1973) injected this virus directly into the brain of fetal monkeys and at birth they had cataracts and hydrocephalus. They review human infected pregnancies when hydroanencephaly has been found (Wenger, 1977).

London, W.T.; Levitt, N.H.; Kent, S.G.; Wong, V.G. and Sever, J.L.: Congenital cerebral and ocular malformations induced in rhesus monkeys by Venezuelan equine encephalitis virus. Teratology 16:285-296, 1977.

Wenger, F.: Venequelan equine encephalitis. Teratology 16:359-362, 1977.

1313 Venom, Snake

Viper venom was injected subcutaneously on various days of the mouse gestation and following treatment on the 7th and 8th days facial anomalies, anencephaly and heart anomalies were produced. Cleft palate in low incidence was produced with treatment on the 8th through 14th day. The dose was 200 microgm of powdered venom which was the LD-50 (Clavert and Gabriel-Robez, 1974.

Clavert, J. and Gabriel-Robez, O.: The effects on mouse gestation and embryo development of an injection of viper venom (Vipera aspis). Acta Anat. 88: 11-21, 1974.

1314 Veratrosine (see Cyclopamine)

1315 Veratrum Californicum

This plant was the dietary source of cyclopamine which caused outbreaks of cyclopia with cleft palate in the fetuses of sheep who fed on it during the 2nd and 3rd week of gestation. The plant grows at relatively high altitudes. A more detailed list of references may be found under cyclopamine. Kalter (1968) has summarized the subject.

1315

Kalter, H.: Teratology of the central nervous system.
Chicago: University of Chicago Press, 1968. pp. 144-146.

1316 Vermox-R (see Mebendazole)

1317 Vibramycin (6-alpha-deoxy-5-oxytetracycline)

Cahen and Fave (1972) in a preliminary report found no
teratogenicity in rats, rabbits and mice. They used dosages
which were more than 100 times those used clinically.
Delahunt et al (1967) found non-teratogenicity in rat,
rabbit and monkey.

Cahen, R.L.; Fave, A.: Absence of teratogenic effect of
6-alpha-   deoxy-5-oxytetracycline.   Fed.   Proc.   31:238
(only) 1972.

Delahunt, C.S.; Jacobs, R.T.; Stebbins, R.B.; Rieser, N.:
Toxicology of vibramycin. Toxicol. Appl. Pharmacol 10:402
(only) 1967.

1318 Vidarabine

This antiviral compound was teratogenic when given
intramuscularly in the rat (30 mg per kg) and in the rabbit
(5 mg per kg) (Schardein et al, 1977). The defects included
orofacial clefts, skeletal and renal malformations.
Application a 10 perent ointment topically to 5 or 10
percent of the body surface of the rabbit dam also produced
defects.   Of five exposed monkey pregnancies, one had an
enlargement of the tail and abnormally shaped ribs.

Schardein, J.L.; Hertz, D.L.; Petrere, J.A.; Fitzgerald,
J.E. and Kurtz, S.M.: The effect of vidarabine on the
development of the offspring of rats, rabbits and monkeys.
Teratology 15:231-242, 1977.

1319 Vinblastine (Vincaleukoblastine) (see Vincristine)

1320 Vincristine

The vinca alkaloids derived from the common periwinkle plant
Vinca rosea (linn.) include vincristine and vinblastine.
These antineoplastic substances are teratogenic in hamsters,
rats, rabbits and monkeys. Ferm (1963) injected hamsters
intravenously with 0.25 mg per kg of vinblastine or 0.1 mg
per kg of vincristine on the 8th gestational day and
produced skeletal and eye defects as well as spina bifida
and exencephaly.   Demeyer (1964, 1965) used vinblastine
(0.25 mg) and vincristine (0.05 to 0.075 mg) in the pregnant
rat on day 9 of gestation and produced a high incidence of
eye defects with some microcephaly and neural tube closure
defects. Some of the fetuses had midfacial defects with
incomplete development of the prosencephalon. He observed
an accumulation of arrested metaphase figures in the treated
embryos.   Cohlan and Kitay (1965) have observed an increase

page 450

in the number of mitotic figures in fetuses exposed to vinblastine. Ohzu and Shoji (1965) using 2.5 mg per kg daily in the mouse on the 11th through the 14th days produced a few cleft palates. Morris et al. (1967) studied the teratogenesis of vinblastine in the rabbit. In the Rhesus monkey Courtney and Valerio (1967) injected a single daily dose of 0.15 to 0.175 mg of vincristine per kg on the 27th or 29th day of pregnancy and produced one fetus with encephalocele and another with syndactyly. Armstrong et al. (1963) report a normal infant delivered following oral treatment of a mother with 5 mg of vincristine sulfate during her entire pregnancy.

Armstrong, J.G.; Dyke, R.W. and Fonts, P.J.: Vinblastine sulfate treatment of Hodgkins disease during pregnancy. Science 143: 703 only, 1964.

Cohlan, S.Q. and Kitay, D.: The teratogenic action of vincalenkoblastine in the pregnant rat. J. Pediatr. 66: 541-544, 1965.

Courtney, K.D. and Valerio, D.A.: Teratology in the Macaca mulatta. Teratology 1: 163-172, 1968.

Demyer, W.: Vinblastine-induced malformations of face and nervous system in two rat strains. Neurology (Minneap.) 14: 806-808, 1964.

Demyer, W.: Cleft lip and jaw induced in fetal rats by vincristine. Archives of Anatomy 48: 181-186, 1965.

Ferm, V.H.: Congenital malformations in hamster embryos after treatment with vinblastine and vincristine. Science 141: 426 only, 1963.

Morris, J.M.; Van Wagenen, G.; Hurteau, G.D.; Johnstone, D.W. and Carlsen, R.A.: Compounds interfering with ovum implantation and development. I. Alkaloids and antimetabolites.

Fertility Sterility 18: 7-17, 1967.

Ohzu, E. and Shoji, R.: Preliminary notes on abnormalities induced by velban in developing mouse embryos. Proceedings of the Japanese Academy 41: 321-325, 1965.

1321 Vinyl Chloride

Although Infante et al (1976a and 1977b) have reported increased rates of malformations in one city where a vinyl chloride plant was located, subsequent studies by Edmonds et al (1978) found the parents of these children were not workers in the plant nor were they living closer to the manufacturing source than the controls. Infante et al (1976b) found a significant increase in fetal loss among the wives after paternal exposure. As a "control" group they used workers in rubber plants. Sanotsky et al (1980) did not find an increase in spontaneous abortions among the wives of vinyl chloride workers.

1321

Since this compound causes mutations in bacterial systems
there have been a number of dominant lethal studies in
animals. Negative findings in rats exposed to up to 1,000
ppm were reported by Short et al (1977). Anderson et al
(1977) using inhalation doses of up to 30,000 ppm 6 hours
daily for 5 days produced no dominant lethal effects in the
mouse.

John et al (1978) exposed rodents and rabbits to inhalation
of varying doses of 50 to 2500 ppm during major
organogenesis and found no adverse fetal effects. Ungvary
et al (1978) exposed rats to 1500 ppm during pregnancy and
produced increased fetal mortality but no malformations.
Salnikova and Kitsovskaya (1980) exposed Wistar rats during
the entire gestation by inhalation (in a dose of 4.8 mg per
cubic meter). An alteration of blood vessel permeability,
nervous system functional disturbance and other
abnormalities in offspring were found. The dose of 35.3 mg
per cubic meter produced a slight embryotoxic effect.

Anderson, D.; Hodge, M.C.E.; Purchase, I.F.H.: Dominant
lethal studies with halogenated olefins vinyl chloride and
vinylidene dichloride in male CD-1 mice. Environ. Health
Perspect. 21:71-78, 1977.

Edmonds, L.D.; Anderson, C.E.; Flynt, J.W.; James, L.M.:
Congenital central nervous system malformations and vinyl
chloride monomer exposure: a community study. Teratology
17:137-142, 1978.

Infante, P.F.; Wagoner, J.K.; McMichael, A.J.; Waxweiler,
R.J.; Falk, H.: Genetic risks of vinyl chloride. Lancet
1:734-735, 1976.

Infante, P.F.; Wagoner, J.K.; Waxweiler, R.J.:
Carcinogenic, mutagenic and teratogenic risks associated
with vinyl chloride. Mutation Research 41·131-142, 1976.

John, J.A.; Smith, F.A.; Schwetz, B.A.: Vinyl chloride:
inhalation teratology study in mice, rats and rabbits.
Envir. Health Perspec. 171-177, 1981.

Salnikova, L.S. and Kitsovskaya, I.A.: Effect of vinyl
chloride on embryogenesis in the rat. Gig. tr. i prof.
zabol. (USSR)3: 46-47, 1980.

Sanotsky, I.V.; Davtian, R.M.; Glushchenko VI: Study of the
reproductive function in men exposed to chemicals. Gig.
Tr. Prof. Zabol. 5:28-32, 1980.

Short, R.D.; Minor, J.L.; Winston, J.M.; Lee, C.C: A
dominant lethal study in male rats after repeated exposures
to vinyl chloride or vinylidene chloride. J. Toxicol.
Envir. Health 3:965-968, 1977.

Ungvary, G.; Hudak, A.; Tetrai, E.; Lorincz, M.; Folly, G.:
Effects of vinyl chloride exposure alone and in combination
with trypan blue - applied systematically during all thirds
of pregnancy on the fetuses of CFY rats. Toxicology
11:45-54, 1978.

1322 Vinyledine chloride (see 1,1-dichloroethylene)

1323 Viriditoxin

Hood et al (1976) injected mice intraperitoneally on days 7-10 with up to 3.5 mg per kg and observed no adverse effect on the fetuses.

Hood, R.D.; Hayes, A.W.; Scammell, J.G.: Effects of prenatal administration of vitricin and viriditoxin to mice. Fd. Cosmet. Toxicol. 14:175-178, 1976.

1324 VP-16-213

This podophyllotoxin derivative was injected intraperitoneally into mice on days 6,7 or 8 in doses of 1.0, 1.5 and 2.0 mg per kg and defects mainly of the axial skeleton, and dextrocardia, exencephaly and clubfoot were found (Sieber et al, 1978).

Sieber, S.M.; Whang-Peng, J.; Botkin, C. and Knutsen, T.: Teratogenic and cytogenic effects of some plant-derived antitumor agents (vincristine, colchicine, maytansine, VP-16-213 and VM-26) in mice. Teratology 18:31-48, 1978.

1325 VM-26

This podophyllotoxin derivative was injected intraperitoneally into mice in amounts of 0.5 and 1.0 mg per kg on days 6,7 or 8. Numerous malformations were found but dextrocardia, exencephaly and skeletal defects were most common (Sieber et al, 1978).

Sieber, S.M.; Whang-Peng, J.; Botkin, C. and Knutsen, J.: Teratogenic and cytogenic effects of some plant-derived antitumor agents (vincristine, colchicine, maytansine, VP-16-213 and VM-26) in mice. Teratology 18:31-48, 1978.

1326 Virulizing Tumors

Verhoeven et al (1973) reviewed the effect of various masculinizing ovarian tumors on the genitalia of the fetus. Examples of masculinization of the female fetus have occurred with arrhenoblastomas, Lehdig cell tumors, adrenal rest tumors, leuteoma, granulosa cell tumor and Krukenberg tumors. The masculinization was especially common with arrhenoblastomas and krukenberg tumors.

Verhoeven, A.T.M.; Mastboom, J.L.; Leusden, H.A.I.M. and Van der Velden, W.H.M.: Virilization in pregnancy coexisting with an (ovarian) mucinous cystadenoma: A case report and review of virilizing ovarian tumors in pregnancy. Obst. Gynecol. Survey 28: 597-622, 1973.

1327 Vitamin A Deficiency

1327

Hale (1937) using a vitamin A deficient diet was able to demonstrate for the first time that a non-genetic factor could
produce congenital defects. Since then vitamin A deficiency
has been a widely studied teratologic experimental model.
The vitamin A deficient congenital syndrome in the rat
consists of over 90 percent ocular and urogenital anomalies,
50 percent diaphragmatic hernias and 17 percent congenital
heart defects (Wilson et al.; 1953). The eye defects
consist of overgrowth of connective tissue between the
hyaloid vessels in place of the vitreous and coloboma with
retinal eversion (Warkany and Schraffenberger, 1946). Many
of the heart defects simulate malformations in man and
include incomplete interventricular septation and anomalies
of the aortic arch (Wilson and Warkany, 1949). The work by
Millen and Woollam (1956) and Lamming et al. (1954) on
hydrocephalus in the offspring of vitamin A deficient
rabbits has been summarized by Kalter (1968). Increased
intracranial pressure with secondary aqueductal compression
appears to be part of the mechanism underlying the hydrocephalus. Keratinizing epithelial metaplasia, a classic
sign of vitamin A deficiency in postnatal life, was not seen
in the rat fetus before the 18th fetal day (Wilson and
Warkany, 1947). Palludan (1966) has described extensive
work in the pig model. Kalter and Warkany (1959) have
summarized the general topic.

The general lack of evidence that vitamin A deficiency plays
a significant role in human congenital abnormalities is
discussed by Warkany (1971). Giroud and Tuchmann-Duplessis
(1962) briefly illustrate an infant with anophthalmia born
to a deficient mother.

Giroud, A. and Tuchmann-Duplessis, H.: Malformations congenitales. Role Des Facteurs Exogenes. Pathol. Biol. 10:
119-151, 1962.

Hale, F.: Relation of maternal vitamin A deficiency to
microphthalmia in pigs. Texas State J. Med. 33: 228-232,
1937.

Kalter, H.: Teratology of the central nervous system.
Chicago: University of Chicago Press, 1968. pp. 35-40.

Kalter, H. and Warkany, J.: Experimental production of
congenital malformations in mammals by metabolic procedure.
Physiol. Rev. 39: 69-115, 1959.

Lamming, G.E.; Woollam, D.H.M. and Millen, J.W.:
Hydrocephalus in young rabbits associated with maternal
vitamin A deficiency. Br. J. Nutr. 8: 363-369, 1954.

Millen, J.W. and Woollam, D.H.M.: Effect of the duration
of vitamin-A deficiency in female rabbits on incidence of
hydrocephalus in their young. J. Neurol. Neurosurg.
Psychiatry 19: 17-20, 1956.

Palludin, B.: A-avitaminosis in swine: A study on the
importance of vitamin A for reproduction. Copenhagen:
Munksgaard, 1966.

Warkany, J.: Congenital Malformations Notes and Comments.

Chicago: Year Book Medical Publishers, 1971. pp. 127-128.

Warkany, J. and Schraffenberger, E.: Congenital malformations induced in rats by maternal vitamin A deficiency. I.
Defects of the eye. Arch ^phthalmol. 35: 150-169, 1946.

Wilson, J.G.; Roth, C.B. and Warkany, J.: An analysis of
the syndrome of malformations induced by vitamin A
deficiency. effects of restoration of vitamin A at various
times during gestation. Am. J. Anat. 92: 189-217, 1953.

Wilson, J.G. and Warkany, J.: Epithelial keratinization as
evidence of vitamin A deficiency. Proc. Soc. Exp. Biol.
Med. 64: 419-422, 1947.

Wilson, J.G. and Warkany, J.: Cardiac and aortic arch a-
nomalies in the offspring of vitamin A deficient rats
correlated with similar human anomalies. Pediatrics 5:
708-725, 1950.

1328 Vitamin A Excess (see Hypervitaminosis A)

1329 Vitamin B Deficiency (see Riboflavin, Folic acid,
Nicotinamide or Pyridoxine Deficiency)

1330 Vitamin B-12 Deficiency

A series of papers on the teratogenic effects of a diet
deficient in folic acid and B(12) indicated that a low
percentage of fetal hydrocephalus could be produced
(Grainger et al.; 1954). Using a Steenbock-Black
rachitogenic diet supplemented with viosterol and riboflavin
11.7 percent of the rat offspring developed hydrocephalus,
14.4 had bone defects and 6.7 had eye defects. When the
same diet was supplemented with B(12) virtually no defects
were observed. Woodard and Newberne (1966) confirmed the
findings using a better defined basal diet.

They reported finding hydronephrosis, cleft lip and neural
closure defects. The hydrocephalus is thought to be due to
intermittant obstruction of the cerebral aqueduct
(Overholser et al.; 1954). Kalter (1968) has summarized
this subject.

Grainger, R.B.; O'dell, B.L. and Hogan, A.G.: Congenital
malformations as related to deficiencies of riboflavin and
vitamin B(12), source of protein, calcium to phosphorous
ratio and skeletal phosphorous metabolism. J. Nutr. 54:
33-48, 1954.

Kalter, H.: Teratology of the central nervous system.
Chicago: University of Chicago Press, 1968. pp. 28-32.

Overholser, M.D.; Whitley, J.R.; O'dell, B.L. and Hogan,
A.G.: The ventricular system in hydrocephalic rat brains
produced by a deficiency of vitamin B(12) or of folic acid
in the maternal diet. Anat. Rec. 120: 917-934, 1954.

Woodard, J.C. and Newberne, P.M.: Relation of vitamin b(12) and one-carbon metabolism to hydrocephalus in the rat. J. Nutr. 88: 375-381, 1966.

1331 Vitamin C Deficiency

Kalter and Warkany (1959) have reviewed work which has been done on scorbutic guinea pigs during pregnancy. The animals did not become pregnant on a standard vitamin-C deficient diet; with daily supplements of 5 ml of orange juice abortions or resorptions occurred (Kramer et al.; 1933). Harman and Warren (1933) reported that when the pregnant guinea pigs were started on a vitamin C-deficient diet on the 21st day of gestation the fetuses were smaller than controls and retarded in development of skin and muscle. Martin et al (1957) studied a large group of women during pregnancy and did not find increased malformation rates in those with low serum and intake levels. The lowest group had the highest prematurity rate.

Harman, M.T. and Warren, L.E.: Some embryologic aspects of vitamin C-deficiency in the guinea pig (Cavia cobaya). Trans. Kans. Acad. Sci. 54: 42-57, 1951.

Kalter, H. and Warkany, J.: Experimental production of congenital malformations in mammals by metabolic procedure. Physiol. Rev. 39: 69-115, 1959.

Kramer, M.M.; Harman, M.T. and Brill, A.K.: Disturbances of reproduction and ovarian changes in guinea-pig in relation to vitamin C deficiency. Am. J. Physiol. 106: 611-622, 1933.

Martin, M.P.; Bridgforth, E.; McGanity, W.J. and Darby, W.J.: The Vanderbilt cooperative study of maternal and infant nutrition 10. Ascorbic acid. J. Nutrit. 62: 201-224, 1957.

1332 Vitamin D

Friedman (1968) has reviewed the evidence that vitamin D may produce the syndrome of supravalvular aortic stenosis with elfin facies and mental retardation (Garcia et al.; 1964). The virtual absence of this cardiac lesion before the years of routine institution of vitamin D prophylaxis and the high incidence of the syndrome in Gottingen, Germany where rickets prophylaxis during pregnancy consisted of huge doses of vitamin D, may be circumstantial evidence of the vitamin's role in supravalvular aortic stenosis. The great difficulty in measuring vitamin D in serum and the frequent absence of hypercalcemia in patients with supravalvular aortic stenosis have made it impossible to definitely implicate vitamin D in the etiology of supravalvular aortic stenosis. Forbes (1979) has commented on the lack of evidence that vitamin D is related to Williams syndrome.

Friedman and Roberts (1966) in rabbits have shown that 1.5 million units to the mother produced abnormalities of the aorta in 14 of 34 offspring. Many of these aortic lesions resembled the form seen in children. In addition to the aortic lesion the rabbits exhibited a reduction defect in dentition which was similar to the maxillary changes in patients with the syndrome (Friedman and Mills, 1969).

Ornoy et al (1972) gave 20,000 or 40,000 IU of vitamin D-2 to rats by gavage from day 10 through 21 of gestation and produced growth retardation, neonatal death, and postnatal impairment of ossification with fractures. Later Ornoy (1981) reported that 1,2,5(OH)2-D-3 was the metabolite causing the adverse effects.

Makita et al (1977) administered 1-alpha-hydroxy cholecalciferol (D-3) to rabbits on days 6 through 18. Embryolethality was increased at doses of 0.8 microgm per kg. Three malformations (cleft palates and absence of gall bladder) occurred at 0.02 and 0.2 microgm per kg and one grossly malformed fetus at 0.5 microgm per kg. The total number of fetuses examined in the 3 dose level groups was 134.

Friedman, W.F.: Vitamin D and the supravalvular aortic stenosis syndrome. In, Woollam, D.H.M. (ed.): Advances in Teratology, Vol. 3. New York: Academic Press, 1968. pp. 83-96.

Friedman, W.F. and Mills, L.F.: The relationship between vitamin D and the craniofacial and dental anomalies of the supravalvular aortic stenosis syndrome. Pediatrics 43:12-18, 1969.

Friedman, W.F.; Roberts, W.C.: Vitamin D and the supravalvular aortic stenosis syndrome: the transplacental effects of vitamin D on the aorta of the rabbit. Circulation 34:77-86, 1966.

Forbes, G.B.: Letter to the editor: Vitamn D in pregnancy and the infantile hypercalcemic syndrome. Pediat. Res. 13:1382, 1979.

Garcia, R.E.; Friedman, W.F.; Kaback, M.M. and Rowe, R.D.: Idiopathic hypercalcemia and supravalvular aortic stenosis: documentation of a new syndrome. N. Engl. J. Med. 271:117-120, 1964.

Makita, T.; Kato, M.; Matuzawa, K.; Ojima, N.; Hashimoto, Y. and Noguchi, T.: Safety evaluation studies on the hormonal form of vitamin D-3. 3. Teratogenicity in rabbits by oral administration. (Japanese) Iyakuhin Kenkyu 8:615-624, 1977.

Ornoy, A.; Kaspi, T. and Nebel, L.: Persistent defects of bone formation in young rats following maternal hypervitaminosis D-2. Israel J. Med. Sc. 8:943-949, 1972.

Ornoy, A.; Zusman, I.; Hirsh, B.E.: Transplacental effects of vitamin D-3 metabolites on the skeleton of rat fetuses (abstract). Teratology 23:55A, 1981.

1333 Vitamin D Deficiency

Warkany (1943) produced a congenital malformation consisting of curvatures of the long bones in rat offspring after chronic feeding of a rachitogenic diet. The histologic appearance of the bones was similar to that seen in rickets except for the absence of large amounts of osteoid tissue. Defective mandibles were produced in chicks whose mothers were maintained on vitamin D deficient diets; 25-hydroxy-vitamin D3 corrected the defect, but feeding of 1,25- di-hydroxyvitamin D3 did not (Sunde et al, 1978).

Sunde, M.L.; Turk, C.M. and DeLuca, H.F.: The essentiality of vitamin D metabolites for embryonic chick development. Science 200:1067-1069, 1978.

Warkany, J.: Effect of maternal rachitogenic diet on skeletal development of young rat. Am. J. Dis. Child. 66: 511-516, 1943.

1334 Vitamin E

Momose et al (1972) administered vitamin E in amounts of 150 or 300 mg per kg per day to pregnant mice subcutaneously on days 6, 8 and 10 of gestation. Growth retardation and fetal survival were increased in the treated group. The incidence of cleft palate was increased. Studies with the rat (75 mg per day) were negative (Sato, 1973).

Momose, Y.; Akiyoshi, S.; Mori, K.; Nishimura, N.; Fujishima, H.; Imaizumi, S. and Agata, I.: On teratogenicity of vitamin E. Reports from the Department of Anatomy, Mie Perfectural University School of Medicine 20: 27-35, 1972.

Sato, Y.: Study of developmental pharmacology on vitamine E. (Japanese). Folia Pharmacol. 69: 293-298, 1973.

1335 Vitamin E Deficiency

Kalter (1968) has reviewed the experimental literature dealing with the teratogenicity of a diet deficient in vitamin E. Rats were reared from about 3 weeks of age on a deficient diet. By supplementing the deficient diet with 2 to 4 mg of vitamin E once on the 10th to the 13th day surviving offspring with congenital defects were produced. Exencephaly or hydrocephalus was found in about 30 percent of the fetuses (Cheng and Thomas, 1953; Cheng et al.; 1960). Hook et al (1974) found no significant teratogenicity when they gavaged pregnant mice with 591 IU on days seven through eleven. An equivalent dose in the human would be about 1 million IU.

Steele et al (1974) using the explanted rat embryo system were able to show that vitamin E acts directly on the conceptus. N,N-diphenyl-P-phenylenediamine had a similar effect to vitamin E but ethoxyquin was inactive in vitro.

Cheng, D.W.; Bairnson, T.A.; Rao, A.N. and Subbammal, S.: Effect of variations of rations on the incidence of teratogeny in vitamin E-deficient rats. J. Nutr. 71: 54-60,

1960.

Cheng, D.W. and Thomas, B.H.: Relationship of time of therapy to teratogeny in maternal avitaminosis E. Proceedings of the Iowa Academy of Science 60: 290-299, 1953.

Hook, E.B.; Healy, K.M.; Niles, A.M. and Skalko, R.G.: Vitamin E: A teratoen or antiteratogen? Lancet 1:809, only, 1974.

Kalter, H.: Teratology of the central nervous system. Chicago: University of Chicago Press, 1968. pp. 41-43.

Steele, C.E.; Jeffery, E.H. and Diplock, A.T.: The Chicago: University of Chicago Press, 1968. pp. 41-43. vitro of explanted rat embryos. J. Reprod. Fert. 38: 115-123, 1974.

1336 Vitamin K-(2) [Menaquinone-4]

Suzuki et al (1971) gave this vitamin to mice and rats on the 7th through the 14th day of gestation respectively. The maximum doses were 1,000 mg per kg orally and 100 mg per kg intraperitoneally. No growth inhibition, teratogenicity or post-natal effects were observed. Some delay in appearance of ossification centers was found in the mice fetuses.

Mikami et al (1981) gave this agent orally to rats in amounts of up to 1000 mg per kg daily either before pregnancy and during the first 7 days or on days 7-21 of gestation. No adverse effects on fertility or fetal postnatal function were observed.

Mikami, T.; Mochida, H.; Osumi, I.; Gioto, K.; Suzuki, Y.: Fertility study and perinatal and postnatal study of menatetrenone in rats. Kiso to Rinsho 15:1143-1159, 1981.

Suzuki, Y.; Yayanagi, K.; Okada, F. and Furuuchi, M.: Toxicological studies of menaquinone-4 on development of fetuses and offsprings in mice and rats (Japanese). Oyo Yakuri 5: 469-487, 1971.

1337 Vitamin K-3 [Menadione]

Kosuge (1973) fed 15 mg and 150 mg per day to rats and at both levels fetal resorptions were increased but no increase in defects was found. A marked retardation of skeletal ossification was observed.

Kosuge, Y.: Study of developmental pharmacology on vitamin K-3 part 1 effect of vitamin k-3 on the rat fetus. Folia Pharmacol. Japon 69: 285-291, 1973.

1338 Water, Drinking

Chernoff et al (1979) and Staples et al (1979) could find no fetal changes in mice drinking municipal water.

1338

Chernoff, N.; Rogers, E.; Carver, B.; Kvalock, R.; Gray, E.:
The fetotoxic potential of municipal drinking water in the
mouse. Teratology 19: 165-170, 1979.

Staples, R.E.; Worthy, W.C. and Marks, T.A.: Influence of
drinking water - tap versus purified on embryo and fetal
development in mice. Teratology 19:237-244, 1979.

1339 Western Equinine Encephalitis

Medovy (1943) reported two infants who had encephalitis
during the first week of life after the mothers had mild
febrile illnesses. Both infants developed spastic diplegia
with either cortical atrophy or microcephaly. London et al
(1982) injected intracerebral virus into monkey fetuses and
produced hydrocephalus in 12 of 16.

London, W.T.; Levitt, N.H.; Altshuler, G.; Curfman, B.L.;
Kent, S.G.; Palmer, A.E.; Sever, J.L.; Houff, S.A.:
Teratological effects of Western Equine Encephalitis virus
on the fetal nervous system of Macaca mulatta. Teratology
25:71-79, 1982.

Medovy, H.: Western equinine encephalomyelitis in infants.
J. Pediatr. 22: 308-318, 1943.

1340 Wl-27 (see O-Chloro-beta-phenylethylhydrazine Dihydrogen
Sulfate)

1341 Workplace (see Occupation)

1342 Xanthinol Niacinate

Taniguchi et al (1974) gave this compound orally and
subcutaneously to mice and rats from the 7th through the
14th day of gestation. In mice the maximum oral dose was
5,000 and subcutaneous dose 1,250 mg per kg. In the rats
oral doses to 10,000 mg and subcutaneous doses to 1,250 mg
per kg were used. No teratogenicity was found, but some
growth retardation of the fetus was seen.

Taniguchi, S.; Yamada, A. and Morita, S.: Teratogenic
studies of xanthinol nicotinate. (Japanese) Oyo Yakuri 8:
1145-1156, 1974.

1343 Xenon (see Nitrous Oxide)

1344 Xenytropium Bromide

This anticholinergic was given intraperitoneally to rats and
mice on the 7th through the 14th day of gestation and no
teratogenicity or postnatal functional changes were found.
The rats received up to 1000 mg per kg per day and the mice
500 mg per kg per day (Aono et al, 1970).

Aono, K.; Mizusawa, H.; Oketani, Y. and Masuda, N.: Teratogenic study of xenytropium bromide in mice and rats. Oyo Yakuri 4: 725-739, 1970.

1345 Xylene

Kucera (1968) reports studies in chick embryos exposed for 60 to 240 minutes to a xylene atmosphere at developmental periods up to the 10 somite stage. A high malformation rate was found and nearly one-half of the defects were rumplessness, a defect resembling caudal regression syndrome. In mice, Marks et al (1982) found fetal deaths increased when they gavaged 3.6 ml of xylene mixtures er kg on days 5 through 14 of gestation. This dose was close to the LD-50 for the dams. Increased defects (mostly cleft palate) were found at dose levels of 2.4 3.0 and 3.6 ml per kg per day.

Among nine pregnancies producing offspring with caudal regression syndrome five mothers had exposure to fat solvents (Kucera, 1968). These included acetone, trichloroethylene, methylchloride and xylene. Hudak and Ungvary (1978) exposed rats to 1000 mg per square meter of air during days 9 through 14 and found no teratogenic results although minor skeletal anomalies occurred.

Hudak, A. and Ungvary, G.: Embryotoxic effects of benzene and its methyl derivatives: toluene, xylene. Teratology 11:55-63, 1978.

Kucera, J.: Exposure to fat solvents: A possible cause of sacral agenesis in man. J. Pediat. 72: 857-859, 1968.

Marks, T.A.; Ledoux, T.A.; Moore, J.A.: Teratogenicity of a commercial xylene mixture in the mouse. J. Toxicol. Envir. Health 9:97-105, 1982.

1346 Beta-D-xylosides

Gibson and Doller (1978) using p-nitrophenyl-beta-D-xyloside and 4-methylumbelliferyl-beta-D-xyloside and their derivatives in doses of 5-10 mg into the amniotic sac of 9 day chick embryo produced generalized stunting of the skeleton.

Gibson, K.D. and Doller, H.J.: Beta-D-sylosides cause abnormalitie of growth and development in chick embryos. Nature 273:151-153, 1978.

1347 X-ray (see Irradiation)

1348 Ytterbium

in the hamster, Gale (1975) found damage to the axial skeleton of the fetus when doses of 50 to 100 mg per kg were given intravenously on the 8th day. A few nervous system defects and ventral body wall openings were also found.

Gale, T.F.: The embryotoxicity of ytterbium chloride in golden hamsters. Teratology 11: 289-296, 1975.

1349 Zearalenone

This is an estrogenic mycotoxin produced by Fusarium. Ruddick et al (1976) treated pregnant rats orally with 1 to 10 mg per kg. At the higher doses there was some fetal growth retardation and some dely or absence of ossification centers. No visceral defects occurred.

Ruddick, J.A.; Scott, P.M. and Harwig, J.: Teratological evaluation of zearalenone administered orally to the rat. Bull. Envir. Contam. Toxicol. 15:678-681, 1976.

1350 Zeranol

The anabolic agent was tested in rats with oral doses of up to 4.0 mg per kg on days 6-18 of gestation. No adverse fetal effects were found except for increased resorptions at the 4.0 mg level. Tibial length was not altered (Wardell et al, 1982).

Wardell, R.E.; Seegmiller, R.E.; Bradshaw, W.S.: Induction of prenatal toxicity in the rat by diethylstilbestrol, zeranol, 3,4,3,4-tetrachlorobiphenyl, cadmium and lead. Teratology 26:229-237, 1982.

1351 Zerontin-R (see Ethosuximide)

1352 Zinc Chloride

Chang et al (1977) injected 20 mg per kg intraperitoneally on day 8, 9, 10 or 11 of the mouse pregnancy and produced a delay and some malformations in fetal ossification. Ferm and Carpenter using 2 mg per kg intravenously on the eighth day in the hamster did not find increased malformations.

Chang, C-H; Mann, D.E. and Gautieri, R.F.: Teratogenicity of zinc chloride, 1,10-phenanthroline and a zinc-1,10-phenathroline complex in mice. J. Pharm. Sc. 66:1755-1758, 1977.

Ferm, V.H. and Carpenter, S.J.: Teratogenic effect of cadmium and its inhibition by zinc. Nature 216:1123 (only), 1977.

1353 Zinc Deficiency

Hurley and Swenerton (1966) reared rats on a marginally deficient Zn diet and at the onset of gestation placed them on a Zn deficient diet. Nearly all of the surviving fetuses exhibited one or more congenital malformations. Cleft palate, skeletal defects, hydrocephalus (65 percent), eye, heart, lung and urogenital (49 percent) abnormalities were found. A reduction of Zn content in the fetuses was found.

Hurley et al. (1971) after exposing rats to only a few days of Zn deficiency were able to produce fetal defects. Purichia and Erway (1972) produced a reduction in the otoliths of rat fetuses whose mothers were maintained on deficient diets. Evidence that a 3 day period of zinc deficiency can produce abnormal rat blastocysts and morulae has been published by Hurley and Shrader (1975).

Sever and Emanuel (1973) have pointed out that zinc deficiency is clinically prevalent in Egypt and that the incidence of cns defects there is high (7.88 per 1,000 births). Cavdar et al (1980) have reported from Turkey that maternal serum Zn levels are significantly lower in those giving birth to anencephalics than in controls. Warkany and Petering (1973) have provided detailed descriptions of the central nervous system defects in the rat model. Warkany and Petering (1973) have provided detailed descriptions of the central nervous system defects in the rat model.

Hambridge et al (1975) raised the question that zinc deficiency in patients with acrodermatitis enteropathica might account for two major defects occurring among seven pregnant patients with the disease. The two defects were anencephaly and fatal achondrogenesis.

Cadvar, A.O.; Arcasoy, A.; Baycu, T.; Himmetoglu, O.: Zinc deficiency and anencephaly in Turkey. Teratology 22:14 (only) 1980.

Hambridge, K.M.; Neldner, K.H. and Walravens, P.A.: Zinc, acrodermatitis enteropathica, and congenital malformations. Lancet 1: 577-578, 1975.

Hurley, L.S. and Shrader, R.E.: Abnormal development of preimplantation rat eggs after three days of maternal dietary zinc deficiency. Nature New Biology 254: 427-429, 1975.

Hurley, L.S.; Gowan, J. and Swenerton, H.: Teratogenic effects of short-term and transitory zinc deficiency in rats. Teratology 4: 199-204, 1971.

Hurley, L.S. and Swenerton, H.: Congenital malformations resulting from Zn deficiency in rats. Proc. Soc. Exp. Biol. Med. 123: 692-696, 1966.

Purichia, N. and Erway, L.C.: Effects of dichloro-phenamide, zinc and manganese on otolith development in mice. Dev. Biol. 27: 395-405, 1972.

Sever, L.E. and Emanuel, I.: Is there a connection between maternal zinc deficiency and congenital malformations of the central nervous system in man. Teratology 7: 117-118, 1973.

Warkany, J. and Petering, H.G.: Congenital malformations of the central nervous system in rats produced by maternal zinc deficiency. Teratology 5: 319-334, 1972.

AUTHOR INDEX

Name			
Durel, J.			877
Dushkin, V.A.			995
Dyar, E.			702
Dyban, A.P.	30	81	265
	403	973	1216
Dyer, D.C.			741
Dyke, I.L.	37	376	1070
Dyke, R.W.			1320
Dzierzawski, A.		280	417
Earl, F.L.			224
Easterday, C.L.			1106
Eastwood, D.W.			942
Eayrs, J.T.			1152
Ebbin, A.J.		710	1122
Ebert, J.D.		104	589
Ebino, K.			245
Ebi, Y.			746
Edmonds, L.D.	650	695	1321
Edwards, J.H.			1188
Edwards, L.E.			541
Edwards, M.J.			695
Efimenko, L.P.			424
Egler, J.M.			402
Eguchi, K.			714
Eguchi, M.			535
Ehlers, K.H.			1281
Ehrenbard, L.T.			485
Eibs, H.G.		364	800
Eichenberger, E.			329
Einhorn, A.			725
Ekert, H.			828
Elbe, H.U.			1150
Elger, W.			364
Elhassani, S.			810
Elhassani, S.B.			810
Elian, I.			1179
Elis, J.			38
Elledge, W.			825
Ellington, A.C.			793
Elliott, M.			1106
Ellison, A.C.	6	158	303
	545	673	1061
Elshove, J.			485
Elton, R.L.		542	812
Elwood, J.M.			1062
El-Karim, A.H.B.			752
El-Sebae, A.H.			629
Emanuel, I.	1	315	370
	574	1062	1353
Ema, M. 59	517	611	842
Emerson, J.L.		666	1035
Emery, H.			344
Emi, Y.			879
Emmerson, J.L.	578	817	1080
		1252	1273
Emmons, R.W.			1122
Endo, A.		50	170
Endo, I.		519	565
Endres, J.			1056
Endres, J.L.			101
Eneroth, G.			326
Eneroth, V.			326
Engelhardt, E.			214
Engfeldt, B.		639	1152

Name			
Enjo, H.	63	582	1007
Enokuya, Y.			1156
Enomoto, H.			531
Epstein, C.J.			602
Erdman, W.J.			885
Erickson, B.H.			68
Erickson, J.D.	589	695	955
Ericksson, W.			402
Eriksson, M.			1130
Erila, T.		765	783
Erkkola, R.			408
Erway, L.C.	427	791	1353
Erwin, H.			782
Esaki, K.	55	122	146	247
	399	487	492	641	754
	777	792	1144	1195	1244
Esher, R.J.			226
Eskaki, K.			122
Essenberg, J.M.			922
Evans, H.M.	606	620	974
			1222
Evans, K.A.			1106
Evans, M.A.			1126
Evans, T.N.			346
Everest, R.P.			1100
Everett, G.			361
Everson, G.J.		342	791
Ezami, Y.			801
Ezumi, Y.	446	587	772	880
Fabro, S.	42	119	222	380
	543	706	782	994	1024
		1059	1216	1281
Fabro, S.M.			922
Fagerstone, K.A.			154
Faigle, J.W.			1216
Fainstat, T.D.		26	343
Fairweather, D.V.I.			91
Falchetti, R.			494
Falek, A.			1067
Falk, H.			1321
Falk, H.L.			1273
Fallon, J.F.		526	741
Falterman, C.G.			162
Fancher, O.E.	209	222	607
Fanelli, D.			191
Fanelli, O.			571
Fantel, A.G.	3	13	23
	42	332	362	696	928
			1113	1130
Farias, E.			900
Farquhar, J.W.			402
Farwell, J.W.			1187
Faucounau, N.			1243
Faustman-Watts, E.			13
Fave, A.			1317
Favre-Tissot, M.			493
Fayerweather, W.E.			662
Fazekas-Todea, I.			1004
Fechter, L.D.			228
Fedorova, E.A.			180
Fedrick, J.	144	485	1062
Feild, L.E.			91
Feldman, G.L.			1281
Feldman, H.A.			1261

Fukui, Y.		646	704	Genieser, N.B.			344
Fukunishi, K.			605	Gennaro, J.F.			1291
Funatsu, H.			275	Georges, A.		79	142
Funatsu, I.			275	Gerber, G.B.			763
Funatsu, T.			275	Gerbig, C.G.		1035	1273
Furakawa, E.			810	German, J.			1281
Furasawa, S.			886	Gershon, A.A.		656	1310
Furuhashi, T.	146	244	255	Gershon, R.			1112
			915	Gersony, W.M.		900	1079
Furukawa, S.			1166	Gianutsos, G.			793
Furuoka, R.		256	674	Gibbon, J.			696
Furuta, H.		350	467	Gibson, J.E.	359	362	478
Furuuchi, M.			1336		480	705	1217
Fuste, F.			1123	Gibson, J.P.	149	431	506
Fuyita, I.			420				876
Fuyita, M.			675	Gibson, K.D.			1346
Fuyuta, M.			204	Gibson, W.R.		578	1252
Fyler, D.C.			958	Gidley, J.T.			542
Gabriel-Robez, O.			1313	Gift, H.C.		101	942
Gachon, J.			228	Giknis, M.L.A.			1091
Gage, C.			1112	Gilbert, C.	173	848	1291
Gaines, T.B.	62	409	426	Gilbert, D.L.			577
		660	814	Gilbert, E.F.	217	526	741
Galbreath, C.			793				1219
Gale, T.F.		312	1348	Gilkeson, M.R.			1123
Galina, M.P.			725	Gillet, C.			52
Galloway, T.M.			900	Gillman, J.	173	848	1291
Gal, I.			1067	Gillman, T.	173	848	1291
Gamm, S.H.			214	Gill, W.B.			443
Gandelman, R.			1066	Ginsberg, M.D.			228
Gandier, B.			1005	Ginsburg, B.E.			42
Ganter, P.		877	1125	Gioto, K.			1336
Garau, A.			163	Girakawa, T.			981
Garcia, J.D.			810	Giroud, A.	170	343	606	696
Garcia, R.E.			1332		974	1243	1327
Gardner, K.A.			315	Giroud, J.			217
Gardner, L.I.	726	782	793	Giroud, M.			345
Gareis, F.J.			726	Giroud, P.			345
Garro, F.			1200	Gitterman, C.O.			1202
Gaskin, J.M.			900	Givelber, H.M.			782
Gasset, A.R.			729	Gjeruldsen, S.T.			986
Gaston, J.			696	Glade, G.			316
Gatling, R.R.	526	665	913	Gladstone, G.R.			1079
			950	Glebatis, D.M.		946	958
Gaub, M.L.			942	Gleich, J.			118
Gaudry, R.		539	1073	Globus, M.	144	414	456	635
Gaulme, J.			1308		822	930	1000	1209
Gauter, P.			881	Gluck, L.			1123
Gautieri, R.F.	102	123	185	Glushchenko VI			1321
	899	1140	1352	Gnezdilova, A.J.			1130
Gautier, M.			52	Goda, S.			540
Gavrilenko, E.V.			62	Gofmecler, V.A.			942
Gaylor, D.W.			1273	Gofmekler, V.A.		153	612
Gaynor, M.F.			828	Gofni, J.			335
Geber, W.F.	102	334	793	Gofuku, M.			936
	811	899	1218	Gojo, T.			936
Gebhardt, D.O.E.			1078	Golberg, L.			1206
Geelen, J.A.G.			696	Golbus, M.S.			602
Gefter, J.W.			729	Golby, M.			131
Gehring, P.J.	229	294	421	Goldberg, A.			763
	719	849	851	988	1207	Goldberg, I.D.			315
			1271	Goldberg, L.			363
Geiger, J.F.		791	1291	Goldblatt, A.			958
Gellert, R.J.			380	Goldenthal, E.I.			405

Howell, J. 798
Ho, O.L. 366
Hsia, D.Y. 1005
Hsieh, F-S. 652
Huber, J.J. 751
Hudak, A. 153 1258 1321 1345
Huebner, R.J. 370
Huel, G. 269 408 485 803 1002
Hughes, C.R.T. 308
Hughes, J.P.W. 900
Hultquist, G.T. 639 1152
Humphrey, R.R. 510
Hung, W. 1240
Hunter, C.M. 315
Hunter, J.R. 149 946
Huntley, C.C. 1005
Hunt, D.M. 1086
Hunt, V.R. 955
Hunt, W.H. 209
Hurley, L.S. 510 786 791 1209 1353
Hurni, H. 612
Hurteau, G.D. 335 1320
Hutchings, D.E. 696
Hwang, L-Y 652
Hytten, F.E. 315
Ichibana, T. 580
Ichija, M. 675
Ichikara, T. 295
Ichikawa, A. 674
Ichikawa, K. 936
Ichikawa, N. 1254
Ichikawa, Y. 479 1084 1270
Ichio, Y. 1254
Idanpaan-Heikkila, J. 485 710
Idanpaan, J. 144
Iffy, L. 1216
Igali, S. 3 42
Igarashi, N. 245 628
Ignatyeva 635
Ignatyeva, T.V. 3 42
Ignatyev, V.M. 810
Ihara, T. 240 720 904 961 1102 1194 1223
Iida, H. 63 113 287 451 608 1048
Iijima, M. 1248
Iijime, S. 920
Iizuka, H. 147
Ikeda, M. 527
Ikeda, T. 767 1106
Ikega, E. 244
Ikemori, M. 141
Ikeya, E. 146 255
Ikka, T. 854
Ikuzawa, M. 72
Imada, O. 953
Imagawa, D.T. 656 721 1304
Imaizumi, S. 1334
Imai, K. 122 459 503
Imai, M. 810
Imamichi, T. 245

Imamura, H. 73 159
Imamura, S. 119
Imamura, T. 37 766
Imanishi, M. 236 569 883 891 927
Imprei, J. 493
Imrei, J. 3 42
Imura, Y. 570
Inaba, J. 12 249 1191
Inaba, K. 55 1144
Inaba, Y. 40
Inamoto, M. 646
Infante, P.F. 1321
Ingalls, T.H. 77 702 721
Ingall, D. 1190
Ingle, L. 268
Ingram, S. 315
Innes, J.E. 1126
Innes, J.R.M. 342
Inoue, A. 1106
Inoue, K. 884 1253
Inoue, N. 714
Inoue, S. 199 561
Inoue, Y. 289
Inouye, M. 120 405 810 857 897
Ino, T. 317
Inst. of Medicine 1
Inui, H. 1046
Ioset, H.D. 428
Irikura, T. 213 232 843 953
Iritani, I. 426
Isaac-Mathy, M. 233
Isa, Y. 83 925
Ishihara, H. 781 1285
Ishihara, T. 324
Ishii, H. 514
Ishii, K. 1123
Ishii, Y. 729
Ishikawa, J. 1248
Ishikawa, K. 200
Ishikawa, S. 217 1219
Ishisaka, K. 878
Ishizaka, K. 755
Ishizaki, O. 203 636 1074 1085 1133
Ison, J. 408
Isuruzaki, T. 207
Itani, I. 540
Itoi, M. 729
Itono, Y. 936
Ito, 275
Ito, C. 884 1253 1263 1300
Ito, H. 5
Ito, M. 1013
Ito, N. 290
Ito, R. 231 520 992 1294
Ito, T. 277 1006
Ito, Y. 190 275
Iuliucci, J.D. 899
Ivankovic, S. 564 1008 1070
Ivanova-Tchemishanska, L. 496
Iverson, F. 555 845 940

Ivy, A.C.   98 384 443 530
                               1203
Iwadare, M.   459 748
Iwaki, M.   1038
Iwaki, R.   458
Iwaki, T.   247
Iwasaki, K.   1256
Izaki, K.   291
Izumiyama, K.   55 146 754
                      777 792
Izumi, T.   588
Izutsu, M.   1138
Jackson, A.J.   512
Jackson, B.A.   888
Jackson, C.W.   1083
Jackson, D.   335
Jackson, R.A.   150
Jackson, W.P.U.   308
Jacobsen, L.   1106
Jacobsohn, D.   364
Jacobson, B.D.   539
Jacobs, R.M.   304 622 711
                          1293
Jacobs, R.T.   1317
Jacob-Muller, U.   362 800
Jacquet, P.   763
Jaffe, P.   958
Jagiello, G.   958
Jago, R.H.   1293
Jakobovits, A.   1216
James, L.F.   107 114 175
                 342 361 775
James, L.M.   149 1321
James, N.   606
James, W.H.   326
Janerich, D.T.   946 958
Janerich, E.T.   958
Janisch, W.   564
Jansons, R.A.   922
Janz, D.   485
Jarman, J.A.   726
Jeffery, E.H.   1335
Jenkins, D.H.   787 1094
Jensen, B.   593
Jensen, N.M.   160
Jensh, R.P.   1287
Jeyasak, N.   820
Jick, H.   149 946
Jida, T.   525
Jirasek, J.   134
Jochmann, G.   856
Johannesson, T.   899
Johansen, K.T.   773
Johnson, A.R.   206
Johnson, E.M.   606 696 917
Johnson, J.M.   1070
Johnson, M.L.   1130
Johnson, R.H.   576
Johnson, W.E.   760
Johnstone, D.W.   1320
Johnstone, E.E.   539 1073
Johnston, D.W.   335
Johnston, M.C.   42   383 514
John, J.   1310

John, J.A.   25 153 418 659
              719 1165 1174 1204 1321
Jolly, H.   793
Jolou, L.   881
Joneja, M.G.   793
Jones-Price, C.   1181
Jones, A.M.   371
Jones, H.W.   197 534
Jones, K.L.   42
Jones, M.H.   656 721 1304
Jones, T.W.   101 942
Jongbloet, P.H.   385
Jonson, K.M.   695
Jonsson, N.A.   1216
Jordan, H.C.   1106
Jordan, R.L.   512 989 996
                               1216
Jost, A.   51   91 364 526
               539 702 868 1203 1311
Juchau, M.R.   13 362 1130
Julou, L.   877 1125
Juma, M.B.   474
Junkmann, K.   539 683 800
                               1073
Jurand, A.   817 935 1275
Juriloff, D.M.   1243
Juszkiewicz, T.   280 417
Kaan, H.W.   621
Kaback, M.M.   1332
Kaczka, E.A.   1202
Kadama, N.   446
Kadota, T.   200
Kadota, Y.   20 509
Kadoya, K.   336
Kado, Y.   254 879 1039
Kagan, Yu. S.   1031
Kageyama, M.   1275
Kagiwada, K.   203 636 1074
Kahi, S.   309
Kahrs, R.F.   184
Kaihara, N.   204
Kai, S.   200
Kajima, N.   295
Kajiwara, S.   1294
Kakemoto, Y.   20
Kakishita, T.   774
Kalb, J.C.   735
Kallen, B.   1067 1308
Kalow, W.   788
Kalter, H.   26   50 179 307
               342 358 514 574 606
               674 695 702 720 935
               974 1106 1112 1130 1181
              1315 1327 1330
Kamada, K.   325 336
Kamata, J.   525
Kamata, K.   21   56 398
Kamata, S.   196
Kamata, T.   981
Kambara, K.   135
Kamei, T.   311
Kameyama, Y.   160 702 763
                           810 1106
Kamimura, K.   277 1006

Matumoto, M.	40	745	Mellman, W.J.	1070
Matuo, M.		1225	Melman, W.J.	1281
Matuura, M.		295	Melnick, J.L.	1123
Matuzawa, K.		1332	Meltzer, H.J.	81
Matzilevich, B.		344	Melville, H.A.H.	1
Maurer, R.R.		117	Mendelson, G.F.	436
Mau, G.	800	1073	Mendizabal, A.	657
Maxwell, M.	1136	1235	Mendoza, G.R.	370
Mayor, G.H.		60	Mendoza, L.A.	514
Mays, C.W.		215	Menges, R.W.	262 922
Mayumi, T.		186	Mennel, H.D.	564 1008
Mazue, G.		193	Mennuti, M.T.	1070
Mazze, R.I.	520	942	Menser, M.A.	1123
Mazzoncini, V.		191	Menvet, J.C.	42
McBride, J.G.		25	Mercier-Parot, L.	30 82
McBride, W.G.	710	1216	104 131 233	298 308
McCallion, D.J.		104	335 351 396	510 630
McCarthy, J.F.		226	646 723 798	815 837
McCarthy, W.V.		433	853 896 918	958 998
McClain, R.M.	485 763	1296	1070 1085 1112	1255
McClure, H.M.		362	Meredith, P.A.	763
McColl, J.D.	144 414	456	Merker, H.J.	786 986 1206
	635 822 1000	1209	Meshorer, A.	885
McConnell, J.M.		621	Metcalf, R.L.	933
McCormack, K.M.	60	480	Meyers, J.D.	1122
McCormack, S.		326	Meyer-Wendecker, R.	390 590
McCoy, T.A.	75 1136	1235	Meyer, H.M.	1123
McCreadie, S.R.		197	Meyer, J.G.	485
McCue, C.M.		1114	Michaelis, H.	695
McCulley, L.B.		485	Michaelis, J.	695
McDonald, J.S.		782	Michaelson, S.M.	885
McFadyen, I.		958	Micheals, R.H.	1123
McGanity, W.J.		1331	Michida, K.	194
McGarrity, C.		1130	Miike, T.	709
McGlothlin, W.H.		782	Mikami, T.	126 1336
McIlhenny, H.M.		773	Mikami, Y.	48
McIntyre, M.S.		763	Mikhailova, E.G.	94 959
McKee, A.P.		721	Mikita, I.	63
McKendrick, D.M.		1062	Mikita, T.	1231
McKendry, J.B.J.		1310	Mikiver, L.	1216
McKenzie, B.E.		946	Miki, T.	309
McLachlan, J.A.	160	443	Milaire, J.	644
McLaren, D.A.		763	Miles, B.E.	782
McLaughlin, J.	62 222	448	Miles, V.N.	104
	607 1027	1212	Milham, S.	825
McLean, M.		687	Milkovich, L.	144 269 353
McMichael, A.J.		1321	400 798 803	999 1002
McNamara, D.G.		400		1072 1282
McPadden, A.J.		343	Millar, J.H.D.	223
McRee, D.I.		885	Millen, J.W.	1243 1327
McRorie, M.M.		1132	Miller, E.J.	761
McVie, R.		1308	Miller, H.C.	315
Meader, R.D.		310	Miller, J.	710
Meadow, S.R.		485	Miller, J.R.	574 602 697
Medearis, D.N.		721		958 1103
Medovy, H.		1339	Miller, M.	402 574
Mehrizi, A.		1216	Miller, M.H.	606
Meigs, J.W.		1187	Miller, P.	695
Meise, W.	1029	1032	Miller, R.K.	214 315 408
Mele, J.M.		1287	Miller, R.P.	408
Melish, M.E.		370	Miller, R.W.	275 1106
Mellin, G.W.	1002 1072	1123	Miller, T.J.	574 728
	1179	1216	Mills, L.F.	1332
Mellitis E.D.		315	Mills, R.F.N.	703

Milunsky, A.		402	828	Monroe, B.L.			1077
Minami, J.			1071	Monson, R.R.	144	217	485
Minami, Y.			527		722 958	1002 1130	1181
Mineshita, T.		289	1080	Montagne, J.			435
Minesita, T.			528	Montenegro, J.E.			1005
Minor, J.L.	419	1001	1321	Moodie, C.A.			38
Minsker, D.H.	617	713	763	Moore, B.S.			1123
			882	Moore, J.A.		669 1206	1273
Minton, P.D.			1025				1345
Miranda, D.			344	Moore, M.R.			763
Mirkes, P.E.	23	264	362	Moore, W.			660
Mirkin, B.L.		450	485	Moosa, A.			1310
Misson, C.			217	Moran, J.			322
Mitarai, H.			458	Moreau-Stinnakre, M.			51
Mitchell, A.A.	144	217	485	Moreland, A.F.			900
Mitchell, I.			1273	Morelock, S.			149
Mitchell, J.M.			920	Morgane, P.J.			574
Mitchell, M.			402	Morganti, J.B.			257
Mitchell, M.D.			906	Morgan, N.F.			485
Mitchell, S.			1062	Morgareidge, K.			8
Mitchell, S.J.			1062	Moriarity, A.J.			1276
Mitchener, M.	894	920	1135	Moriguchi, K.			785
Mitsumori, T.	314	598	605	Moriguchi, M.	432	614	1076
Mitsuzona, T.			936	Moriji, H.			616
Miyagawa, A.			119	Morimoto, K.			141
Miyagawa, E.			784	Morioka, M.			147
Miyahara, M.			275	Morita, H.	194 317	1245	1262
Miyaji, S.			638	Morita, K.		1186 1198	1210
Miyaji, T.		141	618	Morita, S.			1342
Miyake, H.			294	Morita, T.			776
Miyake, J.			294	Moritoki, H.		147	1286
Miyakubo, H.			784	Moritoki, M.			147
Miyakubo, T.			44	Moriyama, I.			675
Miyame, Y.			238	Mori, H.			774
Miyamoto, I.			48	Mori, K.			1334
Miyamoto, K.		231	1294	Mori, N.		196 230	323
Miyamoto, M.	285	360	594	Mori, S.			1294
	984	991	1050	Mori, T.			560
Miyamoto, S.			1148	Morobushi, A.			5
Miyamoto, T.			638	Moro, A.D.			174
Miyata, T.			324	Morriss, F.C.			720
Miyazaki, E.	500	601	766	Morriss, J.H.			104
Miyazaki, H.			121	Morris, C.R.			656
Miyazaki, K.			290	Morris, J.M.		335	1320
Miyoshi, K.		146	915	Morris, N.			1310
Mizuno, T.			1210	Morse, L.M.			403
Mizusawa, H.			1344	Mortoki, H.			147
Mizutani, M.	240	720	904	Moscarella, A.A.			100
	961 1102	1138 1194	1223	Moser, H.W.			344
Mjolnerod, O.K.			986	Mosher, H.P.		964	1103
Mochida, H.			1336	Mosier, H.D.			922
Mochida, K.		194	1245	Moskalski, N.			763
Modlin, J.F.			1122	Mots, M.N.			300
Moffett, B.C.		696	1113	Mottet, N.K.			810
Moisand, C.			875	Mounoud, R.L.			696
Molello, J.A.		37	376	Moxon, A.L.			1135
Moloshok, R.E.	521	539	1203	Moya, F.			942
Momiyama, H.	504	1090	1237	Mukaikawa, H.		246	619
			1249	Mukumoto, K.			1042
Momose, Y.			1334	Muller, D.			553
Moncrieff, A.			1203	Muller, M.			935
Monie, I.W.		264	606	Mulvihill, C.G.			958
Monif, G.R.G.			1123	Mulvihill, J.E.			214
Monnet, P.			735	Mulvihill, J.J.		217	958

Penny, R.H.C. 695
Penn, G.B. 115
Pentschew, A. 1200
Peralta, H. 900
Percy, D.H. 371 729
Pereira, G.R. 316
Pero, R.W. 58
Perry, M.M. 127 156 600
Persaud, T.V.N. 91 144 663
    698 765 793 1083 1230
Pershin, G.N. 180
Pessonnier, J. 435
Petering, H.G. 1353
Peterson, R.G. 1130
Peters, J.M. 955
Peters, P.W.J. 1128
Peters, R.L. 652
Peter, C.P. 763
Peter, D.W.J. 351
Petrere, J.A. 485 1318
Petreve, J. 510
Petrova-Vergieva, T. 496
Petrova, L. 94
Petter, C. 702
Pettiflor, J.M. 344
Pettit, M.D. 1240
Pfaltz, H. 1222
Pharoah, P.O.D. 725
Phelan, D.G. 638
Phelps, N.E. 344
Phillips, C.A. 1123
Phillips, F.S. 81
Phillips, P.E. 1123
Pierce, E.C. 578
Pierleoni, P. 1276
Pierro, L.J. 30 260
Pineda, R.G. 1123
Pinsent, K. 1130
Pinsent, R.J. 269 408 803
Pinsky, L. 77 399 674 1065
Piper, E.M. 958
Piper, J.M. 958
Pirskanen, R. 765 783
Pitel, M. 947
Piton, Y. 1226
Pizzarello, D.J. 977
Plank, J.B. 209
Platner, W.S. 14 123 1034
Platzek, T. 9 11
Pleet, H.B. 695
Plotkin, S.A. 1122
Plummer, G. 1106
Poland, B.J. 958
Polani, P.E. 1106
Polednak, A.P. 946
Poley, W.E. 1135
Ponte, C. 1005
Popova, N.V. 70
Popov, V.B. 3 362 403
Popov, V.G. 42
Populaire, P. 877 1125
Porter, J.B. 946
Port, R. 344
Poskanzer, D.C. 443

Posner, H.S. 58 798
Possamai, A.M. 1062
Poswillo, D.E. 695 1062
Potworowski, M. 540
Poulson, E. 292 671 732
    997 1140
Powell, H.R. 828
Powell, J.G. 578 720
Powers, H. 793
Pozanski, A.K. 485
Pozharsky, K.M. 1110
Poznakhirev, P.R. 995
Prahalada, S. 800
Pras, M. 335
Preston-Martin, S. 955
Preussmann, R. 4 564 740
    852 875 1008
Price, K.R. 1062
Prindle, R.A. 702
Pringle, J.L. 557
Printz, R.H. 810
Pritchard, J.A. 606
Prochazka, J. 265
Proffit, W.R. 541
Proinova, V.A. 180
Proll, J. 280
Prywes, R. 958
Puchkov, V.F. 3 42 81
    362 602
Pueschel, S.M. 589
Pujol, M. 735
Purchase, I.F.H. 419 1321
Purichia, N. 427 1353
Purmalis, B.P. 322
Pushkina, N.N. 153 612
Quimby, E.H. 726
Rabe, A. 840
Rachelefsky, G.S. 710
Rader, M. 514
Radovskaya, T.L. 331
Radow, B. 42
Rahm, U. 9 11
Rakalska, Z. 280 417
Ramel, C. 810
Ramer, R.M. 729
Rampy, L.W. 153 419
Randall, C.L. 42
Rao, A.N. 1335
Rao, K.S. 418 480
Rao, K.V. 1121
Rao, R.R. 1278
Rapaka, R.S. 670
Rassmussen, K. 986
Rating, D. 1308
Raushenbakh, M.O. 682
Ravenholt, R.T. 315
Rawls, W.E. 656
Raynaud, A. 1203
Raynaud, E-J. 1308
Readshaw, M.A. 1184
Read, A.P. 606
Recavarren, S. 702
Record, R.G. 1188
Rector, G.H.M. 942

SUBJECT INDEX

        page 511

page 513

DEVELOPMENTAL EVENT

	MAN
20 Somites	27-28
Metanephric Bud Appears	28
Lung Bud Appears	28
Crown-Rump Length, 5 mm	29-30
• Lower Limb Bud Appears	29-30
Spiral Septum Begins	34
Herniation of Gut	34
Eye Pigment	34-35
⦂ Digital Rays-Upper Extremity	35
Crown-Rump Length, 10 mm	37
⦂ Ossification Begins	40-43
Müllerian Duct Appears	40
Cloaca Divided by Urorectal Septum	43
△ Testes, Histological Differentiation	43
Digit Separation	43-47
Heart Septation Complete	46-47
o Eye Lids Closed	56-58
◊ Palate Closed Completely	56-58
Herniation of Gut Reduced	60
Urethral Groove Closed in Male	90
References-Number (see pp. xvi – xvii)	3, 10, 13, 17, 19, 24-27